Voice Therapy

Clinical Case Studies

Third Edition

Voice Therapy

Clinical Case Studies

Third Edition

Joseph C. Stemple and Lisa Fry

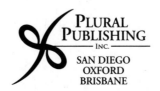

PLURAL
PUBLISHING
INC.

SAN DIEGO
OXFORD
BRISBANE

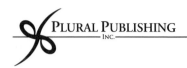

PLURAL PUBLISHING
INC.

5521 Ruffin Road
San Diego, CA 92123

e-mail: info@pluralpublishing.com
Web site: http://www.pluralpublishing.com

49 Bath Street
Abingdon, Oxfordshire OX14 1EA
United Kingdom

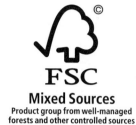

FSC
Mixed Sources
Product group from well-managed
forests and other controlled sources

Cert no. SW-COC-002283
www.fsc.org
© 1996 Forest Stewardship Council

Typeset in 11/13 Palatino by Flanagan's Publishing Services, Inc.
Printed in the United States of America by McNaughton and Gunn, Inc.

Library of Congress Cataloging-in-Publication Data:

Voice therapy : clinical case studies / [edited by] Joseph C. Stemple and Lisa Thomas
Fry. -- 3rd ed.
    p. ; cm.
  Includes bibliographical references and index.
  ISBN-13: 978-1-59756-344-4 (alk. paper)
  ISBN-10: 1-59756-344-7 (alk. paper)
  1. Voice disorders--Treatment. I. Stemple, Joseph C. II. Thomas Fry, Lisa.
  [DNLM: 1. Voice Disorders--therapy--Case Reports. WV 500 V8896 2010]
  RF510.V68 2010
  616.85'5606--dc22
                                     2009036442

Contents

Preface

We have had many opportunities over the years to write research articles, book chapters, and other texts. Preparing this particular text is always a joy. As clinical voice pathologists, the suggestions made for treatment of various voice disorders by our colleagues and friends are so meaningful to our own clinical development. We are all challenged daily by difficult clinical questions. It is our hope that the expertise offered in these pages will serve the reader well in answering some of these questions.

Our knowledge and understanding of clinical voice disorders continues to evolve, making this type of communication disorder an exciting and dynamic area of practice. Indeed, the science of voice production, as well as the evaluation and management of its disorders, is a formidable specialty within the professions of speech-language pathology and otolaryngology. One of the most exciting aspects of practicing clinical voice pathology is the opportunity to participate in the interdisciplinary team approach to the care of patients with voice disorders. Voice scientists and physiologists have greatly advanced our techniques for objectively evaluating voice production and treating voice disorders. Laryngologists are concerned with the medical and surgical management of voice disorders and utilize appropriate pharmacologic and surgical treatments to aid patients with voice disorders. Voice pathologists are concerned with discovering the causes of the voice problem and eliminating and modifying these causes to improve overall voice production. Finally, other specialists, such as singing teachers and vocal coaches, are concerned with maximizing the use of the performance voice. Interdisciplinary voice clinics utilize many or all of these professionals in a multidisciplinary team approach for management of clinical voice disorders to enhance patient outcomes.

As the knowledge of voice production continues to expand, so, too, have the publications dedicated to describing this knowledge. Currently, there are excellent texts and journals dedicated to describing the scientific understanding of voice. Other publications are available to help prepare students to evaluate and manage clinical voice disorders. By necessity, these texts must include great quantities of didactic information so that the student learns not only "how" but "why." To utilize a management approach without understanding the underlying basis of the approach is inappropriate. Nonetheless, because of the breadth of material necessary in these texts, therapeutic methods for voice disorders often are given only a cursory and generalized discussion.

The purpose of this text is to provide both the student and the working clinician with a broad sampling of management strategies as presented by master voice clinicians, laryngologists, and other voice care professionals. The text is meant to serve as a practical adjunct to the more didactic publications.

Utilizing the format of case studies, complete descriptions of diagnostic and therapeutic methods are provided for a full array of voice disorders. Chapter 1 includes information on the various philosophies of treatment. With the maturation of the voice care specialty, different schools of thought have evolved regarding treatment designs. These philosophical orientations include hygienic, symptomatic, psychogenic, physiologic, and eclectic orientations. Each orientation is discussed and illustrated with a representative case study.

Chapter 2 comments on various voice evaluation techniques. These techniques include the formal questionnaire, the patient interview, perceptual voice analysis, patient self-assessment and instrumental assessment of voice production. The role of the evaluation process as a part of the overall management plan is also discussed.

Chapter 3 discusses treatment approaches for voice disorders caused by vocal hyperfunction. This chapter provides information regarding the types of behaviors that lead to the development of common laryngeal pathologies. Management approaches for both children and adults including hygiene programs, symptomatic modifications, attention to psychosocial issues, and direct physiologic exercises are presented in illustrative case studies.

Treatments for various etiologies of glottal incompetence are described in Chapter 4. Management for voice fatigue, presbylaryngeus, and vocal fold paralysis are described, including direct voice therapies, surgical intervention, and a combination of these approaches. Many voice facilitating techniques are discussed.

Chapter 5 presents management strategies for various functional voice disorders. These include disorders caused by environmental stress, muscle tension dysphonia, functional aphonia, and male and female functional falsetto.

Because of the voice pathologist's unique blend of knowledge regarding upper respiratory physiology and behavior modification, we have become the caregivers for complex respiratory and laryngeal disorders. Chapter 6 provides several detailed case studies regarding the various etiologies, patient profiles, evaluation and treatment approaches used with those diagnosed with irritable larynx syndrome. Included in this category are chronic cough and vocal cord dysfunction (VCD). These cases include treatments for laryngopharyngeal reflux and VCD in the young child, young athlete, and elite athlete.

The professional voice user may present with any or all of the wide variety of voice disorders that also may be experienced by nonprofessional voice users. The consequences of a voice disorder on the professional's life and livelihood, however, create unique difficulties and the need for specialized treatment. For this reason, Chapter 7 presents case studies for the full range of professional voice users—from the elite vocal performer to the student in training. In addition, cases also are described from the perspective of a singing voice specialist and an acting voice coach.

Chapter 8 discusses management approaches for neurogenic voice disorders including spasmodic dysphonia, Tourette syndrome, and Parkinson disease. Although the incidence of these insidious disorders is low, the impact of the conditions on those who suffer from them is immeasurable. Direct voice therapy, surgical intervention, Botox injections, and combination management approaches are described.

The final chapter is devoted to a discussion of successful voice therapy and patient compliance. What makes therapy successful or unsuccessful? This chapter looks at both the therapist and the patient and describes the pitfalls that may influence the ultimate goal of therapy: improved vocal function.

As with the first two editions, the most exciting element in the preparation of this text was the support received by the master clinicians who graciously submitted these case studies. What a wonderful opportunity it is to learn from those who are in the trenches, experts who embody not only superior clinical skills, but a wonderful insight as to why they do what they do. We are deeply indebted to all of them and proudly offer their collective expertise. We are certain that the reader will benefit from their vast clinical experiences.

Text preparations are extremely time-consuming and require many hours of tedious work. Checking and preparing references, organizing tables, figures, and their legends, reading and rereading in an attempt to make the intent clear to those we are trying to reach are only a few of the tasks involved. We were so very fortunate in the preparation of this text to have the invaluable editorial assistance of Whitney Casey-Heatherman and Caroline Banks, graduate students in Communication Disorders at Marshall University. They graciously offered multiple hours completing the final edits. Their wonderful good humor and "can do" attitudes are greatly appreciated. We would also like to acknowledge the support, guidance, and encouragement of the Plural professionals including Stephanie Meissner, Sandy Doyle, Angie Singh, and Brian Phillips. It is always a pleasure to work with a supportive, creative team.

Finally, with deep appreciation, we thank our patients and clients who have taught us so much.

Joseph C. Stemple, PhD
Lisa Fry, PhD

Contributors

Moya L. Andrews, PhD
Professor of Speech and Hearing
  Sciences Emerita
Indiana University
Bloomington, Indiana
United States
Chapter 3

Mary V. Andrianopoulos, PhD
Associate Professor
Department of Communication
  Disorders
Clinical Consultant, Center for Speech,
  Language and Hearing
University of Massachusetts
Amherst, Massachusetts
United States
Chapter 6

Julie M. Barkmeier-Kraemer, PhD
Associate Professor
Department of Speech, Language,
  Hearing Sciences
University of Arizona
Tucson, Arizona
United States
Chapter 4

Mara Behlau, PhD
Director of Specialization Program in
  Voice
Center for Voice Studies (CEV)
São Paulo, Brazil
Chapter 4

Andrew Blitzer, MD, DDS
Professor of Clinical Otolaryngology
Columbia University College of
  Physicians and Surgeons
Director, New York Center for Voice
  and Swallowing Disorders
New York Head and Neck Institute
New York, New York
United States
Chapter 8

Osíris Brasil, MD
Associate Professor
Specialization Program in Voice
Center for Voice Studies (CEV)
São Paulo, Brazil
Chapter 4

Maria Dietrich, PhD
Post-Doctoral Scholar
Division of Communication Sciences
  and Disorders
College of Health Sciences
University of Kentucky
Lexington, Kentucky
United States
Chapter 4

Cynthia Fox, MA, CCC-SLP
National Center for Neurogenic Voice
  Disorders
Department of Speech and Hearing
  Sciences
University of Arizona-Tucson
Tucson, Arizona
United States
Chapter 8

Jacqueline L. Gartner-Schmidt, PhD
Assistant Professor of Otolaryngology
University of Pittsburgh School of
  Medicine
Associate Director, University of
  Pittsburgh Voice Center
Pittsburgh, Pennsylvania
United States

Chapter 3

Leslie Glaze, PhD
Adjunct Faculty
Department of Speech-Language-
    Hearing Sciences
University of Minnesota
Minneapolis, Minnesota
United States
Chapter 3

Stephen J. Gorman, PhD
Voice Pathologist
Blaine Block Institute for Voice
    Analysis and Rehabilitation
Dayton, Ohio
Professional Voice Center of Greater
    Cincinnati
Cincinnati, Ohio
United States
Chapter 4

Edie R. Hapner, PhD
Assistant Professor
Emory University School of Medicine
Department of Otolaryngology Head
    and Neck Surgery
Director of Speech Language
    Pathology
Emory Voice Center
Atlanta, Georgia
United States
Chapter 8

Sara Harris, FRCSLT
Specialist Speech and Language
    Therapist, Voice
Queen Mary's Hospital, Sidcup
Kent, United Kingdom
Chapter 3

Bari Hoffman Ruddy, PhD
Associate Professor
Department of Communication
    Sciences and Disorders
University of Central Florida
Director, The Voice Center

The Ear Nose & Throat Surgical
    Associates
Orlando, Florida
United States
Chapter 7

Barbara H. Jacobson, PhD
Assistant Professor
Vanderbilt Voice Center
Department of Otolaryngology
Vanderbilt University Medical
    Center
Nashville, Tennessee
United States
Chapter 7

Michael M. Johns III, MD
Director, Emory Voice Center
Assistant Professor
Emory University
Atlanta, Georgia
United States
Chapter 8

Lisa N. Kelchner, PhD
Associate Professor
Communication Sciences and
    Disorders
College of Allied Health Sciences
University of Cincinnati,
Cincinnati, Ohio
United States
Chapter 4

Aliaa Khidr, M.D., PhD
Professor of Phoniatrics
Department of Communication
    Disorders, Human Services Division
Curry School of Education
University of Virginia,
Charlottesville, Virginia
Department of Phoniatrics,
    Otolaryngology Division, School of
    Medicine
University of Ain Shams
Cairo, Egypt
Chapter 4

Mary McDonald Klimek, MM, MS
Senior Speech Pathologist, Professional
    Voice
Voice and Speech Laboratory
Massachusetts Eye and Ear Infirmary
Boston, Massachusetts
Certified Voice Instructor of Estill
    Voice Training
Partner, Vocal Innovations
Pittsburgh, Pennsylvania
United States
Chapter 7

Wendy DeLeo LeBorgne, PhD
Voice Pathologist and Singing Voice
    Specialist
Clinical Director
The Blaine Block Institute for Voice
    Analysis and Rehabilitation
Dayton, Ohio
The Professional Voice Center of
    Greater Cincinnati
Adjunct Assistant Professor
College Conservatory of Music
University of Cincinnati
Cincinnati, Ohio
United States
Chapter 7

Linda Lee, PhD
Professor Emeritus
Department of Communication
    Sciences & Disorders
University of Cincinnati
Cincinnati, Ohio
United States
Chapter 3

Jeffrey Lehmann, MD
Otolaryngologist
The Ear, Nose and Throat Surgical
    Associates
Winter Park, Florida
United States
Chapter 7

Nicole Yee-Kee Li, MPhil, PhD
University of Pittsburgh
Pittsburgh, Pennsylvania
United States
Chapter 3

Dawn B. Lowery, PhD
Ohio ENT Surgeons
Columbus, Ohio
United States
Chapter 4

Stephen C. McFarlane, PhD
Dean Emeritus, School of Medicine
University of Nevada
Reno, Nevada
United States
Chapter 4

Claudio F. Milstein, PhD
Head and Neck Institute
Cleveland Clinic
Associate Professor
Cleveland Clinic Lerner College of
    Medicine
Case Western Reserve University
Cleveland, Ohio
United States
Chapter 5

Murray Morrison, MD
Professor Emeritus
Past Head of the Division of
    Otolaryngology
Active Staff, Vancouver Hospital and
    Health Sciences Centre
Vancouver, Canada
Chapter 6

Gisele Oliveira, MSc
Associate Professor of the
    Specialization Program in Voice
Center for Voice Studies (CEV)
São Paulo, Brazil
Chapter 4

Rita Patel, PhD
Assistant Professor
Communication Sciences and
  Disorders
Director, UK Clinical Voice Center
University of Kentucky
Lexington, Kentucky
United States
Chapter 3

Robert C. Peppard, PhD
Associate Professor and Graduate
  Coordinator
Department of Communication
  Sciences and Disorders
California State University–East Bay
Hayward, California
United States
Chapter 5

Brian E. Petty, MA
Clinical Speech Pathologist and
  Singing Voice Specialist
UW Voice and Swallowing Center
University of Wisconsin School of
  Medicine and Public Health
Madison, Wisconsin
United States
Chapter 7

Bruce Poburka, PhD
Professor
Department of Speech, Hearing &
  Rehabilitation Services
Minnesota State University
Mankato, Minnesota
United States
Chapter 4

Sharon L. Radionoff, PhD
Director
Singing Voice Specialist
Sound Singing Institute
Houston, Texas
Voice Care Team Member

Singing Voice Specialist
Texas Voice Center
Houston, Texas
United States
Chapter 7

Lorraine Ramig, PhD
Professor
Department of Speech, Language, and
  Hearing Sciences
University of Colorado–Boulder
Boulder, Colorado
Senior Scientist, National Center for
  Voice and Speech
Denver, Colorado
Adjunct Professor,
Columbia Teacher's College
New York, New York
Founder/President of the LSVT®
  Foundation
United States
Chapter 8

Linda Rammage, PhD
Director, Provincial Voice Care
  Resource Center
University of British Columbia
Vancouver, Canada
Chapter 6

Bonnie N. Raphael, PhD
Professor, Department of Dramatic Art
University of North Carolina at Chapel
  Hill
Resident Voice, Speech, and Text
  Coach
Play Makers Repertory Company
Chapel Hill, North Carolina
United States
Chapter 7

Nelson Roy, PhD
Associate Professor
Department of Communication
  Sciences and Disorders

Division of Otolaryngology-Head &
    Neck Surgery
Department of Surgery, School of
    Medicine
University of Utah
Salt Lake City, Utah
United States
Chapter 5

Stephen Salloway, MS, MD
Assistant Professor
Department of Clinical Neuroscience
Brown University
Director of Neurology
Butler Hospital
Providence, Rhode Island
United States
Chapter 8

Mary J. Sandage, MA
Adjunct Clinical Faculty
Auburn University
Auburn, Alabama
United States
Chapter 6

Christine Sapienza, PhD
Chair, Department of Communication
    Sciences and Disorders
University of Florida
Gainesville, Florida
United States
Chapter 7

**Robert Thayer Sataloff, MD, DMA,
FACS**
Professor and Chairman
Department of Otolaryngology–Head
    and Neck Surgery
Senior Associate Dean for Clinical
    Academic Specialties
Drexel University College of Medicine
Philadelphia, Pennsylvania
United States
Chapter 7

Susan Shulman, MS
Co-Director
Speech Pathology Services
Dallas, Texas
United States
Chapter 6

Martin Spencer, MA
Ohio ENT Surgeons
President, Ohio Voice Association
Columbus, Ohio
United States
Chapter 7

Celia F. Stewart, PhD
Associate Professor
Chair, Department Speech-Language
    Pathology and Audiology
Steinhardt School of Culture,
    Education, and Human Development
New York University
New York, New York
United States
Chapter 8

R. E. (Ed) Stone, Jr, PhD
Retired, Vanderbilt Voice Center
Nashville, Tennessee
United States
Chapter 5

Edie Swift, MA
Previously Clinical Supervisor
University of Wisconsin Voice Clinic
Currently Private Practice
Mexico City, Mexico
Chapter 6

Jennifer B. Thompson, MA
Clinical Voice Therapist
JamesCare Voice and Swallowing
    Disorders Clinic
The Ohio State University
Columbus, Ohio
United States
Chapter 6

Lyn R. Tindall, PhD
Speech-Language Pathologist
Department of Veterans Affairs
  Medical Center
Lexington, Kentucky
United States
Chapter 8

Michael D. Trudeau, PhD
Associate Professor
Department of Speech and Hearing
  Science
Department of Otolaryngology/Head
  and Neck Surgery
Arthur G. James Cancer Hospital Voice
  and Swallowing Disorders Clinic
The Ohio State University
Columbus, Ohio
United States
Chapter 6

Eva van Lear, MS, MFA
Research Fellow
University of Wisconsin
Department of Communicative Disorders
Department of Surgery, Division of
  Otolaryngology/Head & Neck
  Surgery
Madison, Wisconsin
United States
Chapter 9

Katherine Verdolini Abbott, PhD
Professor
Communication Science and Disorders
  and Otolaryngology
University of Pittsburgh
Member, McGowan Institute for
  Regenerative Medicine
Member, Center for the Neural Basis of
  Cognition, University of Pittsburgh
  and Carnegie Mellon University
Pittsburgh, Pennsylvania
United States
Chapter 3

Shelley Von Berg, PhD
Assistant Professor
Communication Sciences and Disorders
California State University-Chico
Chico, California
United States
Chapter 4

Miriam van Mersbergen, PhD
Clinical Speech Pathologist and
  Singing Voice Specialist
UW Voice and Swallowing Center
University of Wisconsin School of
  Medicine and Public Health
Madison, Wisconsin
United States
Chapter 7

Barbara D. Weinrich, PhD
Professor
Department of Speech Pathology
Miami University
Oxford, Ohio
United States
Chapter 7

Richard Zraick, PhD
Associate Professor
Department of Audiology and Speech
  Pathology
University of Arkansas for Medical
  Sciences/University of Arkansas at
  Little Rock
Little Rock, Arkansas
United States
Chapter 3

1

Principles of Voice Therapy

Introduction

In preparing the third edition of this text it was necessary to review almost 80 years of history related to voice therapy techniques and approaches. It is a rich and interesting history that gives an excellent understanding of how the treatment of voice disorders has grown and evolved to our present practice. Some of the therapy approaches developed by early speech pathologists continue to be used successfully in the remediation of voice disorders to this day. Because of the growth in our knowledge and understanding of voice production, other therapy approaches once commonly used were proven to be ineffective. The past 30 years have yielded tremendous growth in our knowledge and understanding of vocal function. Computer models of phonation,[1-6] histologic studies of the vocal folds,[7-10] analysis of the vocal fold cover and tissue engineering,[11-19] and

genetic issues associated with voice disorders[20-23] are but a few of the many advances in voice science. Furthermore, consider the rapidly evolving ability to measure and describe normal and pathologic voice function objectively through sophisticated acoustic and aerodynamic instrumentation, as well as the ability to observe vocal fold vibration. All of these scientific advancements have provided voice clinicians with the tools to confirm the efficacy of their approaches.

The number of traditional therapy approaches that continue to be used in voice therapy today is a strong statement of appreciation and admiration for the voice pedagogues, clinicians, and scientists of earlier days. The accuracy of their practical observations regarding voice function has proved to be uncanny. The efficacy of many of these traditional voice therapy techniques is now being tested through systematic outcomes research.[24] Proof of the worthiness of many of these techniques, however, has been well established by the clinical results of skilled voice pathologists.

The major difference in voice therapy today compared with even 10 to 15 years ago is the ability to diagnose a problem quickly and accurately and to confirm the efficacy of our management approaches through objective measures. These objective measures may also be used as patient feedback during the therapeutic process. Although our management approaches have remained rather constant, voice therapy has truly become a blend of "art" with "science."

The artistic nature of voice therapy is dependent on the human interaction skills of the clinician. Compassion, understanding, empathy, and projection of credibility, together with listening, counseling, and motivational skills are essential attributes of the successful voice clinician. Philosophically, we might make these statements about the artistic nature of voice:

- When considering the voice, we must consider the whole person.
- To examine a voice disorder is to examine a unique individual.
- The way that individual feels, both physically and emotionally, may be directly reflected in the voice.
- To remediate a voice disorder, we must have the skills to counsel and motivate the patient and instill action for change.

The scientific nature of voice therapy involves the clinician's knowledge of several important areas of study. These areas include the anatomy and physiology of normal and pathologic voice production; the nuances of laryngeal pathologic conditions; the acoustics and aerodynamics of voice production; and the etiologic correlates of voice disorders,

including patient behaviors, medical causes, and psychological contributions.

- When considering the voice, we are considering the most widely used instrument on earth.
- To understand the voice disorder, we must understand the instrument's physical structure and functional components.
- We must have the skills to measure these components objectively and to relate these measures to our management choices.
- In addition, we must possess a broad knowledge of the common causes of voice disorders and the nuances of laryngeal pathologic conditions.

The successful voice clinician will combine attributes of the artistic approaches toward voice therapy with the objective scientific bases to identify the problem and plan and carry out appropriate management strategies. Nonetheless, possession of a solid base of didactic information cannot replace experience. Experience continues to teach even the masters. It is hoped that the experiences of others provided in this text will prove helpful in the development of superior voice clinicians.

Historical Perspective

In examining the evolution of the treatment of voice disorders, we find it was not until around 1930 that a few laryngologists, singing teachers, instructors in the speech arts, and a fledgling group of speech correctionists became interested in retraining individuals with voice disorders. This group used drills and exercises borrowed from voice and diction manuals designed for the normal voice in an attempt to modify disordered voice production. Many of these rehabilitation techniques were and remain creative and effective, but they were not necessarily based on scientific principles. Indeed, the "artistic" portion of voice treatment was the strong point of the early clinicians.

Out of this artistic approach came the general treatment suggestions of (1) ear training, (2) breathing exercises, (3) relaxation training, (4) articulatory compensations, (5) emotional retraining, and (6) special drills for cleft palate and velopharyngeal insufficiency.[25,26] These treatment suggestions became the foundation of vocal rehabilitation.

Several general management philosophies have arisen from the early foundations of voice rehabilitation. These philosophical orientations are based primarily on the clinician's mindset and previous training regarding voice disorders that directs the management focus. For the sake of discussion, we classify these management philosophies as:

- hygienic voice therapy
- symptomatic voice therapy
- psychogenic voice therapy
- physiologic voice therapy
- eclectic voice therapy.

In short, *hygienic voice therapy* focuses on identifying inappropriate vocal hygiene behaviors, which then are modified or eliminated. Once modified, voice production has the opportunity to improve or return to normal. *Symptomatic voice therapy* focuses on modification of the deviant vocal symptoms identified by the voice pathologist, such as breathiness, low pitch, glottal attacks, and so on. The focus of *psychogenic voice therapy* is on the emotional and psy-

chosocial status of the patient that led to and maintains the voice disorder. The *physiologic orientation* of voice therapy focuses on directly modifying and improving the balance of laryngeal muscle effort to the supportive airflow, as well as the correct focus of the laryngeal tone. Finally, the *eclectic approach* of voice therapy is the combination of any and all of the previous voice therapy orientations.[27] Indeed, none of these philosophical orientations is pure. Much overlap is present, often leading to the use of an eclectic approach. With this introduction, let us examine the orientations of voice therapy in greater detail.

Hygienic Voice Therapy

Hygienic voice therapy often is the first step in many voice therapy programs. Many etiological factors contribute to the development of voice disorders. Poor vocal hygiene may be a major developmental factor. Some examples of behaviors that constitute poor vocal hygiene include shouting, talking loudly over noise, screaming, vocal noises, coughing, throat clearing, and poor hydration. When the inappropriate vocal behaviors are identified, then appropriate treatments can be devised for modifying or eliminating them. Once modified, voice production has the opportunity to improve or return to normal.

Poor vocal hygiene may also include the habitual use of voice components in an inappropriate manner. Often, changes in these components are the compensatory results of the vocal pathology. In the case of poor vocal hygiene, however, use of an inappropriate pitch or loudness, reduced respiratory support, poor phonatory habits (glottal attacks, fry), or inappropriate resonance are simply functional vocal behaviors that may contribute to the development and maintenance of a voice disorder. Hygienic voice therapy presumes that many voice disorders have a direct behavioral cause. This therapy strives to instill healthy vocal behaviors in the patient's habitual speech patterns. Good vocal hygiene also focuses on maintaining the health of the vocal fold cover through adequate internal hydration and diet. Once identified, poor vocal hygiene habits can be modified or eliminated leading to improved voice production.

Symptomatic Voice Therapy

Symptomatic voice therapy was a term first introduced by Daniel Boone.[28] This voice management approach is based on the premise that modifying the symptoms of voice production including pitch, loudness, respiration, and so on will improve the voice disorder. Once identified, the misuses of these various voice components are modified or reduced using *voice therapy facilitating techniques.*

> In the voice clinician's attempt to aid the patient in finding and using his best voice production, it is necessary to probe continually within the patient's existing repertoire to find the best one voice which sounds "good" and which he is able to produce with relatively little effort. A voice therapy facilitating technique is that technique which, when used by a particular patient, enables him easily to produce a good voice. Once discovered, the facilitating technique and resulting phonation become the symptomatic focus of voice therapy ... This use of a facilitating technique to produce a good phonation is the core of what we do in symptomatic voice therapy for the reduction of hyperfunctional voice disorders.[28(p11)]

Boone's original facilitating approaches included:

1. altering tongue position
2. change of loudness
3. chewing exercises
4. digital manipulation
5. ear training
6. elimination of abuses
7. elimination of hard glottal attack
8. establishing new pitch
9. explanation of the problem
10. feedback
11. hierarchy analysis
12. negative practice
13. open mouth exercises
14. pitch inflections
15. pushing approach
16. relaxation
17. respiration training
18. target voice models
19. voice rest
20. yawn-sigh approach.

Many if not all of these facilitators remain useful and popular in the treatment of voice disorders and are described in greater detail in cases throughout this text.

The main focus of symptomatic voice therapy is direct modification of vocal symptoms. For example, if the patient presents with a voice quality characterized by low pitch, breathiness, and hard glottal attacks, then the main focus of therapy is to directly modify the symptoms. The facilitating approaches used to modify these symptoms might include items 9, 5, 8, 7, and 17 (as listed above). The voice therapist constantly probes for the "best" voice and attempts to stabilize that voice with the various appropriate facilitating techniques. Symptomatic voice therapy assumes voice improvement through direct symptom modification.

Psychogenic Voice Therapy

Early in the study of voice disorders, the relationship of emotions to voice production was well recognized. As early as the mid-1800s, journal articles discussed hysteric aphonia.[29,30] West, Kennedy, and Carr[26] and Van Riper[25] discussed the need for emotional retraining in voice therapy. Murphy[31] presented an excellent discussion of the psychodynamics of voice. Friedrich Brodnitz,[32] as an otolaryngologist, was uniquely sensitive to the relationship of emotions to voice. These early readings are most interesting and remain informative to those treating voice disorders.

Our understanding of psychogenic voice therapy was further expanded by Aronson,[33] Case,[34] Stemple,[35] and Colton and Casper.[36] These authors discussed the need for determining the emotional dynamics of the voice disturbance. Psychogenic voice therapy focuses on identification and modification of the emotional and psychosocial disturbances associated with the onset and maintenance of the voice problem. Pure psychogenic voice therapy is based on the assumption of underlying emotional causes. Voice clinicians, therefore, must develop and possess superior interview skills, counseling skills, and the skill to know when the treatment for the emotional or psychosocial problem is beyond the realm of their skills. A referral system of support professionals must be readily available.

Physiologic Voice Therapy

Physiologic voice therapy includes voice therapy programs that have been devised to directly alter or modify the physiology of the vocal mechanism. Normal voice production is dependent on a balance among airflow, supplied by the respiratory system; laryngeal muscle balance, coordination, and stamina; and coordination among these and the supraglottic resonatory structures (pharynx, oral cavity, nasal cavity). Any disturbance in the physiologic balance of these vocal subsystems may lead to a voice disturbance.[37]

These disturbances may be in respiratory volume, power, pressure, and flow. Disturbances also may manifest in vocal fold tone, mass, stiffness, flexibility, and approximation. Finally, the coupling of the supraglottic resonators and the placement of the laryngeal tone may cause or may be perceived as a voice disorder. The overall causes may be mechanical, neurologic, or psychological. Whatever the cause, the management approach is direct modification of the inappropriate physiologic activity through exercise and manipulation.

Inherent in physiologic voice therapy is a holistic approach to the treatment of voice disorders. They are therapies that strive to at once balance the three subsystems of voice production as opposed to working directly on single voice components, such as pitch or loudness. Examples of physiologic voice therapy include Vocal Function Exercises,[38] Resonant Voice Therapy,[39] and the Accent Method of Voice Therapy,[40] all of which are presented in this text.

Eclectic Voice Therapy

Adherence to one philosophical orientation of voice therapy would not be advisable. Indeed, successful voice therapy depends on utilization of an approach that happens to work for the therapist and the individual patient. The more management approaches understood and mastered by the clinician, the greater the likelihood for success. Management techniques that prove successful for one patient may not be successful for a similar patient. The clinician, therefore, must possess the knowledge to adjust the management approach.

On the other hand, some techniques that work well for one therapist may prove to be difficult for another. In whatever management approach you choose, you must have supreme confidence in your understanding of the technique and your ability to make that approach work successfully. Your confidence is one factor that will determine the success or failure of therapy. Using a typical case, let us examine how each therapy orientation might be used to treat the vocal difficulties of this composite patient.

Case Study: Patient A

Patient A, a 52-year-old woman, was referred by her laryngologist to the voice center for postsurgical evaluation and treatment. Large bilateral draping polyps were first identified by an anesthesiologist while intubating the patient for a laminectomy 6 months prior to her voice evaluation. Because of the large polyps, intubation had been difficult. The problem was reported to her family physician, who in turn referred the patient to an otolaryngologist for a laryngeal examination.

Indirect mirror examination revealed bilateral polypoid degeneration, worse on the left than the right. Audible inspiratory stridor was noted by the physician, and the patient reported shortness of breath during even limited physical exertion. Therefore, two surgeries (one for each vocal fold) were scheduled 6 weeks apart for aspiration of fluid and laser vaporization of redundant tissue.

The surgeries were performed without complication, and the patient was seen for voice evaluation 5 weeks after the second surgery.

History of the Problem

The patient reported that she had always had a "deep" voice, which had lowered even more over the past several years. Her presurgical voice quality had not been a concern to her, however. Instead, it was the shortness of breath that led her to agree to surgery. She reported that voice quality following the first surgery (left fold) was a little "hazy" but returned to "normal" within 1 week. The second surgery left her with significant, bothersome hoarseness that made her "wish I had never had surgery."

Medical History

The patient reported undergoing two previous surgeries: removal of her gall bladder 10 years earlier and the laminectomy performed earlier this year. Even with the difficult intubation and the risk of vocal fold paralysis inherent in laminectomy, her presurgical voice quality was maintained. In addition to surgeries, she had been hospitalized 3 years before for 3 weeks and treated for chronic depression.

Chronic medical disorders included frequent upper respiratory infections including bronchitis, high blood pressure, circulatory problems in her legs, elevated blood sugar; and chronic neck and back pain. Daily medications were taken for blood pressure, chronic pain, depression, and sleep. She continued a 30-year history of smoking 1½ to 2 packs of cigarettes per day. Her liquid intake consisted mostly of 6 cups of caffeinated coffee per day. Chronic throat clearing and a persistent cough were noted throughout the evaluation.

Social History

Patient A had been married for 12 years to her second husband, following a first marriage of 18 years and divorce. She had two adult children from her previous marriage. Her elderly mother-in-law lived with her and her husband, a situation that often caused friction and conflict with her husband. Indeed, she was not shy in reporting her unhappiness with her marital relationship. This unhappiness was said to be a major factor in her history of depression.

Both the patient and her husband were employed by the local automobile assembly plant. She had worked as an assembler for 14 years in an environment described as "noisy, dusty, and full of fumes" and was on a temporary medical disability because her back problems precluded her working in the plant. Present activities included shopping with her daughter, talking on the telephone, caring for her home (back permitting), watching daytime television "talk" shows, and bowling two nights per week in two different leagues. The latter activity appeared somewhat inconsistent with her report of current back problems.

Voice Evaluation

Perceptually, the patient's voice quality was described as moderately dysphonic, characterized by low pitch, inappropriate loudness, strained raspiness, and intermittent glottal fry phonation. Acoustic and aerodynamic analyses revealed the following:

- fundamental frequency
  150 Hz (low) *180–220 is normal*
- frequency range
  118–290 Hz (limited)
- jitter percent
  1.18% (high)
- intensity (habitual)
  76 dB (high)
- airflow volume
  2300 mL H_2O (normal)
- airflow rate
  <80 mL H_2O/sec (low) *hyperfunctioning the mech.*
- maximum phonation time
  <12 sec all pitches (low) *86/2300 = 30*

Should be able to sustain at 30 sec

Laryngeal videostroboscopic observation revealed mild-to-moderate bilateral true vocal fold edema and erythema. Glottic closure demonstrated an irregular glottal chink with a moderate ventricular fold compression. The edges of the vocal folds were rough and irregular, worse on the left than on the right. The amplitude of vibration was severely decreased bilaterally. The mucosal waves were barely perceptible. The closed phase of the vibratory cycle was strongly dominant, whereas the symmetry of vibration was generally irregular. No mass lesions, paresis, or paralysis was evident. In short, the patient had an edematous *swollen*, stiff, hyperfunctioning vocal fold system.

Impressions

Patient A presented with a voice disorder that derived from the following possible causal factors:

- cigarette smoking
- harsh employment environment
- talking over noise at work
- large caffeine intake
- frequent upper respiratory infections
- prescription medications

- coughing and throat clearing
- emotional instability
- talking too loudly (suggesting possible hearing loss, which later proved not to be present)
- using a low pitch
- laryngeal muscle tension
- postsurgical vocal fold mucosal changes.

Recommendations

Hygienic Voice Therapy. The general focus would be to identify the primary and secondary vocal misuses and then to modify or eliminate these nonhygienic behaviors. The primary etiologic correlates include:

- smoking
- laryngeal dehydration from caffeine and drugs
- voice abuse, such as coughing, throat clearing, and talking loudly over noise at work.

Secondary precipitating factors that result from the pathologic condition include:

- laryngeal area muscle tension and hyperfunction caused by vocal fold stiffness
- low pitch caused by increased mass; and
- increased loudness caused by effort used to force stiff vocal folds to vibrate.

Therapy would focus on modification or elimination of the primary causes. The patient would be aided in her attempt to stop smoking, encouraged to begin a hydration program, and given vocal hygiene counseling to aid in elimination or reduction of the vocally abusive behaviors. The secondary causes most likely would improve spontaneously as the primary causes were modified and the vocal fold condition improved.

Symptomatic Voice Therapy. General focus would use facilitating techniques to:

- raise pitch
- reduce loudness
- reduce laryngeal area tension and effort.

This direct symptom modification would follow an explanation of the problem and would run concurrently with modification of vocally abusive behaviors, including:

- smoking
- caffeine intake
- coughing and throat clearing.

Psychogenic Voice Therapy. General focus would explore the psychodynamics of the voice disorder. Techniques would include:

- detailed interview with the patient to determine the cause and effects of depression
- determination of the relationship of emotional problems and voice problem
- counseling the patient regarding the effects of emotions on voice production
- reduction of the musculoskeletal tension caused by emotional upheaval
- referral for marital counseling as deemed appropriate.

Secondary focus would deal with modification or elimination of the abusive behaviors including:

- smoking
- caffeine and medications

■ coughing and throat clearing.

Inappropriate use of pitch and loudness would most likely be viewed as obvious symptoms of the problem. These symptoms would likely improve as the psychodynamics were improved.

Physiologic Voice Therapy. The general focus would be on evaluating the present physiologic condition of the patient's voice production and developing direct physical exercises to improve that condition. We know that the patient presented with extreme laryngeal tension. Irregular vocal fold edges caused a glottal chink. In addition, her vocal folds were extremely stiff, both in amplitude and mucosal wave.

   Normal voicing is dependent on near total closure of the vocal folds, permitting air pressure to build below the folds. As the pressure builds, it eventually overcomes the resistance of the approximated folds, permitting the release of one puff of air. As the air rushes between the vocal folds, subglottal, supraglottal, and intraglottal pressures, along with the static position of the vocal folds, draw them back together to complete one vibratory cycle. Air gaps, or glottal chinks, change the physical dynamics of vocal fold vibration requiring an increased subglottic pressure. Patients such as this woman often make physical compensations in an attempt to push out the "best" voice by hyperfunctioning the supraglottic structures. Add vocal fold muscular and mucosal stiffness to this mix and the patient presents with a significant muscle tension dysphonia with associated respiratory, laryngeal, and resonance dysfunctions.

   Direct physiologic voice therapy would focus on exercises designed to rebalance the three subsystems of voice production: respiration, phonation, and resonance. Therapy methods chosen to accomplish this task might include Vocal Function Exercises, Resonant Voice Therapy, or the Accent Method of Voice Therapy. (All methods are described in subsequent chapters.)

Eclectic Voice Therapy. In this review of philosophical orientations of voice therapy, you have seen the various strengths of each management orientation, as well as the difficulty in subscribing to any one philosophy. All patients will be treated best by a voice pathologist with knowledge and understanding of all possible management strategies and alternatives. As you read and study the many case presentations of this text, it is beneficial to evaluate the philosophy behind the treatment approach as a means of better understanding the reasons for the approach. The successful voice pathologist is both an artist and a scientist with an eclectic point of view. Therapy for Patient A should focus on:

■ vocal hygiene counseling
■ symptom modification
■ attention to the psychodynamics of the problem
■ direct physiologic vocal exercise.

Voice Care Professionals

Thus far we have discussed the treatment of voice disorders in terms of direct voice therapy. Voice care, however, is a shared province, with contributions from the primary care physician, laryngologist, voice pathologist, neurologist, allergist, gastroenterologist, pulmonologist, psychologist, vocal coach, singing instructor, and others. Case studies presented in all chapters of this text describe the unique interdisciplinary and complementary relationships of each of these professionals with the others and with their patients.

References

1. Alipour F, Berry DA, Titze IR. A finite-element model of vocal-fold vibration. *J Acoust Soc Am.* 2000;108(6):3003–3012.

2. Hunter EJ, Titze IR, Alipour F. A three-dimensional model of vocal fold abduction/adduction. *J Acoust Soc Am.* 2004; 115(4):1747–1759.

3. Story BH, Titze IR. Voice simulation with a body-cover model of the vocal folds. *J Acoust Soc Am.* 1995;97(2):1249–1260.

4. Titze IR. The human vocal cords: a mathematical model. I. *Phonetica.* 1973; 28(3):129–170.

5. Titze IR. The human vocal cords: a mathematical model. II. *Phonetica.* 1974; 29(1):1–21.

6. Titze IR, Hunter EJ. A two-dimensional biomechanical model of vocal fold posturing. *J Acoust Soc Am.* 2007;121(4): 2254–2260.

7. Kersing W, Jennekens FG. Age-related changes in human thyroarytenoid muscles: a histological and histochemical study. *Eur Arch Otorhinolaryngol.* 2004; 261(7):386–392.

8. Kahane JC. Histologic structure and properties of the human vocal folds. *Ear Nose Throat J.* 1988;67(5):322, 324–325, 329–330.

9. Hirano M. Morphological structure of the vocal cord as a vibrator and its variations. *Folia Phoniatr (Basel).* 1974;26(2): 89–94.

10. Gray SD, Titze IR, Alipour F, Hammond TH. Biomechanical and histologic observations of vocal fold fibrous proteins. *Ann Otol Rhinol Laryngol.* 2000;109(1): 77–85.

11. Duflo S, Thibeault SL, Li W, Shu XZ, Prestwich GD. Vocal fold tissue repair in vivo using a synthetic extracellular matrix. *Tissue Eng.* 2006;12(8):2171–2180.

12. Hansen JK, Thibeault SL. Current understanding and review of the literature: vocal fold scarring. *J Voice.* 2006;20(1): 110–120.

13. Hansen JK, Thibeault SL, Walsh JF, Shu XZ, Prestwich GD. In vivo engineering of the vocal fold extracellular matrix with injectable hyaluronic acid hydrogels: early effects on tissue repair and biomechanics in a rabbit model. *Ann Otol Rhinol Laryngol.* 2005;114(9):662–670.

14. Chen X, Thibeault SL. Novel isolation and biochemical characterization of immortalized fibroblasts for tissue engineering vocal fold lamina propria. *Tissue Eng Part C Methods.* 2009;15(2): 201–212.

15. Schweinfurth JM, Thibeault SL. Does hyaluronic acid distribution in the larynx relate to the newborn's capacity for crying? *Laryngoscope.* 2008;118(9): 1692–1699.

16. Thibeault SL, Duflo S. Inflammatory cytokine responses to synthetic extracellular matrix injection to the vocal fold lamina propria. *Ann Otol Rhinol Laryngol.* 2008;117(3):221–226.

17. Thibeault SL, Klemuk SA, Smith ME, Leugers C, Prestwich G. In vivo comparison of biomimetic approaches for tissue regeneration of the scarred vocal fold. *Tissue Eng Part A.* 2009;15(7):1481–1487.

18. Hirschi SD, Gray SD, Thibeault SL. Fibronectin: an interesting vocal fold protein. *J Voice.* 2002;16(3):310–316.

19. Ward PD, Thibeault SL, Gray SD. Hyaluronic acid: its role in voice. *J Voice.* 2002;16(3):303–309.

20. Duflo SM, Thibeault SL, Li W, Smith ME, Schade G, Hess MM. Differential gene expression profiling of vocal fold polyps and Reinke's edema by complementary DNA microarray. *Ann Otol Rhinol Laryngol.* 2006;115(9):703–714.

21. Rousseau B, Ge PJ, Ohno T, French LC, Thibeault SL. Extracellular matrix gene

expression after vocal fold injury in a rabbit model. *Ann Otol Rhinol Laryngol.* 2008;117(8):598–603.

22. Thibeault SL, Hirschi SD, Gray SD. DNA microarray gene expression analysis of a vocal fold polyp and granuloma. *J Speech Lang Hear Res.* 2003;46(2):491–502.

23. Thibeault SL, Smith ME, Peterson K, Ylitalo-Moller R. Gene expression changes of inflammatory mediators in posterior laryngitis due to laryngopharyngeal reflux and evolution with PPI treatment: a preliminary study. *Laryngoscope.* 2007; 117(11):2050–2056.

24. Thomas L, Stemple J. Voice therapy: Does science support the art? *Comm Disord Rev.* 2007;1(1):51–79.

25. Van Riper C. *Speech Correction Principles and Methods.* Englewood Cliffs, NJ: Prentice-Hall; 1939.

26. West R, Kennedy L, Carr A. *The Rehabilitation of Speech.* New York, NY: Harper & Brothers; 1937.

27. Stemple J, Glaze L, Klaben B. *Clinical Voice Pathology: Theory and Management.* 3rd ed. San Diego, CA: Singular; 2000.

28. Boone D. *The Voice and Voice Therapy.* Englewood Cliffs, NJ: Prentice-Hall; 1971.

29. Goss F. Hysterical aphonia. *Boston Med Surg J.* 1878;99:215–222.

30. Russell J. A case of hysterical aphonia. *Brit Med J.* 1864;8:619–621.

31. Murphy A. *Functional Voice Disorders.* Englewood Cliffs, NJ: Prentice-Hall; 1964.

32. Brodnitz F. *Vocal Rehabilitation.* Rochester, NY: American Academy of Opthalmology and Otolaryngology; 1971.

33. Aronson A. *Clinical Voice Disorders: An Interdisciplinary Approach.* New York, NY: Brian C. Decker; 1980.

34. Case J. *Clinical Management of Voice Disorders.* 3rd ed. Austin, TX: Pro-Ed; 1996.

35. Stemple J. *Clinical Voice Pathology: Theory and Management.* Columbus, OH: Charles E. Merrill;1984.

36. Colton R, Casper J. *Understanding Voice Problems: A Physiological Perspective for Diagnosis and Treatment.* Baltimore, MD: Williams & Wilkins;1996.

37. Stemple JC, Glaze L, Klaben BG. *Clinical Voice Pathology: Theory and Management.* San Diego, CA: Singular; 2000.

38. Stemple JC, Lee L, D'Amico B, Pickup B. Efficacy of vocal function exercises as a method of improving voice production. *J Voice.* 1994;8(3):271–278.

39. Verdolini K. *Resonant Voice Therapy.* Iowa City, IA: National Center for Voice and Speech; 1998.

40. Kotby MN, Shiromoto O, Hirano M. The accent method of voice therapy: effect of accentuations on F_0, SPL, and airflow. *J Voice.* 1993;7(4):319–325.

2

Comments on the Voice Evaluation

Introduction

Voice clinicians use a variety of tools to evaluate and document voice disorders. Traditional components of the voice evaluation have included the medical examination to diagnose the disorder, systematic interviewing of the patient to determine causes, and a perceptual voice evaluation to describe the vocal symptoms. Other tools include acoustic and aerodynamic measures of voice production, along with observation of vocal fold vibration through laryngeal videostroboscopy,[1] kymography,[2,3] and high speed digital imaging.[4–7] Information gathered through these evaluation tools will provide:

■ understanding of the perceptual symptoms
■ a means of systematically describing the vocal condition

■ pretreatment and post-treatment measures used to describe the efficacy of intervention
■ patient education and feedback.

Many of the case studies presented in this text use instrumental measures of voice production. Although instrumental measures are an important adjunct to the traditional components of voice evaluation, they are not meant to replace any other component. The eyes and ears of the physician and the clinician cannot be replaced. The most important aspect of the diagnostic voice evaluation is the ability to talk to one's patients, that is, to conduct a patient interview that will yield the necessary diagnostic information. If only one evaluation component was available to me, the patient interview would be my choice.

Another important aspect of the evaluation process is to gain an understanding of the functional impact of the voice disorder on the individual in daily life. Those in clinical practice know that individual patients will perceive similar voice disorders differently. For example, a professional voice user with vocal nodules may be devastated by the effect that nodules have on the voice, whereas a computer programmer may not consider the mild hoarseness to be a problem. One method of gaining this functional measure is through the use of validated tools that measure the patient's self-assessment of the voice disorder.[8,9]

The primary objective of the diagnostic voice evaluation is to discover etiologic factors specific to the development of the voice disorder. Voice pathologists will use all of their artistic and scientific skills in a systematic evaluation to determine these specific causes. In addition, a detailed analysis of the vocal symptoms, both subjective and objective, will be completed. A systematic management approach will be the result.

Secondary objectives of the diagnostic evaluation include education and motivation of the patient and the establishing of credibility and trust in the voice pathologist. Most patients have little knowledge or understanding of the normal voice, to say nothing of their own voice disorders. During the voice evaluation, the voice pathologist will find it useful to explain, in simple terms, normal voicing and how it relates to the patient's current problem. Videostroboscopy, when available, is invaluable as a patient educator and often encourages patients to become partners in their own care. The better understanding patients have of their voice disorders, the more helpful they can be in answering questions designed to discover the causes of their voice disorders. In addition, the well-informed patient generally is more moti-

vated to follow a therapy regimen and resolve the disorder.

It is essential that the credibility of the voice pathologist be established early during the evaluation. Many probing questions regarding the patient's personal life must be asked in seeking etiologic factors. The patient must trust the voice pathologist's intent to use this information appropriately. The voice pathologist who projects a casual yet professional demeanor may develop credibility and trust at the initial patient contact. This type of relaxed demeanor will reduce anxieties and establish an atmosphere for easy discussion.

Once the primary etiologic factors have been discovered, the vocal symptoms have been subjectively and objectively described, the impact of the disorder has been determined, the patient has been educated, and the clinician has established credibility, the management plan can be outlined. When patients understand the causes of the problem and are presented with a systematic management approach, along with a reasonable estimated time for completion, a positive therapeutic attitude usually is developed.

Management Team

Evaluation and management of patients with voice disorders increasingly have been accomplished through the teamwork of several professionals. These include the laryngologist and voice pathologist and other medical professionals including pulmonologists, gastroenterologists, and neurologists, among others. In addition, speech/voice trainers and singing teachers or coaches may be required. The laryngologist is trained to examine the laryngeal mechanism and to determine the need for medical, surgical, or behavioral intervention. The voice pathologist is trained to identify the causes of voice disorders, evaluate the vocal symptoms, and establish improved vocal function through various therapeutic methods. The speech/voice trainer or singing teacher judges the efficiency and correctness of performance technique and suggests modifications as deemed necessary. This complementary professional relationship has significantly improved the care of the voice-disordered population.

Medical Evaluation

A laryngologic examination involves examination of the entire head and neck region, as well as a detailed medical history. It includes otoscopic examination of the ears; observation of the oral and nasal cavities; palpation of the salivary glands, lymph nodes, and thyroid gland; and a visual examination of the larynx. The visual examination of the larynx may be performed in the office using indirect mirror observation, a fiberoptic nasal endoscope, or a rigid oral endoscope. The fiberoptic or rigid scopes may be attached to a digital camera, permitting the vocal folds to be viewed on a monitor. A laryngeal stroboscope also may be used with the digital video equipment and endoscopes to provide a simulated, slow-motion view of vocal fold vibration.

The vocal folds also may be viewed directly through direct laryngoscopy. During this surgical procedure, the patient receives general anesthesia, and a magnifying laryngoscope is placed into the oral cavity and pharynx to yield a direct view of the larynx. Biopsies and surgical excisions also may be performed through the laryngoscope.

The medical examination also may include special radiographs of the head and neck, as well as blood analysis and swallow studies. The final result of the medical examination is a diagnosis of the problem and recommendations for treatment including medical, surgical, voice evaluation, and voice therapy, or any combination thereof.

Voice Pathology Evaluation

When referral is made for a diagnostic voice evaluation, the three major objectives of the voice pathologist are to:

1. identify the causes of the disorder;
2. describe the present vocal components; and
3. develop an individualized management plan.

Various methods have been used to identify the causes of voice disorders. These methods include the formal interview with the patient or a predeveloped case history form to be completed either by the patient or by the patient and clinician together. This author finds prepared forms to be restrictive and prefers to use the patient interview format. Beginning clinicians may find prepared questionnaires useful, however. The following interview procedure (reprinted from Stemple, Glaze and Klaben [2009], *Clinical Voice Pathology: Theory and Management*, 4th ed.) describes specific goals for each component of the patient interview, as well as pertinent areas of investigation.

Referral

The goal is to establish the referral source, which should be clearly understood at the beginning of the evaluation. The primary referral source will be the otolaryngologist, but referrals may also come from other speech pathologists, singing teachers, voice coaches, the patient's relatives and friends, or the patient may be self-referred.

Reason for the Referral

The goals are to:

1. establish the exact reasons for patient referral;
2. establish patient understanding of the referral;
3. develop the patient's knowledge of his or her voice disorder; and
4. establish the credibility of examiner.

It is important to have adequate information regarding the exact reason the patient was referred. When a physician refers a patient, the specific medical diagnosis should be reported along with the physician's expectations. There are many reasons for patient referrals. These may include preoperative objective measures of voice, evaluation without management, baseline description of present voice, preoperative trial therapy, postoperative follow-up therapy, or a complete diagnostic voice evaluation with appropriate vocal management. Understanding the physician's expectations will avoid confusion and help maintain the necessary working relationships.

It is also desirable at this time to establish the patient's understanding of the referral for "speech therapy." A typical dialogue between a patient (*PT*) and voice pathologist (*VP*) might be:

VP: "Do you understand why the doctor referred you here?"

PT: "Not really. The doctor just said I needed speech therapy, but I really don't understand what it is all about. My speech is OK; I'm just hoarse."

This is an excellent opportunity for the voice pathologist to explain in some detail the three major goals he or she intends to accomplish during the evaluation. The more patients understand the procedures, the more reliable they will be in communicating pertinent information to the clinician throughout the evaluation.

It also is helpful to establish and develop the patient's knowledge of the voice disorder before proceeding. This may be accomplished by explaining briefly how the normal laryngeal mechanism works and how it is affected by the disorder. With this information, patients will better understand where certain questions are leading and may be able to give more reliable information. Some patients even volunteer pertinent information following this discussion and before other questions are asked. For example:

VP: "Do you understand what vocal nodules are?"

PT: "They're some kind of growths on my vocal cords, aren't they?"

VP: "Something like that. Do you know what your vocal cords look like?"

PT: "No, not really."

VP: "Well, when the doctor looked down your throat at your vocal folds, she or he was essentially looking at two solid shelves of muscle tissue, one on each side. (Draw a diagram, show pictures, or use a video.) Those shelves are the vocal folds, or cords, and we're looking down on top of them. The point here where they meet is your Adam's apple. Can you feel yours? (Gives patient spatial orientation.) Now, the space between the vocal folds is the airway where air travels to the lungs as we breathe.

Attached to the back of each vocal fold we have two cartilages: one here, and one here. The reason we have these cartilages is so that other muscles that work the vocal folds may have a place on which to attach. Some muscles separate the folds, whereas other muscles draw them together. This is certainly a simplified explanation, but I think it will give you the basic idea of how the system works.

To move the vocal folds together, we have muscles attached to each cartilage pulling in opposite directions. These pull the vocal folds to the middle where they vibrate, giving us our voices.

If these muscles pull too hard, such as when we shout, talk loudly for a long time, or clear our throats, this excessive pull will cause the vocal folds to rub and bang together. (Demonstrate with clapping hands.) If this rubbing and banging occurs too frequently, it eventually will cause some swelling of the tissues that usually causes temporary hoarseness. The hoarseness may go away after a day or so, but if whatever caused the swelling persists, the folds will remain swollen and eventually attempt to protect themselves from further damage. In your case, they've done this by developing, layer by layer, small callouslike structures, which are called vocal nodules.

As you've experienced, the nodules cause a change in your voice. Because of the swelling and the nodules, your voice is deeper in pitch; and because the nodules are holding your folds apart when you try to vibrate them, your voice is breathy. You've also probably noticed that when you do a lot of talking your voice fatigues, and it becomes quite an effort just to talk. Sometimes by the end of the day, you may be worn out from the effort, and you simply don't feel like talking anymore.

One final point. Vocal nodules are not cancer, are not related to cancer, and do not lead to cancer. Many people do not understand this, and I think it's important to mention. So do you now understand basically what the vocal folds are like and what vocal nodules are?"

PT: "Yes, now I do. I'm glad you mentioned cancer. I was worried about that. But what do you think caused the nodules?

I don't raise my voice very much."

VP: "That's what we're here today to find out. I'm going to ask you many questions. I need to get to know who you are and how you use your voice. From that information, we will try to determine what specifically has caused your nodules. Any questions?"

It also should be noted that this type of discussion goes far in developing your credibility as an "expert" in this area. You usually will have managed to develop a high level of trust before you begin questions regarding the history of the problem.

History of the Problem

The goals are to:

1. establish the chronologic history of the problem;
2. seek etiologic factors associated with the history and
3. determine patient motivation.

This section of the evaluation is designed to yield a chronological history of the voice disorder from the onset of vocal difficulties, through the development of the problem over time, and ending with the patient's present vocal experiences. All questions are designed to yield information regarding the causes of vocal difficulties. Finally, the patient's motivation for seeking vocal improvement is determined. A list of appropriate questions may include the following:

■ When did you first notice you were having some difficulties with your voice?

■ Was this the first time you ever experienced vocal difficulties?
■ How did the problem progress from there?
■ What finally made you decide to see your doctor about it?
■ How did the doctor treat the problem?
■ Did your family doctor refer you to the otolaryngologist?
■ Has anyone else in your family ever had voice problems?
■ Is your voice better in the morning than in the evening or vice versa?
■ Have you ever totally lost your voice?
■ Do you have any occasion at all to raise your voice, to shout, or to talk loudly over noise?
■ Do you talk often to anyone who is hard of hearing?
■ Do you have a pet?
■ Not knowing you prior to your vocal difficulties, I don't know what your normal voice is like. I have a scale of 0 to 5. How hoarse are you right now if 0 is normal and 5 is very hoarse?
■ How much does this problem actually bother you?
■ Are you interested in doing something about it?

Medical History

The goals are to:

1. seek medically related etiologic factors; and
2. help establish awareness of patient's basic personality.

Taking the medical history is the process of seeking out any medically related etiologic factors regarding the presenting disorder. Questions are asked regarding past surgeries and hospitalizations. Chronic disorders are probed, along with the use of medications. Smoking history and alcohol and drug use are explored. The patient's hydration habits also are discussed. The medical history also helps to establish in the clinician's mind how patients "feel" about their physical and emotional well-being. This may be accomplished by asking patients whether, on a day-to-day basis, they feel "excellent, good, fair, or poor." The response to this question will provide the voice pathologist with insight into how patients feel about themselves. Some patients report lengthy medical histories with many chronic disorders, but they indicate that they feel "good" on a day-to-day basis. Other patients with unremarkable medical histories may report feeling "fair" or "poor." This information is helpful in learning patients' basic personalities.

Social History

The goals are to:

1. know the patient's work, home, and recreational environments;
2. discover emotional, social, and family difficulties; and
3. seek more etiologic factors for the disorder.

The social history finalizes in the clinician's mind a perception of the patient. It yields information regarding work, home, recreational and social lifestyles and whether these lifestyles contributed to the development of laryngeal disorders. All questions probe for answers to possible etiologic factors. For example:

- Are you married, single, divorced, or widowed?
- How long have you been married?
- Do you have children?

- What are their ages?
- How many are still at home?
- Does anyone else live in your home? Parents? Others?
- Do you work? Where? How long?
- Specifically, what do you do in your work?
- How much talking is required?
- What is the work environment?
- Does your husband or wife work? Where? How long? What shift?
- When you're not working, what do you enjoy doing? (Include clubs, groups, hobbies, organizations, and so forth.)
- Sometimes voice problems arise out of upsetting events. Has anything occurred that has been particularly upsetting to you recently or that has caused you to have increased anxiety?

As you begin the social history questions, it often is helpful to explain to patients that you need to get to know who they are and what they do to find the causes for their vocal difficulties. You want patients to "excuse" you if some of the questions seem personal. This questioning is necessary to discover all possible causes. Do not be surprised when patients open up to you with many personal, family, social, marital, or work problems. If you have developed your credibility and gained their trust, you often will be entrusted with this important information.

Oral-Peripheral Examination

The goals are to:

1. determine the physical condition of oral mechanisms;
2. observe laryngeal area tension;
3. check for swallowing difficulties; and
4. check for laryngeal sensations.

A routine oral-peripheral examination also should be conducted to determine the condition of the oral mechanism in its relation to the patient's speech and voice production. Also included is observation of the patient's laryngeal area tension utilizing visual observation of posture and neck muscle tension, as well as digital manipulation of the thyroid cartilage. The patient also should be asked whether any swallowing difficulties are present to determine whether this function has been affected by or is affecting vocal production. Finally, the patient should be asked whether any laryngeal sensations are present. The laryngeal sensations most often associated with voice disorders include aching, dryness, tickling, burning, and a feeling of a "lump in the throat."

Voice Evaluation

The goals are to:

1. describe the present vocal components; and
2. examine inappropriate use of the vocal components.

Following the patient interview, the perceptual and instrumental voice evaluations are conducted. Through the patient interview, the examiner has had an adequate sample of conversational voice to make a subjective description of the patient's voice quality. Several formal voice rating scales have been developed and utilized for perceptually judging voice quality.[1-3] One method used to report the degree of baseline dysphonia uses a 6-point, equal-appearing interval scale where 0 = normal, 1 = mild, 2 = mild to moderate, 3 = moderate, 4 = moder-

ate to severe, 5 = severe dysphonia. This scaled description is followed, for the future reference of the examiner, by a descriptive characterization of the voice, including descriptive terms such as hoarseness, harshness, breathiness, raspiness, glottal fry, low pitch, and so on.

A more formalized scale for evaluating hoarseness, GRBAS, was developed by the Committee for Phonatory Function Tests of the Japan Society of Logopedics and Phoniatrics.[10] This scale evaluates five components of voice production: grade (G), roughness (R), breathiness (B), aesthenia (A), and strained (S). Each component is rated on a 4-point scale where 0 = normal, 1 = slight, 2 = moderate, and 3 = extreme.

Grade (G) represents the degree of hoarseness or voice abnormality. Rough (R) represents the perceptual impression of the irregularity of vocal fold vibrations. It corresponds to the irregular fluctuations in the fundamental frequency, the amplitude of vibration, or both. Breathy (B) represents the perceptual impression of the extent of air leakage through the glottis. Aesthenic (A) denotes weakness or lack of power in the voice. Strained (S) represents the perceptual impression of vocal hyperfunction.

In an attempt to further improve the perceptual evaluation of voice, a committee of the American Speech-Language-Hearing Association Special Interest Division 3, Voice and Voice Disorders, developed the Consensus Auditory-Perceptual Evaluation of Voice (CAPE-V).[11,12] The CAPE-V uses a 100-mm visual analog scale to assess voice quality at the vowel, sentence, and conversational speech levels. The parameters of voice assessed include overall severity, roughness, breathiness, strain, pitch, and loudness. Areas for describing additional features such as diplophonia, fry, falsetto, asthenia, aphonia, pitch instability, tremor, wet/gurgly, or other relevant terms are provided.

The perceptual voice evaluation is conducted to describe the current condition of voice production and to determine whether any vocal components— such as pitch, loudness, breathiness, and so on—are inappropriate to the degree of contributing to the development or maintenance of the disorder. Beyond the formal scales described above, each vocal component may be examined separately as follows:

Respiration

This includes a description of conversational breathing patterns, including supportive or nonsupportive, clavicular, thoracic, or abdominal-diaphragmatic breathing patterns. Speaking on a poorly supported airstream is determined through observation. The s/z ratio is formally tested when the diagnosis is vocal nodules.

Phonation

Subjective observations regarding vocal function are made through critical listening. These include the presence of hard glottal attacks, glottal fry, diplophonia, and breathiness. These vocal characteristics may be observed conversationally throughout the evaluation. The clinician may also recheck by listening for specific phonatory behaviors while the patient says the alphabet at a normal conversational rate.

Resonance

Observation regarding the type of resonance quality is made. These qualities may include normal, hypernasality, denasality, assimilative, and cul-de-sac nasality. In addition, observations of tone focus (forward or back) are made.

Pitch

The patient's present pitch range is tested by having the patient sing up a scale from the lowest note to the highest note and from highest to lowest and matching the extremes to a pitch pipe or a keyboard. Conversational inflection and pitch variability are also important to describe.

Loudness

The appropriateness of the patient's speaking loudness level during the evaluation is described. It is also important to test the patient's ability to increase subglottic air pressure. This may be accomplished by asking the patient to shout "hey." The ability to produce a more solid phonation during a shout is a good indicator of the severity of the problem. If the patient is able to override the dysphonia with increased loudness (which is determined by the ability the folds to approximate tightly to increase subglottic air pressure), the disorder is perhaps not as severe as when a patient cannot easily increase loudness.

Rate

The rate of the patient's speech may contribute to the development of the vocal disorders. This is especially true for the individual who speaks with an exceptionally fast rate. During the diagnostic work-up, the rate of conversational speech is described as normal, fast, or slow.

Instrumental Voice Analysis

Instrumental measures of vocal function, sometimes called laryngeal function studies or phonatory function tests, may be conducted if the appropriate instrumentation is available. Acoustic, aerodynamic, and laryngeal imaging analyses are used to objectively describe vocal function. Common acoustic measures include:

- fundamental frequency
- frequency range
- frequency perturbations (jitter)
- habitual intensity
- intensity range (maximum/minimum)
- intensity perturbations (shimmer)
- signal-to-noise ratio
- spectral analyses.

Useful aerodynamic measures include:

- airflow volume
- airflow rate
- maximum phonation time
- subglottic air pressure
- glottal efficiency
- phonation threshold pressure
- laryngeal airway resistance.

Laryngeal videostroboscopy demonstrates a simulated, slow-motion view of the vocal fold vibration. This view provides much additional diagnostic information, including:

- configuration of glottic closure
- degree of supraglottic activity
- vertical level approximation of the vocal folds
- condition of the vocal fold edge
- amplitude of vibration
- integrity the mucosal wave
- nonvibrating areas of the vocal folds

- phase and symmetry of the vibratory pattern of the vocal folds.

Impressions

The goal is to summarize the etiologic factors associated with the development and maintenance of the individual's voice disorder. This section of the diagnostic procedure is used as a summary for the causes of the voice disorder discovered throughout the evaluation. These causes are listed in order of perceived importance, relating first to the initiation of the problem and second to the maintenance of the problem. Remember that the precipitating factor may not be the maintenance factor.

Prognosis

The goal is to analyze the probability of improvement through voice therapy. The prognosis for improving many voice disorders through voice therapy is generally good. Nonetheless, many factors influence prognosis (see Chapter 9), including the motivation, interest, and time of the patient; ability of the patient to follow instructions; the physical and emotional conditions of the patient; and the general condition of the vocal folds. The prognosis section permits the voice pathologist to give a subjective opinion regarding the chances for successful remediation based on the diagnostic information. A reasonable time frame for expected completion of the management program also should be stated.

Recommendations

The goal is to outline the management plan. This management plan is then briefly outlined based on the etiologic factors discovered during the evaluation. The plan includes the therapy approaches to be used and additional referrals to be made.

Additional Considerations

The evaluation format presented here may be classified as semistructured. The basic questions remain the same from patient to patient, but the answers given by individual patients dictate the direction in which the questioning will proceed and the order in which each diagnostic section is reviewed. This format favors the more experienced voice pathologist. The beginning clinician may feel the need for a more structured format. As experience is gained, the structured formats may prove limiting, and the semistructured method is often the method of choice. Some voice pathologists also feel most comfortable audio or video recording the entire diagnostic session for later review. This may help in determining the exact vocal components produced during the evaluation and serves as a record of the baseline voice quality. Even if the entire diagnostic session is not recorded, recording of a standard speech sample is necessary for later comparison. It is not unusual for the voice pathologist and the patient to forget the actual severity of the baseline quality. Audio recordings serve as an objective reminder and should be used liberally.

Finally, the American Speech-Language-Hearing Association mandates that patients who undergo speech, voice, and language evaluations must have had a current hearing screening. Audiometric evaluation is important for the patient with a voice disorder. The

inability to monitor one's voice may result in the use of inappropriate vocal components. Severe voice disorders are often observed in the hard-of-hearing and deaf populations.

Summary

Successful voice therapy is totally dependent on an in-depth and accurate diagnostic evaluation. Indeed, this author views the voice evaluation as a primary therapy tool. The evaluation determines the causes for the disorder, teaches the patient about the disorder, and describes the vocal function that must be modified for voice improvement to occur.

The remainder of this text is devoted to management techniques for voice disorders. You will realize in studying the many case presentations that selecting the appropriate treatments depends on the multidisciplinary evaluations of management team members. For organization purposes, the remaining chapters are organized to describe management strategies for disorders of vocal hyperfunction, glottal incompetence, functional voice disorders, respiratory/laryngeal disorders, professional voice disorders, and neurogenic voice disorders. Many crossovers in management approaches are evident and useful for the various disorders. All successful voice therapy, however, begins with accurate diagnosis and planning through the medical examination and voice evaluation.

References

1. Hirano M, Bless, D. *Videostroboscopic Examination of the Larynx.* San Diego, CA: Singular Publishing Group; 1993.

2. Larsson H, Hertegard S, Lindestad PA, Hammarberg B. Vocal fold vibrations: high-speed imaging, kymography, and acoustic analysis: a preliminary report. *Laryngoscope.* 2000;110(12):2117–2122.

3. Wittenberg T, Tigges M, Mergell P, Eysholdt U. Functional imaging of vocal fold vibration: digital multislice high-speed kymography. *J Voice.* 2000;14(3): 422–442.

4. Patel R, Dailey S, Bless D. Comparison of high-speed digital imaging with stroboscopy for laryngeal imaging of glottal disorders. *Ann Otol Rhinol Laryngol.* 2008;117(6):413–424.

5. Bonilha HS, Aikman A, Hines K, Deliyski DD. Vocal fold mucus aggregation in vocally normal speakers. *Logoped Phoniatr Vocol.* 2008;33(3):136–142.

6. Deliyski DD, Petrushev PP, Bonilha HS, Gerlach TT, Martin-Harris B, Hillman RE. Clinical implementation of laryngeal high-speed videoendoscopy: challenges and evolution. *Folia Phoniatr Logop.* 2008;60(1):33–44.

7. George NA, de Mul FF, Qiu Q, Rakhorst G, Schutte HK. New laryngoscope for quantitative high-speed imaging of human vocal folds vibration in the horizontal and vertical direction. *J Biomed Opt.* 2008;13(6):064024.

8. Hogikyan ND, Wodchis WP, Terrell JE, Bradford CR, Esclamado RM. Voice-related quality of life (V-RQOL) following type I thyroplasty for unilateral vocal fold paralysis. *J Voice.* 2000;14(3): 378–386.

9. Jacobson B, Johnson A, Grywalski C, Silbergleit A, Jacobson G, Benninger MS. The Voice Handicap Index (VHI): Development and validation. *Am J Speech Lang Pathol.* 1997;6:66–70.

10. Hirano M. *Clinical Examination of Voice.* New York, NY: Springer-Verlag; 1981.

11. American Speech-Language-Hearing Association. Consensus Auditory-Perceptual Evaluation of Voice (CAPE-V) Purpose and Applications. Available from http://www.asha.org.

12. Kempster GB, Gerratt BR, Verdolini Abbott K, Barkmeier-Kraemer J, Hillman RE. Consensus auditory-perceptual evaluation of voice: development of a standardized clinical protocol. *Am J Speech Lang Pathol.* 2009;18(2):124–132.

3

Management of Vocal Hyperfunction and Associated Pathologies

Introduction

Knowledge of the common causes of voice disorders is essential when planning appropriate management programs. Many voice disorders and associated laryngeal pathologic conditions are caused by hyperfunction of the laryngeal mechanism. At times, this hyperfunction is behavioral, causing harmful mechanical impact to the tissue lining of the vocal folds. Examples of potentially harmful vocal behaviors include shouting, loud talking, screaming, vocal noises, coughing, throat clearing, and inappropriate singing technique. Inappropriate use of the components of voice production, including faulty breathing patterns and breath support, and poor phonatory

habits (such as the use of glottal attacks and glottal fry, restricted resonance, and improper pitch, loudness, and rate) also may lead to a hyperfunctional voice disorder. The condition of the vocal fold mucosal lining and underlying muscular relationships also may cause vocal compensations that are implicated in the hyperfunctioning of the vocal mechanism. For example, a dehydrated mucous membrane lining caused by lack of adequate liquid intake, drying medications, and smoking may create inefficient vocal fold vibration.[1–3]

Inefficient vibration requires greater effort to initiate and maintain vocal fold oscillation. This increased effort may lead to vocal hyperfunction, causing laryngeal fatigue and subsequent compensatory muscle tension. Indeed, most hyperfunctional voice disorders have multiple causes and, therefore, have multifaceted management approaches.

This chapter is devoted to the treatment of vocal hyperfunction in both children and adults. Management strategies include an eclectic array of techniques involving vocal hygiene, psychosocial considerations, symptom modifications, and direct physiologic manipulations of the voice subsystems. We begin with several presentations of the treatment of vocal hyperfunction in children.

Vocal Hyperfunction in Children

Vocal hyperfunction can occur at any age and is the most common cause of voice disorders in children.[4] Children with hyperfunctional voice problems pose a challenge because they traumatize their vocal mechanisms in various ways. The following cases illustrate some important issues when dealing with vocal hyperfunction in children.

Therapy with Limited Parental Interaction

Joseph C. Stemple, PhD

Case Study: Patient B

In discussing the treatment of children's voice disorders with public school speech-language pathologists, one of the primary treatment problems identified is the lack of interaction with and cooperation from parents. Because most parents work outside the home, interaction with schools is often limited and difficult to schedule. Behavior modification voice therapy therefore may be difficult. This

was the case with Patient B, a 9-year-old, fourth-grade child who was identified as hoarse during the fall speech screening. A form letter was sent to his home describing the voice problem and suggesting that either his family physician or an ear, nose, and throat physician check the problem.

Patient B's parents did not respond to the letter, and as school progressed, he became more dysphonic. His classroom teacher became concerned and invited the school's speech-language pathologist (SLP) to discuss the problem with the parents during a parent-teacher conference. The patient's mother confirmed receiving the form letter but indicated that her son had "always had a husky voice." She and his father were neither alarmed nor overly concerned. The patient's teacher indicated that her own concern focused on how it was affecting the child in the classroom. He could not speak softly, so he had to talk loudly to be heard. This was somewhat embarrassing to him, and he had become reticent to participate in class. In addition, his chronic throat clearing was annoying and occasionally had been disruptive during "quiet periods."

The speech pathologist explained the common causes of hoarseness and the possibilities of edema and vocal nodules, the common childhood laryngeal disorders. Patient B's mother left the conference promising to discuss the matter with her child's pediatrician.

Patient B's mother followed through with her promise. The pediatrician placed the boy on antibiotics for 10 days, which did not modify his symptoms. A referral was made to a laryngologist in December. Indirect laryngoscopy revealed the presence of bilateral vocal fold nodules. Voice therapy was recommended and then scheduled to begin in January. Thus, between identification of the problem in

September and referral for therapy, half of the school year had been lost.

Public school speech pathologists often ask if they must wait for laryngologic examination and therapy recommendation. The answer is yes. From both medical and legal standpoints, we need to know what we are treating. Personal examples of this rule include the 10-year-old child who was indeed treated for "hoarseness" without improvement for 3 years in the school. When an indirect laryngoscopic examination was finally performed, a congenital web was found to be the cause of her voice problem. Any amount of therapy would have been of little use. In another case, persistent hoarseness was identified in a 9-year-old girl. An immediate laryngologic examination and subsequent direct laryngoscopy with biopsy revealed a carcinoma, a shocking and highly unusual diagnosis in a child. Imagine the implications had medical management not been implemented. As it was, this child required a total laryngectomy.

In January, Patient B's speech pathologist evaluated his voice production. She described his voice as moderately dysphonic, characterized by breathy, husky, hoarseness and loud volume. He had a pitch range of less than one octave and could sustain the /a/ sound for only 5 seconds. The s/z ratio was 11 seconds to 4 seconds.[5] His phonation was characterized by hard glottal attacks.

Many phonotraumatic behaviors also were identified. They included the following:

■ shouting at or with his 6- and 11-year-old brothers (arguing, playing, fighting)
■ shouting during sporting events (the patient played soccer, baseball, and basketball on organized teams)
■ chronic, habitual throat clearing

■ production of vocal noises while pretending to be a professional wrestler; engine noises while playing with toy cars, trucks, and motorcycles; various vocal sounds while playing with action figures
■ shouting with an extremely high pitch
■ habitual loud talking.

It was decided to focus therapy on the issues that could be best addressed in school. Parental support would be sought, but realistically was not expected or subsequently received. Patient B's speech pathologist developed a program that consisted of four components:

1. *Education.* Photographs, line drawings, and videos of vocal nodules obtained from the Web were used with the patient to describe his vocal folds and to describe how vocal nodules are developed. The boy's inability to talk softly was discussed as it related to the inability of the vocal folds to totally approximate. With the nodules holding his vocal folds apart, this patient was required to force a greater amount of air between the vocal folds to initiate and maintain vibration, increasing the amplitude of vibration. This increased effort made him talk louder and caused constant voice strain.

Audio recordings of clear voices, hoarse voices, and his own voice were used to demonstrate the voice qualities being discussed. Finally, vocally traumatic behaviors (such as shouting, loud talking, vocal noises, and throat clearing) were discussed and related to the causes of hoarseness. Substitutions for various vocal noises were described, as well as suggestions for eliminating the most vocally traumatic. Shouting for "play" was contrasted with shouting in nonplay activities. Nonplay shouting (such as calling for another family member from one part of the house to another, yelling for the dog, and arguing with his brothers) was discussed, and an appeal was made to "think before you shout." Again, without parental cooperation, modifying nonplay shouting may be difficult.

2. *Behavior modification.* Utilizing his classroom teacher, a best friend, and the speech-language pathologist, Patient B was taught the "forceful swallow" method for eliminating throat clearing (forceful swallow will be described later in this chapter). A method of charting throat clearing during school was devised, and the occurrences decreased significantly within 3 weeks.

A chart also was used for shouting activities in school. These included shouting on the playground, during gym class, in the hallway, and in the cafeteria. An appropriate reward system was developed.

3. *Direct voice therapy.* Patient B's increased loudness level, breathiness, and hard glottal attacks all were symptoms of his vocal nodules and not causes of the problem. Direct therapy using Vocal Function Exercises (described later) was initiated as a means of indirectly teaching easy onset, respiratory support, and frontal focus while balancing respiration, phonation, and resonance.

4. *Teach an appropriate method of shouting.* This patient was an active, vocally enthusiastic child. His coaches encouraged him to shout during organized sporting events. In addition, it was evident that he lived in a loud, active household. It was impractical to expect elimination of all shouting behaviors, and thus the speech pathologist decided to teach him "how" to shout.

As the boy's voice quality began to improve with the previous three meth-

ods, the SLP taught him a less traumatic manner of shouting. When the patient shouted, his pitch level went to an unusually high pitch. Production of this high pitch required the vocal folds to be stretched and tensed. He was, therefore, taught to shout using a low pitch, with improved abdominal breath support and a forward tone focus. The vocal folds thus would be less abused when absorbing the impact of shouting because the vocal folds were thicker and less tense at lower pitches.

Integrating education, behavior modification, direct voice manipulation, and instructions for less vocally traumatic shouting, Patient B was able to improve his voice quality and stabilize his voice by the end of the school year to a mild dysphonia characterized by a slight dry hoarseness. More important was his increased participation in the classroom. The speech-language pathologist did not have the opportunity of a follow-up laryngologic examination. Nonetheless, even without the parent's active participation, Patient B's voice therapy could be judged successful.

Psychosocial Aspects of Children's Behaviors and the Development of Voice Disorders

Moya Andrews, Ed.D

Case Study: Patient C

> *In the following case study, Moya Andrews explores the psychosocial aspects of a child's behavior related to the development of a voice disorder and introduces voice facilitating techniques including storytelling, role-playing, and others.*

Patient History. Patient C, aged 4 years and 6 months, was referred by her teacher at a Montessori preschool because of "hoarseness, loud talking, and frequent attention-getting behaviors in class." She was brought to the speech and hearing clinic by her mother, who had taken the patient from school in time for their 11 AM appointment. The mother apologized for the fact that the child insisted she needed to bring a large, "fast-food" milkshake into the diagnostic room with her. "She always has to have a shake," said the mother with a shrug, while the little girl smiled complacently and toyed with her straw. When the speech pathologist suggested that Patient C should sit in the waiting room until she had finished her shake, the mother looked distressed and said, "Oh no, she wouldn't like that at all." The patient's smile widened, she tossed her head, did a little dance around the room, and spilled some of the shake on the floor. "Oh dear," said the mother helplessly, "she's just so full of energy."

During the interview, the mother reported that Patient C was the youngest of three children. Her two older brothers, aged 14 and 16 years, attended the local high school. The mother, a homemaker, said that the patient had been born in Germany during the time that her husband had been in the U.S. military service. The father was currently employed at a local hospital. "My husband always wanted a daughter, so I suppose we spoil her," said her mother.

Patient C demonstrated many of the classic behaviors associated with vocal abuse: inefficient respiratory pattern; tension in the shoulder, neck, and jaw; phonation breaks; hard glottal attacks; loud conversational level; hoarse vocal quality; weak resonance; limited vocal variety; and frequent throat clearing. She

could prolong a vowel for only 3 seconds and exhibited hearing sensitivity within normal limits bilaterally. The results of an examination of her peripheral speech mechanism were unremarkable. The otolaryngological report noted small bilateral vocal nodules and redness of laryngeal structures but no evidence of allergies or infections. The school psychologist's report noted above-average intelligence, frequent temper tantrums and episodes of crying, and use of manipulative interpersonal strategies. The child was involved in after-school programs such as ballet, swimming, an art class, and a neighborhood play group.

The mother characterized her daughter's behavior in the following way: "She is quite a handful at times, but she's intelligent and has had more opportunities than other children her age because we lived abroad. Also, she has had to be assertive or her brothers ignore her. She is a live wire and can be difficult, but she is so cute and talented that we can never stay angry with her for long." It appeared that the psychodynamics in the patient's family merited further attention.

Further questions resulted in the information that when the patient's vocal behavior was loud and forceful, she usually got what she wanted at home. The patient's teacher reported that the child's interpersonal strategies did not help her succeed in her school environment, however. Rather, she needed to develop more effective interpersonal and vocal strategies to establish satisfying relationships with her peers and teachers. Therefore, the therapy program was designed to include work on relevant psychosocial issues, as well as modification of abusive vocal behaviors.

General Awareness Phase. Voice therapy programs for children usually begin with a general awareness phase. During this phase, the child is oriented to the general area of voice and taught basic concepts and the background information that is necessary before the clinician targets specific symptoms. For example, Patient C needed a general awareness of respiration because it was an area of her behavior that needed to be modified. The clinician used a "science project" format to teach the girl general information about breathing. Activities were designed to achieve two sets of goals.

1. I can talk about breathing.
   - I can describe some different ways people and animals breathe.
   - I can describe how air is used (for example, to sustain life, to make sound, to pant, and so forth).
   - I can label the body parts used during breathing (such as lungs and windpipe).
   - I can tell my teacher how to breathe in without tensing her shoulders and neck.
   - I can time the number of seconds it takes for my teacher to breathe out air.
2. I can talk about what happened in stories my teacher reads to me.

Another general awareness goal for Patient C was for her to develop an understanding of psychosocial factors relevant to vocal communication. The clinician used a "story format" to teach the patient some general principles of communication. The following activities were designed to achieve this:

- I can guess what might happen when storybook characters act in certain ways (utilization of cause and effect).
- I can make up different endings to some stories (analysis of choices).

- I can explain why some things go wrong for some children in our stories (identification of unproductive strategies).
- I can suggest some other ways the characters may handle situations (problem solving).

Sample Stories

1. Jennifer and Mary were both doing puzzles at preschool. Mary finished her puzzle and started to watch Jennifer, who was having trouble with hers. Mary picked up two of the pieces of Jennifer's puzzle, shrieked loudly, and ran across the room. Jennifer ran after Mary and tried to grab the pieces from her, but Mary quickly threw them under a storage cabinet. It took Jennifer a long time to crawl under the low cabinet and find them.

Answer these questions:

- How did Mary feel?
- How did Jennifer feel?
- Why do you think Mary threw the pieces away?
- What would you suggest Mary should do next?
- Does Mary like Jennifer? Explain why or why not?
- What would you do if you were the teacher?

2. Ann told Cathy that she was mean and no one wanted to play with her anymore. Cathy felt very bad, but she didn't want Ann to know, so she knocked over the glue and then screamed loudly that Ann had knocked the glue over on purpose and ruined Cathy's work. Cathy screamed so much she got red in the face, and the teacher had to tell her to have a drink of water to calm

down. The teacher also told Ann to go and work on the other side of the room. Cathy felt she had paid Ann back.

Answer these questions:

- What do you think the other children in the class were thinking during the uproar?
- Why do you think Ann said Cathy was mean?
- How do you think Cathy could have solved the problem differently?
- What would Cathy wish Ann had said instead?

3. During recess, Emily was playing by herself. A new girl named Lindy stood nearby. Emily asked Lindy if she wanted to play with her in the sandbox. Lindy was pleased when Emily quietly asked her about her family and where she lived. Lindy thought Emily was a really friendly girl.

Answer these questions:

- Why did Lindy think Emily was friendly to her?
- Why didn't Emily talk more about herself?
- Describe how it feels on the first day at a new school.
- What advice would you give to someone who wanted to make friends?

4. Mrs. Brown's class was having a discussion about different ways to talk. They had two boxes. One box was labeled "loud talking," and one box was labeled "soft talking." The children had to think of times when they talked in loud or soft voices. The teacher wrote their ideas on pieces of paper, and they put them in the correct box. Here are some of their ideas. You decide which

box they go in! In the library; at a ball game; telling secrets; visiting a sick relative; calling the dog; saying goodnight; fighting with my brother; making friends; calling for help; calming a frightened animal; when I'm not getting my fair share; when my mom has a headache.

Specific Awareness Phase. During the specific awareness phase of therapy, the child is taught to focus on specific behaviors, discriminate between behaviors, and describe pertinent behavioral characteristics. This creates a perceptual and linguistic framework that prepares the child to modify critical behaviors during the subsequent production phase of therapy. Four goals for Patient C included:

1. Identification of abusive vocal behaviors exhibited by others;
2. Description of the salient characteristics of vocal behaviors;
3. Discrimination of differences between appropriate and inappropriate behaviors; and
4. Explanation of ways inappropriate behaviors can be avoided or changed.

Targets

Respiration

- Use lower chest breathing
- Use more replenishing breaths
- Eliminate unnecessary upper torso movement.

Phonation

- Use easy onsets
- Use easy breathy quality (clear quality is not realistic until the nodules are resolved)
- Decrease tension
- Decrease loudness level in conversational speech

- Employ vocal variety (not only increased loudness).

Interpersonal

- Increase question asking
- Improve listening-to-talking ratio
- Use "other" referenced statements in addition to "self" referenced ones.

Resonance

- Improve resonance
- Increase articulatory precision.

Because Patient C needed to modify a number of different behaviors subsumed under four different areas, the clinician decided to present the behaviors as a set or a gestalt. Consequently, the appropriate behaviors were associated with one storybook character and the inappropriate behaviors with another. The "beautiful ballerina's" voice was relaxed and "airy" and her lips danced when she used them. She made music by a humming on the front of her face, and the music was carried over into the voice as she chanted words. The ballerina voice was characterized by appropriate breathing patterns, easy onsets, resonance, and lack of laryngeal tension. The voice was light and musical and easy to listen to. Listeners felt relaxed and pleased when they heard it.

In contrast, laryngeal effort, hard glottal attacks, excessive loudness, and inefficient breathing patterns characterized "tense Tessie's" voice. Patient C was given ample opportunity to identify the two patterns and their effects on listeners during discussion of stories.

Sample Stories

1. The beautiful ballerina came onto the stage wearing a frothy white tutu. She breathed deeply and her lower chest swelled with the air. She stood with her lovely head, neck, and shoulders relaxed and poised. The audience admired her patient, restful posture and relaxed expression. As she began to dance she hummed to the music and the bones of her face vibrated. "Hmmmm" she hummed as she glided smoothly across the flower-strewn stage under the glittering chandelier.

Answer these questions:

- Describe how the ballerina breathes.
- How does she hum?
- Explain how she keeps her body relaxed.

2. Tense Tessie tightens her jaw and neck and raises her shoulders when she breathes in. She pushes hard with her throat and makes a little click or grunt on phrases such as:

I'm always eager.

But everywhere I go.

I jerk instead of glide.

I feel all stiff, you know!

Answer these questions.

- Can you tell Tessie what she must do to breathe more efficiently?
- How can she relax her neck?
- Can you tell which words Tessie makes with a hard start?

Sample Activity. When your teacher tells you an action, do it the way tense Tessie would do it and then do it the way the beautiful ballerina does it. Explain the difference.

Production Phase. During the production phase of therapy, Patient C learned to produce and monitor target vocal behaviors in structured and controlled situations. Initially, cues and monitoring were provided by the clinician. Gradually, however, the patient learned to assume more and more of this responsibility. For this patient, the production goals were sequenced as follows:

1. Produce each target behavior correctly (in isolation):
   - with instructions, cues, and presentation of the model
   - with instructions and cues
   - with instructions
   - spontaneously.

2. Prolong and repeat the target behavior.

3. Stop and start the target behavior at will.

4. Demonstrate both the appropriate and inappropriate forms of the behavior (negative practice).

5. Produce the target behavior, varying length of utterance:
   - isolated sounds
   - syllables
   - words
   - phrases
   - sentences

6. Produce the target behavior, varying the complexity of processing:
   - imitation
   - automatic responses
   - limited repertoire of responses
   - simple self-generated responses
   - complex self-generated responses

7. Produce the target behavior, varying the timing of the response:
   - predictable response time
   - unpredictable response time

8. Describe the characteristics of one's own production in terms of the following:
   - preparatory set
   - strategies used
   - reactions of self
   - reactions of others

9. Monitor one's own production:
   - when cued verbally
   - when cued nonverbally
   - after practicing aloud
   - after thinking about it first
   - spontaneously

Sample Materials

Facilitating Techniques

- Yawn-sigh
- Humming
- Chanting.

Facilitating Contexts

- Minimal pairs to teach breathy onset. "Think" the [h] in the second word of the following pairs:

whose	ooze
hear	ear
hair	air
has	as
his	is
how	ow
ha	ah
hoe	oh
heel	eel
high	eye
hobo	oboe

- Words and phrases containing only vowels and voiced continuant consonants for continuity of tone and maximum vibration of facial structures:

/z/	/l/	/m/
zulus	lovely	Maisie
zoo	lazy	Molly
Zoro	long	mowing
Zelma	lions	money
zero	lying	Moses

/v/	/th/
Vivian	them
violin	those
Vera	there
vision	these
Volvo	then

■ Sentences:

Mow the lawn.

Move the Volvo.

Vivian is lazy.

The lions were lying in the zoo.

Molly loves violins.

My mom never loses money.

Noses are nozzles.

I was living in Germany then.

Zionsville is near there.

Nellie is never nosy.

■ Words, phrases, and sentences loaded with "front" sounds to promote articulatory movement and forward tone focus:

Words:

1. whirl
2. bounce
3. jump
4. wobble
5. tap
6. tumble
7. topple
8. toddle
9. pretty
10. dainty

Sentences:

1. Pop goes the weasel.
2. Pitter patter water splatters.
3. Fit as a fiddle.
4. Tap with your toes.
5. Pearl buttons to button up.
6. Touch Tilly's white tulle tutu.
7. Leap up and down.
8. Tiptoe through the tulips.
9. Puppies snap and yip and yap.
10. You yell at little lizards

Sample Activities

1. Be the dancing teacher and "sing" as you count for the ballerinas to practice at the bar: "One and two and three and four."
2. Play "singing Simon says," and sing the instructions for dance movements.
3. Look at this stack of cards with the names of foods (ie, eggs, apples, onions). Use the carrier phrase "I eat" and make a sentence with each card in the stack. You get 1 point for each word you say with an easy onset. Try lengthening the vowel sound.
4. Find the sounds that will help you vibrate your voice on the front of your face. ("I'll say some words, and you tell me which sounds helped you when you repeated the words.")

The Carryover Phase. The clinician arranged with the teacher for Patient C to present some of her "science projects" in her school classroom. Patient C enjoyed the opportunities for attention as she explained and demonstrated some of the information she had learned about respiration. The teacher also implemented a unit on "voice pictures" into her classroom curriculum and provided opportunities for Patient C to be the "expert" on how to make pictures with her voice without talking loudly or in a tense manner. The patient demonstrated "high jumps," and "broad jumps," and "long worms," and "soft fur" using vocal variety, and she served as the judge when the teacher organized a "voice-picture" competition. The patient also starred in another classroom activity where picture cards were used. For example, two cards, one with a bird (blue jay) and one with a letter (blue J), were held up. The listeners had to identify to which card Patient C was referring.

The patient's mother routinely observed therapy sessions and observed the ways in which the clinician insisted on mature, direct interpersonal interactions. The mother also met for several sessions alone with the clinician and the school psychologist so that she could talk about ways to help the patient at home. The teacher and the parents agreed to give the patient lots of attention and praise when she used mature, nonabusive vocal strategies.

Patient C's father agreed to read stories with his daughter each evening before bedtime and to reinforce appropriate voice use. For example, he used phrases such as "I really like these times when we talk quietly together. You make me see the pictures in my head, and the stories come alive for me," and "you have the prettiest 'quiet voice' I know." The parents set up rules during mealtimes to ensure that everyone had a turn to talk and that loud interruptions and shouting down other siblings was not reinforced. When Patient C lapsed into her immature, manipulative patterns of interacting, the parents calmly said, "Let's replay that in a more grown-up way."

Fortunately, Patient C's p understood the importance of addressing the psychosocial issues underlying their daughter's vocal behavior. Their commitment to change and, not coincidentally, Patient C's progress were remarkable. From the outset, their interest in their daughter's well-being was reinforced, and the clinician served as a facilitator encouraging them to expand their range of parenting skills. Patient C attended therapy for 2 years, twice weekly for 45-minute sessions. After she was dismissed from therapy, she was followed for 1 year to ensure that gains were maintained.

Use of Patient-Family Education and Behavior Modification to Treat Vocal Hyperfunction

Leslie Glaze, PhD

Case Study: Patient D

In the following case study of vocal hyperfunction in a 7-year-old child, Leslie Glaze advocates for supplemental patient-family involvement to support traditional treatment strategies, including voice conservation and a vocal exercise regimen.

Patient History. Patient D, a 7-year-old girl, was referred for voice evaluation and treatment by the otolaryngologist, who had diagnosed bilateral vocal fold nodules. Her mother described her daughter as active, energetic, and frequently "difficult," based on "temper tantrums" and episodes of yelling and screaming with her younger brother. Her second-grade schoolwork was average and she did not pose behavior problems at school.

Her parents divorced 2 years ago and the patient lived primarily with her mother, but spent extended summer vacations at her father's home. Patient D, her mother, and her brother were receiving family counseling sessions weekly to resolve problems with discipline and communication at home. The patient reported that her favorite activities were watching videos, playing outside with neighbor friends, riding her bicycle, and Scouts. She was also active in a summer softball league, spring gymnastics team, and a winter hockey league.

Patient D had a normal, healthy medical history, with very infrequent middle ear infections during the first 4 years of life. She had no history of allergies, postnasal drip, chronic colds, sinus infections, or other upper respiratory infections. She had not had any injury to the throat, nose, or neck, and had no evidence of hearing loss. She had never been hospitalized and was not on any medication. The patient reported that she drank approximately three cans of caffeinated soda per day and drank milk with meals, but consumed little or no water regularly. Her favorite foods were spaghetti, pizza, and "McDonald's." She denied any symptoms of burping, "hot spit-up," burning throat, or stomach aches.

History of the Problem. Initially, Patient D's first- and second-grade teachers noticed that she had frequent hoarseness with approximately four episodes per year of complete voice loss. The patient had no evidence of other speech or language problems, but they reported this concern to Patient D's mother, the school speech-language pathologist, and the school nurse. The child did not qualify for school services, but the school nurse asked the family to seek a medical evaluation and treatment for the voice problem. The otolaryngologist examined her larynx with a mirror and observed "soft-appearing, moderate-sized, bilateral vocal fold nodules." The remainder of the head and neck examination was negative, including normal appearing ears, nose, mouth, pharynx, and neck.

The patient's mother reported that she believed her daughter's voice had worsened gradually over about a 3-year period, beginning during the time when she and her ex-husband were separating. Patient D and her younger brother were upset about the transition and the mother reported a general increase in vocal arguments, crying, and tantrum behavior by both children during that time. However, her mother also noted that in two consecutive summers, her daughter's voice had improved following vacations with her father. Her mother believed this improvement was attributable to the fact that the patient's father is a psychologist who manages the children's behavior differently, such that fewer tantrums or vocally abusive episodes occur. In fact, the principal goal of the ongoing family counseling sessions was to learn different behavior management styles, to create a calmer, more communicative home environment.

Evaluation Procedures. Patient D received a standard battery of vocal function testing in the voice laboratory. These assessments included:

1. *Visual-perceptual.* A stroboscopic examination was conducted using a rigid 70-degree endoscope without need for topical anesthesia. The recording revealed moderate-sized, bilateral vocal fold nodules at the anterior two-thirds junction of the vocal folds with no evidence of edema or hemorrhage. Mucus stranding between the vocal nodules was

persistent. The nodules appeared to vibrate with the vocal folds, although mucosal wave and amplitude were reduced at the midline bilaterally, presumably as a result of stiffness at the lesion sites. Phase symmetry and periodicity were always irregular. Supraglottic hyperfunction was evident throughout sustained vowel productions because of a mild, but consistent, medial compression and "bulging" of the ventricular folds. There was no evidence of tissue irregularity or irritation anywhere else on the vocal folds or in the posterior larynx.

2. *Acoustic analysis.* Patient D's recorded mean fundamental frequency was 237 Hz during sustained vowel /i/, following the elicitation cue, "start counting and when you get to three, hold out the 'ee' sound." Following cues for pitch glide on /i/ from lowest to highest sounds, Patient D produced a range from 157 Hz to 314 Hz. Perturbation values were also obtained during sustained vowel /i/ using the CSL software program (KayPENTAX), with results for jitter measuring 1.68% (normal = <1.0%); shimmer .56 dB (normal = <.35 dB); and signal to noise ratio of 14 dB (normal = 20 dB or greater). All of these measures represented subnormal performance based on the expected acoustic measures for a 7-year-old girl. Patient D produced a maximum loudness of 87 dB SPL following the cue to "yell 'Hey!' as loudly as possible." Her minimum loudness was 62 dB SPL on a sustained /a/ produced "as quietly as possible." Her habitual loudness was 70 dB SPL, measured during conversational speech. All of Patient D's loudness productions were within typical expectations.

3. *Aerodynamic measures.* Airflow measures were taken during sustained vowel productions; intraoral pressure measures were estimated from repeated productions of /pi/. Mean airflow rate was 270 cc/sec, which exceeds the normal range of approximately 120 to 200 cc/sec, suggesting "air leak" through the laryngeal valving mechanism. Intraoral pressure was measured at 8.3 cm H_2O, which is also greater than the expected norm of approximately 5 cm H_2O.

4. *Audio-Perceptual.* Patient D's voice quality was judged perceptually by the voice pathologist during informal conversation and sentence productions, using the CAPE-V (Consensus Auditory Perceptual Evaluation of Voice) protocol and form developed by Special Interest Division 3 of the American Speech-Language-Hearing Association.[6] On the day of the evaluation, Patient D exhibited consistently moderate vocal roughness (55 mm) and strain (42 mm) with a mild amount of intermittent breathiness (23 mm) and intermittent aphonia of one- to two-syllable duration occurring about once each sentence. Her habitual loudness level was appropriate and she did not exhibit any signs of hard glottal attack during casual conversation. She also sang "Happy Birthday to You" to assess pitch-changing ability in song and demonstrated five pitch breaks.

Description and Rationale for Therapy Approach. The patient's history, medical diagnosis of bilateral nodules, and evaluative findings all corroborated the clinical impression that Patient D has developed a hyperfunctional voice disorder due to her frequent phonotraumatic behaviors, aggravated by chronic, ongoing stress in the family setting.

Accordingly, the initial treatment need was to eliminate the vocal behaviors that contribute to vocal nodules and modify the communicative environment that produced stressful or aggressive communications. To address these concerns comprehensively, both Patient D *and her mother* agreed to work together to identify, then reduce or eliminate aggressive vocal behaviors *in each other* that injure vocal fold tissue, such as crying, screaming, and speaking with excessive tension or loudness. This shared approach to detecting and modifying faulty voice patterns was designed to increase mutual awareness and responsibility for establishing healthy vocal communication patterns. Because some arguments occurred between Patient D and her mother, the family counselor also supported Patient D and her mother in this aspect of voice therapy. Counseling emphasized the need to resolve conflicts at home without screaming, arguing, and yelling, thereby avoiding further vocal damage. In working together on this challenge, Patient D and her mother strengthened their mutual support for voice goals. The treatment program involved both voice conservation strategies, to maximize vocal fold tissue health, and active therapy exercises, to restore and stabilize improved voice quality. Five specific treatment goals were established for the patient, focusing on patient and family education, eliminating vocal abuse, increasing hydration, achieving healthy voice through active vocal exercises, and increasing Patient D's vocal self-awareness and personal responsibility for voice quality.

Goal 1. Patient D, her mother, and her brother learned about the origin and recovery patterns for vocal nodules, including the effects of vocally abusive behaviors on vocal fold structure and function and the risks of future tissue deterioration with prolonged vocally aggressive behaviors.

Rationale. Teaching children and families about the pathologic impact of problem vocal behaviors is essential to ensure compliance with a conservation component of voice therapy. When children develop a proprietary sense of responsibility for the voice problem, it can motivate the child to control behaviors that influence vocal health. Visual aids and other demonstrations help convey this information to children. For Patient D, viewing the videostroboscopy recordings of her larynx was particularly illustrative. Another example of vocal fold injury was simulated by having the patient and her brother rub their hands together for a 3-minute period so that they could feel how tired and hot their hands were after clapping hard together for that time. Pictures of just a few other benign structural pathologies (eg, hemorrhagic nodules, polyps, and cysts) sparked her further interest in vocal fold tissue health. From session to session, the voice pathologist asked Patient D to answer a game show style question we called "Treatment Knowledge Check," such as "For 5 stickers, Patient D, please describe how drinking more water might help your vocal folds get better!" or "Why is it helpful to rest your voice after speaking loudly?" Patient D appeared to enjoy displaying her new knowledge, as the voice pathologist reinforced the cause-and-effect relationship between voice behaviors and the rehabilitation plan.

Goal 2. Patient D and her mother participated in a home program designed to identify and reduce their instances of vocal abuse and to provide "recovery" time for each occurrence. Patient D and her mother monitored and recorded every vocally abusive production on a chart at home, including screaming, yelling, excessive crying, and "tantrum" behavior. Each time, Patient D (or her mother) agreed to be silent for a 10-minute recovery period, spent in a pleasant, relaxed, quiet activity, such as reading or taking a walk. Each week, Patient D and the voice pathologist predetermined a target maximum of vocally abusive episodes, for example, no more than twice per day. If, at the end of the week, Patient D stayed at or below the weekly target, she earned a specific reward, such as a video rental or a trip to the park.

Rationale. Home programming allows the greatest potential for treatment success and generalization, especially when the goal is to reduce vocally aggressive behaviors. In my experience, without home compliance, the prognosis for improvement with therapy is limited. Moreover, home programming is family therapy; if other family members exhibit vocally aggressive behaviors (as in the case of Patient D's mother), these members must also participate in treatment, if possible.

To clarify the incidence and severity of problem behaviors, it is helpful to implement a token charting system, to reinforce self-awareness and motivate patients to change. When vocally aggressive behaviors occur, patients can experience success and control by applying a defined alternative response, such as a 10-minute silent recovery time, immediately afterward. This recovery time is never intended to be punitive; rather, it provides a specific reminder that tissue damage requires a recovery period. For Patient D, it was especially important

that her mother participate, so that both were able to distinguish their voice program responsibilities from their other work, school obligations, household chores, and disciplinary events. As Patient D developed increasing compliance, she successfully reduced vocal abuse incidents in five out of seven regular treatment sessions.

Goal 3. Patient D eliminated all colas and caffeinated beverages from her diet and drank a minimum of five 8-oz glasses of water per day.

Rationale. Evidence of mucus stranding and reports of Patient D's typical caffeine consumption raise questions about sufficient vocal fold hydration. By increasing water intake and avoiding caffeine, she increased the possibility of adequate hydration, without modifying her age-appropriate milk consumption. Because caffeine also can be associated with hyperactive behavior and laryngeal reflux, minimizing or eliminating caffeine is a useful adjunct to most voice care routines for children.

Goal 4. In conjunction with her family therapy, Patient D kept a daily journal of pictures, drawings, or written material describing her voice use that day, based on feelings and events that created opportunities for positive or negative voice use.

Rationale. The family counselor began this journal project earlier with the patient and her brother to encourage greater self-awareness of their feelings. With the counselor's permission, a voice use component was added for the patient to allow her to relate everyday stress responses to her vocally abusive behaviors. She made schematic drawings of the nodules in her throat, drew pictures for her room to remind her not to yell (such as a drawing of a lion "roaring" with a big X over the mouth), and wrote large signs to use instead of yelling (eg, "LEAVE ME ALONE"). Her journal contained pictures she drew or cut from magazines to describe her feelings whenever she was sad, angry, or upset. Initially, Patient D received a small reward (eg, a quarter or sticker) every time she used these graphic cues instead of a vocally aggressive response. Quickly, these rewards ceased as she learned to describe her feelings in conversational exchanges with her mother. Moreover, Patient D's mother reported that as the frequency of aggressive vocal behavior lessened, the overall level of household calmness, behavioral cooperation, and positive communication increased.

Goal 5. Patient D and her mother both attended voice therapy sessions, where they learned to perform a series of direct vocal exercises, including a warm-up routine and Stemple's vocal function exercises. They received a 10-minute CD recording of home practice cues to allow them to practice therapy tasks twice daily. The warm-up consisted of "vocal play" cues for relaxed breathing, gentle sighs and pitch glides, humming nursery rhymes and other simple tunes, and short conversational phrases. The vocal function exercise segment contained pitch cues for sustained resonant tones, according to that protocol.

Rationale. Besides learning about voice care and addressing the psychosocial contributors to the patient's voice problems, it is essential for patients and their families to learn to produce healthy voice independently, outside the treat-

ment room. Audio-recorded exercises conducted at home are a useful adjunct to therapy time, because they create opportunities for consistent and accurate vocal practice. For Patient D, the home exercises provided a fun and relaxing opportunity for her and her mother to talk, sing, and play quietly using audio cues to progress through the warm up and vocal function exercise routine.

Results of Therapy. Patient D received seven sessions of voice therapy over the course of 3 months and attended two follow-up sessions at 1 and 3 months following treatment. At the final session (approximately 6 months from initial diagnosis), we collected posttreatment data.

Visual-Perceptual. Patient D's vocal fold nodules resolved as judged by the patient and her voice pathologist from visual records of her pre- and posttreatment stroboscopic recordings. The otolaryngologist confirmed this judgment during a follow-up indirect mirror examination, which revealed no evidence of any midline vocal fold lesion or supraglottic hyperfunction. Under stroboscopic light, vibratory movement exhibited normal phase closure, with normal mucosal wave and amplitude. Phase symmetry and periodicity were still irregular.

Acoustic Analysis. Using the same sustained vowel /i/ protocol measured at pretesting, Patient D reduced jitter to .89% and shimmer to .31 dB. She also increased signal-to-noise ratio to 25 dB SPL. Her maximum pitch increased to 547 Hz. All of these posttest acoustic measures were within expected norms for her age. Habitual pitch and loudness tasks did not change.

Aerodynamic Measures. Mean airflow rate decreased to a final mean rate of 150 cc/sec, which was within expected normal limits. Mean intraoral pressure was measured at 5.7 cm H_2O, which is also decreased from initial measures and within expected limits.

Audio-Perceptual. Patient D's voice quality improved markedly as judged perceptually by the patient, her mother, and the voice pathologist. She eliminated pitch breaks and intermittent aphonia entirely during a repeat perceptual assessment using the CAPE-V. Both the patient and therapist rated conversational voice productions as normal overall with only mild, intermittent evidence of roughness (11 mm), and no evidence of breathiness, or strain. She sang "Happy Birthday to You" again without any pitch breaks.

The positive outcome of this treatment plan is attributable to the patient and family compliance with the home programming effort. The concurrent family counseling process undoubtedly assisted with creative problem-solving strategies to mitigate angry or emotional vocal outbursts. During the course of voice treatment, Patient D developed a sense of self-awareness and responsibility toward her voice problem, as evidenced by her willingness to report her weekly progress and to display some of her creative journal entries when she came to therapy. The behavioral modification program of effort and reward did seem to reinforce her "control" over vocally abusive behaviors. Certainly, not all children can eliminate vocally aggressive behaviors. Fortunately, Patient D enjoyed the positive attention and support she received from her mother and brother for her compliance with vocal

exercises and voice conservation strategies. Thus, her decisions about good voice use were motivated by her own sense of self-determination and satisfaction, and the entire household benefitted from improved communication patterns. Both she and her mother were pleased with the outcome.

Treatment of Vocal Nodules in a Child with Associated Laryngopharyngeal Reflux

Edie Swift

Case History: Patient E

Patient E was 6 years and 8 months old when initially seen at the combined Voice and Pediatric Otolaryngology Clinic. His mother reported that he "has always been hoarse" and she could identify him in a group of children by his voice. At the time of his initial evaluation, he had begun to experience periods of aphonia and dysphonia marked by pitch breaks. Teachers had noticed his dysphonia and his choir teacher had asked him to "mouth the words" and not to sing. He reported that this was embarrassing. Additionally, his voice was beginning to be a source of negative attention from his peers.

Patient E was the youngest of three children. His oldest brother had been diagnosed with attention deficit disorder (ADD) and the second child with autism. Patient E's mother reported that he frequently shrieked and spoke loudly. She indicated that she felt this was a strategy to help him "hold his own" in the household. The mother holds a full-time job. Patient E's father is generally in charge of the household. He often has trouble tolerating the chaos and frequently leaves the children unmonitored while he goes outside to smoke and calm himself. The parents had approached the school district about therapy but were told they could not complete the necessary paperwork before the end of the school year and needed a medical diagnosis. No school-based summer therapy was available. Additionally, it was the mother's opinion that the school clinician had seen only a few voice cases and was a bit unsure about how to proceed.

Voice Evaluation. Perceptually, the staff described Patient E's voice as moderately hoarse with intermittent pitch breaks. If ranked on a 7-point scale (with 7 equaling aphonia and 1 equaling normal), severity of hoarseness was 5. Only three pitch beaks were observed in a 2-minute free speech sample. The history, however, indicated considerable fluctuation in this parameter.

Flexible fiberoptic nasopharyngoscopy and videostroboscopy showed large bilateral lesions on the medial aspect of the membranous vocal folds. During phonation, there was considerable hyperfunction evidenced by both anterior-posterior constriction and lateral compression of the ventricular folds. Mucosal wave was evident but dampened at the site of the lesions. The tissue was sufficiently stiff that a differential diagnosis between nodules and a possible cyst was impossible. Both lesions were white in color with no evidence of translucency. Both were well defined and conical in shape. Thick, tenacious mucus tended to adhere to the lesions. Additionally, erythema of the supraglottic area, as well as edema on the infraglottic margins of both vocal folds, was observed, suggesting possible laryngopharyngeal reflux (LPR). This was supported by Patient E's report that his stomach often hurt after eating and that he frequently had "vomity burps." The voice team suggested 2 months of therapy. Additionally, Cisapride .3 mg/kg qid with meals plus 10 mg/qid of Prilosec were prescribed. Although we seldom remove nodules surgically, it was possible that Patient E was presenting with a cyst; the nature of his lesions made him a possible surgical candidate if behavioral management failed.

Voice Therapy. Therapy was initiated at the end of the diagnostic visit. A behavioral program intended to reduce the effects of possible LPR was discussed. The stroboscopic videorecording was reviewed with the patient so that his questions could be reviewed and the mechanics of the problem were repeated for Patient E and his mother. Weekly therapy was scheduled and he was reassured that visualization would not be necessary when he returned the next week. It was decided to videorecord all of the therapy sessions so that any helpful techniques could be shared with his speech pathologist at school in the fall.

Session 1: Vocal Hygiene. Recommendations for Patient E and his family were tailored for his situation. He and his mother reported success in eliminating pop with caffeine and most carbonated beverages in general. Additionally, he had stopped his "late-night snack." Increased hydration had also been encouraged in an effort to thin the observed mucus. The behavioral changes he was recommended to make, in addition to changes in his diet, were then introduced. Each was discussed, and a plan for implementation was either decided on, or the problem was referred to a planned family conference that would be used for ideas about the most difficult things for him, such as yelling during sibling disputes.

Patient E's personal hygiene list included trying to:

- Drink lots of water
- Talk with his family about alternatives to screaming and arguing
- Let his friends know that he would clap or whistle for their attention for a while; (He was given a video-print of his nodules to help him explain nodules to his friends)
- Give his voice a nap after it gets tired (This translated into a 5-minute silent period after a period of abuse.)

He was also asked to try not to use vocal "play" noises or be around smoke.

Patient E indicated that he would like to make a video recording the following week to explain how nodules are formed and how one should take care of the voice. It was agreed that he would work on his script during the week and that he would get a copy of his tape to take to school the following year.

Session 1, Part 2: Changes in Phonatory Pattern. Resonant voice was introduced to Patient E by having him bend over from his waist with his head and neck relaxed and initiate an /m/. He used tactile feedback with his hands by his nose to confirm that vibration was present above the larynx. He also tried to initiate what was labeled his "buzzy" voice by sitting on his knees with his head on a mat and feeling the vibration in his head. During both of these activities, he was asked to try to move to standing or sitting, respectively, maintaining the "buzz" and breathing as often as needed. He was given verbal feedback about the sound of his voice ("that sounded loose and buzzy" or "that

sounded tighter and in your throat") and feedback about perception was checked by asking him how the production felt. At the end of the session, he was extending his "buzzy" voice into syllables using /m/, /n/, and lower, more relaxed vowels. His homework was extended to include "playing with his humming" to see what parts of his head he could make vibrate and trying 10 syllables each night. His mother felt she had time to do this with him at bedtime. She did not feel confident that she heard the difference between his "usual" voice and his target voice, so it was decided she would just praise him for practicing and following the hygiene suggestions and help him with the video script.

Session 2: The First Problems. Patient E returned after an "out-of-control" weekend and was quite hoarse. Resonant voice was reintroduced. The filming of his "commercial" was done last because it was hoped that his voice quality could be improved during the session. He responded well, and although he needed cuing for each production, he could correct himself consistently. Resonant voice was maintained in phrase-length productions, and his tape was filmed. He reported that his brothers frustrated him and that he was still yelling at them. He decided to try walking out of the room if they started yelling and to see what happened. The other components of the hygiene program were reportedly going better. There was less yelling for mutual attention between Patient E and his parents. He indicated that he would be going to camp soon, and it became clear that work on "safer yelling" (see Patient E Appendix) would have to start more quickly than was ideal. His homework that week was limited to extended work on resonant voice, and his mother gave him the feedback the last 5 minutes of the clinic session. Her perceptions were generally the same as the clinicians, but Patient E's tactile perceptions were the "final word."

Session 3: Coordinated Voice Onset. Patient E came in sounding encouragingly improved. He practiced using his resonant voice in phrases, and the coordination of breath support with the initiation of voice was introduced. The use of Coordinated Voice Onset (CVO) was taken from Linda Rammage's book, *Vocalizing with Ease*.[7] Although he could do this while on his back, he tended to use a tense, shallow respiratory pattern when sitting or standing. Calling attention to his breathing was making his whole phonatory pattern worse. We worked alternately for 5 minutes at a time on CVOs and extending resonant voice. He was asked to do 10 CVOs using syllables at the beginning of each hour unless he was outside with his friends. Two weeks until camp!

Session 4: Teaching Safer Yelling. At the following session, Patient E was coordinating breath support with vocal initiation and work on louder production. We picked likely "scripts," such as the names of friends, "my turn," or "throw me the ball." Practice was limited to 5 minutes at a time with multiple requests for him to evaluate whether productions were "buzzy" or "tight." His first revisualization would be the day after he returned from camp.

Session 5: Revisualization. Fortunately, Patient E returned from camp sounding much as he had before he left. Mildly hoarse, with some pitch breaks,

but quality was judged improved by him, his mother, and the clinician. He reported that he had not received negative feedback from peers at camp and that his voice had not restricted any of his activities. He was experiencing improvement in the function of his voice.

Revisualization was again done with the flexible fiberoptic endoscope and videostroboscopy. A reduction in the prominence of the lesions was evident. Mucosal wave clearly moved through the lesions and, while still well defined, the concern that he had a cyst was eliminated. His medications were unchanged.

Session 6: Ready for School. Patient E returned after 2 weeks for one additional therapy session before starting school. During the 2-week break, he had forgotten his "internal standard." His judgments of productions seemed inconsistent, and he expressed some confusion. This was a long session with considerable review of his "buzzy" voice, CVOs, and his techniques for safer yelling. This entire session was put on his tape to take to school.

Session 7: Clinical Follow-Up. Patient E was next seen in the clinic in November. There had been several phone calls to the school clinician working with him. She had seen him weekly for 6 weeks and then removed him from her caseload indicating that she no longer perceived him as hoarse. Calls to his mother were consistent with these perceptions. On the phone, Patient E said using his "new voice" had become easy, and he didn't think about it too much. He now was able to sing with his class.

Last Session. Patient E had one additional clinic visit and was visualized with the rigid endoscope. There continued to be some edema of the folds, which was quite diffuse. Edema of the infraglottic area suggested that reflux was an ongoing problem. He was told to finish the medication prescribed, then to rely on his behavioral changes. If hoarseness returned, the pediatric otolaryngologist indicated that consultation by a pediatric gastroenterologist would be appropriate. A telephone call to the family instigated by writing this report was made. The mother reported that Patient E is still sometimes hoarse after school, but the functional concerns that led to the original request for help were no longer an issue.

Patient E Appendix
Safer Yelling

Every typical child screams. This is a universal truth of childhood, and it is unreasonable to expect them to stop. A sensible goal for voice therapy is the modification of this behavior.

Basic Introduction

1. A screaming-awareness program is initiated with input from the client and the caretakers.
2. A temporary alternative to screaming is put in place. An agreement between the child, parents, and clinician is reached that includes the time span likely to be required and a reward that will accompany improvement.
3. Implement the vocal hygiene program while the client is working to reduce screaming.
4. Teach the fundamentals of Resonant Voice, Accent Technique, or both in the speaking voice. Some elements of Resonant Voice and controlled breath support will be required.

Specific Techniques

1. Select a meaningful single word (syllable) as a target. (names, mom, hey). Monitor the phonetic context to avoid /i/ and glottals.
2. Monitor the respiratory pattern so that abdominal muscles contract before voicing is initiated. Pair the start of exhalation with the onset of voice. Feel the stomach move firmly.
3. Monitor the focus of the vocal energy. Ask, "Does it feel buzzy?" or "Does it feel tight?" after the understanding of these questions is established.
4. Throughout the therapy, the child will have been asked to monitor their productions. Be sure to continue the training of this awareness when the context moves from speech to yelling.
5. Expand to two syllables, still monitoring the context. The clinician needs to be sure there are two "stomach pulses" for the two syllables. Continue to monitor tension and focus of energy.
6. Continue expansion until the client can manage three or four syllables.

Three- to four-syllable productions are the final goal as longer productions will always be a problem.

Vocal Hyperfunction in Adults

Vocal hyperfunction may take many forms and result from many causes in the adult. Sometimes the hyperfunction may be the result of phonotraumatic habits; at other times, the hyperfunction may be secondary to compensatory voice behaviors caused by pathology. In the following case, Joe Stemple describes a complex voice disorder requiring an eclectic treatment approach.

Vocal Hyperfunction in a Second-Grade Teacher

Joseph C. Stemple, PhD

Case Study: Patient F

Patient F, a 26-year-old second-grade teacher, was referred by a laryngologist to the voice center for a complete diagnostic voice evaluation, with the diagnosis of large bilateral vocal fold nodules and a left vocal process ulcer. Patient F first became symptomatic in the fall of her first year of teaching. In October of that year, she became dysphonic. When the hoarseness persisted, she sought the opinion of the referring physician, whose examination revealed mild bilateral vocal fold edema. The physician instructed her to reduce caffeine intake and to increase intake of water and briefly counseled her regarding voice misuse. The patient followed these instructions, and her voice quality improved.

Between fall and late winter, the patient experienced intermittent hoarseness. She thought the mild hoarseness was fairly normal considering her level of voice use in the school setting. In late February, however, she became moderately hoarse during an upper respiratory infection. Like most teachers, she continued to work a normal schedule during her illness. She began to notice not only hoarseness but also voice fatigue and a burning sensation on the left side of her "throat." When the upper respiratory infection resolved and her voice symptoms persisted, she sought the opinion of the laryngologist.

On seeing the vocal nodules and the ulcerated tissue located on the vocal process of the left arytenoid cartilage, the laryngologist prescribed reflux medication (proton pump inhibitor [PPI]) and referred the patient for a voice evaluation and therapy. The PPI was prescribed as a precaution because of the implications of acid reflux on the development of contact ulcers and granulomas.

The information gathered during the voice evaluation confirmed the nature of the voice trauma that had significantly increased the patient's symptoms in February. Patient F had indeed experienced a mild hoarseness since school began that fall. She reported that her voice quality typically was better on Monday and much worse by Friday but that she always had some level of hoarseness. On a daily basis, she was more symptomatic during the early morning. The hoarseness would clear somewhat by midmorning and worsen again by afternoon.

With the onset of the respiratory infection, Patient F began coughing and throat clearing. By the time of the voice evaluation, the coughing had decreased, but chronic throat clearing was noted. Her voice use was typical for a second-grade teacher. Students of this age require much instruction and nonspeech times in the classroom were reported to be minimal. In addition, the patient was assigned playground and school-bus duty, which required occasional shouting and raising the voice above noise to be heard.

There was no evidence that the patient misused her voice away from her work environment. She was married and had a 2-year-old daughter. She denied any direct vocal trauma or environmental contributions, such as inhaled dust, fumes, chemicals, or paints. She reported that her voice improved on weekends and always returned to normal during the summer months. The remaining social history was unremarkable as related to this problem.

The patient's medical history also was unremarkable. She was free of any chronic illnesses or disorders; took only the PPI, although she was not symptomatic with "heartburn;" and was a nonsmoker, living and working in a nonsmoking environment. Her liquid intake was not adequate. She drank two cans of caffeinated soda and two glasses of iced tea per day. Patient F reported that she "loved" teaching and felt "great" on a daily basis.

During the voice evaluation, Patient F presented with a moderate dysphonia characterized by dry, breathy hoarseness. The laryngeal videostroboscopic examination revealed large bilateral vocal fold nodules, worse on the right than on the left; bilateral edema and erythema; and an apparent resolving left contact ulcer. The nodules caused glottic closure to demonstrate an hourglass configuration with a slight ventricular fold compression. Both the amplitude of vibration and the mucosal waves were severely decreased bilaterally. The open phase of the vibratory cycle was dominant, whereas the symmetry of vibration generally was irregular. In other words, she presented with significant tissue changes that would present a challenge to functional voice therapy.

Acoustic measures demonstrated a limited frequency range of 147 to 562 Hz. Her fundamental frequency remained appropriate at 211 Hz. Although her jitter measures for sustained vowels were normal at .87%, her shimmer measures were high at .46 dB.

Aerodynamic measures yielded significantly high airflow rates for high pitches averaging 305 mL/H_2O. Comfort and low pitches were borderline high at 180 and 189 mL/H_2O respectively. The patient was required to push more air through her vocal system to support the vibration because of increased vocal fold mass and the hourglass glottal chink. Her subsequent phonation times at all pitch levels were only 11 seconds or less.

Patient F also completed the Voice-Related Quality of Life (V-RQOL), a self-assessment scale to demonstrate the effect the voice disorder was having on her life.[8] Results demonstrated a moderate life impact.

Following the voice evaluation and testing, a treatment plan was proposed. The plan included:

- temporary reassignment from playground and school-bus duties
- site visit to determine environment and teaching style
- elimination of the abusive behavior of throat clearing
- oral hydration program
- symptom modification
- Vocal Function Exercises designed to rebalance respiration, phonation, and resonance.

Temporary Reassignment. It was decided to immediately eliminate the potential for the most obvious vocal traumas. The patient therefore requested to be assigned to other duties away from the playground and school buses where voice would not be a factor and she would not be required to raise her voice. If therapy proved to be successful, reassignment would be temporary. Otherwise, it would continue until the end of the school year.

Site Visit. Site visits are time consuming and not always practical, but the value of seeing the patient in the implicated environment cannot be overemphasized. Other useful options to site visits are video or audio recordings of the patient in the speaking environment. Recordings can be viewed or listened to during therapy.

Patient F's school was convenient to the voice center, so a 1-hour site visit was arranged. Observations made during the visit included:

- large room
- unusually high (16–18 feet) acoustical tile ceilings
- sound was lost in space
- only 24 students spread throughout the large room at different "stations"
- all sounds (scooting chairs, dropped books, and so forth) were magnified by glass and plastic
- speech was hard to discriminate.

It was obvious that Patient F indeed "loved" her work. She was enthusiastic and had complete control of the classroom. Observations made regarding her teaching style included:

- vocally enthusiastic, but does not shout
- room requires that she speak loudly and precisely, not to be heard but to be understood
- spends a good deal of time "directing" children when not actually teaching

- uses high pitch, limited inflection, and back focus; constantly strains voice

An audio recording was made during the visit that was reviewed later in therapy.

The opportunity to visit the patient's classroom led to several suggestions. These included:

- Decrease the physical space by rearranging seating and using approximately two-thirds of the classroom. With a class size of only 24 students, this was easy to accomplish. The patient herself suggested an additional change. She physically decreased the room size by using large, freestanding display boards (which were normally in school storage) as temporary walls.
- Soften the acoustics of the room by using the window blinds, pulled halfway down. Use fabric in a work display area by hanging a sheet on the wall to display student papers, pictures, tests, and similar exhibits. The large display boards also functioned well as an acoustic barrier.
- Build into the schedule a vocal "timeout" for both the teacher and the students. Learn to respect and appreciate the silent time as a chance to rest the voice and as a reminder to talk only as loudly as necessary in the newly configured classroom.
- Develop a sign system for common instructions and requests. It was noted during the site visit that the patient was constantly correcting and directing students' actions while instructing. When this was brought to her attention, she decided to implement an interesting sign-symbol system that would preclude voice commands. She listed the names of the students on a large magnetic board in the corner of the classroom. Signs were then

made with picture symbols depicting the most common corrections and directions that she made. They included symbols representing such directions as the following: be quiet, don't tilt your chair, slow down, stop talking, talk softer, and pay attention. These symbol pictures were attached to magnets. When the need arose, the patient would place the symbol next to the name of the offending child, all the while continuing her teaching. A list of consequences for receiving more than one symbol correction was established by the teacher and well understood by the children.

Elimination of Throat Clearing. The previous suggestions proved successful in immediately decreasing the daily laryngeal fatigue and voice struggle. The patient, of course, remained dysphonic. The therapy plan then introduced a behavior modification approach for eliminating the phonotraumatic behavior of throat clearing. Until brought to her attention by the therapist, the patient was not aware of the frequency of her throat clearing. Throat clearing may be extremely abusive to the tissue lining of the vocal folds and arytenoid cartilages. Once brought to her attention, the patient was surprised by the number of times she cleared her throat during the session. To modify this behavior, she was told the following.

Throat clearing is one of the most abusive things you can do to your vocal folds. When you clear your throat like this (demonstrate), you create an extreme amount of movement of your vocal folds, causing them to slam and rub together (demonstrate using your hands). You should understand that it is not unusual to have developed this habit. The vast majority of patients we

see with your type of voice problem also have this habit. Sometimes people do not even know that they are doing it, but often they say that they feel something in their throat, such as a lump or mucus. The majority of the time, however, when you clear your throat, there is nothing there. Often, patients only feel a sensation of thickness from chronic strain. The only thing you have accomplished is to create more vocal fold abuse.

We have demonstrated to you with the audio recording from your class that, most of the time, you clear your throat right before you begin to speak. We call that a preparatory throat clear. Also, you are clearing many more times than you realized. This is a sign that throat clearing is a habit. As with all habits, it is difficult to break. We are, therefore, going to try to make it easier by giving you a substitute habit that will (1) take the place of throat clearing, (2) accomplish the same thing as throat clearing, and (3) is not abusive. This substitute, nonabusive habit is a hard, forceful swallow.

If you do, in fact, occasionally have increased amount of mucus on your vocal folds, a forceful swallow will accomplish the same thing as throat clearing, minus the abuse. The only difference is that throat clearing feels good. It psychologically gives you more relief than the forceful swallow, even though it physically accomplishes no more. It is your goal to overcome the psychological dependence. Understand that this habit is harmful and that it must be broken.

To break this habit, you need to tell everyone in your family and any friends who are often around you (and whom you feel comfortable telling) that you're not permitted to clear your throat anymore. When these "helpers" hear you clear your throat, and they will, they are to immediately point it out. You may even consider using your students as helpers. Your task, then, is to swallow forcefully. Obviously, it will not be necessary to swallow because you just cleared your throat, but this is your first step in substituting the hard swallow for the throat clearing.

After your family, friends, or students have pointed out your throat clearing to you several times, you will begin to "catch" yourself. You will clear your throat and almost immediately think, "Oops! I am not supposed to do that." Your response again should be to swallow forcefully.

When you have caught yourself clearing your throat several times, you begin to halt yourself just prior to clearing. Once again, you will substitute the hard swallow, but this time the throat clearing was stopped. By the time you have reached this point, you will be close to breaking the habit totally. The final goal will be met when you realize that you are swallowing many fewer times than the number of times you previously were clearing your throat.

I want you to work hard on this problem. I think you will be surprised just how quickly you are able to break this habit. As a matter of fact, the majority of our patients have significantly reduced the habit within 1 to 2 weeks. Most patients, however, cannot do it alone. So please, find other people to help you by having them point out when you are doing it. Any questions?" (Reprinted from Stemple, Glaze and Klaben [2009], *Clinical Voice Pathology: Theory and Management*, 4th edition.)

Following this explanation, the patient typically will clear his or her throat more times than usual. The voice pathologist immediately points this out, and the patient initiates a forceful swallow substitution. Often, patient's make great gains in habit modification during this initial session. Patient F received help from her husband, mother, and a friend and was able to totally eliminate the habit of throat clearing within 2 weeks.

Oral Hydration Program. The superficial layer of the vocal folds must be well lubricated to decrease the heat and friction of vibration. A thin, slippery mucus secreted onto the vocal folds serves the same purpose as oil serves to the engine of car. It was explained to Patient F that what she swallows does not touch her vocal folds but is diverted around them. Therefore, the amount and type of liquid intake will either permit or inhibit the normal mucus flow to the vocal folds. Caffeine, alcohol, and many medications are drying agents. Many times, when patients feel as if they have too much mucus on the vocal folds, they actually have increased mucous viscosity, which is thicker and stickier than is desirable.

This patient's liquid intake was minimal and caffeinated. She therefore was placed on a hydration program that required a minimum intake of six, 8-ounce glasses of water or fruit juice per day. In addition, she was asked to decrease her caffeine intake but was not required to totally eliminate caffeine from her diet.

Symptom Modification. Direct symptom modification also was introduced. These tasks included the following:

- The patient enhanced her awareness of appropriate pitch and loudness used during teaching. The initial audio recording was used to demonstrate problems with pitch, loudness, and focus.
- Direct practice using feedback from a Visi-Pitch instrument was helpful in introducing more appropriate pitch and loudness.

■ The patient was instructed to talk only as loudly as was absolutely necessary in the classroom. A combination of these approaches returned her teaching style to a more conversational mode.

■ Reconfiguring the classroom and improving the acoustics was also a factor in making positive changes in voice production.

Vocal Function Exercises. An important part of this patient's voice therapy program was the use of Vocal Function Exercises. These exercises, first described by Barnes[9] and modified by Stemple,[10] strive to balance the subsystems of voice production. The exercise program has proven successful in improving and enhancing the vocal function of speakers with normal voices and disordered voices.[11,12] In addition Sabol, Lee, and Stemple[13] demonstrated the effectiveness of Vocal Function Exercises in the exercise regimens of singers.

The program is rather simple to teach and, when presented appropriately, seems reasonable to patients. Indeed, many patients are enthusiastic to have a concrete program, similar in concept to physical therapy, during which they may plot the progress of their return to vocal efficiency. The program is as follows.

Describe the problem to the patient, using illustrations as needed or the patient's own stroboscopic evaluation video. The patient is then taught a series of four exercises to be done at home, twice each, two times per day, preferably morning and evening. These exercises include:

1. Sustain the /i/ vowel for as long as possible on a musical note F above middle C for all female patients and boys and F below middle C for mature male patients. (Notes may be modified up or down to fit the needs of the patient. Seldom are they modified by more than two notes in either direction.)

   Goal: based on airflow volume. (In our clinic the goal is based on reaching 80 to 100 mL/sec of airflow. So, if the flow volume is equal to 4000 mL, then the goal is 40 to 50 seconds. When airflow measures are not available, the goal is equal to the longest /s/ that the patient is able to sustain. Placement of the tone should be in an extreme forward focus that is almost, but not quite, nasal. All exercises are produced as softly as possible, but not breathy. The voice must be "engaged." This is considered a warm-up exercise.)

2. Glide from your lowest note to your highest note on the word "knoll."

   Goal: no voice breaks. (The glide requires the use of all laryngeal muscles. It stretches the vocal folds and encourages a systematic, slow engagement of the cricothyroid muscles.) The word "knoll" encourages a forward placement of the tone as well as an expanded open pharynx. The patient's lips are to be rounded and a sympathetic vibration should be felt on the lips. (May also use a lip trill, tongue trill or the word "whoop.") Voice breaks typically will occur in the transitions between low and high registers. When breaks occur, the patient is encouraged to continue the glide without hesitation. When the voice breaks at the top of the current range and the patient typically has more range, the glide may be continued without voice as the folds will continue to stretch. Glides improve muscular control and flexibility. This is considered a stretching exercise.)

3. Glide from a comfortable note to your lowest note on the word "knoll."

   Goal: no voice breaks. (The patient is instructed to feel a half-yawn in the throat throughout this exercise.) By keeping the pharynx open and focusing the sympathetic vibration at the lips, the downward glide encourages a slow, systematic engagement of the thyroarytenoid muscles without the presence of a back-focused growl. In fact, no growl is permitted. (May also use a lip trill, tongue trill, or the word "boom.") This is considered a contracting exercise.

4. Sustain the musical notes C, D, E, F, and G for as long as possible on the word "knoll" minus the "kn." (Middle C for all female patients and boys, an octave below middle C for mature male patients.)

   Goal: remains the same as for exercise 1. (The "oll" is once again produced with an open pharynx and constricted, sympathetically vibrating lips. The shape of the pharynx to the lips is likened to an inverted megaphone. The fourth exercise may be tailored to the patient's present vocal ability. Although the basic range starting at middle C, an octave lower for mature male patients, is appropriate for most voices, the exercises may be customized up or down to fit the current vocal condition or a particular voice type. Seldom, however, are the exercises shift-

ed more than two notes in either direction. This is considered a low-impact adductory power exercise.)

Quality of the tone is also monitored for voice breaks, wavering, and breathiness. Quality improves as times increase and pathologies begin to resolve.

All exercises are done as softly, but engaged. It is much more difficult to produce soft tones; therefore, the vocal subsystems will receive a better "workout" than if louder tones were produced. Extreme care is taken to teach the production of a forward tone that lacks tension. In addition, attention is paid to the glottal onset of the tone. The patient is asked to breathe in deeply with attention paid to training abdominal breathing, posturing the vowel momentarily, and then initiating the exercise gesture without a forceful glottal attack or an aspirate breathy attack. It is explained to the patient that maximum phonation times increase as the efficiency of the vocal fold vibration improves. Times do not increase because of improved "lung capacity." Indeed, even aerobic exercise does not improve lung capacity but rather the efficiency of oxygen exchange with the circulatory system, thus giving the sense of more air.

The patient is provided with an audio CD of live voice doing the exercises which is used to guide the home exercise sessions. We have found that patients who complain of "tone deafness" often can be taught to approximate the correct notes with practice and guidance from the voice pathologist.

Finally, patients are given a chart on which to mark their sustained times, which is a means of plotting progress (see Patient F Appendix). Progress is monitored over time and, because of normal daily variability, patients are encouraged not to compare one day with the next. Rather, weekly comparisons are encouraged. Estimated time of completion for the program is 8 to 10 weeks.

When the patient has reached the predetermined therapy goal and the voice quality and other vocal symptoms are improved, a tapering maintenance program is recommended. Although some professional voice users choose to remain in peak vocal condition using the exercises, many of our patients desire to taper the program. The following systematic taper is recommended:

- Full program 2 times each, 2 times per day
- Full program 2 times each, 1 time per day (morning)
- Full program 1 time each, 1 time per day (morning)
- Exercise 4, 2 times each, 1 time per day (morning)
- Exercise 4, 1 time each 1 time per day (morning)
- Exercise 4, 1 time each, 3 times per week (morning)
- Exercise 4, 1 time each, 1 time per week (morning).

Each taper should last one week. Patients should maintain 85% of their peak time, otherwise they should move up one step in the taper until the 85% criterion is met.

In short, Vocal Function Exercises provide a holistic voice-treatment program that attends to the three major subsystems of voice production. The program appears to benefit patients with a wide range of voice disorders both hyper- and hypofunctional. The daily exercises require a reasonable amount of time and effort. In addition, it is similar to other recognizable exercise programs; the concept of "physical therapy" to improve muscle function is understand-able; progress may be easily plotted, which is inherently motivating; and it appears to balance airflow, laryngeal activity, and supraglottic placement. (Reprinted from Stemple, Glaze and Klaben [2009], *Clinical Voice Pathology: Theory and Management*, 4th edition.)

Vocal Function Exercises were helpful in improving the overall condition of Patient F's vocal folds and helped to retrain frontal focus. The patient's baseline mean phonation time for sustaining the appropriate notes was 8.5 seconds. This measure improved to a mean of 18 seconds during 6 weeks of therapy.

Significant improvement was noted during 6 weeks of therapy for both subjective observations of voice quality and objective measures of vocal function. The patient was experiencing much less vocal fatigue and laryngeal discomfort. Audio recordings made while teaching demonstrated stabilization of new voicing habits and only very occasional throat clearing. She did, however, remain mildly dysphonic, characterized by a slight breathy hoarseness.

Objective measures demonstrated a fundamental frequency of 196 Hz and an expanded frequency range of 165 to 720 Hz. Jitter and shimmer measures were within normal limits. Airflow rates for comfort and low-pitched voices were decreased to 136 and 150 mL/sec, respectively. Airflow rate for high-pitched voice was also decreased to 240 mL/sec but was still above the normal limit of 200 mL/sec.

Videostroboscopy also demonstrated improvement. The edema and erythema were resolved, and there was no evidence of the contact ulcer. A slight thickness was noted where the left nodule had been. The right nodule was still present but appeared much more cyst-like. Glottic closure retained an hourglass shape; however, the glottal chinks were much smaller. The amplitude of vibration was only slightly decreased left and moderately decreased right. The mucosal wave was normal on the left and moderately decreased around the right lesion. The open phase of the vibratory cycle was slightly dominant, while the symmetry of vibration remained irregular.

The results of the therapy program were discussed with Patient F's physician. Considering the cystlike nature and stiffness of the right vocal fold lesion, it appeared unlikely that the lesion would resolve with therapy. It was decided to extend therapy for an additional month to be certain that this was the case. When the remaining lesion did not resolve, surgery was scheduled for the second week in June.

The pathologist's report confirmed the lesion to be a cyst. Following surgery, the patient continued Vocal Function Exercises for 1 month and began a maintenance exercise program for the remainder of the summer. Maximum phonation times improved and stabilized at an average of 32 seconds. The voice quality improved to normal. Changes in objective measures included a higher frequency range (+900 Hz) and a normal airflow rate at high pitch (160 mL H_2O/sec). Videostroboscopic examination performed just prior to the fall opening of school revealed all observations to be within normal limits except for the symmetry of vibration, which remained irregular at higher pitches.

Patient F was followed monthly to confirm her symptom-free status. Her voice remained normal. The combination of medical and surgical treatment and a holistic voice therapy program proved successful in remediating a long-term voice disturbance in this patient.

Patient F Appendix
Vocal Function Exercise

Daily Record

Name _____   Begin Date _____

		MON	TUE	WED	THU	FRI	SAT	SUN
	Date							
	E/F	/	/	/	/	/	/	/
	C	/	/	/	/	/	/	/
AM	D	/	/	/	/	/	/	/
	E	/	/	/	/	/	/	/
	F	/	/	/	/	/	/	/
	G	/	/	/	/	/	/	/
	E/F	/	/	/	/	/	/	/
	C	/	/	/	/	/	/	/
PM	D	/	/	/	/	/	/	/
	E	/	/	/	/	/	/	/
	F	/	/	/	/	/	/	/
	G	/	/	/	/	/	/	/

		MON	TUE	WED	THU	FRI	SAT	SUN
	Date							
	E/F	/	/	/	/	/	/	/
	C	/	/	/	/	/	/	/
AM	D	/	/	/	/	/	/	/
	E	/	/	/	/	/	/	/
	F	/	/	/	/	/	/	/
	G	/	/	/	/	/	/	/
	E/F	/	/	/	/	/	/	/
	C	/	/	/	/	/	/	/
PM	D	/	/	/	/	/	/	/
	E	/	/	/	/	/	/	/
	F	/	/	/	/	/	/	/
	G	/	/	/	/	/	/	/

> *The importance of appropriate voice resonance to sustain vocal health is not new. Indeed, many techniques have been used by voice pathologists to gain appropriate tone focus in their patients. In the following case study, Linda Lee describes the history of refocusing laryngeal tone, along with management techniques for facilitating a more appropriate frontal focus in a case of voice fatigue.*

Refocusing Laryngeal Tone

Linda Lee, PhD

Case Study: Patient G

Patient History. Patient G, a 21-year-old female college senior, came to the University of Cincinnati Speech and Hearing Clinic because of vocal fatigue and periodic loss of voice. She reported that her voice had always been what she described as "rough" and would "give out" after long periods of talking, but daily fatigue had coincided with the start of student teaching in her major area of elementary education. Her voice production became increasingly effortful as the day of teaching progressed and improved on weekends.

The patient was a nonsmoker in good health, with the exception of allergies that caused sinus congestion in the spring. She used an antihistamine during this period and took no other medication. Her daily fluid intake included orange juice and caffeinated tea at breakfast, iced tea during the day, and diet cola at dinner. Water intake was limited to occasional sips at the school water fountain or following exercise.

Patient G's teaching schedule consisted of 5 hours in the classroom. She had a 1-hour preparation break late in the morning, 30 minutes for lunch (shared with a group of teachers in a lounge), and two breaks in the afternoon (6 minutes each). The patient lived with two nonsmoking roommates and described herself as socially outgoing. Her interests included dining out, biking, and traveling. Singing activities had been eliminated several years previously.

Laryngeal Examination. Patient G was examined by an otolaryngologist, who found edema of the vocal folds. An expectorant (Humibid) was prescribed on an as-needed basis. Thyroid function tests were performed because some patients with these symptoms have hypoactive thyroids; hers was normal.

Voice Evaluation

Perceptual Observations. Patient G's voice production during conversation consisted of 60 to 75% glottal fry. Phonation during the initial portion of most sentences was at the lower end of her frequency range but had good tonal quality. Mild laryngeal and jaw tension was noted during conversation. The focus of the voice was low and back. Respiration was characterized by shallow breathing during conversational speech.

Objective Analysis. Fundamental frequency was determined with a Visi-Pitch (KayPENTAX, Lincoln Park, NJ). During production of sustained vowels /i/, /a/, /u/, the fundamental frequencies averaged 192 Hz for comfortable pitch, 405 for high pitch, and 182 for low pitch. The total frequency range was 168 to 525 Hz. The average fundamental frequency during reading was 185 Hz.

Maximum phonation times for vowels averaged 11 seconds at comfortable pitch, 7.5 seconds at high pitch, and 9 seconds at low pitch.

Impressions. Patient G had a voice disorder characterized by the frequent use of glottal fry phonation and a low, back focus. The disorder was further complicated by a lack of hydration of the system, poor breath support, and a vocally demanding schedule.

Prognosis. The prognosis for eliminating the voice disorder was considered good, based on the patient's recognition of the problem, motivation, and willingness to assume the responsibility for change.

Recommendations. Patient G was enrolled in voice therapy. Her goals consisted of the following:

- perform physiologic exercises once daily to improve vocal function, as described by Stemple.[10]
- improve vocal hygiene by increasing hydration and reducing laryngeal tension
- improve respiratory support for speech
- use a forward, frontal focus for her voice
- eliminate the use of glottal fry phonation.

Management Program. Following initial counseling and introduction to therapy, Patient G was trained in the use of the Vocal Function Exercises. These exercises were reviewed at the initial part of each therapy session. The patient immediately switched from caffeinated to noncaffeinated beverages and increased her intake of water to eight glasses per day by carrying a thermos of ice water to school with her. She also substituted fruit juice for some of her colas. Changes were made in the arrangement of her room at school so that the environment was as free of competing background noise as possible. She also found ways to incorporate more vocal rest into her breaks during the school day.

The mechanics of speech breathing and importance of respiratory support for speech were explained. The patient learned to inspire to a higher lung volume by placing one hand on her chest and one on her abdomen during speech. This tactile cue was enough to remind her to take a deeper breath at the beginning of sentences and at phrase boundaries. Occasionally, the tactile cue was supplemented by marking breathing places on her reading passages. The tactile cue was dropped as soon as the pattern began to habituate.

The majority of the therapy sessions were aimed at changing the focus of the voice. Therefore, this aspect of management is described in detail.

Philosophy of Treatment for Altering Tone Focus. Focus refers to the resonance of the voice in the airways. Forward focus allows the voice to resonate fully throughout the pharyngeal, oral, and nasal cavities. When an obstruction, such as the presence of laryngeal or upper airway tension, impedes resonance, the focus of the voice is shifted away from its ideal placement. The result is a voice that tires easily and lacks flexibility and vibrancy.

The concept of altering focus has been addressed in two bodies of literature: voice disorders and singing. Techniques for altering focus in both disciplines are similar, although terminology varies and some authors rely more heavily on imagery than physiologic information. Singers most often refer to "placing the voice" in their attempts to control focus. Lamperti [14(p40)] is probably the most poetic in his address of the subject:

> Noise is a naked skeleton. Tone is fleshed in its own harmonics, and clothed in the overtones of surrounding space.
> When the top and bottom of the lungs are equally full of compressed air, the voice will focus in the head, and awake all the resonance in the head, mouth, and chest. Diction then is master over all."[14(p43)]

Constriction at any point alters focus. Christy[15] talked about moving focus away from the larynx by releasing it of tension. He stated that the voice places itself if resonance is free and balanced. A common technique of singing teachers is to ask the student to place the voice "into the mask" behind the eyes, out in front, behind the teeth, and so forth. Although this imagery will work for some, Christy believed that the voice should not be "put" anywhere. He felt this concept leads to fixing or setting of the muscles of phonation or articulation, thereby moving the constriction from one part of the airway to another. The resonance tends to be "imprisoned," and the individual pushes the voice, leading to even tighter muscles and a more deteriorated tone.[16,17]

Improper focus is rarely an isolated problem. Nevertheless, when focus is moved forward, improvements may be seen in other aspects of phonation. Tetrazzini[18] stated that if breathing and the focus of the tone are correct, other problems probably will resolve. This was the philosophy applied to the present case. Therapy was aimed at altering Patient G's focus rather than the glottal fry production, assuming that tone would improve as a secondary effect.

Orientation to the Management Approach. The concept of resonance is not an easy one to communicate to the patient. It is often preferable to rely on sensation than the ear when teaching focus. Patients typically have an "ah-ha!" experience, when the perception of focus suddenly becomes meaningful. Always searching for new and better ways to explain this concept, patients are asked to describe the difference between the back focus and the more forward placement. Each has said it "feels different," that the energy now is experienced anywhere from the alveolar ridge to the front of the mouth. They typically state that phonation is easier or more comfortable to produce. When a patient hears his or her voice on an audio recorder, most recognize that it sounds brighter and louder. One patient said, "Oh, that's my bedroom voice!" When we managed to stop laughing and her face returned to its normal color, she explained that she uses that voice when she and her husband are talking in bed and they do not want to wake the children in the next room. What she did not realize is that her properly focused "bedroom voice" probably carried farther than the disordered one!

The importance of providing a model for each stage of treatment cannot be overemphasized. Adding a bit of tension in the laryngeal and back tongue area without altering fundamental frequency results in a more back-focused tone that can be used for demonstration. Audio-recording is a part of every session and often is used as a form of feedback. Homework is also assigned. In addition to the Vocal Function Exercises, Patient G was given drills to complete at home. Sometimes she was asked to record these drills, provided she did not need cues or feedback to complete them.

Treatment Stages. Traditional programs for management of resonance have been a part of voice treatments since the early days of our profession. Many patients respond to one concept or approach better than they respond to others, and clinician flexibility is important. The treatment program developed for Patient G was an eclectic combination of techniques that evolved from these traditional approaches.

Step 1. The resonance program began by asking Patient G to read a passage while concentrating on where she felt the most sensations and where she felt the "energy" of her speech. Invariably, patients with low, back focus point to the throat. The need to pull that energy forward was discussed, explaining that sound is restricted when it is confined in the laryngeal area. Patient G was told that the voice receives its quality or character by resonating through the passages above the throat, and she needed to open these cavities to take advantage of them.

Following this orientation to the treatment approach, Patient G was instructed to hum at a comfortable pitch. She was encouraged to relax, enjoy the process, and phonate without pushing. Some patients may need stretching or relaxation exercises to loosen the jaw, tongue, and laryngeal area prior to this activity.

Patient G then produced the nasal consonants /m/ and /n/ with vowels in consonant-vowel (CV) combinations. These were repeated slowly, using a comfortable pitch so that one sound dissolved into the next and the nasal was emphasized. Patient G was encouraged to feel the vibration created at the sides of her nose and on the facial bones.

Other clues that may help bring focus forward at this stage include the following:

- Pretend to have a comb with a tissue over it. Put the comb in front of the lips and make a vibrating noise on it. Pretend to move the place of sound vibration from the vocal folds to the front of the lips.
- Make a "motorcycle noise" by vibrating the lips together. Extend phonation and change vowels (for example, bbbrrr /i/, bbbrrr /o/).
- Trill the tongue on the top of the alveolar ridge. Move the lips to shape different sounds. With all three of these techniques, extend the forward placement of vibration by moving into CV combinations with frontal placement.
- Produce a rather loud, well-supported sigh on the vowel /o/ or /a/, beginning at the higher end of the frequency range and phonating without break into lower mid-range. This technique should extend the more forward focus usually produced at the higher pitches into the comfortable frequency range.
- A singer who uses forward focus during song but not in speech may be asked to sing a few sentences of a piece that lies in midrange (eg, the first few phrases of "America the Beautiful," started at a comfortable pitch). Immediately mimic the sung passages, using a speaking voice. If a forward focus was used while singing, it should carry over into speech.

■ Finally, a kazoo cannot be played without forward focus—a reminder that therapy procedures should be fun!

Step 2. Using the humming procedure, Patient G produced CVCV combinations. Initially, the consonants were all nasals (such as /mona/). Later, one /z/ (not /s/) was added, such as /mozo/ or /mizi/. Combinations were repeated, combined, produced on one pitch, inflected, and changed in loudness as the patient progressed.

Step 3. Patient G read short sentences that were loaded with nasal and many voiced consonants. The sentences were chanted slowly on a comfortable pitch, connecting the sounds together to make the sentence "legato." She was reminded to take an adequate breath at the beginning, relax, and concentrate on the feelings of vibrations. Examples of the sentences used are:

■ My mother makes much money.
■ Nana made some lemon jam.
■ Many mice munch on melons.
■ Mary meets me at the market.
■ Mudpies are made in mud.
■ Meet me at the market on Monday.
■ Mickey meets Minnie in the movies.

Some patients prefer using shorter phrases first; however, the sentence often gives the patient time to sense and develop the feeling of resonance.

Step 4. This stage usually proves to be the most difficult because it is the transition from chanting to speaking. Using the same sentences as in step three, Patient G first chanted the whole sentence. Next, following clinician model at Patient G's comfortable pitch, she chanted the first word and spoke the sentences as a question with rising intonation. At first, as soon as she ended the chanted word, she dropped into back focus. She was reminded to emphasize the nasal sounds just as she had during the chanting and take her time producing the sentence. Occasionally, she needed reminders to take an adequate breath or to relax her jaw. Patient G spent 1 week at this stage. When she could produce the questions without first chanting the entire sentence and with 90% success, she followed the same procedure but used falling intonation. It was at this stage that the Patient had her "ah-ha" experience and began to show consistency.

Negative practice was employed to emphasize the differences between forward and back focus. This is a powerful technique that provides the patient the opportunity to feel the differences between the two placements. The technique also assures the patient of his or her ability to alter productions.

Step 5. Patient G was ready to move into longer utterances, but she needed the nasal context to keep the focus forward. The following paragraph was used. Initially, breath groups were marked.

Minnie mariner loved the water. Many members of her family had been in the navy. Her uncle was a fisherman. He remembered many moments netting tuna in the pouring rain. When Minnie was a little girl, she dangled slimy worms to catch sunfish. Nothing was more fun than watching the sunfish nibble the worms. When she was seventeen, Minnie learned to sail. She named her boat Minerva. Sometimes her best friend Norman went with her. Their mothers never minded their sailing. When the dinner bell rang, Norman and Minnie always came home.

Step 6. Patient G's maximum phonation times on the Vocal Function Exercises had increased to an average of 20 seconds at all pitch levels. Inspiring to higher lung volumes was more automatic, and signs of tension were gone during practice. Exercise sentences were free of glottal fry, although it still entered into conversational speech. Patient G was now aware of its occurrence in all contexts.

Nonnasal sentences with many forward consonants were introduced (eg, "Ted bought a baby bed"). A light articulatory contact was encouraged. If this patient had experienced difficulty with this step, questions containing nasals in the initial word only would have been used, followed by statements.

Step 7. As Patient G became accustomed to sentences and paragraphs that were not controlled for phonetic context, short segments of conversation were added. Whenever she slipped into old patterns, she was reminded to take a deeper breath, hum for a moment to regain focus, drop her jaw, and so forth as she repeated the phrase. Short periods of conversation were extended outside the therapy room by establishing specific times, places, and conversation partners.

Step 8. When the patient could converse without losing focus the majority of the time, background noise was added with a radio in the therapy room. Conversations held outside the therapy room and with different people also were conducted.

Step 9. Finally, Patient G role played some of her teaching activities in a large classroom. Here, she sometimes needed reminders about breath support. She audio-recorded parts of her lessons at school so they could be evaluated in therapy.

Results of Therapy. Patient G improved the quality of her voice production by creating a more forward focus, increasing breath support, and releasing tension. These changes resulted in an elimination of glottal fry. She was dismissed after 7 weeks of therapy, with the advice that she continue the Vocal Function Exercises once a day and maintain her present level of fluid intake. She no longer experienced laryngeal fatigue and was happy with her new manner of speaking.

Resonant Voice Therapy (Precursor to *Lessac-Madsen Resonant Voice Therapy*)

Katherine Verdolini Abbot, PhD and Nicole Yee-Key Li, PhD, MPhil

Case Study: Patient H

This case is presented to illustrate the use and principles of an early version of what is now called "Lessac-Madsen Resonant Voice Therapy" (LMRVT). A key feature of both earlier and current versions of LMRVT is its contrast with voice therapy approaches that emphasize voice conservation in the treatment of patients with phonotrauma. LMRVT is founded in the opposing notion that people with phonotrauma probably have the condition because they need to speak often and loudly due to life circumstances, personality, or both. Since the time of the initial description of Patient H in 2000,[19] biomechanical data on resonant voice in LMRVT have been joined by biological data, which *illuminate molecular mechanisms through which resonant voice not only may optimize voice output while protecting from injury, but may also generate actual healing effects in the larynx. Moreover, since 2000, LMRVT has undergone further elaboration with respect to motor learning principles, based on new data published in the interim. However, the basic structure of the program has remained unchanged. Comments about some of the key new developments in LMRVT since the original case description are embedded in the text that follows. This text describes Patient H's symptoms, her clinical history, initial observations, treatment goals, and treatment course as well as foundational concepts for LMRVT. Findings from larger data are forthcoming.*

History and Complaints. Patient H was a 19-year-old female college student, an avid debater, and tour guide. She was referred to our clinic by an outside hospital. The referring diagnosis was bilateral nodules and mild laryngopharyngeal reflux (LPR). History suggested her nodules were chronic.

Patient H complained of hoarseness and voice loss brought on by extended voice use or upper respiratory tract infection. She had experienced the problem for about 2 years. Our initial evaluation was conducted at a clinical satellite equipped with minimal instrumentation; standardized procedures were used.[20,21] Results are shown in Figure 3–1.

Summary of Results. The overall impression was a recurring voice problem that ranged from mild (eg, on the day of the evaluation) to severe (outright voice loss following vocal loading or upper respiratory tract infection). For Patient H, one of the most functionally distressing aspects of her condition was the debilitating effect it had on her debating, which she took very seriously.

Observations from vocal performance tests were consistent with the referring diagnosis of vocal fold nodules.[21] History and observations suggested that the following factors contributed to Patient H's nodules, recurring hoarseness and voice loss.

1. Voice use patterns
   a. Adducted hyperfunction in general and during debating in particular [The biomechanical result would be large intercordal impact stresses, producing nodules and hoarseness.[22–24]].
   b. Reactive nonadducted hyperfunction
   [Such hyperfunction can contribute to voice problems[25] and in the extreme, episodic voice loss.]
2. Medical factors
   a. Laryngopharyngeal reflux (LPR)
   [Speculatively, reflux can predispose vocal fold tissue to phonotrauma or slowed tissue recovery following trauma, although the mechanisms for a link between LPR and nodules are unclear in the literature.[26–29]].
   b. Relative dehydration
   [Dehydration may predispose laryngeal tissue to injury or slow recovery from injury, as well as increased phonatory subglottic pressure.[30–32]].
   c. History of chronic nodules
   [Prior laryngeal injury may biologically predispose the tissue to further injury.[30,31]]

Patient: H
Referring Diagnosis: Soft nodules and gastric reflux

Date: 10/22/98
Clinician: Verdolini

		POOR			NORMAL			SUPERIOR	
GENERAL									
VHI									
Functional	40	30	20	10	0				
Physical	40	30	20	10	0				
Emotional	40	30	20	10	0				
Effort	X4	X3	X2		X1				
Voice									
Grade	SEV	MOD	MIL		NORMAL				
Roughness	SEV	MOD	MIL		NORMAL				
Asthenia	SEV	MOD	MIL		NORMAL				
Breathy	SEV	MOD	MIL		NORMAL				
Strain	SEV	MOD	MIL		NORMAL				
Tremor	SEV	MOD	MIL		NORMAL				
Nasality	SEV	MOD	MIL		NORMAL				
Speech	SEV	MOD	MIL		NORMAL				
Language	SEV	MOD	MIL		NORMAL				

FIGURE 3–1. Patient H's results from formal voice testing at the outset of therapy.

In the General Voice Index, the Physical subscale of the Voice Handicap Index[68] indicated mild impairment. She rated phonatory effort as moderately elevated, using a Direct Magnitude Estimation scale.[122,123] Auditory-perceptual evaluation of voice, based on the GRABS scale[91] (G = overall Grade of dysphonia; R = Roughness; A = Asthenia; B = Breathiness; S = Strain) adding the dimensions "T" for tremor and "N" for nasality indicated a mild overall grade of dysphonia and moderate voice strain on the day of the evaluation. Other parameters of the auditory-perceptual evaluation were judged normal. Also articulation and language were normal, informally assessed based on conversational speech. *continues*

Treatment Goals and Treatment. Specific information about Patient H's treatment goals and her treatment is provided in Tables 3–1 and 3–2. Here, I would like to make some general comments that may help to interpret the details.

Treatment Goals. As for all of my patients, I established with Patient H three levels of treatment goals:

1. Functional goals, which are the ultimate target of treatment and are determined by the patient.

ACOUSTIC								
Fo ave (Hz)			175					
ST range (z)	-3.0	-2.0	-1.0		0	+1.0	+2.0	+3.0
I ave (dB 3')	50 80	55 75	60 70		65			
I range (dB)	10	20	30		40	50	60	70
PHYSIOL								
L-D rate (z)	-3.0	-2.0	-1.0		0	+1.0	+2.0	+3.0
L-D str	SEV weak SEV tight	MOD weak MOD tight	MIL weak MIL tight		NORMAL			
L-D con	SEV	MOD	MIL		NORMAL			
S:Z (z)	+3.0 -3.0	+2.0 -2.0	+1.0 -1.0		0			

FIGURE 3–1. *continued* The Acoustic Index indicated abnormally low fundamental frequency in spontaneous speech, as compared with normative data. Also average intensity in speech and dynamic range were low compared with norms. The semitone pitch range was normal or superior, however, suggesting that the lesions did not necessarily impair physiologic capabilities, at least not in all dimensions. Perturbation measures were not made because of my belief that they reveal little about the acoustic status of voice in the best cases, and may be misleading in the worst cases.

The Physiologic Index was modeled after a framework that distinguishes characteristic "profiles" associated with a range of laryngeal and vocal pathologies.[21] This framework distinguishes between measures that generally reflect vocal fold posturing capabilities (laryngeal diadochokinetic or L-DDK rate, strength, and consistency) and vocal fold oscillatory closure (s/z ratio). The patient's profile was typical for patients with nodules.[21] Although her L-DDK performance was normal or superior, because of apparent intact functioning of the recurrent laryngeal nerve, her s/z ratio was greater than one standard deviation above the norm and thus was abnormal based on our criteria.

Table 3–1. Goals for Patient H's Treatment

Functional	Medical	Biomechanical
Normal or near-normal voice, without dysphonia, hoarseness, or voice loss during debating or tour-guiding, without constant vigilance	Reduction or resolution of nodules	Hygiene • Hydration • Behavioral control of LPR Voice training • Use of slightly abducted vocal fold configuration for most speech, especially loud speech, to replace hyper- and hypoadducted hyperfunction

Table 3–2. Therapy for Patient H. "BTG" Refers to Resonant Voice "Basic Training Gesture" Exercises in LMRVT and Its Precursor. BTG Exercises Involve Explorations in Resonant Voice During All-Voiced Consonant Productions, Modeled after Lessac's "Consonant Orchestra" Exercises.[46,47] (It is assumed clinicians are familiar with other acronyms used in the table.)

Session	Status at Start of Session	Therapy Provided During Session	Patient's Performance Within Session	Home Tasks and Exercises	Time to Next Session
Initial evaluation	Intermittent hoarseness and voice loss	• *Hygiene:* hydration, reflux management • *Voice training:* stretches; RV BTG exercises; words	• Hygiene instructions understood • Produced RV relatively well to word level on 80% of trials with models	• 2–3 qt water daily; steam inhalations 5 min bid; behavioral reflux precautions • Stretches; RV foundation exercises and RV words 10 min bid	10 days
Therapy #1	Voice unchanged	• *Voice training:* stretches; RV BTG exercises; words-sentences	• Produced RV relatively well to sentence level without models; hyperfunction decreased particularly when models indicated increased airflow	• Continue hygiene • Stretches; RV BTG-words-sentences 10 min bid	1 wk
Therapy #2	Voice good during past week, but had not been challenged	• *Voice training:* stretches; RV BTG-words-sentences; video feedback used; loudness variations practiced to sentence level with models	• Produced RV well to sentence level without models following video feedback; produced loudness variations to sentence level without hyperfunction with models	• Continue hygiene • Stretches; RV BTG-words-sentences including loudness variations, 10 min bid	3 wk (Thanksgiving with family and friends)

66

Session	Status at Start of Session	Therapy Provided During Session	Patient's Performance Within Session	Home Tasks and Exercises	Time to Next Session
Therapy #3	No voice problems occurred over break	• *Voice training:* stretches; RV BTG-reading-conversation; "deep" practice with loudness variations on vowels	• Produced relatively good RV without hyperfunction to conversational level; needed to continue to purposefully expand pharynx	• Continue hygiene • Stretches; RV BTG-words-sentences, including loudness variations on vowels, 10 min bid	2 mo; patient reported doing exercises 3–4 times/wk
Therapy #4	Voice fine. No voice changes subsequent to long debate tournament. Patient noted recalling and using sensations from training during debates.	• *Voice training:* stretches; RV BTG-words-conversation; headphones used for audiofeedback	• Produced RV without hyperfunction to conversational level at nearly 100% with prompts and models	• Continue hygiene • Stretches; RV BTG-words-sentences, including loudness variations on vowels, 10 min bid	2 wk
Therapy #5	Voice generally feeling not only "OK," but "actually good." No voice changes during debate tournament.	• *Voice training:* stretches; RV BTG adding "structure" (inverted megaphone, after Lessac), to phrase and conversation level	• Produced completely hyperfunction-free voice on 30–40% of conversational trials and good approximations on remainder of trials, with some models	• Continue hygiene • Stretches; RV BTG-words-sentences, adding "structure;" use "minis" as needed during day	5 wk

continues

Table 3–2. *continued*

Session	Status at Start of Session	Therapy Provided During Session	Patient's Performance Within Session	Home Tasks and Exercises	Time to Next Session
Therapy #6	Voice has been fine; patient has been symptom-free. She had a cold 2 wk prior without any voice loss. RV generally automatic in debate setting; less automatic socially.	• *Voice training:* stretches; "structural" exercises, to phrase and conversational level	• By end of session patient produced hyperfunction-free voice on about 65% of trials during structured conversation, with minimal cues	• Continue hygiene • Continue exercises as previously, adding "structural" words and sentences, followed by /h/ to /m/ sentences to integrate structure and RV	1 wk to final evaluation

2. Medical goals, which pertain to medically relevant conditions and are implied by the medical referral.
3. Biomechanical goals, which are subdivided into (a) education in basic tenets of voice care ("vocal hygiene") and (b) voice training, and are directly addressed in voice therapy.

Biomechanical goals are the primary ones directly addressed in therapy. If those goals are properly identified and pursued, medical and functional gains should be byproducts of changes in the biomechanics of the patient's voice use.

Specific to Patient H, she indicated her functional goal was "normal voice," without dysphonia, hoarseness, or voice loss during debating and tour guiding, without requiring "constant vigilance." The implicit medical goal was improvement or resolution of nodules. Biomechanical goals suggested by the patient's history and observations were: (a) increased hydration and LPR control, and (b) the acquisition of a voice production pattern associated with barely ad/abducted vocal folds. In greater detail, although hydration and LPR control relate to medical issues, they were identified under the rubric of "biomechanical goals" in voice therapy because, by addressing them in behavioral therapy, they should have ultimately influenced the biomechanical properties of the vocal folds and thus phonatory biomechanics. With respect to the voice production goal, data have indicated that the barely ad/abducted vocal fold configuration that was targeted in this case tends to generate an optimized relation of voice output intensity (strong) to vocal fold impact intensity (relatively small), ideally allowing people to phonate relatively loudly, at the same time protecting the laryngeal tissue from (further) injury.[22]

Perceptually, this phonatory setup has been found to be associated with what has been called "resonant voice," perceptually defined as "easy" voice involving perceptible anterior oral vibrations during phonation.[33–35] In sum, for this patient who presented with phonotrauma and, simultaneously, a need to use her voice frequently and loudly, this biomechanical target seemed rationally favorable.

Treatment. Details regarding Patient H's treatment are shown in Table 3–2. After her initial evaluation, H received a total of six 45-minute voice therapy sessions over an 18-week period. Usually, I see patients for about 8 sessions over 4 to 8 weeks, but H's scheduling constraints dictated more time between visits. Her rapid gains in therapy also indicated fewer treatments would be needed than usual.

A synopsis of the overarching therapeutic framework—for Patient H and for LMRVT in general—is shown in Table 3–3. This basic framework identifies three factors that I hold are necessary—and in the extreme "sufficient" to address in physical training of any type, including voice training. Those factors are (a) the "what," (b) the "how," and (c) the "if" of voice training or therapy. The "what" of therapy refers to the behaviors and biomechanical targets that will be addressed in therapy. "What" do we want our patients to be doing differently behaviorally (eg, drink more water) and biomechanically (eg, using a barely abducted vocal fold configuration during phonation) by the end of therapy? The "how" of voice therapy refers to the approach to training, independent of the biomechanical target. That is, "how" will patients acquire the behaviors and biomechanical targets we identify for them? The "if" of voice therapy refers to patient compliance, for lack of a better term: "if" the patient will do what we suggest, especially outside the clinic.[34]

The "What" of Voice Therapy. As noted, in LMRVT, and in most approaches to voice therapy for that matter, the "what" piece of therapy is subdivided into two parts: voice care education and voice training. A concept I introduced from the earliest versions of LMRVT was that voice care education ("vocal hygiene") ideally should limit the number of parameters we ask patients to address rather than asking them to adhere to a large list of "do's and don'ts," which can be overwhelming and moreover generally lack specificity for a given patient. I believe that the "short list" of key targets to consider in a hygiene program are those relating to (a) hydration, (b) inflammation control (from LPR, environmental pollutants, illness and medications, smoke, etc), and (c) patent phonotraumatic behaviors even under ideal conditions, such as out-and-out uncontrolled, unskilled screaming. Key in Patient H's program and in LMRVT in general was the identification of *only* those hygiene parameters relevant to her case, based on history and observations. Recent data from our laboratory indicate patient compliance with *targeted* hygiene programs can be excellent,[36] in contrast to poorer compliance with hygiene programs reported in less enthusiastic reports about elaborate," one size fits all" hygiene programs.[37] Moreover, new, as yet unpublished evidence suggests slimmed down, targeted hygiene interventions can help to prevent the onset of new voice problems in at-risk populations (eg, teachers[36]), although they may indeed be ineffectual as self-standing programs for individuals with existing phonogenic voice problems.[36,37]

With respect to actual voice training, in LMRVT for this patient and others, most sessions initiate with exercises to stretch extrinsic and intrinsic structures related to phonation. This approach is based on the notion that skilled perceptual-motor behavior in most domains fundamentally involves inhibition of musculature that is irrelevant to the task at hand, and activation of relevant musculature. Support for this approach is found in the developmental motor learning literature that points to selective activation as a hallmark of skilled performance. [38] Accordingly, I initiated all therapy sessions for Patient H with a series of "deactivation" stretches targeting the thorax, cervical region, oropharynx, and vocal folds in an attempt to deactivate musculature involved in the phonatory substrate.[39] Selective activation exercises followed (Table 3–3).

The selective activation piece of therapy may proceed according to any one of a number of specific therapy interventions, including Vocal Function Exercises described elsewhere in this text and in the literature.[40,41] For Patient H, this intervention was a primitive form of what, as noted, would later be called LMRVT.[39,42]

Table 3–2 describes the specific contents of Patient H's therapy, which arose from the overarching framework described. Detailed information about the contents of current LMRVT can be obtained through Plural Publishing,[39,42]

Table 3–3. General Model of Voice Therapy

"What"	"How"	"If"
Biomechanics	Learning	Compliance

coupled with hands-on training in seminar format. Here, I limit my discussion to general "philosophical" comments around LMRVT and to newer findings and speculations pertinent to LMRVT for this patient and others.

As already noted, in LMRVT, the target voice production modality is defined both productively and perceptually. Productively, the target involves voicing with barely adducted or slightly abducted vocal folds.[33,35] This configuration, and specifically a configuration involving an approximately 0.5- to 1.0-mm separation between the vocal processes, appears to generate an optimized ratio of voice output intensity versus vocal fold impact intensity under constant subglottic pressure (Ps) and fundamental frequency (F_0) conditions.[22] Not incidentally, the same general vocal fold configuration requires relatively small subglottal pressure to initiate and maintain vocal fold oscillation,[43] and thus should be physiologically "easy." Perceptually, one correlate of this laryngeal setup is "resonant voice" (RV), which involves vibratory sensations in the anterior oral cavity in the context of "easy" phonation.[33–35] Thus far, reliable noninvasive tools have not been identified to detect instrumentally what is recognized perceptually as "resonant voice" (eg, Verdolini, Kobler, Conversano, Walsh, Xiu, Milstein, Hillman, unpublished data, 2000), although one instrumented approach, involving a laryngeal resistance measure (estimated phonatory subglottic pressure divided by glottal airflow[44]) may have potential to identify the target *laryngeal* configuration, at least within a given subject on a given day.[45] Interestingly, in that latter data set, laryngeal resistance quantitatively distinguished pressed, normal/resonant, and breathy voice types across and within vocally healthy subjects, but failed to distinguish normal and resonant voice, which were reliably distinguished perceptually. The implication is that differences between resonant and "normal" voice, at least in healthy vocalists, reside in production parameters not assessed by laryngeal resistance, and that is vocal tract parameters. In fact, the Lessac work as well as LMRVT involve vocal tract manipulations to optimize anterior facial vibratory sensations and also voice output intensity,[22,46,47] Stated differently, resonant voice is *one* voicing modality that likely signals the target laryngeal configuration, adding to laryngeal posturing also vocal tract manipulations that should increase oral vibratory sensations and output intensity. Also a voicing pattern that judges would consider "normal" (for healthy individuals) appears to be associated with the target laryngeal posture, although intensity may be lower as compared to "resonant voice." In summary, various data sets have indicated the perception of anterior oral vibrations during "easy" voicing—and also more simply, "normal voice"—are general indicators of the target biomechanical configuration for both healthy subjects and subjects with nodules who have been described in the literature thus far.[33,35]

Recent observations have suggested that the advantages of resonant voice in voice therapy may not only be linked to its likely connection to a biomechanical setup that favors strong voice production (when needed), while at the same time protecting from laryngeal injury.[22] Preliminary data from biological studies indicate this voicing approach may have actual "medicinal" therapeutic properties. Specifically, some data indicate that, in some cases, resonant voice exercises may help to reduce acute vocal fold inflammation even more than voice rest.[48] Speculatively, the reason is related to findings reported for other tissue domains, that tissue stretching—in this case associated with relatively large-amplitude vocal fold oscillations in resonant voice, coupled with pitch manipulations in LMRVT exercises—deforms cells within the tissue, thereby altering their mechanical signaling in a way that is favorable for the wound healing process.[49-52] Thus far, a favorable result from resonant voice and its experimental correlates has been seen in human subjects, in in vitro data, and in computer modeling of vocal fold inflammation.[48,53,54] Further verification is needed. However, clinical anecdotal as well as formal biological observations point to some optimism that, in some cases, resonant voice may have actual healing properties.

LMRVT is similar in emphasis to traditional "forward focus" approaches used by many clinicians. Further, the laryngeal goal is essentially identical to the goal implicitly targeted in Vocal Function Exercises.[40,41] The distinguishing characteristics of LMRVT as I have developed it are as follows:

1. *LMRVT connotes a specific approach to the training of resonant voice, involving a specific set of training exercises that aim to link basic resonant voice exercises (partly found in Lessac's "consonant orchestra" work)[46,47] to everyday speech by way of special "bridging exercises."* Specifically, the exercises start with all-voiced utterances exploring resonant voice, and proceed to resonant voice discovery in utterances with voiced-voiceless contrasts, prosodic variations, conversational interjections, "pull-outs," intensity training, and finally to increasingly challenging real-life communication tasks, using RV.

2. *LMRVT arises from a synthesis of quantitative biomechanical and biological voice science, cognitive neurophysiological learning science, health care compliance literature, and artistic tradition.* The biomechanical piece of LMRVT focuses on the slightly abducted vocal fold configuration and minimal subglottic pressure already described. The biological underpinnings of the program relate to healing mechanisms that may be triggered by specialized forms of vocal exercises. Cognitive neuroscience contributions to LMRVT have to do with the learning aspect of therapy. Specifically, emphasis is placed on a single focus for the *patient* in training, and that is resonant voice, as well as on exploration rather than prescription in training, attention to sensory processes, attention to detail, specificity of practice, and flexibility in the use of the approach by individual clinicians.[55-57] More recently, learning elements in LMRVT have further underscored the importance of variability (specificity) of practice variability throughout the program[58] as well as patients' attention to production gestures' *effects* rather than biomechanics in training.[59-63] The artistic portion of LMRVT is derived from the work of theatre trainer Dr. Arthur Lessac, whose decades-long traditions in actor training inspired much of LMRVT at its origin.[46,47] (http://www.lessacinstitute.com/bio.html) and from the work of singer trainer Dr. Mark Madsen (University of Missouri-St. Louis (http://www.midnightsunburstmusic.com/).

3. LMRVT is founded in the principle that voice conservation is not a necessary or pervasive component of treatment for phonogenic problems.

Instead, LMRVT emphasizes the notion that people with such problems need to learn to produce strong voice *safely*.

A further word is in order regarding the "singular training focus" in LMRVT, which was instituted with Patient H as it is with most patients who receive LMRVT. Clinicians often express consternation over the proposal that a therapy program can proceed emphasizing one central notion, such as resonant voice, without addressing corollary parameters such as breathing, alignment, oropharyngeal factors, and so forth. Certainly, all of these parameters are important in determining phonation patterns. However, in LMRVT, if they are addressed, they are addressed only if their manipulation is required for the patient to achieve resonant voice. Moreover, they are addressed in the context of resonant voice, without directing the patient's attention away from this central construct, as opposed to addressing them as separate, independent parameters. The emphasis on a singular training focus is similar to the approach taken in Lee Silverman Voice Treatment, a program clinicians use in the treatment of patients with voice and speech problems due to Parkinson disease.[64–67]

Treatment Outcome and Recommendations. Patient H's formal posttherapy status 1 week following therapy termination is reflected in Figure 3–2, and can be compared to her pretherapy status in Figure 3–2. In summary, her phonatory discomfort was alleviated following treatment (see results for Voice Handicap Index,[68] Physical Subscale, Fig 3–2). My unblinded, unverified perceptual evaluation of her voice quality during conversational speech in the clinic indi-

cated an improvement from mild overall dysphonia (and moderate strain) to normal. Although her fundamental frequency in speech was not addressed in therapy, it improved from low (pretherapy) to normal (posttherapy). Similarly, her conversational intensity improved from mildly weak to normal. Her physiologic measures improved from reflecting potentially poor glottal closure (s/z ratio[69]) before therapy to normal after therapy.

Most important were Patient H's results relative to specific therapy goals. Biomechanically, by my evaluation, she produced the target voice production type—perceptually evaluated—on about 65% of words in structured conversation within therapy sessions. Her own judgments were more optimistic, indicating automatic use of RV in formal (eg, debate) settings but less automatic use socially.

Medically, Patient H's vocal folds appeared pearly white with razor-straight free edges except at high pitches, for which a barely perceptible bulge was noted at the midfold on the left. She did still exhibit thick secretions that probably were either an artifact of topical anesthesia administered for the laryngovideostroboscopy or persistent gastric reflux.

Functionally, Patient H felt that she had obtained her goals of speaking normally, without discomfort during most speech. In particular, she had been involved in several demanding debates over the preceding months without voice loss or other vocal sequelae even in the presence of upper respiratory tract infection.

Based on medical and biomechanical findings at treatment termination, I recommended that Patient H increase oral fluid intake and seek medical re-evaluation for possible persistent reflux.

Patient: H

Referring Diagnosis: Soft nodules and gastric reflux

Date: 3/29/99

Clinician: Verdolini

	POOR				NORMAL		SUPERIOR	
GENERAL								
VHI								
Functional	40	30	20	10	0			
Physical	40	30	20	10	0			
Emotional	40	30	20	10	0			
Effort	X4	X3	X2		X1			
Voice								
Grade	SEV	MOD	MIL		NORMAL			
Roughness	SEV	MOD	MIL		NORMAL			
Asthenia	SEV	MOD	MIL		NORMAL			
Breathy	SEV	MOD	MIL		NORMAL			
Strain	SEV	MOD	MIL		NORMAL			
Tremor	SEV	MOD	MIL		NORMAL			
Nasality	SEV	MOD	MIL		NORMAL			
Speech	SEV	MOD	MIL		NORMAL			
Language	SEV	MOD	MIL		NORMAL			
ACOUSTIC								
Fo ave (Hz)			175					
ST range (z)	-3.0	-2.0	-1.0		0	+1.0	+2.0	+3.0
I ave (dB 3')	50 / 80	55 / 75	60 / 70		65			
I range (dB)	10	20	30		40	50	60	70
PHYSIOL								
L-D rate (z)	-3.0	-2.0	-1.0		0	+1.0	+2.0	+3.0
L-D str	SEV weak / SEV tight	MOD weak / MOD tight	MIL weak / MIL tight		NORMAL			
L-D con	SEV	MOD	MIL		NORMAL			
S:Z (z)	+3.0 / -3.0	+2.0 / -2.0	+1.0 / -1.0		0			

FIGURE 3–2. Patient H's posttherapy status on formal voice measures, 1 week following therapy termination, compared with pretherapy status.

She was instructed to continue using stretches and RV exercises once weekly, prophylactically, and as warm-ups prior to any vocal loading as might occur in debating.

Conclusion. A precursor of Lessac-Madsen Resonant Voice Therapy (LMRVT) was used as part of a larger "what-how-if" model of voice therapy to address the functional concerns of a female college student who presented with chronic vocal fold nodules and functional consequences thereof. An abbreviated program of what later would be called LMRVT resulted in markedly improved vocal function in public speaking (debating) and a significant reduction in nodules. Principles described for this patient may be applicable to other patients with voice disorders associated with hyper- or hypoadduction of the vocal folds.

Acknowledgments. The writing of this section was partly supported by Grants No. K08 000139, R01DC005643, and R01 DC008290-01A1 (Verdolini Abbott, Principal Investigator) from the National Institute on Deafness and Other Communicative Disorders.

The Accent Method in Clinical Practice

Sara Harris

Case Study: Patient I

Another voice therapy program, which is popular in Great Britain, Scandinavia, Europe, and the Middle East, is the Accent Method. In this study of a young singer, Sara Harris describes in detail the rationale and the management plan for this approach.

This case study discusses the Accent Method of Voice Therapy and describes its benefits in restoring efficient vocal function to a young singer with midthird vocal fold thickening and a muscular tension pattern of dysphonia.[70] The Accent Method is a holistic therapy regime designed to coordinate the muscles of respiration, phonation, and articulation to produce efficient voice production and clear, resonant, well-modulated speech.

Svend Smith, a Danish phonetician designed the Accent Method in the 1930s. It is used widely in Europe including the Scandinavian countries. Smith was keen to develop a dynamic technique for voice and speech skills that emphasized the whole communication process, including nonverbal aspects such as eye contact and gesture. He was influenced greatly by the rhythmic patterns produced by the bongo drummer Joe Bogdana who accompanied the entertainer Josephine Baker. He saw a potential use of these rhythms to reinforce intonation and prosody, as well as to provide a framework in which to practice voice and articulatory skills. Smith and Bogdana worked together to devise the three tempos—largo, andante, and allegro—that are still used in the technique today.

The theoretical underpinning of the Accent Method is based on the following:

1. the myoelastic-aerodynamic model of vocal fold vibration
2. conditioning (the unconscious process of learning)
3. focus on normal vocal function rather than the pathology.[71,72]

The myoelastic-aerodynamic theory of vocal fold vibration was described in the 1950s by van den Berg[73] and relies on the concept of the Bernoulli effect.

Although recent research has demonstrated that this effect cannot explain all the factors involved in sustaining vocal fold vibration, the need to establish and maintain a satisfactory subglottic pressure and transglottal airflow remains essential to efficient voice production.[74]

The conditioning of the desired phonation pattern takes place during long periods of repetition of the Accent Method exercises. The exercises include all the vowels and consonants used in spontaneous speech from which the patient produces sequences of sustained sounds and syllables to sentence level. These meaningless babbled sentences incorporate prosodic features such as rhythmic stresses, intonation, and loud-soft vocal dynamics. The practice sessions may range from anywhere between 10 and 30 minutes. Although concentration is needed in the early stages as patients establish the desired patterns, the unconscious processes of learning and overlearning take over as they practice. Carryover of the newly learned skills into spontaneous, continuous speech then occurs easily and reliably, decreasing the likelihood of relapse. This is in stark contrast to other methods in which patients are asked to produce a sustained sound or short utterance but then discuss the effects of it using their habitual pattern of voice production.

The Accent Method exercises concentrate on establishing efficient vocal fold closures for speech in modal voice using simultaneous vocal onset coordinated with a stable, well-controlled expiratory airflow. Initially, the exercises deliberately encourage breathy phonation with gradual increase of vocal fold adduction until comfortable, clear voice is achieved. Recent research suggests that this phonation pattern made with the vocal folds barely touching produces efficient and particularly resonant voicing.[75,76] It allows the therapist to work equally effectively with patients who are hyperadducted or hypoadducted and explains why the Accent Method exercises have been reported as being successful with a wide range of vocal disorders.

Specific Features. Establishing abdominal breathing is a specific feature of the Accent Method. Inspiration relies on contraction of the diaphragm, which has been described as the major muscle of inspiration,[74] allowing the speed and amount of inspired air to be controlled easily and effectively. Expiration is controlled in part by elastic recoil and in part by contraction of the abdominal musculature. Contractions of the latter may be smooth for sustained vocalization and unstressed utterances or punctuated by smaller, faster contractions that alter the subglottic air pressure to produce changes in vocal intensity associated with stressed words or utterances of increased vocal loudness. Although research has shown that there are a number of different patterns of breathing and breath control,[77] it may be argued that diaphragmatic-abdominal control is most economical of muscular effort. Diaphragmatic-abdominal breathing displaces soft tissue and the abdominal contents, rather than pulling against the semirigid structure of the rib cage.

The development of modal voice is also a specific feature of the Accent Method. Modal voice is produced by short, thick vocal folds with relaxed cricothyroid muscles. Good vocal fold closure can be achieved easily and, provided there is sufficient subglottic pressure, satisfactory mucosal waves are generated. The larynx lies neutrally in the neck, and the pharyngeal and supraglottic musculature is less likely to constrict. By contrast, production of a technical falsetto or head voice requires thinned vocal folds and contracted cricothyroid muscles. When the vocal ligaments are stretched, mucosal waves are smaller, and the vocal fold closure may be harder to maintain over long periods. The larynx is raised to shorten the vocal tract and adjust the resonators appropriately for higher pitches, which may lead to constriction in the supraglottic and pharyngeal musculature. In every way, head voice requires more muscular effort on the part of the laryngopharynx. Many of our English patients adopt this type of phonation pattern for speech, and it is especially common in singers who are used to producing head voice for singing. Some singing teachers even encourage a higher speaking voice by suggesting it is more appropriate for sopranos. Unfortunately, clinical evidence suggests that long periods of this pattern of vocal use may result in bowing of the vocal folds as they become unable to maintain closure against the stretching produced by powerful cricothyroid muscle contraction.[78]

The initial focus on fricatives and close vowels during the Accent Method exercises is also an important feature of the method. These sounds all produce narrowing of the vocal tract within the oral cavity and are believed to create back pressure,[79] which assists fast closure of the vocal folds and may influence the length of the closed phase. They also encourage a high, forward tongue position, opening space between the back of the tongue and the pharynx, which may be associated with the "forward resonance" described by singers. The high tongue position has also been associated with enhancement of the 250 kHz region in the vocal spectrum, providing extra brightness and penetration to the vocal tone and allowing it to be heard through background noise.[80]

Case History. Patient I presented in the ear, nose and throat (ENT) clinic at the request of her general practitioner and her singing teacher. She was 22 years old and studying singing at a well-known music college in London. She planned to be a professional mezzo-soprano, specializing in classical and early romantic styles of singing. At the time she was seen, she was in her final year at college with only 3 months remaining before her final examinations and recital.

Patient I had been noticing a problem with her voice for approximately 6 months. She reported that it sounded breathy and immature in her singing and that there were "dead patches" in her upper pitch range where the voicing broke into audible air escape. Her singing teacher was particularly concerned because Patient I was no longer responding to the usual singing techniques designed to resolve these problems. She reported that her speaking voice was "mostly OK" but became breathy and hoarse both when she was tired and following prolonged voice use.

Patient I's case history revealed that she was fit and well with no previous or family history of voice problems. In particular, she had no symptoms of gastroesophageal reflux and no asthma, allergies, or other ENT problems.

As with many students, Patient I needed to work to support herself at college. She worked in a noisy restaurant that was air conditioned and often smoky. She was aware of how much she had to shout in her job, and she also had to do shift work that often involved late nights. In addition to her work and her singing, she ran a youth group at a local church that also involved protracted voice use and shouting. Patient I was the youngest of three sisters and described herself as "small but noisy" as a child. She was aware of stress induced by her college work.

Assessment. Initially Patient I was seen by an otolaryngologist specializing in voice disorders, who carried out video-strobolaryngoscopy. Examination revealed that she had an average to large larynx with significant midthird polypoid thickening of both vocal folds. The right fold thickening was more prominent than the left. There was a wide interarytenoid chink, and the anterior third of the vocal folds failed to close during phonation. Mucosal waves were present but poorly developed, largely because of inefficient voice production. The laryngologist diagnosed Patient I's vocal pathology as a type-2 muscular tension dysphonia, [81] later named laryngeal isometric disorder.[70] The laryngologist referred Patient I for voice therapy with a speech-language therapist who specialized in voice.

Perceptual Analysis. This was carried out informally in clinic and from the patient's initial audio recording of a standard reading passage.

Pitch. Patient I's speaking pitch and intonation range appeared to be well within the norm for her age and gender. Sirening through her full pitch range for singing showed a characteristic break in the upper register where she could no longer sustain phonation. Efforts to overcome this problem area resulted in a breathy "squeak" and visible effort in the extrinsic laryngeal muscles.

Intensity and Volume. Patient I's speaking voice was normal in intensity

for quiet conversation with no obvious signs of increased laryngeal effort. She was able to shout, but this produced extrinsic laryngeal muscle effort and led to early vocal fatigue. She reported that the intensity of her singing voice had decreased and that she no longer had control over her dynamic range. High-intensity singing tired her voice more quickly and felt effortful.

Quality. The patient's speaking voice was rated as mildly-moderately hoarse. She used a thin fold phonation type with audible air escape.

Comfort. Patient I reported no discomfort when speaking or singing but described a sense of increased effort or tiredness with high-intensity voice use, whether singing or speaking.

Stamina. The patient reported that her speaking voice felt "tired" and became increasingly breathy and weak by the evening. Fatigue developed after an hour of singing or speaking loudly. Her voice responded to rest and had usually recovered by morning, although after a heavy week of voice use in the restaurant, the recovery period increased to several days of normal voice use and voice rest.

Patient I had no malocclusion, dental problems, or articulatory disorders. She produced a good range of articulatory movement in speech with normal oral-nasal resonance balance. Her tongue position appeared to be reasonably neutral and her lip set in speech was rated as neutral and slight rounding.

Assessment of Breathing Patterns. Airflow measures are not available to this clinician for routine use. The assessment therefore was carried out on informal observation in the clinic. The breathing pattern at rest was produced in the upper chest. There was little observable movement of the abdomen during quiet breathing. During speech, this pattern of breath control continued. Expiration was controlled by the upper chest, which was observed pushing inward, particularly when words were stressed. "Top-up" breaths were also upper chest or clavicular. Observation of breath control for singing revealed that Patient I was able to produce a more central pattern and was attempting to recruit the abdominal muscles to help control expiration for sustained notes. The pattern was erratic and hampered by poor fold closure and air escape, however. As a result, she frequently used residual air and produced signs of increased effort, both in the upper chest and extrinsic laryngeal muscles. She reported that her singing training had provided relatively little guidance on breathing, and she was uncertain about the meaning of the term "breath support."

Palpation of the Extrinsic Laryngeal Musculature. Assessment of the external laryngeal musculature is standard practice in the author's clinic, and a shortened form of the Lieberman protocol is used.[82,83] As yet, there are no international norms for palpatory findings; however, Jacob Lieberman, a qualified osteopath specializing in laryngeal manipulation, has trained this clinician, and practitioner agreement has been reached for the following tasks.[84]

■ *Jaw:* There was some asymmetry of jaw opening to the right, and the left temporomandibular joint appeared to be more active than the right. This was apparent during the jaw open-

ing assessment tasks and during spontaneous speech. The patient had no awareness of the asymmetry and did not suffer from temporomandibular joint discomfort. Her singing teacher had commented that she felt Patient I's jaw tended to be "tight" during singing.

■ *Suprahyoid and base of tongue musculature:* The suprahyoid and base of tongue musculature was assessed as tighter than average on palpation. Patient I did not report any tenderness in these muscles, but there was strong contraction of the geniohyoid muscles during speech and singing. The anterior aspect of the hyoid bone was aligned with the anterior aspect of the thyroid cartilage.

■ *Thyrohyoid musculature:* Palpation of the thyrohyoid musculature revealed that these muscles were judged to be "held" tightly with a reduced thyrohyoid space area. They contracted briskly when speech was initiated and remained contracted throughout the utterance. The normal contractions usually observed during speech were reduced. Patient I was able to release this musculature using the yawn-sigh technique to lower the larynx and was able to maintain a greater thyrohyoid space successfully when the laryngeal position returned to its rest position. She did not report tenderness when these muscles were palpated.

■ *Cricothyroid musculature:* The cricothyroid muscles were judged to be held more tightly on the right than on the left, and the patient reported some tenderness when these muscles were palpated. The cricothyroid visor (the anterior space between the lower border of the thyroid cartilage and the upper border of the cricoid cartilage) appeared to open and close as expected with changing vocal pitch (yawn-sigh contrasted with a high-pitched "squeak"); but it was habitually held at rest in a closed neutral position. The alignment between the lower border of the thyroid cartilage and the upper border of the cricoid cartilage showed that the cricoid was held in a more anterior position relative to the thyroid. This suggested the possibility of some anterior sliding at the cricothyroid joint.[78,85]

- *Strap musculature:* These muscles were judged to be tight, particularly on the right on palpation and laryngeal shift. The larynx moved easily to the right but was anchored by the tight right strap muscles, restricting laryngeal shift to the left.
- *Laryngeal position in speech:* The patient's larynx maintained a neutral position in the neck for breathing and raised normally for swallowing. It returned easily to a neutral position in the neck following swallowing, but as Patient I anticipated speech, the larynx rose in the neck and maintained the raised position reliably throughout the utterance. It returned to neutral as soon as phonation ceased.

Treatment Plan. The assessment findings were explained and discussed with Patient I in the clinic. Vocal rest was not an option because of her need to earn money and the fact that her final recital was only 3 months away. Therefore, we agreed that she would continue with her normal vocal commitments but try to schedule her restaurant work during the day or on weekday evenings to avoid the greatest levels of background noise at the weekends. She also agreed to try to reduce some of the talking at her youth club. Her singing lessons

would continue as a priority.

Six, 1-hour sessions of voice therapy, once weekly, were agreed on, using audio-recorded exercises made during the sessions for home practice. Patient I stated her voice therapy aims as:

1. restoring her full vocal range without her voice breaking or hitting a "dead patch"
2. restoring her clear vocal quality in singing and speaking
3. restoring vocal stamina and comfort for singing and speech.

The therapist's treatment aims were to:

1. facilitate full and uniform vocal fold closure
2. establish modal (thick fold) phonation during speech
3. establish a higher subglottic air pressure and better breath control supported by the abdominal musculature
4. reduction of supraglottic muscular effort during speech.

The therapist decided to use the Accent Method as the main treatment technique for Patient I to establish the above aims. In addition, it would be supported by:

1. discussion on vocal hygiene and the use of a "voice diary" to highlight vocal trauma in daily life
2. techniques such as sirening[34] to facilitate better control of the cricothyroid mechanism, improving vocal range and register changes
3. the introduction of some work on "twang" voice quality[34] for specific use in the restaurant where shouting was inevitable

4. specific laryngeal massage to reduce excess tension in the extrinsic laryngeal muscles.

Early Accent Method Exercises: Establishing Abdominal Breathing. The patient was seated in a comfortable, upright chair for back support and her posture checked and aligned. She was encouraged to drop her shoulders down and to allow her abdominal muscles to relax. She then observed and monitored the movement of her abdominal wall, placing her hand on her abdomen, low down, below the level of her waist. The therapist sat beside her and placed the back of her own hand over Patient I's hand to monitor the movement. The patient, likewise, placed the back of her hand over the therapist's abdomen to feel the therapist model the desired breathing pattern. As the therapist breathed in, Patient I observed her lower abdomen expand and then contract, moving inward on expiration. Gradually, the patient began to produce the same pattern, and the therapist synchronized her own breathing rate to Patient I's, having reminded her not to breathe too quickly or too deeply.

As a singer, Patient I had little difficulty establishing abdominal breathing. When patients have difficulty, the early Accent Method exercises may be carried out with the patient lying supine so that the abdominal musculature can relax because these muscles are no longer required for postural support. This has the advantage of allowing patients to lie on their sides, which facilitates contraction of the abdominal musculature on expiration, once abdominal breathing has been established.

Patient I was asked to repeat sounds modeled by the therapist. The initial sounds recommended are the voiceless fricatives /k/ (bilabial) /s/, /sh/, and /f/, repeated to form a rhythmic sequence designed to increase transglottic airflow. Gradually, the voiced counterparts /g/, /z/, /zs/, /v/, and close vowels such as /i/ and /u/ were introduced into the repeated sequences with emphasis on deliberately gentle, breathy phonation. At this stage, patients are encouraged not to breathe in more deeply than they would for the previously established rest breathing, and the fricatives are made on elastic recoil rather than recruiting the abdominal musculature for controlling either the length or intensity of the sound.

Traditionally, little explanation is given to patients treated with the Accent Method; if errors occur, the therapist simply returns the patient to tasks he or she manages easily before gently increasing the complexity again. This therapist, however, does provide more guidance to patients, depending on their level of knowledge, experience, and skill because it is vital to maintain the patient's cooperation for a conditioning activity that can appear eccentric and mindless. At this early stage, if a patient continues to produce a low flow for fricatives, an overly long and controlled expiration, or both, this could be drawn to their attention. It also can be helpful for patients to notice that expiration stops naturally as lung pressure equalizes with the air pressure outside and that expiration pushed past this point requires muscular effort. This observation allows patients to locate any increased effort in the upper chest and strap muscles when they push past the rest position, which they can then correct.

The therapist monitors the vocal quality to ensure that the patient uses modal phonation. Voice onset may need to begin with breath before tone (ssssszzzzss) but should gradually become simultaneous with exhalation and phonation coordinated together. The vocal quality should become clearer but remain somewhat breathy. Phonation should be reliable and consistent as vocal fold closure becomes uniform, with the midthird swelling displaced upward and away from the vibrating edge of the fold by increased subglottic air pressure and airflow. If these changes are not achieved, the therapist may need to return to an earlier stage, drawing the patient's attention to any problems that have developed.

Other techniques can be incorporated if necessary to provide a bridge from one stage to another, depending on the problem. For example, staying with "breath before tone" onset for longer periods ensures that the patient does not return to his or her previous hyperadduction patterns, and introducing nasal consonants /m/, /n/, /ng/ usually resolves closure problems and the wide glottic chink. Problems of continued supraglottic tension often may be overcome using palpatory monitoring of the thyrohyoid space or the general laryngeal movement. Very rarely is it necessary to resort to gentle glottal onsets to ensure modal voice because this can usually be achieved using palpatory monitoring of the cricothyroid visor.

Gradually, Patient I was encouraged to produce gentle contractions of her abdominal musculature on expiration. The *largo* tempo (Fig 3–3) was introduced, in which expiration is punctuated by shorter, sharper rhythmic contractions of the abdominal muscles to produce stressed or "accented" beats. The largo tempo is slow, allowing the patient time to coordinate expiration and the activity of the abdominal mus-

cles. It also allows time for a relatively slow inspiration. The therapist and Patient I continued to monitor the excursions of the abdominal wall while sitting and standing. Gentle rocking of the entire body may facilitate general relaxation and reinforce the rhythmic structure of the technique. The therapist then works the patient through the *andante* (Fig 3–4) and *allegro* (Fig 3–5) tempos, gradually introducing other vowels and consonants until the patient can maintain the desired phonation pattern for babbling long, prosodic utterances of 20 minutes or more. Work designed to alter tongue position or oral-nasal resonance balance can be incorporated into the sound sequences at this stage. Other prosodic features, such as intonation (pitch contrasts) and dynamic (loud-soft) contrasts, can also be practiced.

As the patient gains confidence, meaningful words are introduced. Initially, repetition of therapist-modeled utterances or rote-learned materials (such as rhymes or poems) are practiced before the patient graduates to spontaneously generated utterances, such as responding to questions from the therapist or describing events.

Results. Patient I completed seven, 1-hour sessions of Accent Method voice therapy, which took place over 3 months between late February and May, with a 2-week break over the Easter holiday. The sessions were audio recorded, and Patient I continued to practice the work at home on a daily basis. Reassessment in early June showed Patient I to have improved significantly in her vocal health and voice production.

Perceptually, the patient's voice continued to be slightly breathy, but the audible turbulent air escape present on her original recording had resolved.

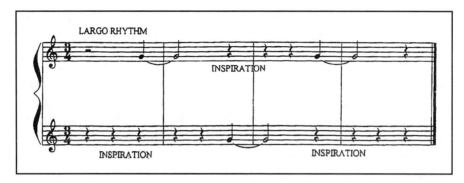

FIGURE 3–3. Largo tempo.

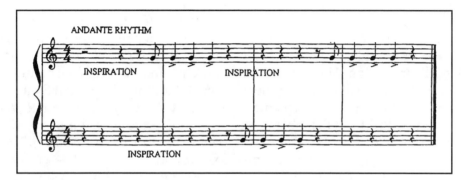

FIGURE 3–4. Andante tempo.

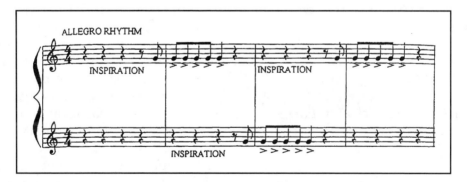

FIGURE 3–5. Allegro tempo.

There were no pitch or voice breaks, and the slow vocal onset initially observed was no longer present. The "dead patch" in her vocal range had disappeared and she was able to siren through her range smoothly and reliably. She still had to be careful to balance the air pressure and transglottal flow correctly while producing high and soft notes in her singing, but otherwise her singing voice no longer gave her trouble. Her teacher reported that she was able to continue developing her singing skills.

Palpation of the extrinsic laryngeal muscles showed that the tightness noted at her first assessment had largely resolved. All her scores had returned to neutral except those for the thyrohyoid muscles. Although these were judged as having reduced in score by half a scalar degree and were not reported as tender, they remained slightly elevated at 3.5 (neutral score 3). Patient I continued a slight tendency to raise her larynx during speech.

Videostroboscopy showed that Patient I was now able to produce full vocal fold closure on phonation and that the midthird swelling had almost resolved. A little minimal thickening remained in the midthird that no longer appeared to be affecting phonation.

Patient I completed her final examination at music college, achieving a good grade. She reported that her final recital had been well received and that she had experienced no difficulty with her voice despite a vocally demanding program.

Flow Phonation

Jackie L. Gartner-Schmidt, PhD

Case Study: Patient J

This case is presented to illustrate the use and concepts of flow phonation. The therapeutic concept was introduced by Stone and Casteel[86] and later instrumentally examined by Gauffin and Sundberg,[87] who coined the term "flow phonation" based on their work with flow glottograms. Flow phonation is a modification of stretch and flow phonation.[86,88–90]

History and Complaints. Patient J, a 17-year-old female high school student, reported a sudden onset of total voice loss approximately 3 months prior to her clinical visit. This loss was precipitated by heavy voice use while playing high school basketball, although "nothing out of the ordinary." Patient J's chief complaints were total voice loss, extreme vocal fatigue, and severe throat constriction when talking. She did not have any prior history of voice loss before this episode. Patient J was taken to the voice lab and laryngeal video endostroboscopy suite. The following noninstrumental and instrumental measures were taken:

Auditory-perceptual evaluation using a modified version of the Consensus Auditory Perceptual Evaluation-Voice (CAPE-V)[6] revealed a Visual Analogue Scale measure of 95/100 for overall severity of voice quality. The following audio-perceptual descriptions of voice were rated with an ordinal scale as done with the GRBAS.[91]: Roughness (0); Breathiness (0); Strain (3); Pitch—high (2); Pitch—low (0); Loudness—loud (0); Loudness—soft (2); Hoarseness (2). It is important to note that the pitch rating was probably due to resonating frequencies of the vocal tract (ie, formant frequencies) as she was aphonic. Patient J's assessment of her overall voice problem was "severe" based on an ordinal scale (none, mild, mild-moderate, moderate, moderate-severe, severe) and her chief complaint included both the sound and feel of her voice. She also described herself as an extremely talkative person.

To quantify the effect of Patient J's perception of her voice problem, two patient-based measures were used. First, a Global Severity Index, which refers to the specific attributes of a patient's voice problem. and second, a Symptom-Specific Severity Measure, which refers to a precise attribute of the patient's voice problem. An example of a Global Severity Index measure that is used in our clinic, the UPMC Voice Center, is the Voice Handicap Index-10(VHI-10).[92] Patient J's score was 36/40. A Symptom Severity Index measure that is used in our clinic is the Reflux Symptom Index[93]; there, her score was 10/45.

Patients J's assessment of her overall vocal effort as measured via a Direct Magnitude Estimation Scale[3,94,95] was 1,000,000. An example of how we have modified the original DME for vocal effort is, as follows:

If I told you that 100 represents an easy amount of vocal effort and 200 is twice that amount and 450 is 4.5 times that amount and 1200 is 12 times . . . there is no ceiling. Pick a number in the hundreds that best indicates how much vocal effort it takes you to voice when you are having a bad day.

Patient J described her feeling of vocal effort as 10,000 times that of "an easy amount of vocal effort." Unfortunately, frequency measures were not valid as the patient had a Type III Signal Typing[96,97] defined as no apparent fundamental frequency as obtained from the Multi-Dimensional Voice Program (MDVP) (KayPENTAX, 2008).

Aerodynamic measures were recorded using the Phonatory Aerodynamic System (PAS, KayPENTAX, 2006) and mean airflow for the center three /pa/ tokens of a five token repetition showed 50 mL/sec with subglottal air pressure estimates of 17.3 H$_2$O at her most comfortable pitch and loudness (MCPL). These measures were interpreted to mean that perhaps she was holding back her airflow (as demonstrated by low flow measures) and using increased thyroarytenoid and lateral cricoarytenoid muscle tension to spike

high indirect subglottal air pressure measures. This appeared to corroborate the voice therapist's audio-perceptual assessment of "severe breath-holding" Phonatory mean airflow rate for a spoken sentence (Peter picked a pound of pickled peppers) was 40 mL/sec. Hence, both of the decreased airflow measures could perhaps be indicative of severe pressed phonation (eg, muscle tension dysphonia). Her intensity range was 11 dB SPL, which is below the norms, perhaps due to the limited vocal agility of her mechanism due to muscle tension.

Psychosocial Screening by the Voice Therapist. Patient J was a product of a split family, although her mother and father were still married. She admitted to being afraid of her father but denied physical abuse. Her father was very competitive when it came to his daughter's basketball playing and was at the game the night she lost her voice. Patient J denied her father's presence as the trigger, given that he often attended her games. However, she admitted that "She did not like him." She and her brother had a very good sibling relationship and were each other's confidantes during their parents' arguments. She said she liked her mother. She divulged that she had been admitted to the hospital for vomiting and dehydration months before her current voice problem; she and the physicians believed that the episode was probably due to stress. In fact, Patient J described herself as always "very stressed." She had never been evaluated by a mental health professional. Other than this information, the patient's medical and speech history were unremarkable. She was a healthy teenager who drank over 64 oz of water a day.

The laryngologist visualized the larynx using a chip-tip flexible endoscope and reported no lesions and bilateral vocal fold motion was normal. Flexible endoscopy is routinely used in the clinic for the diagnosis of muscle tension dysphonia because it allows visualization of speech during the exam. No evidence of larygnopharyngeal reflux was found. The patient was diagnosed with "severe" primary muscle tension dysphonia.

Treatment. After her initial evaluation, Patient J received two voice therapy sessions back-to-back with a 20-minute rest between sessions. The following is a summary of the basic skills of flow phonation and a conceptual diagram (Fig 3–6) of the hierarchical steps of flow phonation. Patients are asked to become aware of frontal energy/airflow while

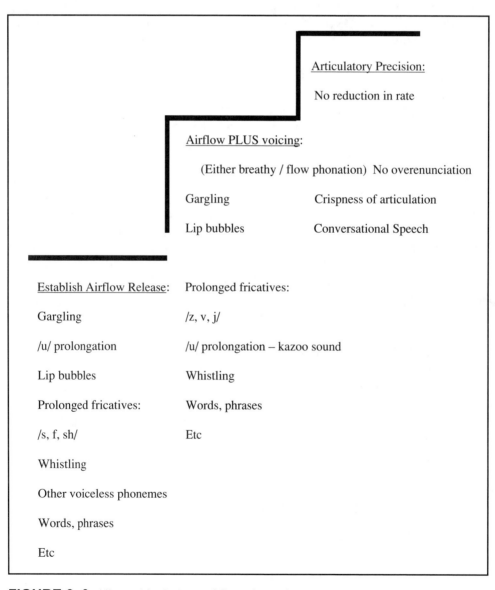

FIGURE 3–6. Hierarchical steps of flow phonation.

feeling no throat tightness. Patients go through the hierarchy but, if problems recur, they go "down a step" until they reach functional performance. It is important to note that patients do *not* have to go through all the steps in order. Also, patients can go back and forth between the "steps" as much as necessary, and because vocal balance is the ultimate goal, it does not matter if each step is used. Finally, this is not a programmatic approach to voice therapy[98]; many times the reader will see the words "et cetera" because the reader is encouraged to invent new stimuli based on the concepts of flow phonation.[99] The examples given are in no way exhaustive.

Skill Levels of Flow Phonation

Skill 1: Airflow Release

1. Unarticulated* airflow (a single oropharyngeal posture for one phoneme)
2. Articulated* airflow

Skill 2: Breathy Phonation

1. Unarticulated breathy phonation
2. Articulated breathy phonation

Skill 3: Flow Phonation

1. Unarticulated flow phonation
2. Articulated flow phonation

Skill 4: Articulatory Precision

Skill 1: Airflow Release— Unarticulated Airflow

Gargling Technique. Patient J was first asked to do the gargle technique. No instructions other than placing the chin upward to the ceiling were given. Patient J was given a glass of water. The therapist modeled the gesture and Patient J was asked to produce plenty of "bubbles" with the water. Patient J responded beautifully and was able to gargle well, which represented the first step toward flow phonation, as gargling is merely airflow in a nonspeech task. Many patients with MTD are noted to have high laryngeal suspension due to tension of the hyolaryngeal sling. Asking a patient to elevate her chin to the ceiling perhaps disrupts an already taut hyolaryngeal sling and stretches out the extrinsic laryngeal musculature so that further laryngeal elevation is impossible. Having a patient gargle initiates airflow release without the maladaptive habits of extra/intralaryngeal tensions.

The next instruction to Patient J was to add the gargle "sound" to the air bubbles, being careful not to use the word "voicing" so as not to introduce any anxiety ridden verbiage. Some patients are so distraught over their lack of voice that the very word may cause increased tensions. Patient J again was successful. The final step in the gargling technique was to have the patient slowly lower her chin while still gargling with sound. Although this request sometimes results in untidiness (tissues should be ready for water dribbling from the mouth), the results can be outstanding. With some patients, once phonation is established with this technique, shaping the sustained gargle into speech is all that is needed. Unfortunately, although Patient J was successful in gaining phonation with the gargle technique, she was unable to transfer the voiced gargle to phonemes,

---

*The terms unarticulated and articulated are defined respectively as a single oropharyngeal posture for one phoneme (eg, /u/) and varying articulatory postures to produce many different phonemes (words, phrases, conversational speech).

words and phrases. Yet, little did she know, I was very encouraged.

/u/ Prolongation. The next instruction I gave Patient J was to produce a /u/ without voicing. A strip of facial tissue was held between her index and third fingers, approximately 2 inches from her nose. I asked her to pucker her lips so as to redirect the airstream into a straight line. The reason a voiceless /u/ is used is because the lip contour for /u/ directs the airflow in a column from the lips and it is easy to move the tissue and hear a steady airflow stream. As Patient J produced the voiceless /u/, I paid attention to any hesitation that could occur at the end of the inhalation just before the exhalation. The cycle of inhalation followed by exhalation on a voiceless /u/ should be produced smoothly and without hesitation. If done properly, the tissue will be uplifted by the airflow and the sound of the airflow will be smooth and consistently steady. Unsteady airflow may be a sign of breath-holding as defined as either constricted intrinsic and extrinsic laryngeal muscles (eg, tight vocal fold closure) and/or constricted thoracic/abdominal muscles. The goal is to achieve the task with minimal throat effort and a feeling of airflow "energy" at the lips. Patient J was asked to take a breath and immediately exhale a sigh on a /u/, as though she had just finished a long, hard day and she was sighing with relief. At first, the tissue only moved with the initial exhalation but then the patient appeared to hold back her airflow; the tissue did not move. She did an audible semi-Valsalva as she stopped the airflow. The instruction was given again and this time the patient released the exhalation for a longer duration but the exhalatory airflow sounds were "jerky" and not consistent. Again, she was asked to pretend

she had just had a really long hard day and sigh but on a /u/ sound. I modeled the sound again while leaning back in my chair and placing my feet on the table to represent a relaxed body posture. Often the therapist will use the following verbiage to instruct her patients: "I want you to pretend that you have had a long day and that you are just letting out a nice, relaxed sigh but on the letter /u/." She performed much better this time. All the while, Patient J was asked if she could feel "airflow energy" at her lips and if her throat felt relaxed. Then she easily produced airflow sirens with no difficulty. She was instructed to hear the pitch changes while she did the airflow sirens. Although not phonatory pitch changes, she was encouraged that at least she could make different pitches.

Lip Bubbles. Wanting to capitalize on her success thus far, I moved on to another airflow-inducing technique by introducing more practice material. I asked her to do an easy lip bubble. Patient J could definitely lip bubble with the aid of placing her two index fingers on the corners of her lips. She lip bubbled for long and short durations, producing high- and low-pitched sirens. All the while, Patient J was asked if she could feel "airflow energy" at her lips and if her throat felt relaxed. Some patients find this very difficult to do; if so, they're asked to move to the next exercise.

Whistle. After the lip bubbles, we changed the airflow inducing maneuver to a whistle but Patient J could not whistle and the exercise was discontinued.

Skill 1: Airflow Release— Articulated Airflow

Voiceless Phonemes. Now that airflow was being released, she was informed that she could produce approximately 31% of the sounds of the alphabet; out of 26 letters, she produced 8 without a problemall the voiceless consonants (c, f, h, k, p, q, s, t). I immediately advanced to prolonging the voiceless fricatives /s, f, sh/. Once she could prolong them, she was asked to do pitch glides, sirens, and be loud and soft with the fricatives. All the while, Patient J was asked if she could feel "airflow energy" at her lips and if her throat felt relaxed.

Voiceless Phrases/Conversation. When it was apparent that Patient J could easily release unvoiced airflow, she was asked to articulate around the airflow. This is a very important instruction to a patient that should be said as follows: "I want you to move your tongue and lips around this steady stream of airflow that you have done so far." Having patients concentrate on airflow versus speech articulation may disentangle the possible maladaptive habits found in speech. The concept of airflow always must be front and center with this therapy. So, keeping the facial tissue in the same position as was done for the voiceless /u/, Patient J was asked to produce phrases with just airflow. The tissue should move with the airflow. Within each phrase, Patient J was asked to connect each of the syllables or words together, so that no separation or pausing occurs. Examples of phrases that direct the airflow to easily uplift the tissue are:

Poo-loo- poo-loo- poo-loo

Who is Lou?

Who is Sue?

Who are you?

At this juncture in the therapy, communications between Patient J and me were done in an easy, breathy unvoiced whisper. First, I wanted to model articulated airflow (ie, efficient whisper) and second, I did not want Patient J to reinforce the old strained whisper in between all her successful trials to establish airflow release done so far. This is an important part of the therapy. During this stage of therapy, often it is a good time to interrupt the structured tasks of therapy and just "talk." This is an opportunity for the therapist to discover any psychosocial issues if she thinks that the voice problem may be secondary to stress-reactivity/personality profiles and/or psychosocial trait or states.[100–104] Furthermore, all patients are asked to adopt this easy unstrained whispering in between sessions if voice reinstatement is not achieved within the first few sessions. Patient J disclosed that she had always been afraid of her Dad because he was "mean" and "big" but denied, for a second time, any physical abuse. When asked if she had any other physical complaints in her past— headaches, irritable bowel syndrome, backaches, hives, and so forth—she said that she used to get severe migraines and has a "nervous stomach."

Skill 2: Breathy Phonation— Unarticulated

/u/ Prolongation. After establishing steady airflow release shaped by the articulators into speech, Patient J was then asked to make voice while continuing to use the tissue as feedback. Patient J was told that the most important part of the exercise was to see and hear the airflow versus produce voice. Patient J was asked to take a breath and exhale on a breathy /u/ in a downward glide like a sigh. The tissue should move with the airflow. The sound she produced was breathy but unsteady

and, at the end, she cut off her airflow. I asked her to do the /u/ on just airflow alone to re-establish the easy feel and see/feel the airflow on the tissue. Then I asked her to try again with sound and this time she was more successful. I modeled sirens and pitch glides on a breathy /u/. As she was a tad too young to really remember the famous: "Happy Birthday, Mr. President," spoken by Marilyn Monroe to President Kennedy in her breathy voice, I modeled it for her.

Voiced Lip Bubbles. Patient J was educated about coordination of airflow with sound and told that these exercises were merely coordinating her airflow with her sound generator. Next she did voiced lip bubbles and was very stimulable, producing a wonderful voice.

Skill 2: Breathy Phonation— Articulated

Voiceless to Voiced Fricatives. Patient J was now asked to do a true vocal balancing technique; that is, to prolong an /s/ and seamlessly add voicing into the cognate /z/. Patient J was asked to pay attention to how little effort was needed to make voice. The transition from voiceless to voiced cognate must be gradual and seamless. She was asked to do an /f/ into a /v/ and back and forth, as well as voiceless[th] to voiced [th] and [sh] to [dz]. She was slowly beginning to coordinate airflow, voicing, and articulation.

Phrases/Conversation. This is the very short section of flow phonation, which is to ask patients to actually converse in breathy phonation. This is very much like Confidential Voice[105] but because we know that breathy phonation actually takes more effort than efficient voicing,[106] this part of therapy is meant only to gradually introduce the

patient to voicing with lots of airflow. Patient J was told that she might need more breaths per phrases because of the breathiness. Also, because airflow is used so much, occasionally patients may need water to hydrate. The same sentences were used as before, but with added voice this time. Patient J was again reminded to feel "airflow energy" at her lips and see that her throat felt relaxed. She was asked to say:

Poo-loo- poo-loo- poo-loo

Fu wu wu

Fu fu sue

Who is Lou?

Who is Sue?

Who are you?

Flow Phonation—Unarticulated

/u/ Prolongation and the Kazoo Sound. Patient J was asked to prolong a /u/ just like in breathy phonation but to make the sound louder and not sound breathy. In other words, produce a nonbreathy sound yet achieve the same movement of the tissue. This manner of voice production is called flow phonation. Often, the only instruction a patient needs to go from breathy to flow phonation is to get louder. Patient J was fairly successful in making the transition to flow phonation but needed much time simply doing pitch glides and sirens on /u/. Finally, she was asked to purse her lips tightly as if to make the kazoo sound while still feeling and seeing the airflow. This is known as a semi-occluded vocal tract technique as well as an airflow technique. Patient J was asked to monitor throat tensions and see/feel the airflow. She was then asked to contrast pressed and flow phonation styles on /u/. First, she was asked to

produce the /u/ again but not to allow any airflow to move the tissue. She was simply instructed to "hold her breath back." Then she was asked to produce /u/ using flow phonation, allowing the tissue to move but without the breathy voice quality. She also was asked to contrast the sensation and degree of effort for the different modes of phonation: breathy, flow, and pressed.[87] Often the voice therapist shows a video clip of an example of rigid stroboscopy depicting someone doing breathy, flow and pressed phonatory postures so that patients can see that a difference is being made at the laryngeal level.

Flow Phonation—Articulated

Voiceless to Voiced Fricatives. Patient J was asked to get louder when doing the seamless transition from the voiceless cognates into the voiced cognates, and to do them on pitch glides. For example, on a siren, Patient J produced /s/→/z/→/s/→/z/, and so forth. This was done on the other fricative cognates. This can be a difficult step for some patients as different pitches are being introduced, different articulatory postures and transitions from voiceless to voiced sounds. Patient J, with some practice, did well.

Phrases/Conversation. Patient J was then asked to say the following phrases in flow phonation and contrast that to pressed phonation (explained as holding back all the airflow):

Poo-loo- poo-loo- poo-loo

Fu wu wu

Fu fu sue

Who is Lou?

Who is Sue?

Who are you?

Patient J did very well and discriminated not only between the difference in the two sounds (pitch lower and rougher for pressed phonation) but between the differences in feeling in the throat (constricted for pressed and "open" for flow phonation).

Articulatory Precision. Up to this point, Patient J was doing all the vocal balancing techniques in fairly structured tasks. However, asking patients to concentrate on flow phonation in conversational speech may be too academic/indistinct when combined with the thought process needed for speech. An easy technique that seems to link cognition to flow phonation in speech is having patients concentrate on articulatory precision in their speech. The final key to using flow phonation in conversational speech is to allow articulation to facilitate the sensation of airflow energy at the front of the mouth. Practice using flow phonation while maintaining awareness of articulatory activity first with sentences that include many phonemes generated in the front of the mouth. The following exercise may be helpful. Patient J was asked to pretend that she was "speaking clearly" to a person who was hard of hearing while she said the following sentences that were loaded with voiceless/voiced consonants and, in particular, voiceless fricatives. The reader is encouraged to invent their own phrases, but here are examples:

Fat Freddy prefers French fries

See Sammy the snake slither in the grass

See Sally sleep soundly by the sea

Zebras zigzag at the zoo

Voices vibrate in Venice

Teachers eat ripe peaches by the beach

Finally, Patient J and the voice therapist had a conversation about a topic chosen by Patient J. The only thing Patient J was asked to do was to use articulatory precision monitoring airflow energy at the lips without any throat constriction. Although the area in the brain that governs speech (speech motor cortex) is different from the area of the brain that governs vocalization, the periacqueductal gray (PAG),[107] the patient was asked to feel the energy of articulation and not be concerned with feeling any constriction in the throat. If not, patients can be very precise in articulation but aphonic at the same time. The patient must produce airflow energy at the mouth but without throat constriction. Patient J did well at using articulatory precision at the beginnings of her phrases but she often let her pitch drop at the end of linguistic strings and, perhaps, used pressed phonation perceived as decreased pitch and increased roughness. This is a very common trait in North American English because of pitch intonation contours. To counter this, she was asked to end every phrase with a voiceless /p/ to offset phonation with abducted vocal folds versus tightly adducted vocal folds. Patient J thought this was "very weird" but seemed to understand the rationale and was successful in monitoring lack of flow at the ends of linguistic strings.

At the end of the session, Patient J's mother was invited into the session. As a rule, the voice therapist usually dissuades parents or caregivers coming to the voice therapy sessions. Their presence may interfere with the trust that needs to develop between a therapist and a patient, as well as consume session time with explanations. The voice therapist likes to invite parents or caregivers after the session and have patients explain to them what they did in therapy. It is not important that Patient J understood how she did something,[108] but rather that she was aware of the effects of different sensations and how it related to the sound and feel of voicing. Patient J nicely demonstrated the difference between breathy, flow and pressed phonation.[87] She was able to adequately relate the four steps in flow phonation and demonstrate some sounds to her mother. She was skeptically happy that her "voice came back." However, when she made that remark, I quickly intervened with "voice production came back." It was important for Patient J to think of herself as an active participant in voicing and not just a victim of "her voice." This is a key point in any type of therapy.

Treatment Outcome and Recommendation. Patient J was fully speaking after being aphonic for 3 months. As is common with many muscle tension aphonic patients, the patient unfortunately did not return for a follow-up clinic. Although this was the first time the patient had lost her voice production, her history and conversations led me to believe that perhaps her aphonia may have been related to stress reactivity. The patient certainly had other known forms of stress-related illnesses, and she described herself as being "always stressed." It is hoped that she will not relapse, but as the literature indicates, 60% of patients are prone to relapse.[103] For now, flow phonation seemed to re-establish vocal balance and give her a conceptual framework for understanding how she could reinstate her voice if needed.

Voice Use Reduction for the Treatment of Chronic Dysphonia

Richard Zraick, PhD, CCC-SLP

Case Study: Patient K

> *Vocal use awareness is important in the rehabilitation of voice disorders. The following case by Richard Zraick describes in detail a step-by-step voice use reduction program. At the core of this program is educating the patient regarding her specific voice use behaviors.*

Patient K, a 23-year-old female graduate student in Speech-Language Pathology, presented with a 2-year history of poor voice quality and vocal fatigue. She was concerned about how her dysphonia might affect her employment opportunities and ability to complete her clinical fellowship year. She desired to work with children, and she also babysat on a regular basis, so thus wished to be able to model appropriate voice quality. She had tried, admittedly unsuccessfully, to self-treat her dysphonia with a loosely defined and applied approach of vocal hygiene.

Patient K's medical history was unremarkable. She reported no history of allergies, postnasal drip, laryngopharyngeal reflux, chronic colds, sinus infections, or other upper respiratory infections. She had not had injury to the throat, nose, or neck, and had no evidence of hearing loss. She had never been hospitalized as an adult, had no chronic medical problems, and was not on any medication or herbal supplements. She reported drinking very little water on a regular basis, and she consumed 1 to 2 cans of caffeinated soda per day.

History of the Problem. Patient K self-referred to an otolaryngologist upon the advice of one of her professors. Indirect laryngoscopy revealed mild edema and erythema of the vocal folds and irregular vocal fold edges, suggestive of vocal hyperfunction. The remainder of the head and neck examination was unremarkable.

Patient K was concurrently enrolled in a graduate-level course on Voice Disorders. She appeared highly motivated to change, had adequate cognitive skills to participate in therapy, and appeared to have an adequate support system— all factors believed to reduce the likelihood of therapy dropout.

Evaluation Procedures. Following is a summary of relevant pretreatment measures for Patient K:

A. *Laryngoscopy:* The Stroboscopy Research Instrument[109] was used to document laryngeal anatomy and physiology. Symmetry of mucosal displacement was normal. Amplitude of horizontal vocal fold excursion was moderately decreased. Vocal fold vibration was moderately aperiodic. There was a nonvibrating mucosal segment near the middle third of each vocal fold. Duration of glottic closure was half closed and half open. The predominant closure pattern was a moderate hourglass.

B. *Acoustic:* The KayPENTAX Computerized Speech Lab (Model 4500) was used to measure various acoustic properties of Patient K's voice. Mean speaking fundamental frequency (F_0) at her most comfortable loudness was 169 Hz, which was low for an adult female. Highest F_0 during reading of the second sentence of the Rainbow Passage was 200 Hz and lowest F_0 was 150 Hz, yielding a range of 50 Hz, which was restricted for an adult female. Mean speaking intensity at her most comfortable pitch was 62 dB, which was low for one-on-one conversation in a quiet room. Maximum speaking intensity during reading of the entire first paragraph of the Rainbow Passage was 70 dB and minimum speaking intensity was 55 dB, yielding a restricted dynamic range of 15 dB. Perturbation measures (ie, jitter, shimmer, and noise) were obtained exclusively from the /a/ vowel sustained at Patient K's most comfortable pitch and loudness for 5 seconds. Pitch perturbation quotient was 0.72%; amplitude perturbation quotient was 2.4%; noise-to-harmonic ratio was .022; voice turbulence index was 0.09; and soft phonation index was 12.0. All the aforementioned perturbation measures were abnormal (high).

C. *Aerodynamic:* The KayPENTAX Phonatory Aerodynamic System (PAS) (Model 6600) was used to measure the patients' laryngeal aerodynamics. Mean expiratory airflow during sustained vowel /a/ was 300 mL/sec. Estimated mean peak intraoral air pressure during production of the syllable train /pi/ was 8.2 cm H_2O. Laryngeal resistance was 50 cm H_2O/(L/s). All the aforementioned speech aerodynamic measures were abnormal (high).

D. *Auditory-Perceptual:* The Consensus Auditory Perceptual Evaluation of Voice (CAPE-V)[110] was used to document the clinician's auditory-perceptual judgments about Patient K's voice. The CAPE-V uses a 100-mm visual analog scale, with "0" indicating no impairment and "100" indicating maximum impair-

ment. Overall severity was rated at 27; roughness was rated at 35; breathiness was rated at 20; strain was rated at 17; pitch was rated at 17; and loudness was rated at 45.

E. *Voice-Related Quality of Life:* Patient K filled out the Voice Handicap Index (VHI).[111] The VHI total score ranges from 0 to 120, with a higher score indicating more self-perceived handicap. Patient K's total score was 60. Her VHI subscale scores (which can range from 0–40) were 20 for the functional subscale, 26 for the physical subscale, and 14 for the emotional subscale. Her primary communication partner completed a companion instrument to the VHI, the VHI-Partner[112] in order to obtain supplemental information about the patient's voice handicap as perceived by others.[113] The VHI-P total score also ranges from 0 to 120, with a higher score indicating more perceived handicap. Patient K's partner's total score was 54. The VHI-P subscale scores (which also can range from 0–40) were 20 for the functional subscale, 24 for the physical subscale, and 10 for the emotional subscale.

Description and Rationale for Therapy Approach. Patient K's background and history, medical diagnosis, and assessment findings were consistent with her chief complaint of chronic dysphonia, likely due to excessive voice use. Consequently, a treatment program was implemented, which at its core, relied heavily on a structured behavior modification approach to the reduction of voice use.[114]

Patient K's voice use reduction program consisted of five design steps, followed by implementation over a 10-week period. In the first design step, the clinician helped the patient identify all vocational, social, and recreational uses of the voice. In the second design step, the clinician helped the patient analyze the voice use situations and determine their cumulative effects on her voice. The criteria to determine the cumulative effects were the degree of self-perceived vocal fatigue, vocal effort, laryngeal pain, level of emotional stress, and the deterioration of the voice quality. This analysis provided a way for the patient to understand the nature of her problem behavior and to target goals. In the third design step, numerical values were assigned to each voice use situation. Each voice use situation was assigned a *voice use unit* ranging from 1 to 6 (Table 3–4). In the fourth design step, the maximum number of *voice use units* that could be used per day and week was determined. This was in preparation for charging the patient with continuously documenting and reporting at subsequent therapy sessions the number of voice use units expended per day and week. The fifth

and final design step was for the clinician and patient to agree upon a *voice use unit*-based definition of severe, moderate, and low voice reduction.

Once the vocal use reduction program was designed as described above, it was implemented using a changing criterion design.[115] This design required initial baseline observations on a single target behavior (voice overuse), followed by implementation of a treatment program in a series of three treatment phases (severe, moderate, and low voice use reduction). Patient K was seen for a 1-hour session once a week for 8 weeks and then again after a 2-week maintenance period. Figure 3–7 shows the maximum number of voice use units allocated per day and the average units used per day by Patient K during the three treatment phases of severe, moderate, and low voice use reduction. As she met criterion at each phase, she was allowed to increase voice use. During each phase, laryngeal health and voice were monitored using the treatment outcome measures described previously.

Table 3–4. Voice Use Situations and the Assigned Units

1	Basic communication (ie, short response to question, giving short instructions in optimum conditions, eg, babysitting)
2	Intermittent phone conversation for 20 minutes in optimum conditions or attending class and chatting with friends against some background noise for 10 minutes
3	Intermittent chatting in small group for 15 minutes in unfavorable conditions or intermittent conversation in favorable conditions for 30 minutes
4	Intermittent conversation in unfavorable conditions for 30 minutes (ie, smoky or loud environment) or uninterrupted voice use for 5 to 10 minutes in unfavorable conditions
5	Uninterrupted professional voice use for 45 minutes with background noise or intermittent professional voice use for 1 hour and 30 minutes with no background noise

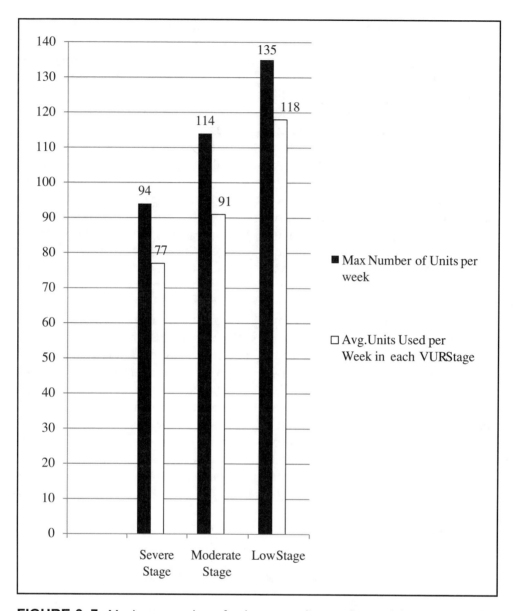

FIGURE 3–7. Maximum number of voice use units per day and the average units used per day during three periods of severe, moderate, and low voice use reduction.

Results of Therapy. Following is a summary of post-treatment measures for Patient K:

A. *Laryngoscopy:* Symmetry of mucosal displacement, amplitude of horizontal vocal fold excursion, and vocal fold vibration were all normal. There were no nonvibrating mucosal segments. Duration of glottic closure remained half closed and half open. The predominant closure pattern was a mild hourglass.

B. *Acoustic:* Mean speaking fundamental frequency (F_0) at her most comfortable loudness was 183 Hz, which was within normal limits. Highest F_0 during reading of the second sentence of the Rainbow Passage was 230 Hz and lowest F_0 was 130 Hz, yielding a range of 100 Hz, which was within normal limits. Mean speaking intensity at her most comfortable pitch was 70 dB, which was adequate for one-on-one conversation in a quiet room. Maximum speaking intensity during reading of the entire first paragraph of the Rainbow Passage was 75 dB and minimum speaking intensity was 50 dB, yielding an adequate dynamic range of 25 dB. Pitch perturbation quotient was 0.39%; amplitude perturbation quotient was 1.5%; noise-to-harmonic ratio was .013; voice turbulence index was 0.05, and soft phonation index was 6.2. All the aforementioned perturbation measures were within normal limits.

C. *Aerodynamic:* Mean expiratory airflow during sustained vowel /a/ was 190 mL/sec. Estimated mean peak intraoral air pressure was 7.4 cm H_2O. Laryngeal resistance was 30 cm $H_2O/(l/s)$. All the aforementioned speech aerodynamic measures were within normal limits.

D. *Auditory-Perceptual:* Using the CAPE-V, overall severity was rated at 3; roughness was rated at 2; breathiness was rated at 2; strain was rated at 0; pitch was rated at 3; and loudness was rated at 4.

E. *Voice-Related Quality of Life:* The VHI total score was 3 (0 for the functional subscale, 3 for the physical subscale, and 0 for the emotional subscale). The VHI-P total score was 2 (0 for the functional subscale, 2 for the physical subscale, and 0 for the emotional subscale).

F. *Patient Satisfaction:* Table 3–5 lists the specific questions posed to Patient K in a posttherapy questionnaire. For

Table 3–5. Questionnaire on the Value of the Voice Use Reduction Program

1. This program was an important part of the voice treatment I received.

2. This program made me aware of the potential danger of speaking in certain situations.

3. This program made me aware of the way I use my voice.

4. This program helped me to reduce the amount of voice use.

5. This program provided me with a method of voice conservation that I can apply in the future.

6. This program made me aware of my voice production errors.

7. This program helped me to understand voice conservation.

8. This program helped me to manage the amount of voice use.

9. This program made me aware that I have to take responsibility for conserving my voice.

10. This program contributed to the improvement of my voice problem.

each question she had five answer choices (Do Not Agree at All, Agree to Some Extent, Agree, Agree to a Large Extent, Agree Fully). For every question, she responded with "Agree Fully."

Voice Therapy Boot Camp

Rita R. Patel, PhD

Case Study: Patient L

> *In her treatment of a 44-year-old male, Rita Patel uses a specific approach of intensive voice therapy, first conceived by Diane Bless, PhD at the University of Wisconsin Voice and Swallowing Center, to create a voice rehabilitation plan that includes components of intensive training and dynamic setup to facilitate carryover.*

Intensive voice therapy is a new treatment approach that is being developed in the field of therapeutic management of voice to maximize behavior change for long-term recalcitrant dysphonia that has poor response to traditional direct voice therapy. Therapy dropout, the ultimate nonadherence, is a common clinical problem in voice therapy.[116] Given the limited availability of resources like Clinical Voice Centers, the limited number of voice clinicians available to provide intensive voice therapy, and the limited number of graduate programs in which voice therapy is a focus of study, this new approach of intensive treatment has benefits, where target behavior change can be accomplished through concentrated practice.

Principles of intensive voice treatment are derived from known literature

in the fields of exercise physiology, intensive psychotherapy, and motor learning, which states that short-term intensive practice results in desirable physiologic changes[117,118] and long-term retention of newly acquired skills.[119,120] It is well known in exercise physiology literature that desirable physiologic changes from training occur primarily from intensity overload.[121] Similar findings have been noted with regard to intensive psychotherapy. The findings from literature in psychotherapy support the notion of positive behavior change due to high levels of personal awareness and intensive practice, which leads to retention of newly learned skills. In the field of voice therapy, Lee Silverman Voice Therapy provides evidence for intensive voice therapy to improve laryngeal function in patients with idiopathic Parkinson disease.[64] Behavior modification of long term refractory dysphonia other than of idiopathic Parkinson disease etiology continues to be challenging for voice therapists.

Like voice therapy, the goal of intensive voice treatment regimen is to maximize vocal effectiveness and behavior modification. However, unique to this approach of intensive treatment is to bring these changes through techniques of concentrated practice, in short-term, in a dynamic setup that involves maximum degree of experiences/challenges to achieve the desired target vocal behaviors.

Intensive voice treatment program, involves a highly structured regime of multiple sessions with a variety of clinicians, incorporating multiple simultaneous voice therapeutic approaches necessary for the client. Part of these therapy sessions can also include additional voice/medical evaluations to clarify the nature of the client's voice disorder. This form of intensive voice therapy provides rigorous practice, involving not only overload, but also opportunities for specificity and individuality, thereby facilitating better transfer of learned skills. Intensive voice treatment program involves voice therapy which is conducted in successive 1- to 4-day sessions, for an average of 5 hours (range 4–6 hours) of voice therapy, with an average of five clinicians (range: 3–7 clinicians) per day. Intensive treatment program is not limited to a particular diagnosis/therapeutic approach. Intensive treatment is particularly beneficial for long-term recalcitrant dysphonia, where voice therapy continues to be indicated; when patient has plateaued with traditional form of individual voice therapy; upcoming vocal performances within short duration of initial assessment; and for clients traveling from longer distances to seek treatment at the Voice Center. Advantages of intensive treatment are that it provides rigorous practice (overload); opportunities for specificity and individuality, simultaneous interventions can be conducted of multiple components involved in voice production, opportunities facilitate transfer of learned skills, and may influence patient compliance. Highly structured voice therapy regimen, team leader, and communication between the clinicians providing treatment are important for successfully conducting intensive voice treatment. The team leader is responsible for setting up of intensive treatment, coordinating team meetings before and after treatments, and creating a plan for transfer of information from one session to the next. The team leader also is responsible for follow-up with the patient after discharge from intensive treatment.

Patient History. Patient L, a 44-year-old male, a native of Iceland was self-referred to the voice center for assess-ment and treatment of long-standing voice difficulty of 10 years. Patient L was accompanied by his wife for the session. The initial assessment was performed both by a voice pathologist and laryngologist. The patient was first examined by the voice pathologist, who obtained a detailed history of the nature and onset of the voice problem, a detailed medical history, and performed stroboscopy, high-speed digital imaging, acoustic analysis, aerodynamic assessment, and auditory perceptual analysis of voice quality. Subsequently, Patient L was examined by the laryngologist, who reviewed the case history, stroboscopy, and high-speed examinations with the voice pathologist, performed indirect laryngoscopy, and performed a detailed head and neck examination.

Patient L reported a gradual worsening of dysphonia since its onset. Voice quality was reported to have reached a plateau in the past 5 years. Patient's chief complaints were weak, strained voice quality and vocal fatigue. Voice quality was reported to deteriorate at the end of the day. Being an industrialist, Patient L had heavy voice use at work and outside of work. Individual meetings and presentations at board meetings constituted voice use at work. Social gatherings at restaurants with increased background noise comprised of additional voice use. Frequent throat clearing was also reported. Throat clearing was reported to be productive during the morning hours. Patient L denied dysphagia or dyspnea.

Over the past 10 years, the patient was examined and treated by different voice centers across the country and internationally. Patient L was examined by one otolaryngologist and one speech pathologist in Iceland, one otolaryngologist in Germany, and by two otolaryngologists in the United States. Impressions from these assessments were of laryngopharyngeal reflux, vocal fold scarring, glottal insufficiency, and vocal fold paresis. Patient L was treated with Omeprazole, 40 milligrams, twice a day, with no improvement of voice quality. At the time of the assessment, patient was still taking Omeprazole, 40 milligrams twice a day for reflux management. Patient L underwent unilateral right sided injection laryngoplasty with Cymetra for glottal insufficiency and vocal fold scarring, in Germany. Due to no improvement of voice quality, Patient L underwent left-sided injection laryngoplasty with cymetra in the United States. Secondary injection laryngoplasty also did not result in improvement of patient symptoms of vocal fatigue and hoarseness. Patient L did not undergo preoperative and postoperative voice therapy during the course of the dysphonia.

Patient L was a nonsmoker and consumed three 8-oz cups of water daily. Intake of two cups of coffee per day was reported. Patient L's medical history did not reveal serious health conditions. He had no history of allergies, postnasal drip, and sinus infections. No evidence of hearing loss and injury to throat or neck region was reported. The patient's medical history was significant for laryngopharyngeal reflux, which was confirmed with laryngeal endoscopy, barium-esophagram, GI endoscopy, and dual pH probe monitoring. Apart from the above mentioned laryngeal surgeries of unilateral injections for medialization, Patient L had not undergone other surgeries. Depression and anxiety were not reported.

Evaluation Procedures. Patient L received a standard battery of vocal function testing in the voice clinic. These assessments included: assessment of structure and vibratory function of the vocal folds with the use of stroboscopy using phonatory tasks of normal phonation, high pitch phonation, loud phonation, soft phonation, glissando, and laryngeal diadochokinesis; detailed assessment of actual vibratory features like mucosal waves, tissue pliability, glottal closure, and cycle-to-cycle periodicity with the use of high-speed digital imaging; acoustic analysis of sustained vowels and sentence production to assess fundamental frequency, loudness, perturbation measurements, and harmonic-to-noise ratio; aerodynamic measurement of respiratory function during speech to assess airflow rate, expiratory volume, phonatory threshold pressure; and perceptual assessment of voice quality on the GRBAS scale.[91] Following is a summary of the relevant pretreatment baseline observations and measures:

1. *Vocal fold structure and function:* Patient L's endoscopic and stroboscopic assessments were performed using a flexible and rigid 70-degree endoscope without need for topical anesthesia. The examination revealed normal movements of the arytenoids cartilages bilaterally. Mass lesions were not observed along the vocal fold margins. Smooth but irregular vocal fold edges were observed. During phonation, mild reduction in vibratory amplitude and mucosal wave of both the vocal folds was observed, suggestive of reduced vocal fold pliability. A small anterior and posterior glottal gap was noted, suggestive of incomplete glottal closure. Phase asymmetry between the vocal folds was not present. Mild lateral compression of the supraglottic structures was observed, suggestive of vocal hyperfunction.

High-speed analysis of vocal fold vibrations was performed at 2000 frames per second using a rigid 70-degree endoscope without application of topical anesthetic to the oral mucosa, to further assess the extent of Patient L's vibratory disturbances. High-speed examination revealed moderate reduction in pliability of the left vocal fold along the anterior margins and mild reduction of vibratory amplitude and mucosal wave of the right vocal fold. Mild phase asymmetry was consistently observed. An irregular glottal closure was observed, which was characterized by a moderate gap along the anterior and mid membranous portions of the vocal folds and a small posterior phonatory gap.

2. *Acoustic analysis:* The patient's acoustic measurements of voice quality were obtained using Multi-Dimensional Voice Profile Module of the KayPENTAX Computerized Speech Lab. The patient's mean fundamental frequency was 147 Hz, mean jitter of 0.90% (norm = 0.59%), mean shimmer of 4.23% (norm = 2.53%), and harmonic-to-noise ratio of 27 (normal = 30). These measurements represented subnormal performance based on the expected acoustic measures for the patient's age and gender. All intensity measurements of the patient's minimum (60 dB SPL), habitual (71 dB SPL), and maximum (89 dB SPL) loudness productions were within expected range for his age and gender.

3. *Aerodynamic measurements:* Airflow measures were taken during sustained vowel productions; intraoral pressure measurements were estimated from repeated productions of /pi/ using the Glottal Enterprise Analysis System. Mean intraoral pressure was measured at 7.1 cm H_2O, which was greater than the expected norm of 5 cm H_2O. Mean airflow rate was 280 cc/s, which is excessive, suggestive of incomplete laryngeal valving mechanism.

4. *Auditory perceptual analysis:* Patient L's voice quality was judged perceptually by the voice pathologist on a 4-point rating scale, known as the GRBAS scale (normal, mild, moderate, severe) for overall grade of hoarseness (G), roughness (R), breathiness (B), asthenia (A), and strain (S). Patient L exhibited moderate amount of hoarseness and strain, and mild amount of breathiness. No evidence of asthenia was noted.

Impression and Rationale for Therapy Approach. Overall the patient's history and examinations revealed reduced pliability of both the vocal folds, left greater than the right; incomplete glottal closure; and vocal hyperfunction. Based on the results of the assessment and nature of the patient's complaints of vocal fatigue and reduced endurance, decision was made that Patient L should undergo intensive voice therapy for three days to reduce hyperfunctional behaviors and improve glottal closure. Successful completion of voice therapy treatment was expected to in turn reduce the degree of hoarseness and enhance vocal stamina. Because the patient was traveling internationally for voice treatments, during the weekly voice clinic team meetings, the decision was made that he would benefit most from concentrated intensive voice therapy. The voice pathologist who performed the initial assessment of Patient L was appointed as a team leader to coordinate patient's intensive voice therapy program during the weekly voice clinic team meeting.

The team leader's responsibilities included:

- scheduling the patient for intensive treatment;
- checking the availability of other voice pathologists for conducting intensive treatment with the patient;

- conducting pretreatment meeting with all voice pathologists to formulate a treatment plan;
- conducting daily meetings with the patient's intensive care team either before the initiation or termination of therapy each day to establish goals for the next day;
- summarizing the patient's status/progress each day;
- formulating a plan for transfer of information between the voice pathologists from one session to the next;
- creating a home program for practice of the voice exercises;
- coordinating patient's care with speech pathologist in patient's home country/state; and
- scheduling a follow-up appointment.

Therapy Goals and Structure. Patient L received 5 hours of voice therapy, conducted by four voice pathologists per day for 3 consecutive days. Pre- and posttherapy measurements were performed at the beginning and end of each therapy day with stroboscopy, high-speed digital imaging, acoustic, aerodynamic, and auditory perceptual analysis of voice quality. The therapy regimen consisted of four different goals focusing on reducing hyperfunctional behaviors, improving glottal closure, building vocal endurance, and increasing hydration. During the 3 days of intensive treatment, Patient L was not provided with additional home practice of the voice exercises.

The above voice therapy goals were achieved using a combination of voice therapy techniques. Patient L's first therapy session each day consisted of performing the vocal function exercises, abdominal breathing, and neck relaxation exercises. During the subsequent sessions, each day the goal was to sys-

tematically progress toward use of resonant voice at conversation level. For this, techniques of resonant voice and flow mode phonation were used at syllable, word, sentence, marked paragraph reading level, paragraph reading level, structured conversation, and conversation.

Patient L attended all scheduled voice therapy sessions. Team meetings were conducted prior to the initiation of voice therapy each day to discuss the patient's response to the targeted voice therapy activities and highlight the therapy plan for each day. During the team meetings, the team leader also summarized the results of the pre- and posttherapy voice measurements for the voice pathologists participating in the patient's care.

Patient L had a breakthrough session with one of the voice pathologists during the early afternoon of the second day, in which the patient was able to maintain resonant voice during structured tasks at sentence and paragraph reading levels. Goals for day 3 were changed to accommodate the progress made during day 2 of the intensive voice treatment. During day 3, Patient L was provided with increased opportunities to practice carryover of the newly learned skills in the voice therapy session to unique situations like ordering at the cafeteria and conversation at the hospital cafeteria with high levels of background noise. The last session during day 3 was geared toward providing a written home practice plan for the patient.

Results of Therapy. Pre- and posttherapy measurements performed during each day consistently revealed significant improvement of voice quality at the end of an intensive voice therapy day. The results from the last therapy session of a 3-day intensive voice treatment regimen are summarized below:

1. *Laryngeal imaging:* Both stroboscopic and high-speed digital imaging revealed improved glottal closure compared to an irregular incomplete glottal closure that was observed during pretreatment recordings. Glottal closure during complete adduction was now characterized by a small posterior phonatory gap. Healthy vibratory amplitudes and mucosal wave was appreciated along the right vocal fold and minimal reduction in mucosal wave was observed along the left vocal fold. Lateral and anterior posterior compression of the glottis was not observed. High-speed analysis inconsistently revealed phase asymmetry between the vocal folds.
2. *Acoustic analysis:* The patient reduced jitter and shimmer measurements and increased the signal-to-noise ratio. Posttest acoustic measurements were grossly within expected norms for the patient's age and gender.
3. *Aerodynamic analysis:* Mean airflow rate was 180 cc/s and mean phonatory threshold pressure was 5.2 cm/ H_2O, which are within the expected limits.
4. *Auditory perceptual analysis:* Conversational speech was rated to have an overall normal grade (G), mild roughness (R), with no evidence of breathiness and asthenia. Patient's voice quality improved markedly as judged by the patient. Even at the end of a 3-day intensive voice therapy regimen, Patient L did not complain of vocal fatigue and hoarseness.

Subsequent follow-up was conducted once every 2 weeks by means of E-mail and by video-voice interface through the World Wide Web. The team leader discussed the maintenance plan with the patient's voice therapist in Iceland by E-mail. Subsequent follow-up at 6 months revealed that Patient L had continued to maintain the improvement achieved during the initial course of intensive voice treatment. At this time, a follow-up in 1year was recommended. The positive outcome of this treatment is attributed to the rigorous concentrated practice of structured therapeutic tasks to bring about a change in target vocal behavior. Intensive therapy with a number of voice clinicians inherently created opportunities for differential practice, which facilitated transfer of learned skills. Because the patient had a long-standing voice problem, the intensive nature of voice treatment also aided in reducing patient's frustration with the therapeutic tasks and enhanced compliance with the voice exercises, by demonstrating success within a short duration.

References

1. Solomon NP, DiMattia MS. Effects of a vocally fatiguing task and systemic hydration on phonation threshold pressure. *J Voice.* 2000;14(3):341–362.
2. Verdolini-Marston K, Titze, IR, Druker, DG. Changes in phonation threshold pressure with induced conditions of hydration. *J Voice.* 1990;4:142–151.
3. Verdolini K, Titze IR, Fennell A. Dependence of phonatory effort on hydration level. *J Speech Hear Res.* 1994;37(5): 1001–1007.
4. Dobres R, Lee L, Stemple JC, Kummer AW, Kretschmer LW. Description of laryngeal pathologies in children evaluated by otolaryngologists. *J Speech Hear Disord.* 1990;55(3):526–532.

5. Eckel FC, Boone DR. The s/z ratio as an indicator of laryngeal pathology. *J Speech Hear Disord.* 1981;46(2):147–149.

6. ASHA. Consensus Auditory-Perceptual Evaluation of Voice (CAPE-V): purpose and applications. Available from: http://www.asha.org/NR/rdonlyres/C6E5F616-972F-445A-AA40-7936BB49FCE3/0/CAPEVprocedures.pdf.

7. Rammage, L. *Vocalizing with Ease: A Self-Improvement Guide.* Vancouver, BC: Available from the author; 1996.

8. Hogikyan ND, Sethuraman G. Validation of an instrument to measure voice-related quality of life (V-RQOL). *J Voice.* 1999;13(4):557–569.

9. Barnes J. *Voice therapy.* Presented at the Meeting of the Southwestern Ohio Speech and Hearing Association. Cincinnati, OH; 1977.

10. Stemple JC. *Voice Therapy: Clinical Studies.* St. Louis, MO: Mosby Year Book; 1993.

11. Stemple JC, Lee L, D'Amico B, Pickup B. Efficacy of vocal function exercises as a method of improving voice production. *J Voice.* 1994;8(3):271–278.

12. Roy N, Gray SD, Simon M, Dove H, Corbin-Lewis K, Stemple JC. An evaluation of the effects of two treatment approaches for teachers with voice disorders: a prospective randomized clinical trial. *J Speech Lang Hear Res.* 2001; 44(2):286–296.

13. Sabol JW, Lee L, Stemple JC. The value of vocal function exercises in the practice regimen of singers. *J Voice.* 1995; 9(1):27–36.

14. Lamperti, G. *Vocal Wisdom.* New York, NY: William Earl Brown; 1931.

15. Christy, V. *Expressive Singing.* Vol 2. Dubuque, IA: WC Brown; 1961.

16. Emil-Behnke K. *The Technique of Singing.* London, England: Williams and Norgate; 1945.

17. Fawcus, M. *Voice Disorders and Their Management.* New Hampshire, England: Croom Helm; 1986.

18. Tetrazzini, L. *The Art of Singing.* New York, NY: Da Capo Press; 1975.

19. Verdolini K. Resonant Voice Therapy. In: Stemple JC, ed. *Voice Therapy: Clinical Studies.* San Diego, CA: Singular Publishing Group; 2000:46–62.

20. Verdolini K. Voice disorders. In: Tomblin JB, Morris H, Spriesterbach D, eds. *Diagnostic Methods in Speech-Language Pathology.* San Diego, CA: Singular Publishing Group; 1999.

21. Verdolini K, Palmer PM. Assessment of a "profiles approach" to voice screening. *J Med Speech Lang Pathol.* 1997;5: 217–232.

22. Berry DA, Verdolini K, Montequin D, Hess MM, Chan R, I.R. T. A quantitative output-cost ratio in voice production. *J Speech Lang Hear Res.* 2001;44(1): 29–37.

23. Jiang JJ, Titze IR. Measurement of vocal fold intraglottal pressure and impact stress. *J Voice.* 1994;8(2):132–144.

24. Verdolini K, Chan R, Titze IR, Hess M, Bierhals W. Correspondence of electroglottographic closed quotient to vocal fold impact stress in excised canine larynges. *J Voice.* 1998;12(4):415–423.

25. Hillman RE, Holmberg EB, Perkell JS, Walsh M, Vaughan C. Objective assessment of vocal hyperfunction: an experimental framework and initial results. *J Speech Hear Res.* 1989;32(2):373–392.

26. Koufman JA, Amin MR, Panetti M. Prevalence of reflux in 113 consecutive patients with laryngeal and voice disorders. *Otolaryngol Head Neck Surg.* 2000;123(4):385–388.

27. Selby JC, Gilbert HR, Lerman JW. Perceptual and acoustic evaluation of individuals with laryngopharyngeal reflux pre- and post-treatment. *J Voice.* 2003;17(4):557–570.

28. Ross JA, Noordzji JP, Woo P. Voice disorders in patients with suspected laryngo-pharyngeal reflux disease. *J Voice.* 1998;12(1):84–88.

29. Jin BJ, Lee YS, Jeong SW, Jeong JH, Lee SH, Tae J. Change of acoustic parameters before and after treatment in laryngopharyngeal reflux patients. *Laryngoscope.* 2009;118(5):938–941.

30. Verdolini K, Sandage M, Titze IR. Effect of hydration treatments on laryngeal nodules and polyps and related voice measures. *J Voice.* 1994;8(1):30–47.

31. Titze IR. Heat generation in the vocal folds and its possible effect on vocal endurance. In: Lawrence VL, ed. *Transcsripts of the Tenth Symposium: Care of the Professional Voice. Part I: Instrumentation in Voice Research.* New York, NY: The Voice Foundation; 1981:52–65.

32. Jiang J, Verdolini K, Aquino B, Ng J, Hanson D. Effects of dehydration on phonation in excised canine larynges. *Ann Otol Rhinol Laryngol.* 2000;109(6): 568–575.

33. Verdolini K, Druker DG, Palmer PM, Samawi H. Laryngeal adduction in resonant voice. *J Voice.* 1998;12(3):315–327.

34. Verdolini-Marston K, Burke MK, Lessac A, Glaze L, Caldwell E. Preliminary study of two methods of treatment for laryngeal nodules. *J Voice.* 1995;9(1): 74–85.

35. Peterson KL, Verdolini-Marston K, Barkmeir JM, Hoffman HT. Comparison of aerodynamic and electroglottographic parameters in evaluating clinically relevant voicing patterns. *Ann Otol Rhinol Laryngol.* 1994;103(5 pt 1):335–346.

36. Najundeswaran C, Li NYK, Chan K, Wong R, Trovarelli A, Verdolini K. *Prevention of voice problems in student teachers: a pilot study.* In preparation.

37. Roy N, Weinrich B, Gray SD, et al. Voice amplification versus vocal hygiene instruction for teachers with voice disorders: a treatment outcomes study. *J Speech Lang Hear Res.* 2002;45:625–638.

38. Lee TD, Swinnen SP. Three legacies of Bryan and Harter: automaticity, variability and change in skilled performance. In: Starkes JL, Allard F, eds. *Cognitive Issues in Motor Expertise.* Amsterdam: Elsevier; 1993:295–315.

39. Verdolini Abbott K. *Lessac-Madsen Resonant Voice Therapy: Clinician Manual.* San Diego, CA: Plural Publishing; 2008.

40. Stemple JC, Lee L, D'Amico B, Pickup B. Efficacy of vocal function exercises as a method of improving voice production. *J Voice.* 1994;8(3):271–278.

41. Sabol JW, Lee L, Stemple JC. The value of vocal function exercises in the practice regimen of singers. *J Voice.* 1995; 9(1):27–36.

42. Verdolini Abbott K. *Lessac-Madsen Resonant Voice Therapy: Patient Manual.* San Diego, CA: Plural Publishing; 2008.

43. Gauffin J, Sundberg J. Spectral correlates of glottal voice source waveform characteristics. *J Speech Hear Res.* 1989; 32(3):556–565.

44. Smitheran JR, Hixon TJ. A clinical method for estimating laryngeal airway resistance during vowel production. *J Speech Hear Disord.* 1981;46(2): 138–146.

45. Grillo EU, Verdolini K. Evidence for distinguishing pressed, normal, resonant, and breathy voice qualities by laryngeal resistance and vocal efficiency in vocally, trained subjects. *J Voice.* 2008;22(5): 546–552.

46. Lessac A. *The Use and Training of the Human: A Biodynamic Approach to Vocal Life.* Mountain View Ca: Mayfield Publishing Co; 1997.

47. Lessac A. *The Use and Training of the Human Voice.* 2 ed. New York, NY: DBS Publications; 1967.

48. Verdolini K, Li NYK, Branski RC, Rosen CA, Urban EG, Hebda PA. *The effect of targeted vocal exercise on recovery from acute inflammation.* In preparation.

49. Agarwal S. Low magnitude of tensile strain inhibits IL-1 beta dependent induction of pro-inflammatory cytokines and induces synthesis of IL-10 in human periodontal ligament cells in vitro. *J Dental Res.* 2001;80(5):1416–1420.

50. Long P, Hu J, Piesco N, Buckley M, Agarwal S. Low magnitude of tensile strain inhibits IL-1 beta-dependent induction of pro-inflammatory cytokines and induces synthesis of IL-10 in human periodontal cells in vitro. *J Dental Res.* 2001;80(5):1416–1420.

51. Agarwal S, Deschner J, Long P, et al. Role of NF-kappaB transcription factors

in antiinflammatory and proinflammatory actions of mechanical signals. *Arthritis Rheum.* 2004;50(11):3541–3548.

52. Deschner J, Hofman CR, Piesco NP, Agarwal S. Signal transduction by mechanical strain in chondrocytes. *Curr Opin Clin Nutr Metab Care.* 2003;6(3): 289–293.

53. Branski RC, Perera P, Verdolini K, Rosen CA, Hebda PA, Agarwal S. Dynamic biomechanical strain inhibits IL-1 beta-induced inflammation in vocal fold fibroblasts. *J Voice.* 2007; 21(6):651–660.

54. Li NYK, Verdolini K, Clermont G, Mi Q, Hebda P, Vodovotz Y. *A patient-specific in silico model of inflammation and healing tested in acute vocal fold injury.* Presented at the 8th International Conference on Systems Biology. Long Beach, CA; 2007.

55. Verdolini-Marston K, Balota DA. Role of elaborative and perceptual integrative processes in perceptual-motor performance. *J Exper Psych Learn Mem Cog.* 1994;20(3):739–749.

56. Schmidt R, Lee T, eds. *Motor Control And Learning: A Behavioral Emphasis.* Champaign, IL: Human Kinetics Publishers; 2005.

57. Verdolini K. Principles of skill acquisition applied to voice training. In: Hampton M, Acker B, eds. *The Vocal Vision: Views on Voice by 24 Leading Teachers, Coaches and Directors.* New York, NY: Applause Books; 2000:65–80.

58. Verdolini K, Rosen CA, Branski RC, Hersan R, Scheffel L. *Effect of associational versus sensory processing instructions on the outcome of resonant voice therapy.* In preparation.

59. Wulf G, Prinz W. Directing attention to movement effects enhances learning: a review. *Psychol Bull Rev.* 2001;8(4): 648–660.

60. Wulf G, Shea CH. Principles derived from the study of simple skills do not generalize to complex skill learning. *Psychol Bull Rev.* 2002;9(2):185–211.

61. Schmidt RA. A schema theory of discrete motor skill learning. *Psychol Rev.* 1975;82:225–260.

62. Wulf G, Lauterbach B, Toole T. The learning advantages of an external focus of attention in golf. *Res Q Exerc Sport.* 1999;70(2):120–126.

63. Wulf G, McNevin NH, Fuchs T, Ritter F, Toole T. Attentional focus in complex skill learning. *Res Q Exerc Sport.* 2000; 71(3):229–239.

64. Ramig LO, Countryman S, O'Brien C, Hoehn M, Thompson L. Intensive speech treatment for patients with Parkinson's disease: short- and long-term comparison of two techniques. *Neurology.* 1996;47(6):1496–1504.

65. Ramig LO, Fox C, Sapir S. Parkinson's disease: speech and voice disorders and their treatment with the Lee Silverman Voice Treatment. *Semin Speech Lang.* 2004;25(2):169–180.

66. Ramig LO, Fox C, Sapir S. Speech treatment for Parkinson's disease. *Expert Rev Neurother.* 2008;8(2):297–309.

67. Ramig LO, Sapir S, Countryman S, et al. Intensive voice treatment (LSVT) for patients with Parkinson's disease: a 2 year follow-up. *J Neurol Neurosurg Psychiatry.* 2001;71(4):493–498.

68. Jacobson BH, Johnson A, Grywalski C, et al. The Voice Handicap Index (VHI): development and validation. *Am J Speech Lang Pathol.* 1997;6:66–70.

69. Eckel FC, Boone DR. The s/z ratio as an indicator of laryngeal pathology. *J Speech Hear Disord.* 1981;46: 147–149.

70. Morrison MD, Rammage LA, Belisle GM, Pullan CB, Nichol H. Muscular tension dysphonia. *J Otolaryngol.* 1983; 12(5):302–306.

71. Kotby MN, Shiromoto O, Hirano M. The accent method of voice therapy: effect of accentuations on F_0, SPL, and airflow. *J Voice.* 1993;7(4):319–325.

72. Smith S, Thyme K. *Die Akzentmethode.* Vaedbek, Denmark: Danish Voice Institute; 1981.

73. van den Berg J. Myoelastic-aerodynamic theory of voice production. *J Speech Hear Res.* 1958;1:227–244.

74. Titze I. *Principles of Voice Production.* Englewood Cliffs, NJ: Prentice-Hall; 1994.

75. Verdolini K, Titze I. The application of laboratory formulas to clinical voice management. *Am J Speech Lang Pathol.* 1995:62–69.

76. Verdolini K, Druker DG, Palmer PM, Samawi H. Laryngeal adduction in resonant voice. *J Voice.* 1998;12(3):315–327.

77. Hixon TJ. *Respiratory Function in Speech and Song.* San Diego, CA: Singular Publishing Group Inc; 1991.

78. Harris TM, Harris S, Rubin JS, DM. H. *The Voice Clinic Handbook.* London, England: Whurr Publishers Ltd; 1998.

79. Laukkanen AM, Lindholm P, Vilkman E, Haataja K, Alku P. A physiological and acoustic study on voiced bilabial fricative/beta:/as a vocal exercise. *J Voice.* 1996;10(1):67–77.

80. Estill J. *Some Basic Voice Qualities.* Santa Rosa, CA: Estill Voice Training Systems; 1995.

81. Morrison M, Rammage L, et al. *The Management of Voice Disorders.* San Diego, CA: Singular Publishing Group; 1994.

82. Harris TM, Lieberman J. The cricothyroid mechanism, its relation to vocal fatigue and vocal dysfunction. Voice forum. *J Voice.* 1993;2:89–96.

83. Lieberman J. Principles and techniques of manual therapy: applications in the management of dysphonia. In: Harris et al, eds. *The Voice Clinic Handbook.* London, England: Whurr Publishers Ltd; 1998:91–138.

84. Harris TM, Collins SRC, Lieberman J. *The Association Between Head, Neck and Shoulder Girdle Tension and Dysphonia.* London, England: Guy's Hospital; 1992.

85. Vilkman E, Sonninen A, Hurme P, Korkko P. External laryngeal frame function in voice production revisited: a review. *J Voice.* 1996;10(1):78–92.

86. Stone RE, Casteel RL. Intervention in non-organically based dysphonia. In: Filter M, ed. *Phonatory Disorders in Children.* New York, NY: CC Thomas Co; 1982.

87. Gauffin J, Sundberg J. Spectral correlates of glottal voice source waveform characteristics. *J Speech Hear Res.* 1989; 32:556–565.

88. Casteel RL, Stone RE. Maintaining newly acquired normal voice. In: Filter M, ed. *Phonatory Disorders in Children.* New York, NY: CC Thomas Co; 1982.

89. Stone RE. Functional dysphonia (a case report). In: Stemple JC, ed. *Voice Therapy: Clinical Studies.* St. Louis, MO: Mosby-Year Book, Inc; 1993:105–110.

90. Stone RE, Casteel RL. Changing concepts in functional dysphonic patients. *Curr Opin Otolaryngol Head Neck Surg.* 1997;6(6).

91. Hirano M. *Clinical Examination of Voice.* New York, NY: Springer-Verlag; 1981.

92. Rosen CA, Lee AS, Osborne J, Zullo T, Murry T. Development and validation of the Voice Handicap Index-10. *Laryngoscope.* 2004;114(9):1549–1556.

93. Belafsky PC, Postma GN, Koufman JA. Validity and reliability of the Reflux Symptom Index (RSI). *J Voice.* 2002; 16(2):274–277.

94. Brandt JF, Ruder KF, Shipp T, Jr. Vocal loudness and effort in continuous speech. *J Acoust Soc Am.* 1969;46(6): 1543–1548.

95. Solomon NP, Robin DA. Perceptions of effort during handgrip and tongue elevation in Parkinson's disease. *Parkinsonism Relat Disord.* 2005;11(6):353–361.

96. Titze I. *Workshop on Acoustic Voice Analysis: Summary Statement.* Denver, CO: National Center for Voice and Speech; 1995.

97. Ma EP, Yiu EM. Suitability of acoustic perturbation measures in analysing periodic and nearly periodic voice signals. *Folia Phoniatr Logop.* 2005;57(1): 38–47.

98. Stemple J. *Voice Therapy: Clinical Studies.* San Diego: Singular Thomson Learning; 2000.

99. Gartner-Schmidt JL. Flow Phonation. In: Haskell ABJ, ed. *Exercises for Voice Therapy.* San Diego: Plural Publishing, Inc; 2008.

100. Seifert E, Kollbrunner J. An update in thinking about nonorganic voice disorders. *Arch Otolaryngol Head Neck Surg.* 2006;132(10):1128–1132.

101. Seifert E, Kollbrunner J. Stress and distress in non-organic voice disorder. *Swiss Med Wkly.* 2005;135(27–28):387–397.

102. Roy N, Bless DM, Heisey D. Personality and voice disorders: a multitrait-multidisorder analysis. *J Voice.* 2000; 14(4):521–548.

103. Roy N, Bless DM, Heisey D. Personality and voice disorders: a superfactor trait analysis. *J Speech Lang Hear Res.* 2000;43(3):749–768.

104. van Mersbergen M, Patrick C, Glaze L. Functional dysphonia during mental imagery: testing the trait theory of voice disorders. *J Speech Lang Hear Res.* Dec 2008;51(6):1405–1423.

105. Casper JK. Objective methods for the evaluation of vocal function. In: Stemple J, ed. *Voice Therapy: Clinical Studies.* St. Louis, MO: Mosby-Year Book; 1993: 39–45.

106. Berry DA, Verdolini K, Montequin DW, Hess MM, Chan RW, Titze IR. A quantitative output-cost ratio in voice production. *J Speech Lang Hear Res.* 2001; 44(1):29–37.

107. Larson CR. The midbrain periaqueductal gray: a brainstem structure involved in vocalization. *J Speech Hear Res.* 1985; 28(2):241–249.

108. Schmidt, A. R, Lee, TD. *Motor Control and Learning: A Behavioral Emphasis.* 4th ed. Champaign, IL: Human Kinetics; 2005.

109. Rosen CA. Stroboscopy as a research instrument: development of a perceptual evaluation tool. *Laryngoscope.* 2005; 115(3):423–428.

110. Kempster, G, Gerratt, et al. Consensus auditory-perceptual evaluation of voice: development of a standardized clinical protocol. *Am J Speech-Lang Path.* 2009: 18(2):124–132.

111. Jacobson B, Johnson A, Grywalski C, Silbergleit A, Jacobson G, Benninger MS. The Voice Handicap Index (VHI): development and validation. *Am J Speech Lang Pathol.* 1997;6:66–70.

112. Zraick RI, Risner BY, Smith-Olinde L, Gregg BA, Johnson FL, McWeeny EK. Patient versus partner perception of voice handicap. *J Voice.* 2007;21(4): 485–494.

113. Zraick RI, Risner BY. Assessment of quality of life in persons with voice disorders. *Curr Opin Otolaryngol Head Neck Surg.* 2008;16(3):188–193.

114. van der Merwe A. The voice use reduction program. *Am J Speech Lang Pathol.* 2004;13(3):208–218.

115. Satake, EB, Jagaro, V, Maxwell, DL. *Handbook of Statistical Methods: Single Subject Design.* San Diego, CA: Plural Publishing; 2008.

116. Pannbacker, M. Voice treatment techniques: a review and recommendations for outcomes studies. *Am J Speech Lang Pathol.* 1998;7(3):49–67.

117. Peterson MD, Rhea MR, Alvar BA. Maximizing strength development in athletes: a meta-analysis to determine the dose-response relationship. *J Strength Cond Res.* 2004;18(2):377–382.

118. de Vos NJ, Singh NA, Ross DA, Stavrinos TM, Orr R, Fiatarone Singh MA. Optimal load for increasing muscle power during explosive resistance training in older adults. *J Gerontol A Biol Sci Med Sci.* 2005;60(5):638–647.

119. Abbass A. Intensive short-term dynamic psychotherapy in a private psychiatric office: clinical and cost effectiveness. *Am J Psychother.* 2002;56(2): 225–232.

120. Abbass A, Sheldon A, Gyra J, Kalpin A. Intensive short-term dynamic psychotherapy for DSM-IV personality disor-

ders: a randomized controlled trial. *J Nerv Ment Dis.* 2008;196(3):211–216.

121. Saxon K, Schneider C. *Vocal Exercise Physiology.* San Diego, CA: Singular Publishing Group; 1995.

122. Colton RH, Brown J. Some relationships between vocal effort and intraoral air pressure. *J Acous Soc Am.* 1973;53(1):296.

123. Wright HN, Colton RH. *Some parameters of autophonic level.* American Speech and Hearing Association Convention; November 1972.

4

Management of Glottal Incompetence

Normal voicing is dependent on near-total closure of the vocal folds. (The larynges of many women and some men will demonstrate a normal posterior glottal gap of the vocal folds upon adduction.[1]) Subglottic air pressure from the lungs builds and eventually overcomes the resistance of the adducted folds, and a puff of air escapes. This release of air creates a sudden drop of air pressure between the vocal folds that, along with a downward pressure from the supra-glottic structures and the static positioning of the adducted folds, draws the vocal folds back together, completing a vibratory cycle.[2]

When the vocal folds do not totally approximate, as in the case of glottal incompetence, a greater amount of air pressure and airflow is required to create and maintain phonation. The speaker,

therefore, must work harder to produce voice. The perceptual quality of voice and effort required to produce voice will be reflected directly by the size of the glottal gap. The larger the glottal gap, the breathier the voice will be. As the size of the gap may vary from large (as in some cases of vocal fold paralysis) to small (as in cases of small vocal nodules), the voices of individuals with glottal incompetence may range from a mild breathiness to complete whispered aphonia. Interestingly, some patients with glottal incompetence attempt to compensate for the lack of glottic closure by compressing the supraglottic structures. Therefore, this segment of the population may not present not with the expected breathy quality, but with a strained, strangled quality.

Glottal incompetence may result from either functional or organic sources. Functional hypoadduction of the vocal folds may be caused by an imbalance of respiration, phonation, and resonance caused by voice misuse, use-induced vocal fatigue, or emotional concerns.

Voice misuse may lead to laryngeal fatigue in an otherwise medically and emotionally healthy individual, such as patients who report that their voice quality is normal in the morning but becomes weak, hoarse, and breathy as the day progresses. The result of this vocal fatigue may be the development of glottal gaps between the vocal folds,[3] usually with increased supraglottic tension. These patients complain that the harder they try to produce voice, the worse the quality becomes. One might correctly argue that the original cause of laryngeal fatigue was hyperfunctional vocal behavior. Nonetheless, stroboscopic observations of many of these patients made during the fatigued state demonstrate unusual anterior glottal chinks, large posterior glottal chinks, and occasional spindle-shaped chinks.[4]

Lack of glottal closure also may be the result of organic etiology. A variety of diseases and conditions can lead to the concern. A number of neurogenic etiologies, both central and peripheral, have been associated with insufficient glottal closure. Vocal fold paralysis is, perhaps, the most common neurogenic cause of glottal incompetence. Although paralysis may be caused by central neurologic disease, more often it is the result of nerve damage or peripheral disease. Vocal fold paralysis may be unilateral or bilateral. It may be caused by damage to or disease of the vagus nerve anywhere along its course from the brainstem to the target muscle and may, therefore, involve the superior laryngeal nerve (to the cricothyroid muscle), the recurrent laryngeal branch (all remaining intrinsic laryngeal muscles), or both. Location of the lesion along the nerve pathway will determine the type of paralysis, the

degree of glottal incompetence, and the resulting voice quality.

Glottal incompetence also may be secondary to non-neurologic causes. For instance, aging may bring about a characteristic bowing of the vocal fold edge and a resultant lack of glottal closure. Although such changes have been observed across genders, these changes are most commonly observed in males. In cases of reflux, continued irritation of the posterior larynx may result in the formation of additive lesions along the cartilaginous aspect of the vocal folds called granuloma. The firm, granular structures sit between the arytenoid cartilages, preventing closure of the posterior glottis, and creating a glottal gap.

Thus, a variety of functional and organic concerns may lead to glottal incompetence. This chapter highlights management of age-related and neurogenic cases. The studies illustrate the use of direct therapy for improving fold adduction and the use of surgical techniques to decrease the size of glottal gaps. Functional cases of glottal incompetence are discussed separately in Chapter 5.

Management of Presbyphonia

Steve Gorman, PhD

Case Study: Patient M

The aging vocal fold system may be referred to as presbylaryngeus, vocal fold bowing, or senile laryngis. The resulting voice concern is frequently referred to as presbyphonia. In the following case study, Steve Gorman describes a behavioral therapy approach that proves successful in improving the voice quality and quality of life of a 71-year-old man.

History

Patient M, a 71-year-old man, self-employed as an engineering consultant, was referred by an otolaryngologist with complaints of throat irritation, hoarseness, and, in his own words, "distorted speech." According to the patient, he first noticed the degradation of his vocal quality a month prior to his evaluation in the voice laboratory, although his wife noticed it 4 to 5 months prior to that. He was a pipe smoker for 55 years and seldom inhaled, but noticed increased hoarseness after he quit smoking the pipe. At the age of 71, he still worked 40 to 50 hours a week. He spent much of his time either on the phone or meeting with clients in person. He always prided himself on a pleasant, yet authoritative, speaking voice. His voice quality was worse in the morning, improved through midday, then deteriorated through the end of the day.

His medical history was significant for macular degeneration and a history of kidney stones. He was not taking any medications at the time of the evaluation. He reported drinking five glasses of decaffeinated tea, two cups of decaffeinated coffee, and very little water in the course of an average day.

Voice Assessment

Auditory-Perceptual. Voice quality was described as being mildly to moderately dysphonic characterized by a raspy, husky hoarseness. The patient described a feeling of excessive mucus in his throat and admitted to clearing his throat to excess. His voice quality varied throughout the day, with more hoarseness and a feeling of vocal fatigue the more he talked. He demonstrated mildly excessive jaw tension.

Acoustic Analysis. Speaking fundamental frequency was essentially normal, whereas the range of frequency was reduced. Perturbation measures revealed that mean percent jitter and shimmer (dB) were excessive at high and low pitches, and noise to harmonic ratio was excessive at low pitches. Acoustic measurements are summarized in Table 4–1.

Aerodynamic. Airflow rate and maximum phonation time were both below normal limits (Table 4–2). Phonation flow volume was appropriate for his age, physical build, and gender.

Videostroboscopic. Examination of the vibratory characteristics were noted during the examination and are listed in Table 4–3. Most notable was the moderate bowing of the membranous vocal folds during all tasks. A mild-to-moderate decrease in the amplitude of vibration and mucosal wave bilaterally was observed. Symmetry of the phase of vibration was 50% asymmetric. Moderate compression of supraglottic structures in both the lateral-medial and anterior-posterior planes was observed. Furthermore, the patient demonstrated thick mucus in the hypopharynx, giving the appearance of inadequate hydration.

Voice Therapy

Bowing of the vocal folds is often seen in the larynges of the elderly complaining of voice problems. Voice therapy appropriate for this physiologic condition is physiologic voice therapy, supplemented by a formal hydration program and vocal hygiene counseling.

Hydration Program

The patient was instructed to drink at least 64 ounces of water per day and to

Table 4–1. Acoustic Measures for Patient M

Measure	Pretherapy	Posttherapy
Mean F_0, /a/, in Hz		
Comfort pitch	110	122
High pitch	214	250
Low pitch	97	90
Jitter (%)		
Comfort pitch	.87	.61
High pitch	1.03	.73
Low pitch	1.68	.86
Shimmer (dB)		
Comfort pitch	.35	.21
High pitch	.45	.27
Low pitch	.56	.31
N/H (dB)		
Comfort pitch	.14	.09
High pitch	.13	.11
Low pitch	.16	.10
Speaking F_0 (Hz)	116	121
Frequency range (Hz)	83–381	80–611

Table 4–2. Aerodynamic Measurements for Patient M

Measure	Pretherapy	Posttherapy
Phonation Flow Volume (mL)		
Comfort pitch	2190	2450
High pitch	2143	2240
Low pitch	2670	2530
Mean Airflow Rate (mL/sec)		
Comfort pitch	216	112
High pitch	255	124
Low pitch	193	145
Maximum Phonation Time (sec)		
Comfort pitch	10.1	21.9
High pitch	8.4	18.1
Low pitch	13.8	17.4

Table 4–3. Stroboscopic Ratings for Patient M

Parameter	Pretherapy	Posttherapy
Glottic closure	Spindle shape	Slight posterior gap
Supraglottic activity	Mod. L-M and A-P compression	Mild A-P compression
Vertical level	Equal	Equal
Vocal fold mobility	Normal	Normal
Amplitude of vibration	Mild-mod. decrease	Mild decrease
Mucosal wave	Mild-mod. decrease	Mild decrease
Phase closure	Closed phase mildly dominant	Normal
Phase symmetry	50% asymmetrical	Asymmetric, high pitch
Overall laryngeal function	Hyperfunctional	Normal

eliminate all caffeinated beverages from his diet. These steps would increase internal hydration and, thereby, decrease the viscosity of patient's mucous secretions and improve the lubrication of the vocal folds.

Vocal Hygiene

With complaints of a sensation of increased mucus in his throat, the patient had developed the habit of frequent and harsh throat clearing. A simple behavior modification program was devised in which the patient simply tallied on a piece of paper each time he cleared his throat. By increasing his awareness of the habit, he was able to significantly reduce the instances of throat clearing. Additionally, with the increase in systemic hydration, and thus the decrease in viscosity of mucus, the urge to clear his throat subsided.

Vocal Function Exercises

This patient was trying to compensate for the lack of glottic closure by hypercom-

pression of the supraglottic structures. It was determined that a low-impact adductory exercise would be most beneficial to improve glottic closure while reducing the hypercompression. The physiologic voice therapy chosen was the Vocal Function Exercise program,[5] which was described to the patient as "a four-part exercise program similar to physical therapy for the vocal fold muscles." As an engineer, quantitative exercises appealed to this patient because he could objectively measure his own performance by timing how long he could sustain the musical notes for the warm-up and adductory power exercises. He was instructed to do these exercises two times each, two times a day. To aid Patient M in accomplishing his daily exercises, he was given a prerecorded CD of the exercises to use as a guide. (See Chapter 3 for a complete description of the Vocal Function Exercise program.)

During the initial therapy session, Patient M averaged 26 seconds on each of the six timed exercises (warm-up and power). This was described to the patient as his "vocal muscle strength index."

Furthermore, it was explained to him that, as his vocal muscles increased in strength, he would then be able to sustain the notes for increasingly longer periods of time. The patient questioned whether he simply would be improving his lung capacity, whereupon it was explained that the phonation flow volume is basically a static measure. What improves is the ability of the vocal folds to valve the subglottic airstream more efficiently and effectively because of improved glottic closure.

Table 4–4 demonstrates the progression of the patient's improvement in glottic closure over the course of time that he was receiving voice therapy. He achieved a maximum phonation time of 44.8 seconds and during his final therapy session achieved 42 seconds. This final average was achieved after not having performed the exercises in the previous 10 days as he had been on a vacation trip without access to a CD player with which to play his Vocal Function Exercise CD.

Table 4–4. Progression of Vocal Function Exercise Maximum Phonation Times for Patient M

Date	Time (sec)
4/1/08	26.0
4/8/08	29.8
4/22/08	36.2
5/6/08	38.2
5/20/08	37.2
6/12/08	38.8
7/1/08	41.7
7/29/08	44.8
9/9/08	42.0

Summary

Patient M was enrolled in voice therapy once weekly for 2 weeks, once every other week for 6 weeks, once every 3 weeks for 9 weeks, and one more time 6 weeks later. Therapy began with physiologic voice therapy and was supplemented with a systematic increase in systemic hydration, as well as vocal hygiene. The patient maintained a disciplined schedule of performing the exercises twice daily, as well as increasing his hydration and reducing phonotraumatic behaviors. In addition to improving his maximum phonation times from 26 seconds to 44.8 seconds, his vocal quality and vocal stamina improved to a degree such that the patient (or this voice pathologist) did not consider either to be a problem anymore. The auditory, acoustic, and stroboscopic measures taken during the evaluation were repeated at the conclusion of therapy and are listed in Tables 4–1 to 4–3. Acoustic measures of perturbation improved, as did his frequency range. Airflow measurements were also improved. Stroboscopic ratings improved as the spindle-shaped glottic gap changed to a slight posterior gap with significant decrease in supraglottic compression. The patient continued performing his Vocal Function Exercise at the conclusion of formal voice therapy. He followed a maintenance program outlined in Table 4–5. Two months after the conclusion of therapy, the patient was still maintaining phonation times of 43 seconds and performing Vocal Function Exercises three times a week. He remained satisfied with his vocal quality and stamina and reported no vocal complaints. Six months after the conclusion of therapy, performing Vocal Function Exercises three times a week, he had continued to improve his

Table 4–5. Vocal Function Exercise Maintenance Program for Patient M

1. Full exercise program, two times each, two times a day

2. Two times in the morning, one time in the evening, or vice versa

3. One time in the morning, one time in the evening

4. Two times, morning or evening

5. One time a day, 7 days a week

6. One time a day, 6 days a week

7. One time a day, 5 days a week

8. One time a day, 4 days a week

9. One time a day, 3 days a week

10. No vocal function exercises

phonation times even more, reaching an average of 51 seconds. As before, he reported no vocal complaints.

Management of Vocal Fold Bowing

Dawn Lowery, PhD

Case Study: Patient N

Patient N, a 74-year-old retired nurse, was referred by an otolaryngologist with complaints of vocal fatigue, laryngitis "not related to an upper respiratory infection," and "airiness." The otolaryngologist had diagnosed bowed vocal folds but could not find any underlying physiologic cause for the problem. According to the patient, her voice symptoms had progressively increased over several years and were always worse after prolonged use of her voice or later in the day. The patient was active and participated in exercise three times weekly, volunteered twice weekly at the hospital, and routinely participated in numerous social events. Her medical history included osteoarthritis, borderline osteoporosis, and pernicious anemia. Routine medications included aspirin, calcium (1000 mg daily), and vitamin B12 injections (monthly). She also reported being fitted for bilateral hearing aids, which she declined to wear because she found them bothersome.

Voice Assessment

Auditory-Perceptual. Voice quality was moderately harsh and strained. A mild hyponasal resonance was also noted. Visible tension was evident in her face, jaw, and neck. Frequent throat clearing and coughing behaviors were present. Voice quality had deteriorated by the conclusion of the voice testing.

Acoustic. The speaking fundamental frequency was reduced and the phonatory range was reduced for the highest frequency (Table 4–6). In addition, the habitual sound pressure level was elevated, with a normal intensity range. Perturbation measures revealed excessive mean percent jitter and shimmer and a reduced signal-to-noise ratio.

Aerodynamic. The intraoral air pressure and mean airflow were excessive (see Table 4–6). Assessment of air volume revealed subnormal values. In addition, the maximum phonation time was markedly reduced in duration.

Videostroboscopic. Examination of the vocal fold vibratory patterns revealed moderate-to-severe bilateral vocal fold

Table 4–6. Acoustic and Aerodynamic Measures Pre- and Posttherapy for Patient N

Measure	Pretherapy	Posttherapy
Mean F_0 (Hz)	160	190
Highest F_0 (Hz)	370	600
Lowest F_0 (Hz)	120	135
Mean SPL (dB)	75–79	71
Mean jitter (%)	.12	.06
Shimmer (%)	12	4
Signal-to-noise ratio	17	25
Intraoral pressure	17.33	11.43
Mean airflow (cc/sec)	739	110
Max. phonation time (sec)	12	27
Airflow volume (mL)	800	2,050

bowing along the membranous vocal fold during all aspects except low pitch. A moderately decreased amplitude of vibration was noted bilaterally. Mucosal wave movement was similarly decreased. Asymmetric and aperiodic vibration were present across all tasks. These results are shown in Table 4–7.

Laryngoscopic. Other laryngeal conditions were also noted during the examination (see Table 4–7). Moderately compressed ventricular folds (ventricular hyperfunction) were observed during all phonatory tasks. Mild, bilateral vocal fold edema was evident and may be a normal variant for a woman of this age. In addition, excessive and thick mucous stranding and pooling were evident in the glottic region.

Hearing. Patient N was advised to consult with an audiologist about her hearing. Audiometric testing was to be

completed, if necessary, and the hearing aids were to be evaluated to optimize hearing. The patient was informed of the potential effects of poor hearing on voice quality.

Diagnostic Therapy

Diagnostic therapy procedures were used to determine if the vocal fold bowing was modifiable. This was important in determining the prognosis of vocal fold recovery. The rigid endoscope attached to the stroboscopic unit and video monitor were used to assess vocal fold bowing. The patient was asked to sustain /i/ at a comfortable pitch and loudness. Vocal fold bowing again was evident. In addition, marked ventricular fold hyperfunction was apparent. The patient was then asked to produce /i/ on inhalation, producing the sound as soon she began to inhale. Phonatory inhalation was very difficult for this

Table 4–7. Videostrobe and Laryngoscopic Measures Pre- and Posttherapy for Patient N

Measure	Pretherapy	Posttherapy
Videostroboscopic		
Glottic closure	Moderate-severe bowing	Midfold touch closure, posterior glottal gap
Amplitude	Moderately decreased	Slightly decreased
Mucosal wave	Moderately decreased	Normal
Symmetry	Always asymmetrical	Symmetrical
Periodicity	Always aperiodic	Aperiodic at low
Laryngoscopic		
Ventricular fold hyperfunction	Moderately compressed	Absent
Vocal fold edema	Mild, bilaterally	Slight, bilaterally
Laryngeal mucus	Excessive stranding/pooling Thick viscosity	Normal viscosity

patient to perform, and therefore, she was asked to sustain /i/ on exhalation and then reverse the pattern, producing /i/ on inhalation. The exhalation phase was gradually weaned out of the task, and the patient developed the ability to sustain an inhalation sound for a few seconds. This phonatory inhalation task demonstrated that glottal adduction could be improved and that fold hyperfunction could be decreased. Based on this initial voice evaluation, the following recommendations for vocal hygiene and direct voice therapy were made.

Vocal Hygiene Program

Hydration

Steaming. Use of steam as therapy was recommended twice daily to reduce throat dryness, to decrease nasal crusting, and thin the mucus. The patient

was instructed on different ways of steaming. One method included sitting in her bathroom with the door closed and inhaling the steam from the running shower for 10 to 15 minutes. Another method included the use of a commercial facial steamer or simulating a steamer by boiling water, pouring it into a bowl, tenting a towel over the head and the bowl, and inhaling the steam for 10 minutes twice daily. The patient was cautioned about placing her face too close to the water to avoid burns.

Increase Water Consumption. The purpose of this recommendation was to increase internal hydration, which can modify the viscosity of the mucous secretions and result in less throat irritation. Patient N was instructed to increase her water consumption to six to eight 8-ounce glasses of water daily, pending approval from her physician. (It is advised to check with the patient's physician because increasing water consumption in an older individual can be dangerous. The elderly individual has more difficulty handling excessive fluid if blood pressure is high or if other conditions such as cardiac or kidney problems exist.)

Room Humidification. The use of a humidifier in the bedroom at night can provide essential room moisture, especially for a mouth breather who experiences a dry throat in the morning.

Diet. The patient was advised to reduce caffeine consumption and to substitute decaffeinated beverages. The purpose of the suggestion was to facilitate a reduction in muscle tension, as caffeine is a known stimulant. Patient N admitted to drinking the equivalent 250 to 400 mg of caffeinated beverages daily.

Direct Voice Therapy. Voice therapy was recommended to provide education about the laryngeal mechanism and the process of voice production; to eliminate throat clearing and coughing behaviors; to reduce muscular tension, which was most evident in the patient's face, jaw, neck, ventricular vocal folds, and upper chest; to improve breath support for speech; and to improve vocal fold closure. Four of the vocal techniques used for Patient N are described in the list below.

1. *Respiratory training.* Although Patient N was involved in aerobic exercise three times weekly, her air volume was markedly low, coupled with the upper chest breathing and jaw and neck tension. The goals of respiratory training included relaxation and subsequent reduction in visible muscle tension and improv-

ing breath support and control for speech. Training procedures included monitoring respiratory movements by use of a mirror and the placement of the patient's hands. When the appropriate respiratory pattern in this stage is established, the patient can progress to phonatory tasks. Three tasks were emphasized for Patient N.

- *Two-stage breathing.* The patient was asked to place one hand on her upper chest and the other on her lower abdomen. She was asked to inhale and describe which hand (and consequently, which body part) moved first and which hand had the greatest excursion. The goal was to achieve a two-step inspiratory pattern with the lower abdomen moving outward first and most, followed by a less obvious movement of the upper chest.
- *Lower rib expansion.* A second technique required the patient to stand, placing her hands on her lower ribs and extending her fingers toward the spine. She then inhaled, keeping her shoulders low as the fingers passively spread apart due to expansion of the lower rib cage.
- *Breath counting.* When the appropriate respiratory pattern had been established, this technique was used to improve respiratory control. The patient was asked to inhale over five counts and hold the inhalation for five counts, then exhale over five counts and hold the exhalation for five counts. The cycle was then repeated once during this session, and the patient

was asked to practice two cycles of the patterns two to three times daily. When the patient could easily master the pattern at five counts, the task was increased by one count at each stage. Over the course of a few weeks, a patient should be able to eventually master a maximum of 10 counts at each stage.

The patient was advised to practice respiratory exercises throughout the day in a variety of settings. For example, she could practice while driving her car by allowing the lap belt to provide her with kinesthetic feedback.

2. *Relaxation.* Several relaxation techniques should be introduced to patients because they may find only one or two beneficial. The interested clinician should read texts describing various relaxation techniques to understand how to use them in therapy. Techniques include respiratory training, visual imagery, autogenic phrases, and progressive relaxation. Respiratory training was described earlier. Visual imagery is the use of images to invoke physical and mental relaxation. Often, an individual will imagine a peaceful setting, such as a walk along a beach or through a meadow. This can be stimulated by listening to a prerecorded CD that thoroughly describes the relaxing scene. Autogenic phrases, which can be prerecorded, use suggestive phrases to invoke relaxation. These include such sentences as "My breathing is slow and relaxed" and "My right arm is heavy and warm." Finally, progressive relaxation is a technique

that requires a patient to tense, hold, and then relax an isolated body part. Often, a clinician will begin with the top of the body and work down, asking the patient to wrinkle the forehead and hold this posture for 5 seconds and then relax the forehead, noticing the absence of muscle tension during the relaxed state.

Each technique was thoroughly explained to Patient N during therapy and recommended for daily home practice. After 2 weeks, she was asked to select the technique(s) that was most beneficial in achieving relaxation. She chose visual imagery and progressive muscle relaxation, initially using an audio CD as stimulus.

3. *Visual-Auditory Feedback Training.* Biofeedback, using the rigid endoscope and television monitor, were used as described previously in the section "Diagnostic Therapy" to reduce ventricular fold hyperfunction and increase true vocal fold approximation. Visual, auditory, and kinesthetic cues were available to Patient N as she learned the task. The visual stimulus was removed gradually as long as she was able to achieve the appropriate movement patterns.

4. *Phonatory Training.* The first task included sustaining isolated vowels at habitual, highest, and lowest comfortable pitch levels. The patient was asked to vocalize from midrange to highest comfortable pitch, beginning with the easier to produce vowels and progressing to more difficult vowels. The goal is to gradually change pitch at a comfortable intensity level without experiencing voice breaks. Many geriatric patients

have reported that the tense vowel /i/ is easier to produce, noting that the lax vowels reveal excessive voice breaks. Mirror training was used to maintain the appropriate mouth opening during the vowel production. The tendency was to close the jaw at either end of the phonatory range. The mirror was also beneficial for minimizing visible tension in the face, jaw, neck, or shoulders.

Following ascension, the patient was asked to repeat the task, singing from midrange to the lowest comfortable pitch level. The patient was then asked to gradually extend her phonatory range while sustaining a variety of vowels.

The second task in phonatory training was singing, which combines respiratory and phonatory exercises. Songs that the patients enjoy and that are within their vocal range should be selected for practice. The patient can begin by substituting a single vowel for the lyrics to assist in monitoring the respiratory and phonatory patterns. When vowels are mastered, the lyrics can be sung. Again, mirror practice, as well as hand placement on the lower ribs or chest and abdomen, can benefit this technique. The goals developed for the other techniques should be combined during singing to produce phonation that has the appropriate respiratory support, has no voice breaks, is free of visible muscle tension, and maintains the appropriate open posture of the mouth.

Summary. Patient N was enrolled in therapy twice weekly for 3 weeks and then once weekly for 5 weeks. Therapy was initiated with relaxation and respiratory training, which were immediately used for practice. When these techniques were mastered in therapy, visual-auditory feedback and phonatory exercises became the focus of therapy. The patient received audiologic treatment by the second week of therapy and wore her hearing aids consistently following her appointment. She also followed the hydration procedures and felt that the twice-daily steaming was the most beneficial in managing the thick mucous secretions. Patient N noted significant improvement in her voice by the end of the 8th week of therapy. A voice reevaluation was repeated at that time. The posttherapy results are presented in Tables 4–6 and 4–7. All instrumental values improved from the initial evaluation, although the mean percent jitter and intraoral pressure values were above the normal limits. Vocal quality was mildly harsh following prolonged talking but considerably improved over the initial evaluation. Patient N was satisfied with her voice and was discharged from therapy. She was contacted 3 months later by telephone and reported that she continued with the steaming and phonatory exercises and had not noticed regression in her voice.

A major cause of glottal incompetence is vocal fold paralysis. Individual cases of paralysis can present quite differently, pending the type and site of nerve injury, time postonset, and the presence or absence of a compensatory supraglottal response. The case studies that follow reflect a variety of patient profiles and management techniques for vocal fold paralysis.

Unilateral Vocal Fold Paralysis in a Case with a Complex Medical History

Stephen C. McFarlane, PhD, and Shelley Von Berg, MS

Case Study: Patient O

Introduction

Injuries to the vagus nerve anywhere along its path from the medulla to insertion into the larynx inevitably result in paresis or paralysis of those muscles receiving innervation at or below the level of injury. The most frequently observed laryngeal paralysis experienced at this clinic and reported in the literature[6,7] is unilateral vocal fold paralysis (UVFP), with the involved fold fixed in the paramedian position, that is, halfway between the midline and lateral positions.

Unilateral paralyses usually are the result of severing or bruising of the recurrent laryngeal branch of the vagus, the branch responsible for efferent and afferent nerve supply to all of the intrinsic muscles of the larynx except for the cricothyroid muscle, which is innervated by the superior laryngeal branch. At times, the nature of the paralysis is unknown (ie, idiopathic paralysis). Viruses affecting the vagus nerve may be responsible for at least a portion of these idiopathic cases.

McFarlane, Holt-Romeo, Lavorato, and Warner[8] found that behavioral voice intervention produced superior voice quality in patients with unilateral vocal fold paralysis when compared with one group of patients who had received Teflon injections and another group who had undergone muscle-nerve reinnervation surgery. Another study[9] found that voice therapy was instrumental in reducing by half the excessive mean airflow rates in 16 individuals with UVFP. Thus, in the interim period between diagnosis of vocal fold paralysis and the final resolution of the problem, voice therapy has been demonstrated to be an effective intervention for helping many patients achieve normal or near normal voice quality and reducing air wastage.

Patient History

Patient O was a 35-year-old Native American woman, referred to our office by her otolaryngologist, with complaints of dysphagia and poor vocal quality. The patient presented with a complicated and lengthy medical history. Eleven years earlier, she noticed a slight bulge in the neck at the area of the thyroid gland. She underwent total thyroidectomy and partial neck dissection for Hashimoto's thyroiditis, combined with papillary carcinoma of the thyroid with metastasis to three regional lymph nodes. She underwent postoperative iodine 131-treatment. (Iodine is an essential micronutrient; 80% of the iodine present in the body is in the thyroid gland.) Over the years, Patient O underwent 12 additional surgeries to the neck area. Some surgeries involved recurrent tumor removal, but others involved laminectomies and Z-plasty. A number of surgeries involved placement of an electrical implant to reduce chronic pain.

Patient O had never smoked and reported no alcohol use. She drank one cup of caffeinated coffee each day and six glasses of water. A videofluoroscopic swallow examination administered 2 weeks earlier had shown a focal narrowing on the right side of the esophagus at about the level of C5 to C6; however, the course, caliber, and motility of the esophagus were reported to be normal. There was no diverticular formation, hiatal hernia, or mucosal abnormality.

When questioned about her vocal quality, Patient O said that it had deteriorated progressively with successive operations but worsened abruptly after a laminectomy 4 months earlier. She took a fatalistic approach to her dysphonia, stating that she had simply "gotten used to no voice." Speaking behaviors were characterized by a moderate-to-severe degree of neck tension. Routine questioning revealed that the patient was divorced and that her ex-husband had threatened to kidnap their young child. With a wry smile she admitted to having "an element of stress" in her life.

Voice Assessment

Upon examination, the voice was high in pitch, rough, strained, and breathy with phonation breaks and reduced intensity. Patient O said that she now considered this to be her typical voice. Sustained vowel production measured on the Visi-Pitch II (KayPENTAX) revealed a fundamental frequency of 274 Hz with jitter of 2.8% and shimmer of 2.8%. Jitter was considered abnormally elevated, indicating irregular frequency perturbations across vibratory cycles.[7] Fundamental frequency was at the high end of normal for females aged 30 to 40 years.[10]

A rigid endoscope was introduced transorally, and we studied the vocal fold activity by videostroboscopy. Anatomically, the larynx and surrounding structures, including the cricopharyngeal inlet and piriform sinuses bilaterally,

appeared normal. During phonation, the left vocal fold was fixed in the paramedian position. The left vocal fold moved slightly toward the midline during adduction, and a limited mucosal wave was observed for this fold. The reduced mucosal wave was partly responsible for the elevated jitter value and the harsh and breathy quality of the voice.

During vocal fold vibration, glottal closure was adequate for voice production. A glottal gap did exist from the flava to the posterior commissure, but the gap was judged to be less than 3 mm across, and vocal fold medialization was adequate for either contact at the midline or to take advantage of airflow dynamics to set the vocal folds into vibration. The right false vocal fold tended to creep toward the midline during phonation and impinge on the true vocal fold, further contributing to increased vibrational aperiodicity, jitter, and harsh, breathy vocal quality (Fig 4–1).

The Nagashima Phonatory Function Analyzer (Kelleher Medical, Richmond, VA) revealed unstimulated airflow measures of 138 mL/s at 220 Hz. These measures are within normal limits, but they were achieved with abnormally brief phonation times of 4 seconds.

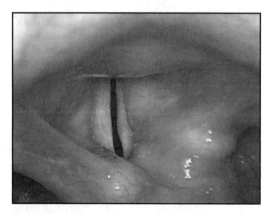

FIGURE 4–1. VF image pretreatment.

In summary, Patient O presented with a unilateral adductor paralysis of the left vocal fold, most likely associated with numerous surgical interventions for cancer of the thyroid gland on the left. Vocal pitch was high and squeaky, and volume was low. Vocal quality was harsh, strained, and breathy. Phonation times were abnormally brief. Endoscopy revealed incomplete vocal fold medialization and limited mucosal wave on the left vocal fold during phonation. Evidence of supraglottal involvement was also observed, characterized by excessive medialization of the right false fold, which was reported as a reactive hyperfunctional response to excessive transglottal airflow. Phonation times were brief, suggesting poor valving of subglottal air.

Swallow Assessment

Review of X-ray film from a barium swallow study confirmed a slight, focal esophageal stricture just below the upper esophageal sphincter. However, sequential X-ray views of swallow revealed adequate esophageal motility and emptying of the bolus into the stomach. No hiatal hernia, diverticular formations or reflux of gastric contents were appreciated. Patient O presented with a robust, volitional cough.

Oral-pharyngeal swallow was assessed via fiberoptic endoscopic evaluation of swallow. A 3-mm flexible endoscope was introduced transnasally and positioned at the base of the tongue. The patient was presented with consistencies of puree, mechanical soft, and solids. For all consistencies, she presented with hyperextensive neck and choking behaviors upon swallow. Hyperfunctional valving of the ventricular folds was appreciated immediately before the onset of swallow. Postswallow, Patient O reported a globus sensation. Nonetheless, oral-pharyngeal transit times were within normal limits and inspection of the hypopharynx postswallow revealed no bolus residue. Moderately thick and stringy mucus was observed at the level of the glottis, and it was suggested that this might be contributing to the globus sensation. Patient O was encouraged to increase water intake to 2 quarts per day to thin the mucus.

Swallow Intervention

Although Patient O presented with normal oral-pharyngeal function and esophageal motility upon swallow, her symptoms of dysphagia needed to be addressed. It is suspected that, over the years, repeated surgery and radiation to the pharynx and larynx had taken their toll and that the patient had gradually developed defensive postures during swallow, which in reality compromised a physiologically normal functioning system. Therefore, swallow strategies were employed to alleviate these defensive postures. Gentle pressure at the anterior aspect of the cricoid cartilage appeared to reduce the sensation of globus and enhance ease of swallow. It was suspected that this midline pressure ameliorated the effects of the stricture. By experimenting with various head turn techniques, it was discovered that the head turned right with chin tucked produced a swallow devoid of hyperextensive posturing. We experimented with several consistencies employing this technique, all which were swallowed with no complications. Patient O was encouraged by these results and was relieved to avoid esophageal dilation or further surgery for cricopharyngeal myotomy.

Voice Intervention

During the initial diagnostic session, it is our practice to devote as much time and effort at attempts to normalize the voice as to documenting the disorder. Therefore, after recording the nonstimulated acoustic, physiologic, and airflow measures of Patient O's voice productions, we introduced facilitating techniques to attempt to improve the voice and acoustic measures. In the case of this patient, we had a dual, simultaneous task: to remove the hyperfunctional component while stimulating the best vocal quality possible by altering glottal activity and phonatory mode.

We normally introduce several facilitating techniques in the first session as the patient invariably responds better to some techniques than to others. In this case, we introduced the following as described in Boone and McFarlane:[11]

- head turning
- lateral digital manipulation of the thyroid cartilage
- half-swallow boom
- facial tone focus with nasal-liquid-glide stimuli
- pitch shifts
- inhalation phonation
- tongue protrusion /i/

(Please refer to Case O Appendix A for complete descriptions of these facilitating techniques.)

Techniques for Establishing Improved Vocal Fold Medialization. Initially, we instructed Patient O to produce half-swallow boom to appreciate the fact that she could generate a stronger voice. We explained that the "boom" is produced "on top of the swallow" to take advantage of the already closed nature of the

vocal folds during the swallowing act. Next, we had her turn her head to one side and then to the other as we gently placed pressure to either side of the thyroid cartilage. Head turned right with pressure to the left thyroid lamina produced the best vocal quality with the strongest vocal intensity and longest phonation time. Patient O was encouraged to develop a kinesthetic sense of the "sound" and "feel" of vocal fold approximation as she slowly brought her head back to midline in steps. Pitch shifts up and down using extended nasal-liquid-glide stimuli were also probed. Patient O produced the strongest intensity with the best vocal quality when phonating between 260 Hz and 300 Hz. During all of the stimulation techniques, the patient's attention was directed to self-monitor airflow, laryngeal configuration, vocal quality, and duration of phonation, as well as to general vocal effort required for phonation.

Reducing Hyperfunctional Behaviors. Throughout therapy, Patient O was gently admonished when she tried to "push" the voice out. We explained that pushing the voice simply tightens the larynx "like a purse-string" and overimpounds subglottal air by bringing the false vocal folds into play. We explained that only by relaxing the system and placing the resonating focus in the nasal and lip area does the voice quality improve with the least effort. Face or "nasal" focus began with sustained nasals, extending to nasal laden phrases (such as *Miami millionaire, man on the moon*).[12] Patient O was stimulable for the auditory and visual feedback displayed on the Visi-Pitch II monitor. Originally, we instructed her to produce the stimuli with the horizontal pitch bars set at 250 Hz to 300 Hz. Slowly, we narrowed the space between the pitch bars until she established good vocal quality at a range of 200 Hz to 240 Hz.

In addition to focus and nasals, tongue protrusion /i/ and inhalation phonation were two techniques highly effective in reducing hyperfunctional behaviors.[11] Tongue protrusion /i/ entails protruding the tongue slightly beyond the lips while producing /mimimi/ in a high pitch. The forward movement of the tongue pulls its root out of the pharynx and opens the laryngeal aditus. The tongue is gradually retracted back inside the mouth and bilabial phonemes (buy baby a bib) and alveolars (tea for two, taking time to talk) are targeted while the improved tone is established.

Inhalation phonation is usually better demonstrated than explained. It involves production of a high-pitched, gentle phonation on inspiration, similar to the sound one might make when caught by surprise (a sharp inhalatory gasp). The high-pitched vocalization produced on inhalation is always produced by true vocal fold vibration, thus eliminating involvement of supraglottal structures. The inhalation is followed by an exhalation equal in vocal intensity and quality but shorter in duration. Duration of the exhalatory phase is gradually extended over the course of therapy until it is lengthier than the inspiratory phase. The pitch of the inhalations is eventually lowered to within normal limits and

productions extend to nonsense syllables and then short phrases.

By session three Patient O's conversational voice was still slightly reduced in intensity, yet the hyperfunctional behaviors, elevated pitch, and phonation breaks had been eliminated (Table 4–8). Acoustic measures using a sustained /i/ on the Visi-Pitch II revealed 243 Hz with jitter of .67% and shimmer of 1.35%. All measures were within normal limits. Maximum phonation time had more than doubled to 9 seconds, indicating enhanced control of transglottal airflow without hyperfunctional overlay (Table 4–9). Rigid videoendoscopy revealed improved vocal fold contact at the midline and normal mucosal wave bilaterally. No ventricular fold hypertrophy was evident (Fig 4–2). Patient O said that she was thrilled with her "new voice," notably because of the improved intensity while retaining quality and the effortless manner in which she was able to speak over the telephone.

Home Program

A videotape featuring Patient O performing the facilitating techniques during the final voice session was made. She was encouraged to view it along with her written home voice program issued by this clinic. The home voice program specified all of the techniques introduced

Table 4–8. Perceptual Measures Pre- and Posttherapy for Patient O

	Pretherapy	*Posttherapy*
Pitch	High and squeaky	Slightly elevated
Vocal quality	Strained, rough, breathy	Fully voiced, pleasant
Loudness	Reduced, soft	Adequate for conversational speech and telephone

Table 4–9. Acoustic Measures Pre- and Posttherapy for Patient O

	Pretherapy	Posttherapy
F_0 (Hz)	274	243
Jitter	2.8%	.67%
Shimmer	2.85%	1.35%
Phonation Time	4 sec	9 sec

Normal values for jitter and shimmer are approximately .80% and 3.8%, respectively.[11] Mean F_0 for women aged 30 to 40 years is 196 Hz and mean phonation times for adult women is 21.34 sec.[10]

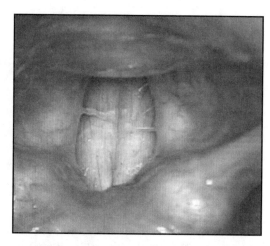

FIGURE 4–2. VF image posttreatment.

above and their rationales. Swallow issues were again addressed, and it was re-emphasized that hypopharyngeal and cricopharyngeal motility was normal, as established by earlier barium and FEES studies. Counseling involved positioning strategies that Patient O found helpful in the clinic environment.

Patient O Appendix A
Facilitation Techniques at a Glance

Half-Swallow Boom

Rationale

Swallow produces as much closure of the glottis and supralaryngeal structures as is physiologically possible. "Boom" is an all-voiced word that is easily produced because air is released from the constricted larynx. Oral opening is minimal, which produces back pressure on the larynx.

Procedure

- Instruct client to swallow and interrupt swallow with "boom."
- Play back louder, stronger voice to client for feedback.
- Instruct client to produce technique with head turned and chin lowered, which essentially "fixes" the desired position of head and neck for optimum voice.
- When best "boom" is produced, transition to longer phrases "boom-one," "boom-me." Gradually phase out the swallow and then the boom. Slowly bring head back to midline and chin up to normal position.

Head Turn

Rationale

Often used with half-swallow boom. A change in head position away from the paralyzed side may improve vocal quality and airflow by stretching the paralyzed vocal fold in an A-P manner, thus improving vocal fold contact at midline. Conversely, head turn to the side of the paralyzed vocal fold has been observed to shorten the effected vocal fold, thus enhancing the extent of the mucosal wave and resulting in improved vibration and better glottal valving.

Procedure

- Instruct patient to slowly turn head first to one side and then to the other side while prolonging vowels /i/, /ɪ/, /ɛ/, /e/, /o/, or /u/ while listening for improved vocal quality, intensity, and airflow.
- When optimum quality is achieved, head is kept in the new position while the client practices nonsense syllables employing vowels and nasal glides. Patient is encouraged to kinesthetically appreciate this new configuration of the vocal folds, as well as attend to the auditory feedback of the improved voice. Nonsense syllables are extended to short phrases and sentences.
- The head is gradually returned to midline while retaining the optimum vocal quality.

Digital Manipulation

Rationale

Often used with half-swallow boom and head turning. Gentle lateral digital pressure to the thyroid cartilage on the affected side helps to medialize the paralyzed vocal fold and improve vocal fold vibration. Likewise, digital pressure to the nonaffected side helps medialize the nonparalyzed fold across the midline, again improving vocal fold vibration.

Procedure

- Instruct client to sustain a vowel while clinician gently applies pressure to the thyroid cartilage, first in one direction, then the other. Continue to manipulate until optimum vocal quality and intensity are achieved.
- When optimum pressure and direction are achieved, instruct client to produce nonsense syllables using voiced phonemes. Extend nonsense syllables to short phrases and sentences.
- Patient is encouraged to kinesthetically appreciate the enhanced vocal fold configuration. Slowly withdraw digital pressure while client retains optimum vocal quality. Patients can also be taught to apply digital pressure to their own thyroid cartilage.

Focus

Rationale

Patients with UVFP often place undue emphasis on the larynx when attempting to phonate. They believe that if they valve more forcefully at the level of the glottis, the voice will emerge stronger. This approach tends to excessively increase glottal and supraglottal resistance during phonation, thus the voice is produced in a strained and strangled manner. Although the voice may indeed be louder, it is almost always rougher in vocal quality with a higher noise-to-harmonic ratio.

The goal of the focus approach is to transfer the patient's focus on the energy of the voice from the larynx to the nose, cheek, and lips. Nasal or facial focus eliminates overvalving at the glottis and supraglottis, thus opening the aditus for enhanced vocal resonance.

Procedure

- The clinician demonstrates focus by placing fingers lightly at the bridge of the nose and gently humming. The patient is instructed to follow the clinician's model. The patient is instructed to feel the amplitude of the clinician's facial focus by placing a finger on the clinician's face and at the same time compare the "buzz" produced by the clinician with his or her own "buzz."
- Once the patient's facial focus amplitude is similar to that of the clinician, the patient is instructed to produce chant talk employing nasals, liquids, and glides ("Miami millionaire"). The patient is encouraged to feel the tingle of vibration in the lips, nose, and cheeks.
- Maintaining focus, the patient is instructed to produce longer phrases using voiced stops.
- After the patient has some success in placing the voice in the face, discuss with the patient the imagery of what is happening to produce good voice.
- Auditory feedback and self-monitoring are highly effective during each phase of this technique.

Pitch Shift with Nasals-Liquids-Glides

Rationale

A shift in pitch either higher or lower than the patient's baseline pitch often will alter the vocal fold configuration sufficiently to trigger better vocal quality. Sliding the pitch up to a slightly higher frequency may help elongate the paralyzed vocal fold, thus enhancing vibration. Likewise, a lower pitch may increase the mucosal wave for the paralyzed vocal fold, again enhancing vibration. An added bonus is a growing awareness on the part of the client that he or she is able to manipulate the vocal fold configuration at will and thus alter the voice.

Procedure

■ Instruct the patient to gently hum up and down the scale, listening for any improvement in vocal quality. When improvement is identified, extend humming to nonsense nasal productions maintaining the desired pitch.

■ Using either a keyboard or a visual feedback instrument (such as the Visi-Pitch from KayPENTAX to monitor pitch), instruct the patient to produce nasal, glide, and liquid productions, generalizing to short phrases. Be sure to establish a range of at least three keyboard notes within which the patient may vary the pitch.

■ Record and play back for the patient various oral reading and conversational samples, analyzing vocal quality at the new pitch range.

Tongue Protrusion /i/

Rationale

The tongue, when protruded, pulls its root out of the pharynx and opens the laryngeal aditus. The production of voice with the tongue protruded is sufficiently novel to break poor habituated vocal habits, such as hyperfunction.

Procedure

■ The clinician models tongue protrusion while producing a high pitched /i/. The jaw is relaxed and open. Patient follows suit. If the patient demonstrates reservation with this technique, explain that it is simply a means to an end, and the tongue will soon be retracted.

■ When patient is comfortable with tongue protrusion /i/, instruct the patient to produce /mimimi/, slowly drawing the tongue back into the mouth.

■ Continue with other voiced bilabials in nonsense syllables, chant talk, short phrases, and sentences. Slowly reduce pitch to normal.[12]

Inhalation Phonation

Rationale

Hyperfunctional behavior secondary to UVFP often indicates the patient has adopted an unhealthy laryngeal configuration or "set" that she or he cannot break. The high-pitch vocalization produced on inhalation phonation is always produced by the true vocal folds. Therefore, patients who develop an odd and inappropriate form of phonation, such as ventricular phonation, are surprised, and usually delighted, to hear true vocal fold phonation with this technique.

Procedure

■ The clinician demonstrates this technique by initiating a gentle intake of air at a high pitch (similar to a gasp of surprise). The inhalation is extended for 1 to 2 seconds, and the exhalation, produced at the same pitch, is relatively short. The patient follows the clinician's model.

■ When the patient is successful with long inhalation and short exhalation, transition to an inhalation followed by longer exhalation that extends from falsetto register to chest register (similar to an extended sigh).

■ If the patient is able to follow these steps, record and play-back the productions, noting how easily the vocal folds are coming together for good voice.

■ Stay at the single-word level until normal voicing is established.

Unilateral Vocal Fold Paralysis Following Complications from a Total Thyroidectomy

Mara Behlau, PhD, Gisele Oliveria, MSc, and Osíris Brasil, MD

Case Study: Patient P

The following case is that of a 72-year-old lawyer with unilateral vocal fold paralysis. In the study, the authors explore the best voice production; changing of the vocal gesture/posture while reinforcing laryngeal mechanics through an active vocal exercise program.

Patient History

Patient P was a 72-year-old retired Appeals Court Judge. At the time of presentation to our clinic, he was working as a professional writer. The patient had recently undergone a total thyroidectomy for papillary thyroid carcinoma. On the first postoperative day, the patient had a spontaneous left cervical hematoma that was treated clinically. At that time, his voice was normal, and an examination showed normal vocal fold mobility. At postoperative day 30, the patient presented to our office for a voice consultation, reporting progressive dysphonia for 15 days. He indicated that his voice had become weaker and lower in recent weeks.

Patient P's medical history included a myocardial infarction in the remote past (>20 years previous). He exhibited good respiration and no report of auditory problems. He denied smoking and alcohol consumption and stated that he had healthy dietary habits. He denied sleep disturbances and other psychiatric problems, such as depression.

Patient P was an extraverted, talkative man who was engaged in multiple social activities. He was a prized poet, novelist, and composer. He considered communication to be one of his main competencies.

History of the Problem

Patient P was referred to the otolaryngologist after a cardiac checkup had pointed out a thyroid lesion. His voice was normal at that time. Laryngeal examination showed mobile vocal folds with complete glottic closure. A total thyroidectomy was performed on January 22. At the first postoperative day (12 hours after the procedure), the patient presented with a spontaneous cervical hematoma, a rare complication probably associated with the surgical intervention.[13,14] Swelling in the neck area was treated with a bedside hematoma evacuation. No respiratory distress, pain, dysphagia or dysphonia occurred. A laryngeal exam performed on the third day postsurgery showed normal laryngeal mobility. On day 15 postsurgery, the patient noticed that his voice was somewhat softer than usual, but he did not bring this concern to anyone's attention. In the days that followed, the symptoms worsened, and the patient noticed increasing shortness of breath. A new consultation revealed a left vocal fold paralysis. The affected fold was bowed and positioned in the paramedian position. Glottic closure was incomplete. Speech-language pathology recommended primary management through voice rehabilitation (conservative treatment). This would be followed by surgical intervention, if needed. Because of the patient's high vocal demand, however, the otolaryngologist advised the patient to undergo thyroplasty type I.[15]

Evaluation Procedures

Patient P received a standard battery of vocal function testing. These assessments included:

- Auditory perceptual analysis using the Consensus Auditory Perceptual Evaluation-Voice (CAPE-V) protocol, Brazilian Portuguese Version[16];
- Visual perceptual analysis with videostroboscopy to assess vibratory pattern of the vocal fold and size of glottal gap;
- Vocal self-assessment using the Voice-Related Quality of Life (V-RQOL)[17] to understand the patient's perspective of the vocal problem;
- Acoustic analysis of sustained vowel and sentence productions to assess frequency, perturbation, and range;
- Laryngeal electromyography (electrophysiologic examination) to confirm the neurologic lesion

1. Auditory Perceptual. In cases of vocal fold paralysis, the degree of vocal impairment is partially related to the position of the paralyzed fold and the degree of muscle atrophy.[18] Patient P's voice quality was assessed perceptually by the speech-language pathologist during the evaluation session using the three speech tasks of the adapted Brazilian Portuguese version of the CAPE-V[16]: sustained vowels, selected sentences, and conversational speech ("Tell me about your voice problem."). Scoring was as follows: moderate overall severity of dysphonia (52/100), mild degree of roughness (26/100), moderate degree of breathiness (47/100) and no noticeable tension (0/100). Modal pitch was judged to be mild low (24/100) for his gender and age, and loudness was judged as moderately reduced (46/100). Asthenia was marked as an additional feature of the voice concern and was rated as a mild to moderate deviation (35/100). Occasional phonatory breaks were also observed. No diplophonia was noticed. Resonance was normal. All voice attributes were consistently present at the assessment session.

2. Visual Perceptual. Patient P had a normal laryngeal evaluation pre- and immediately postsurgery, as well as at the time of his first follow-up consultation. A month after the surgical intervention, Mr. P presented with left vocal fold immobility with bowing. Vocal processes were at the same horizontal plane. A reliable image of vocal fold mucosal vibration was obtained, reinforcing that there was a small phonatory gap.[19] Supraglottic constriction was observed, with a moderate displacement of right ventricular fold. Vocal rehabilitation was then started and the patient was warned about the possibility of surgery to compensate the deficit. Mr. P stated that he preferred voice therapy over an additional surgical procedure, even though the therapy option might suggest a longer period of rehabilitation.

3. Self-Assessment Protocol. The self-assessment of the voice problem was performed using the validated version of the V-RQOL.[17] The total score was 82; physical score was 75, and socioemotional was 93. Lower ratings in the total score and physical score areas clearly showed the nature of the problem.[17,20] Two aspects were particularly deviated per patient report: difficulties in speaking loud and problems at work due to the voice. In the socioemotional domain, the patient identified strongly with only one statement, "I am less extroverted due to my voice problem," an indication that the patient was changing his natural communication habits due to the dysphonia.

4. Acoustic Analysis.

Acoustic measures were obtained from sustained vowel /ae/ using the software Vox-Metria 2.5 (CTS). The main features are summarized on Table 4–10. Jitter, irreg-ularity, and noise component were evidently deviated. The phonatory deviation diagram[21] showed a spread distribution with a predominance of the irregularity axis (Fig 4–3). Spectrographic trace (Fig 4–4) showed predominance of the noise component and irregularity of trace (FonoView 1.0, CTS) as well as

Table 4–10. Acoustic Measures for Patient P at the Assessment Session, After 2 Months and After 6 Months (VoxMetria 2.5, CTS)

Parameters	Assessment Session	After 2 mo	After 6 mo	Normal Values
Habitual fundamental frequency	105 Hz	102.75	114 Hz	80 to 150 Hz
Jitter (PPQ)	0.84	0.27	0.11	0 to 0.6
Shimmer (EPQ)	5.84	5.01	3.23	0 to 6.5
Irregularity	5.78	4.77	3.63	0 to 4.75
GNE (Glottal to noise excitation ratio)	0.35	0.64	0.95	0.5 to 1.0

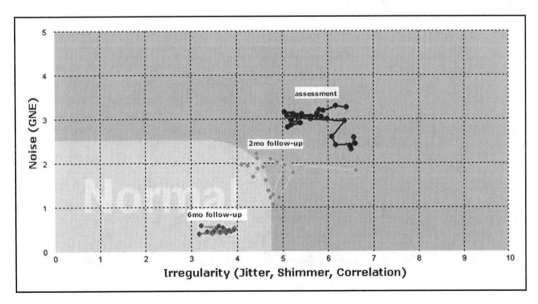

FIGURE 4–3. Phonatory deviation diagram: upper plotting (assessment), middle plotting (after 2 mo therapy) and bottom plotting (after 6 mo therapy); light gray area in lower left corner represents the range of normal (VoxMetria 2.5, CTS).

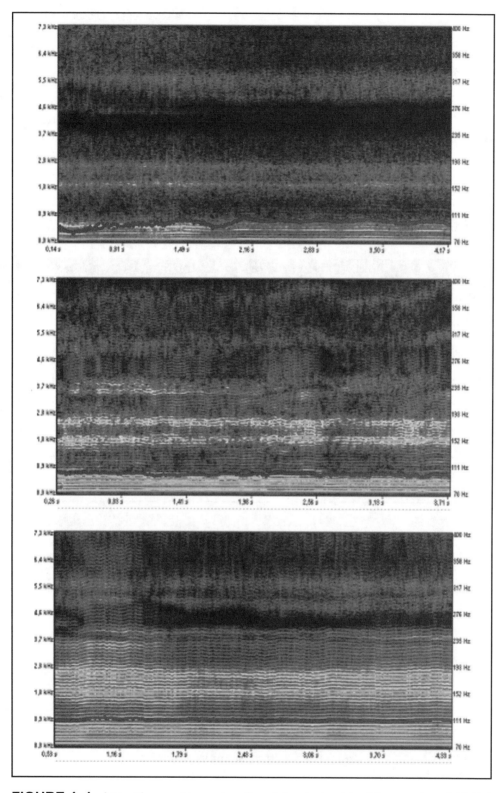

FIGURE 4–4. Acoustic spectrography of sustained vowel /ae/ (narrow band 40 Hz) at assessment (*top*), after 2 months of therapy (*middle*), and after 6 monthys of therapy (*bottom*). (FonoView 1.0, CTS).

unstable fundamental frequency. Maximum phonation time for vowel /ae/ was reduced at 7 seconds. The intensity was estimated from a digital decibel sound pressure level (Realistic, RadioShack) with measurements obtained at 1 meter from the mouth: habitual intensity was 56 dB, minimum 50 dB and maximum 64 dB, measures which clearly show limitations regarding the habitual and maximum values. The phonatory range of 7 semitones was notably reduced.

5. Laryngeal EMG. Electromyography is used to assist in the diagnosis of laryngeal nerves paralysis.[22] In the case of Mr. P, the eletromyography exam was performed 5½ months following the total thyroidectomy. Results showed normal electrical activity of both superior laryngeal nerves and the right recurrent nerve. The left recurrent nerve had reduced activity with signs of acute denervation and reinnervation.

Description and Rationale for Therapy Approach

Postthyroidectomy Vocal Fold Paralysis. Vocal fold paralysis is probably the most frequent neurological problem seen in a voice clinic. The incidence of recurrent laryngeal nerve injury after thyroid surgery is reported to be from 2% to 7% despite a macroscopically intact nerve during the procedure.[23–26] Immobility secondary to thyroid surgery can be transient or permanent and can be due to stretching, traction, compression, ligature entrapment, hematoma, thermal injury, electrical injury, and severing injury.[25] Its presentation can vary significantly, and symptoms can include problems of voicing, breathing, swallowing, airway protection, and proprioception some of which are described below.

Dysphonia resulting from a unilateral paralysis after thyroid surgery is flaccid in nature and relatively constant. The position of paralyzed fold and edge configuration are important in defining vocal rehabilitation. The closer the vocal fold rests to the midline and the straighter the edge, the better the prognosis for improvement with vocal exercise. Potential compensations that may complicate the rehabilitation process include: a shift to falsetto register, vestibular fold interference, tension in the neck, and muscle tension dysphonia. Lack of airway protection is the major concern and should have a central attention during assessment. Other consequences of glottic incompetence are a sensation of breathing problems (with compensatory tachypnea), difficulties with body stabilization in physical activities, and phonatory restrictions such as soft voice, lack of voice projection, limitations in loud voice reading, vocal fatigue, singing restrictions, effortful phonation, intermittent laryngospasms, globus sensation, and nonspecific hoarseness.[27,28] The otolaryngologist and speech-language pathologist must work as a team in the management of vocal fold paralysis, as voice therapy alone or surgery alone may prove ineffective in improving the voice to the desired level.

Treatment Options and Recovery Patterns. The decision for surgical or conservative (ie, behavioral) intervention is driven by patient perception of vocal handicap and the expectations of both the physician and speech-language pathologist regarding potential treatment outcomes.[27] Patients should see the speech-language pathologist soon after the otolaryngologist has diagnosed the paralysis to begin voice rehabilitation. If voice production improves, the patient may be dismissed from therapy. On the other hand, if improvement is not observed, the patient may be referred back for further surgical management.[29] In many cases, therapy alone can result in reasonable improvement in patients with unilateral vocal fold paralysis and eliminate the need for surgical intervention.[30]

Our patient did not present with any swallowing difficulties except for occasional difficulty when drinking liquids too quickly. Thus, swallowing was not a primary clinical concern. The client did evidence a degree of respiratory instability and a sensation of not having enough air to speak. The patient was reassured by the speech-language pathologist that he was getting an adequate amount of air during quiet breathing, and his concerns over the status of his breathing were lessened.

Usually spontaneous recovery can be obtained in 4 to 6 months after paralysis; however, in some rare cases recovery has been reported up to 3 years postinjury. When there is no aspiration, vocal rehabilitation is the primary target of treatment. Surgery usually is performed only after vocal rehabilitation failure.

Goals of Therapy

The general goal of vocal rehabilitation is to reduce aspiration, to improve voice, and to avoid negative compensation (diplophonia, vestibular phonation, paralytic falsetto). The rehabilitation program is an active process, and it requires a cooperative patient. The use of a variety of exercises, different vocal adjustment attempts, and good self-monitoring are some ingredients of successful therapy.

The immediate goal after the assessment session is to explore vocal possibilities and to obtain the best possible voice, usually with a softer voice, frontal resonance, and a higher pitch being preferred. Maximum phonation time assessment can help as a predictor of success; a minimum of 4 seconds is usually required to have chances of positive results with vocal rehabilitation.

There are three basic steps in the vocal rehabilitation for unilateral vocal fold paralysis: (1) to reduce transglottic airflow; (2) to increase vocal fold flexibility; and (3) to increase glottic resistance. Treatment for each of these goals is presented below.

Goal 1. To reduce transglottic airflow

Rationale. Reducing transglottic airflow is an appropriate goal when the patient uses large amounts of air during speech. Patients with vocal fold paralysis show glottic incompetence and difficulties in controlling the air during phonation. This automatic attempt to increase vocal effectiveness may actually work only to exacerbate the loss of air and worsen the vocal problem.[18] Several strategies can be used to help the patient to learn a new physiologic setting. For instance, facilitating sounds (ie, prolonged nasal bilabial "m . . ." or labiodental "n . . .") or glottal attack training may help to produce a sharp onset of vocalization, thereby, reducing airflow. In some cases, postural changes, with the head displaced to the contralateral side of the paralysis can help as well. In the present case, Patient P was instructed to turn his head to the right and to train repeated short "m" followed by repeated short syllables with the same vowel ("ma, ma, ma, ma" and "me, me, me, me" and "mi, mi, mi, mi"), first one syllable per breath, then increasing the number of units per breath group. If the patient presents a hypertonic compensatory muscle involvement, laryngeal manipulation should be used to reduce negative interference.

Goal 2. To increase vocal fold flexibility

Rationale. When the air leakage is not too high and the glottic chink is little, vocal fold flexibility is the main goal. Some patients with the vocal fold paralyzed at median position may not need to address Goal 1 as described above and can move directly into this goal. Several strategies can be used such as modulated sounds (with nasal "m" or voiced fricatives "z" and "v"—it is important to highlight that these latter sounds require a better control) or small and large interval glissandi. After some frequency displacement control has been achieved, larger gaps can be introduced, even using register shifts, such as vocal fry versus high pitch exercises. Several facilitating sounds such as nasal and voiced fricatives are recommended before vowels.

Goal 3. To increase glottic resistance

Rationale. Glottic resistance exercises are used when the voice is acceptable, yet an element of vocal fatigue remains. In this situation, there is usually complete glottic closure but with a short closure quotient. For achieving this goal, mild effort techniques, such as interlocking hands and prolonged sound production can be used. Maximum phonation time exercises can be of great help. A short version of Vocal Function Exercises (VFE)[31] can be administered and it is usually a good conditioning program for concluding the rehabilitation process. Another option is the Lee Silverman Voice Treatment-LSVTR®,[32] a program that shares some of the basic principles of the VFE. In the present case, interlocking hands and sustained vowel production was very important as fundamental frequency was instable.

After mastering this task the patient was submitted to a 2-week VFE program, with positive results.

Summary of Rehabilitation Procedures

Dysphonia was the primary concern of Patient P and the central focus of the treatment. The role of therapy as the primary resource for treating patients with unilateral vocal fold paralysis or a coadjutant of surgery has not been well established,[27] but it is usually seen as beneficial.[28,30,33] The rationale for this case was to reduce translaryngeal airflow, to increase vocal fold flexibility and to enhance glottic resistance. Patient P was highly collaborative and adherent to all requested procedures. For the first 2 weeks this therapy regimen was twice a week with five short sessions of exercises at home. For the following 2 months the patient was seen on a weekly basis and then every 2 weeks. At the close of therapy, all acoustic parameters had shifted to the normal range, and maximum phonation time had clearly increased. During the beginning of rehabilitation the patient quickly learned to change his voice setting to a low loudness, front focus and higher pitch production to appear less dysphonic. The use of short sentences helped him to reduce the sensation of having respiratory distress. The positive outcome was enough to avoid any surgical intervention for the present time.

Results of Therapy

1. Auditory Perceptual. Patient P's voice quality after therapy displayed the following CAPE-V scores: consistently negligible overall severity of dysphonia (13/100), with the same amount of roughness (15/100) and just noticeable degree of breathiness (3/100). Modal pitch and loudness were judged as normal (0/100). Asthenia was not present anymore (0/100). Phonatory breaks were not observed on any task.

2. Visual Perceptual.

A second evaluation was scheduled after 2 months of a series of weekly sessions (8 sessions). On this occasion, the glottal gap was reduced; however, the left vocal fold was still immobile. Voice had a marked improvement, and patient decided to continue with vocal rehabilitation. After 4 months, a new visual evaluation was performed, the gap was minimal, voice production was comfortable, and left vocal fold paralysis remained unaltered. A new control examination after 6 months showed an unaltered image. When reinnervation occurs, it typically is not observed before a 4-month period.[34] It is important to highlight that morphofunctional analysis of the larynx cannot be directly related to treatment results of patients with unilateral vocal fold paralysis. The patient's voice was adapted after rehabilitation despite the vocal fold immobility.[28]

3. Self-Assessment Protocol.

The V-RQOL was administered again after therapy and results showed a remarkable improvement for the total score increased from 82.5% to 100% which clearly showed that there was no impact of the voice on any aspect of the patient's related-communication quality of life. The patient did not show any perception of vocal handicap. A recent study that investigated the effect of voice rehabilitation on 40 subjects with unilateral vocal fold paralysis found significant improvement only in voice quality and quality of life,[30] which reinforces the importance of investigating such aspects.

4. Acoustic Analysis.

Measures taken after 2 months of a series of weekly vocal rehabilitation sessions showed improvement on jitter, shimmer, irregularity and noise component (see Table 4–10). The phonatory deviation diagram (The Gottingen Diagram) showed a closer to normal area distribution (see Fig 4–3). Spectrographic trace (see Fig 4–4) showed higher number of harmonics, but the trace was very irregular (FonoView 1.0, CTS), as was fundamental frequency. After 6 months, the harmonic component had markedly improved (even with some instability), and fundamental frequency trace was more straightforward. Maximum phonation time for vowel /ae/ increased up to almost 16 seconds, allowing normal connected speech at conversational level. The new dynamic range was expanded (dB meter, Realistic, RadioShack) and values were closer to normal; the habitual intensity was 62 dB, minimum 50 dB and maximum 98 dB. Phonatory range seemed to show the most marked improvement in the acoustical analysis, changing from 7 semitones to 24; interestingly, at the assessment session just these few semitones were produced with voicing and as soon as the patient reduced the breathy component the range started to widen. Finally, although number of semitones is not a popular acoustic measure, it does appear to be a good outcome measure for vocal fold paralysis cases.[28]

Conclusions

Vocal fold paralysis after cancer surgery can be seen at the voice clinic, and it is not unusual. However, this patient did not present with vocal fold paralysis soon after the procedure. He showed a rare case of cervical hematoma during the first 24 hours following surgery and the signs and symptoms of laryngeal recurrent paralysis started only after 15 days. Patient P was submitted to vocal rehabilitation, and in spite of only a partial and minimal restoring of laryngeal movement (mainly at the arytenoid cartilage level), vocal function was considered normal, and the patient was fully satisfied with the results. Follow-up was recommended in this case, as the patient was 72 years old and the potential for presbyphonia negatively influencing the rehabilitated voice existed. Moreover, there was a possibility that his laryngeal nerve injury was transient and that the voice would improve further with time.

Although some cases of unilateral vocal fold paralysis have clearly identifiable etiologies, such as those presented above, a significant proportion of paralysis cases are of unknown origin. In the studies that follow, Julie Barkmeier-Kramer and Joe Stemple offer management ideas for individuals with idiopathic paralysis.

Management of Idiopathic Unilateral Vocal Fold Paralysis

Julie Barkmeier-Kraemer, PhD, CCC-SLP

Case Study: Patient Q

Patient History. Ms. Q is a 79-year-old female with onset of voice loss 12 months prior to her voice evaluation. She reported sudden onset of hoarseness associated with an upper respiratory infection. A local otolaryngologist evaluated her 11 months postonset and diagnosed her with left-sided vocal fold paralysis. Subsequently, a CT scan and MRI exam-

ination of the head, neck, and chest areas were completed to rule out the presence of a tumor. Normal findings were reported for both exams. The otolaryngologist recommended Ms. Q consider trial voice therapy prior to surgical intervention due to the medial location of the immobile vocal fold and signs of excessive laryngeal muscle tension during voicing.

Ms. Q underwent a speech-language pathology voice evaluation that included a case history, completion of the Vocal Handicap Index (VHI)[35] and Voice-Related Quality of Life (V-RQOL),[17] examination of the oral mechanism, perceptual evaluation of phonatory-respiratory coordination and voice quality, acoustic and aerodynamic measures, flexible endoscopy, and rigid videostroboscopic recordings.

In addition to information provided from the otolaryngologist's report, Ms. Q confirmed a history of smoking off and on in the past, completely quitting this habit 8 years ago. Her husband also quit smoking 8 years ago. Ms. Q indicated that she did not experience any swallowing problems since onset of her voice problems. However, she noticed an increase in the occurrence of reflux over the past year. She generally eats her dinner 4 to 5 hours prior to bedtime and eats the lunch provided daily at her living complex. Due to a family history of diabetes, she avoids drinking juices and other sugar drinks. Ms. Q reported that she drinks 3 cups of caffeinated beverage daily, 2 to 3 cups of water, and infrequent glasses of wine. She also reported attending an exercise class on a daily basis and sleeping 8 to 9 hours nightly. Ms. Q denied taking any prescription medications at this time, but occasionally takes Tums when she experiences heartburn.

Ms. Q reported her voice quality to be consistent throughout the day. However, she complained of a sensation of strain in her throat and fatigue after prolonged periods of talking beyond 20 minutes. On a scale from 1 (worst voice could be) to 10 (best voice), she rated her voice as a "5" at the time of the voice evaluation. Normally, Ms. Q is a socially active person. She reported that friends had difficulty hearing her during meals, at social events, or in places where there is background noise such that friends appear to avoid talking to her at these times. Consequently, the voice problem makes it difficult for Ms. Q to converse or interact normally. It is also difficult for her to talk on the telephone due to difficulty projecting her voice and because she is embarrassed by her voice quality that she described as sounding like a hoarse "Mickey Mouse." During the interview, Ms. Q was noted to inhale, exhale, and then initiate speaking. Speech rate and phrasing were judged as normal. However, air replenishment occurred after phrase breaks rather than after completion of a sentence.

Hearing Screening. A pure-tone hearing screening was conducted to rule out hearing loss as a contributing factor to Ms. Q's communication problem. She was asked to raise her hand when she heard the testing tones in each ear. Tones were presented to each ear using a 40 dB HL tone at 1000, 2000, and 4000 Hz. She successfully passed this screening for both ears.

VHI and V-RQOL Questionnaires. The Vocal Handicap Index (VHI)[35] and Voice-Related Quality of Life (V-RQOL)[17] were administered to determine the degree of impact Ms. Q's voice problem had on her daily life. The VHI examines three areas of interest identified as functional, physical, and emotional. Ten statements are associated with each domain such as, "My voice makes it difficult for people to hear me," or "I run out of air when I talk," or "I am tense when talking to others because of my voice." The individual must rate each statement on a four-point scale (0 = "never" and 4 = "always") indicating the degree to which each statement applies to them. A total score of 120 is the worst possible score, whereas a score of 0 is the best possible. Ms. Q's total score on the VHI was 62/120 points, with a functional subscore of 23/40, a physical subscore of 30/40, and an emotional subscore of 9/40. Thus, Ms. Q does not exhibit a great deal of emotional impact from her voice problem. However, the physical and functional subscores suggest a moderate to severe impairment due to her voice problem. Thus, Ms. Q's score on the VHI indicated an overall moderate vocal handicap due to her voice disorder.

The V-RQOL is similar to the VHI in that it presents 10 statements that the individual must rate on a 5-point scale (1 = "none, not a problem" and 5 = problem is as "bad as it can be"). Items 4, 5, 8, and 10 represent the Social-Emotional Domain and items 1, 2, 3, 6, 7, and 9 represent the Physical Functioning Domain. Standard scores are determined for each subgroup as well as for the total score. The goal of this scale is to learn how the individual's voice problem interferes with day-to-day activities. Similar to her scores on the VHI, Ms. Q demonstrated a mild impact in the Social-Emotional Domain (standard score of 75) and a moderate to severe impact in the Physical Functioning Domain (standard score of 37.5). Her total score was a 52.5, representing a voice disorder having an overall moderate impact on her day-to-day activities.

Perceptual Examination. The Consensus Auditory-Perceptual Evaluation of Voice (CAPE-V)[36] is a perceptual rating scale of an individual's voice completed by the clinician across various speaking tasks. These include sustained phonation of /a/ and /i/ for 3 to 5 seconds, sentence repetition, and spontaneous conversation in response to the request, "Tell me about your voice problem." or "Tell me how your voice is functioning." The clinician judges the client's voice in terms of overall severity, roughness, breathiness, strain, pitch, loudness using a 100-mm visual analog scale generally categorized as ranging from mild to moderate to severe ratings. Her overall severity during these tasks was rated as 50 mm (moderate to severe). A mild degree of breathiness was also perceived (10 mm) as was a moderate degree of strain (35 mm). Her pitch level was the most aberrant contributor to her ratings of voice quality with an abnormally high pitch during most tasks (83 mm) and a mild to moderately reduced loudness level (8 mm). Pitch breaks also were noted intermittently in the downward direction, particularly during connected speech tasks, in general (rated as 6 mm). There was no consistent type of speech sound associated with these downward pitch inflections. However, the lower pitch achieved during these pitch breaks was perceived as a more normal pitch by the clinician, although diplophonia was perceived at this lower pitch. During conversation, it was noted that the occurrence of downward pitch breaks occurred most frequently toward the end of a phrase, or sentence, or as Ms. Q ran out of air. In summary, Ms. Q received a CAPE-V score of 192 (the total score equals the sum of the measured placement of marks) due to the presence of breathiness, strain, reduced loudness, and an excessively high pitch throughout the speech tasks. These qualities, in addition to the intermittent occurrence of downward pitch breaks, gave the perception of a moderate to severely abnormal voice quality.

Oral Mechanism Examination. Ms. Q exhibited an asymmetric face with greater muscle mass observed in the left cheek and jaw than on the right side. In addition, the mandible appeared to deviate toward the right at rest although there was no detectable reduction in strength during opening or closing. Her tongue also deviated toward the right on protrusion and at rest during mouth opening. However, there was no evidence of impaired tongue strength or mobility. In addition, the soft palate exhibited minimal elevation during sustained "ah." However, during repetition of "ah," normal movement was observed. No evidence of velopharyngeal dysfunction was indicated as speaking and sustained phonation resonance was appropriately oral. During this exam, Ms. Q commented that the left side of her face appeared notably bigger in size to the left side around the age of 14 years. One of her sons also exhibits this trait.

Rigid Videostroboscopy Evaluation. A 70-degree rigid videostroboscopic examination was completed to evaluate laryngeal function during sustained phonation at comfortable, low, and high pitches and at comfortable, soft, and loud levels of production. Throughout this examination, the left vocal fold remained immobile. During phonation at high pitches, vocal fold approximation and vibratory characteristics appeared within normal limits. However, at comfortable pitch and lower, glottic closure was incomplete. Diplophonia was perceived during phonation at low pitch and was associated with intermittent reduced-amplitude periodic vibration of the left vocal fold. The immobile left vocal fold appeared flaccid and varied between aperiodic and periodic patterns of vibration at comfortable and low pitches. The right vocal fold exhibited normal amplitude of vibration and mucosal wave during phonation at all pitches. During loud voice production at comfortable pitch, the right vocal fold crossed midline and made brief contact with the immobile left vocal fold during the closed portion of glottal cycles. The ventricular folds approximated at phonation initiation and then remained adducted, occluding three quarters of the left vocal fold and one half of the right vocal fold. A mild degree of anterior-posterior supraglottal squeeze occurred at comfortable and lower pitches. Thickened white mucus was observed on the superior surface of both vocal folds at rest and migrated toward the vocal fold edges during phonation. Throat clearing and swallowing was not successful at clearing the mucus.

Functional and Acoustic Measures. A maximum phonation time of 8 seconds was achieved. This falls below the expected maximum time of 15 to 25 seconds for normal adult females suggestive of compromised respiratory-phonatory function. Also of interest was a gradual decline in the maximum phonation time across three trials from 8 to 4 seconds. This suggests that the patient experiences fatigue during repetition of a maximum voice performance task. Her maximum s/z ratio was 1.4 indicative of inefficient laryngeal valving during sustained voicing. Laryngeal diadochokinetic testing (repetition of a glottal stop paired with /a/ as quickly and completely as possible) appeared labored and slow in a high-pitched voice. She was unable to perform this task in the lower pitch. The patient also indicated that this task was difficult to perform due to the sensation of strain in the throat. These results support that the larynx is not adequately valving or efficiently valving during phonation.

Her fundamental frequency during sustained voicing of /a/ was 340 Hz with an average intensity of 55 dB SPL. Consistent with the perceptual evaluation, the patient's fundamental frequency was higher than expected and her intensity was lower than expected for an adult female. Her harmonic-to-noise ratio was 10.2 dB, well below the expected value of 20 dB. During spontaneous conversation, her speaking fundamental frequency was 360 Hz with an average intensity of 58 dB SPL. Thus, during speaking, her fundamental frequency and intensity increased slightly. Her minimum and maximum fundamental frequency and intensity were 100 Hz, 500 Hz, 55 dB SPL, and 60 dB SPL, respectively.

Aerodynamic Examination. Airflow and intraoral pressures were obtained during the vowel portion and consonant portion, respectively, during repetition of /pi/. Several practice trials were necessary before the patient could repeat this syllable using her lower pitch. Only four repetitions were produced at this pitch level for measurement due to the patient running out of air quickly. Mean airflow was measured as 300 cc/sec indicative of inefficient laryngeal valving. Intraoral pressure was measured as 9 cm H_2O, higher than the expected value of 7 cm H_2O. Laryngeal resistance was calculated to be 30 cm H_2O/LPS which is below the expected value of 35 cm H_2O/LPS. These measures are indicative of reduced resistance at the level of the larynx and are consistent with observations of incomplete vocal fold approximation during phonation at comfortable and lower pitches during videostroboscopy.

Therapeutic Probes. Therapeutic probes were used to determine whether voice therapy methods could facilitate improved voice production. The patient first was asked to try to purposely speak at a lower pitch to determine how well she could voluntarily change pitch. Her attempts to purposely lower pitch were unsuccessful. The use of yawn-sigh, turning her head toward the left, tongue trill, and kazoo voicing were successful at facilitating lowered pitch during phonation. The clinician also noted that her voice quality at the lower pitch was perceived as mildly lower than expected for an adult female, with diplophonia and moderate to severely breathy voice quality. Finally, laryngeal manipulation was used to palpate the larynx at rest and during phonation. Thyroid compression was associated with increased intensity and strained voice quality. However, posterior and inferior manipulation of the larynx was associated with lowered pitch and breathy voice quality.

Description and Rationale for Therapy Approach. Ms. Q was referred to speech-language pathology with the medical diagnosis of left unilateral vocal fold paralysis. The findings of the voice evaluation were consistent with this diagnosis. Associated with the unilateral vocal fold paralysis were aberrant vocal behaviors consistent with muscle tension dysphonia. That is, the patient complained

of increasing strain in her throat region with prolonged talking. Her sensation of strain likely resulted from two behaviors requiring excessive laryngeal muscle activation: high-pitched phonation and supraglottal squeeze. In addition to excessive laryngeal muscle activation, aerodynamic measures indicate that the larynx was excessively leaky and that indirect measures of tracheal pressures were high. Thus, Ms. Q exhibited increased respiratory drive during voice production, probably to compensate for the leaky laryngeal valving. Increased laryngeal muscle activation and respiratory drive would be associated with increased sense of effort and could explain the strain and fatigue Ms. Q experienced with prolonged talking. Based on the patient's response to therapeutic probes, it was unlikely that her habit of speaking in a high-pitched voice will change voluntarily. However, facilitative techniques were successful in inducing desirable voice production. Thus, her voice treatment was designed primarily to reduce muscle tension associated with high-pitched phonation and to reestablish phonatory-respiratory coordination. In addition, active vocal exercises were incorporated to determine whether voice therapy could also improve strength and flexibility of laryngeal function during voice production.

Goal 1. Ms. Q will learn how to arrange her environment to reduce her vocal demands and improve the ability for others to hear and understand her during conversation.

Rationale. Ms. Q indicated the greatest challenges to successful communication on the telephone and in social situations was background noise. In both situations, she cannot increase her loudness to levels where others can hear her. The telephone is a common challenge for individuals with several different types of voice disorders. One simple solution for projecting her voice on the telephone is to amplify her voice so that listeners can hear her. Most telephones allow control of the listener's amplification. However, if the listener cannot successfully amplify to hear Ms. Q, she can use a microphone amplifier on her phone to increase the intensity of her voice to the listener. Several companies sell headsets with the ability to adjust both the receiver and the microphone. This same approach works for the challenges Ms. Q faces during social situations with background noise. Personal amplification devices are available using either a headset or lapel microphone. Most patients prefer these for group situations rather than as a normal modality of communication. Other simple adjustments to social situations without the use of a personal amplifier would include sitting or standing within arm's reach of her listener facing toward them in a well lit room.

Goal 2. Ms. Q will reduce her intake of caffeinated beverages to 1 cup daily and drink a minimum of eight 8 oz glasses of water daily.

Rationale. The observation of thickened mucus on the vocal folds and Ms. Q's description of her daily liquid intake raise concerns about her systemic hydration of the vocal fold tissues. In addition, she indicated having increasing problems with reflux and heartburn over the past year. By reducing caffeine intake and increasing water intake, Ms. Q might help reduce stomach acid levels and improve vocal fold hydration. Improved vocal fold hydration would

be expected to reduce vocal fold stiffness, thereby reducing vocal effort levels as much as possible in an already compromised larynx.

Goal 3. Ms. Q will learn to reduce laryngeal muscle tension voluntarily so that she can consistently phonate at a comfortable pitch.

Rationale. The primary source of strain associated with the patient's voice production appeared related to the use of an excessively high-pitched phonation. She demonstrated difficulty modifying her pitch voluntarily, but could successfully phonate at a pitch indicated as closer to her normal pitch using facilitative techniques. The techniques of "yawn-sigh," turning her head toward the left (affected side), tongue trill, and kazoo voicing all were successful at facilitating a lower pitch during the voice evaluation. Laryngeal massage was also successful at eliciting reduced pitch. The "yawn-sigh" method is a common relaxation method for promoting reduced laryngeal muscle activation and improving respiratory-phonation coordination. Head positioning in individuals with a unilateral vocal fold paralysis is used to artificially medialize the immobile vocal fold for improved vocal fold contact during phonation. Turning the head toward the affected side, in this case the left, rotates the larynx such that the affected vocal fold is shorter and medial and the unaffected vocal fold is slightly stretched. In some cases, individuals experience improvement by stretching the immobile vocal fold slightly and medializing the mobile fold. Positioning the head by tilting it backward or downward also sometimes helps by either stretching or compressing both vocal folds, respectively. This patient experienced improved pitch by turning her head toward the left. Thus, head positioning technique could be used therapeutically to help promote vocal fold contact during phonation. The tongue trilling method involves rapid obstruction and release of the airstream through the oral vocal tract. This is analogous to creating a smaller vocal tract "tube," on average, through which sound must pass during phonation. It is hypothesized that this functionally smaller vocal tract "tube" increases the acoustic impedance of the vocal tract and is associated with lowering phonation threshold pressures. Thus, trilling is sometimes helpful in promoting more normal sounding phonation in individuals with unilateral vocal fold paralysis, as was the case with this client. Kazoo voicing is a method that typically is used to facilitate voicing with functional voice disorders. The vocal tract configuration might also change when an individual holds a kazoo between the lips. Thus, this method might somehow facilitate forward focus or vocal tract resonance for improved phonation. Finally, laryngeal manipulation is used for palpating and identifying locations of excessive extrinsic laryngeal muscle tension, vertical location of the larynx, and for manipulating laryngeal position or extrinsic laryngeal musculature for the purpose of relaxation or direct laryngeal position modification. Laryngeal compression would be predicted to improve phonation in someone with unilateral vocal fold paralysis as it would reduce the size of the glottis between the mobile and immobile vocal folds. This appeared true for Ms. Q. However, her voice quality also sounded more strained using thyroid compression. Reduced laryngeal vertical height appeared more successful at reducing the strain and

high pitch in this individual. This suggests that high laryngeal carriage may be associated with increased pitch in this patient. Laryngeal manipulation focusing on reducing tension in suprahyoid musculature and the thyrohyoid muscle may be therapeutically beneficial. The clinician can teach the patient how to implement laryngeal massage independently for daily use as needed.

Goal 4. Ms. Q will demonstrate improved respiratory-phonation coordination to ensure an adequate supply of air and efficient use of it during speaking. Excessive laryngeal muscle activity is expected to reduce with improved coordination of the respiratory system due to reliance on respiratory drive during voicing rather than laryngeal squeezing to maintain necessary phonation pressures. Accent therapy will be used to achieve this goal.

Rationale. Ms. Q exhibited inefficient use of air by exhaling her air supply before initiating voicing. This behavior may contribute to excessive laryngeal muscle activation during phonation to prevent further air loss given a reduced air supply and leaky laryngeal valve. Accent therapy helps the patient relearn proper breathing paired with phonation using rhythm and accentuation during voicing and speech tasks.[37,38] The focus on using rhythmic and musical phonation during progressively more complex speech tasks (vowels, voiced consonants, syllables, and so forth) helps shape more efficient voicing using less tension. (A full description of Accent Therapy is provided by Aliaa Khidr later in this chapter.)

Goal 5. Ms. Q will utilize her vocal tract to amplify her voice and improve laryngeal efficiency during voice production.

Rationale. Ms. Q identified reduced loudness as one of the biggest challenges to social interactions. In addition, her abnormally high pitch and excessive laryngeal muscle activation likely occurred in response to the sense of inadequate pressure regulation within the larynx. Resonant voice therapy is helpful for teaching individuals how to get the "biggest bang for their buck," that is, minimizing the amount of laryngeal effort and maximizing the amplification of the voice by utilizing the optimum shape of the vocal tract. Although it is possible that Ms. Q may achieve a more efficient and improved voice quality from implementing resonant voice treatment, the primary goal in using this method is to utilize the vocal tract to amplify the voice and take the patient's focus away from increased respiratory and laryngeal effort. This therapeutic approach will further connect more relaxed phonation methods to speech productions.

Goal 6. Ms. Q will use Vocal Function Exercises to improve vocal pitch flexibility, vocal endurance, and vocal strength once respiratory-phonation coordination and resonance is achieved.

Rationale. Once Ms. Q successfully achieved respiratory-phonation coordination and resonance during speaking, the next step was to determine whether improvements could be made in vocal fold adduction, voicing endurance, and pitch range. Vocal Function Exercises were used to engage the laryngeal musculature that remains innervated or re-innervated and improve laryngeal muscle participation in phonation without strain and increased effort. Individuals may exhibit or report increased effort and strain to produce these exercises as softly as possible during initial training sessions. In such cases, patients can be trained to perform Vocal Function Exercises with a resonant voice until they demonstrate proficiency practicing the exercises. Thereafter, they must learn to perform them as specified by Joseph Stemple,[5] as softly as possible. It is possible that using these exercises will further contribute to Ms. Q's improved voicing endurance, reduced effort levels, and improved voice quality.

Results of Therapy. Ms. Q completed eight therapy sessions over the course of 2 months. She also returned for a follow-up session 3 months after completion of therapy. Posttherapy measures were completed during the eighth therapy session in addition to administration of a patient satisfaction questionnaire.

VHI and V-RQOL Questionnaires. Ms. Q's scores on the VHI and V-RQOL changed significantly. Her total score on the VHI was 14/120 points with a functional subscore of 7/40, physical subscore of 7/40, and an emotional subscore of 0/40. Thus, Ms. Q's scores show that there are still some functional and physical issues associated with her voice disorder and no emotional issues. Her total score on the VHI changed from 62 to 14 points. A therapeutic effect requires a change in score of 18 points or greater. Thus, a total score change of 48 points indicates a significant improvement.

Ms. Q's scores on the V-RQOL also demonstrated improvement posttreatment. Her standard score on the Social-Emotional Domain changed from a standard score of 75 to 93.8. Her Physical Functioning Domain changed from 37.5 to 87.5. Her total score changed from 52.5 to 90. Thus, Ms. Q's scores on this instrument suggest only a slight impact from her voice disorder remaining on her day-to-day activities.

Perceptual Examination. The Consensus Auditory-Perceptual Evaluation of Voice (CAPE-V) was re-administered. Her overall severity during these tasks was rated as 35 mm (moderate). A mild to moderate degree of breathiness remained (35 mm) as did a mildly reduced loudness level (5 mm). Intermittent diplophonia was rated as moderately deviant during sustained phonation (40 mm). However, pitch breaks, strain, and aberrant pitch level were absent features. Ms. Q's total CAPE-V score changed from 192 to 115. Thus, although breathiness and diplophonia remained as a significant feature of Ms. Q's voice problem, the overall score on the CAPE-V indicated improvement.

Rigid Videostroboscopy Evaluation. The videostroboscopic evaluation demonstrated that the left vocal fold remained immobile as during the first recording. The patient was able to produce pitches at low, comfortable, and high levels as well as soft, comfortable, and loud levels on instruction. The primary change in observations from the first evaluation was the reduction in supraglottal activation and the degree of contact between the mobile and immobile vocal fold during comfortable and loud phonations. During comfortable pitch and loudness, the mobile vocal fold crossed midline and approximated with the immobile vocal fold, although contact time appeared brief. During loud phonation, contact time between the vocal folds approached normal limits (almost half of the glottal cycle duration). The left ventricular fold appeared moderately hypertrophied.

However, ventricular fold adduction did not occur at onset of phonation and anterior-posterior supraglottal squeeze was not observed. Thickened mucus observed during the first exam was also absent. These findings demonstrate improved laryngeal efficiency.

Functional and Acoustic Measures. A maximum phonation time of 11 seconds was achieved. This is longer than during the initial evaluation. However, it is still below the expected maximum time of 15 to 25 seconds for normal adult females. In addition, the patient demonstrated consistent maximum phonation times across all three trials, indicating that fatigue no longer occurred. Her maximum s/z ratio was 1.2 indicative of improved, but still slightly inefficient, laryngeal valving during sustained voicing. Laryngeal diadochokinetic testing was performed at a comfortable pitch. However, glottal stops were not produced without air leakage, indicating that laryngeal valving remained impaired.

Her fundamental frequency during sustained voicing of /a/ was 180 Hz with an average intensity of 62 dB SPL. Her harmonic-to-noise ratio was 16 dB. During spontaneous conversation, her speaking fundamental frequency was 190 Hz with an average intensity of 63 dB SPL. Her minimum and maximum fundamental frequency and intensity were 100 Hz, 700 Hz, 55 dB SPL, and 70 dB SPL, respectively. Gains occurred in fundamental frequency and intensity averages and ranges. In addition, the degree of noise present in Ms. Q's voice was significantly reduced posttreatment.

Aerodynamic Examination. Airflow and intraoral pressures were obtained during the vowel portion and consonant portion, respectively, during repetition of /pi/. The patient produced all seven repetitions required for standard measurement. Mean airflow was measured as 220 cc/sec indicative of improved laryngeal valving. Intraoral pressure was measured as 7 cm H_2O, considered normal. Laryngeal resistance was calculated to be 32 cm H_2O/LPS, which is slightly below normal limits. These measures indicate a reduction in intraoral pressure and airflow, although laryngeal efficiency is still slightly compromised.

Patient Satisfaction Questionnaire. A questionnaire was administered to the patient to solicit ratings of her perception as to how much the voice treatment was perceived to improve her voice, how much she liked the therapy, and how much she was able to learn and implement the therapy methods. The patient responded with the highest rating of satisfaction on all of these parameters.

Management for Idiopathic Unilateral Vocal Fold Paralysis

Joseph C. Stemple, PhD

Case Study: Patient R

Controversy regarding the efficacy of direct voice therapy for unilateral vocal fold paralysis is present. Indeed, Colton and Casper[10] argued against the long-held belief that effort closure will strengthen the nonparalyzed fold and encourage the fold to cross the glottal midline, improving closure and voice quality. "Although the notion of the crossover effect is an appealing one, we have been impressed by the lack of its occurrence in patients we have exam-

ined fiberoptically, whether or not they exhibited return of voice."[10(p265)]

Others support the notion of direct therapy for vocal fold paralysis.[10,11,39] My own clinical experience has demonstrated mixed results with these patients. I am never quite sure whether improvement in voice quality can be credited to the management techniques or to natural physiologic changes, such as muscle fibrosis and contractures.[40] It is my belief, however, that the voice pathologist may play a valuable role in helping patients deal with this disorder. This role will include aspects of education, emotional support, environmental manipulation, and direct therapy.

Case History. Patient R was a 42-year-old orthodontist, referred by the laryngologist, with the diagnosis of a left unilateral vocal fold paralysis. The paralysis was idiopathic in that all appropriate diagnostic testing, including a CT scan and chest radiograph, proved negative for disease.

Patient R became symptomatic 1 month prior to the voice evaluation. At that time, he was suffering from a cold and awakened one morning with aphonia. The whispering lasted for 3 days. The patient was not overly concerned because he thought the "laryngitis" was related to the illness. He became concerned when the voice remained weak and breathy following resolution of the cold. Therefore, he sought the opinion of the laryngologist, who diagnosed the left vocal fold paralysis.

It was obvious during the voice evaluation that Patient R was extremely concerned and emotionally distraught as a result of the paralysis. Although his voice quality was moderately to severely dysphonic, characterized by breathiness, strain, pitch, and phonation breaks, he continued to work and follow his normal schedule. He reported that it was increasingly difficult for him to communicate with patients and that his voice was fatiguing significantly by the end of the day.

Most individuals are justifiably concerned about any medical or physical problem. Patient R's response went beyond concern and seemed to border on hysteria. It was evident that solid information regarding this disorder was missing and must be offered quickly to this patient, who knew his test results had shown no serious disorder, but "something" was causing the problem. "What's to stop my other vocal fold from going out? Then what am I supposed to do?" At that point, Patient R broke down emotionally. The implication, of course, was that he would lose his livelihood if he could not communicate.

Videolaryngoscopy, including the laryngeal stroboscope, was used to show Patient R his vocal folds and to demonstrate why his voice quality was dysphonic. (Line drawings also may be used.) The left true vocal fold was paralyzed in a paramedian position, yielding an incomplete closure. The left ventricular fold was strongly compressed toward the midline. The vibratory pattern was extremely distorted, and the left fold seemed to simply flap in the airstream while the right fold could not establish a normal vibratory pattern. It was explained to Patient R that many paralyses are idiopathic and resolve spontaneously within 6 to 12 months. It may be speculated that, because his paralysis began during a cold, the nerve damage may have been the result of viral infection or neuritis. The fact that diagnostic testing was negative, although it didn't give him the answer he sought as to cause, was certainly better than the alternative result.

The likelihood of the right vocal fold becoming paralyzed was extremely slim.

This information appeared to calm the patient somewhat. Objective measures then were completed, which yielded the following results:

- High fundamental frequency (160 Hz)
- Limited downward frequency range (126 to 480 Hz)
- High jitter measures (all pitch levels)
- High airflow rates (all pitch levels +300 mL/sec)
- Low phonation times (all pitch levels).

Once the stroboscopic examination and objective measures were completed, the interview with the patient was conducted. Patient R had practiced dentistry for 12 years as an orthodontist in an upscale neighborhood. He was busy, and his practice was successful. He had developed a personal lifestyle that reflected this success.

Medical History. The patient's medical history included a tonsillectomy and hernia repair as a child, with no other hospitalizations noted. The only chronic disorders reported were frequent sinusitis for which he used a prescription antihistamine and borderline high blood pressure, which was monitored but not medicated. Patient R stopped smoking at age 30 following 12 years of smoking one pack of cigarettes per day. His liquid intake was adequate. He reported that prior to the onset of the paralysis, he "felt great."

Social History. The patient was married for 12 years and had two daughters, aged 9 and 6 years. His wife was a homemaker. His work schedule included office hours from 8 AM to 5 PM 5 days per week and every other Saturday. In addition, he lectured at the medical school for 1 hour, once a month.

Nonwork activities included an active social schedule of parties, dinners, and benefits. His wife was active in volunteer groups, and the patient was obligated to attend many of these activities. In addition, he played tennis three times per week. The patient was distressed because playing tennis made his voice weaker, and he couldn't call out game scores. Other activities involved his daughters' school and extracurricular activities.

Voice Therapy. Following the interview, Patient R continued to express his concerns regarding the paralysis. He was upset not only by the prospect of a permanent paralysis but also by having to wait 12 months for alternative surgical treatments, as explained by the laryngologist. The basic rationale for a trial direct voice therapy program was explained. The concept of effort closure was described, and the following therapy plan was devised:

Goal 1. This patient was hypofunctioning the laryngeal mechanism. There was no evidence of the typical compensatory hyperfunctional behavior. In an attempt to establish some muscular engagement of the nonparalyzed intrinsic laryngeal muscles, Patient R was taught to produce vowels utilizing a glottal attack. Although this form of effort closure is not advised as a primary therapy approach for most paralysis patients, his use of a disengaged, falsetto-type voice quality encouraged its introduction for this particular patient. He was instructed to (a) breathe in, (b) posture the vowel while building air pressure, and (c) release the vowels

and vowel-consonant combinations as follows:

(a, e, i, o, oo, eat, it, ate, etch, at, ooze, oats, ought, out, up, I'm)

Each vowel and vowel/consonant was produced twice each, three times per day, using the glottal attack. The exercise was practiced for 1 week.

Goal 2. Same as week 1, with the addition of stretching the vowel sound for 2 seconds. The exercise was practiced for 1 week.

Goal 3. Same as week 2, with the addition of pushing the palms of the hands together to add an isometric push and to increase effort closure. Again, this exercise was practiced for 1 week.

During the fourth week of therapy, the results of the effort closure approach were reviewed with stroboscopic observation of the vocal folds and objective measures. In addition to direct therapy, Patient R was to build at least three vocal rest periods into his daily work activities, use amplification for an upcoming lecture, and ask his competitor to call out tennis scores.

Only minor improvement was noted during the first 3 weeks of direct therapy. The glottal attack and pushing exercises were simply seen as a possible way of increasing right vocal fold adductory engagement. The patient was not taught to produce conversational voice in this manner. The voice quality remained weak and breathy. It was also evident that the patient continued to be deeply depressed by his vocal condition. This emotional conflict contributed to musculoskeletal tension adding an emotional component to the voice problem. The need for professional counseling was discussed, and the patient agreed to a psychology referral. He was eventually hospitalized for 2 weeks and placed on an antidepressant medication. The patient stabilized emotionally and was able to return to voice therapy with a clearer perspective and realistic expectations.

Because of the patient's acute need, both practically and emotionally, for improved voice, it was decided to offer temporary relief and improvement of voice through a gel foam injection. This was accomplished by the laryngologist on an outpatient basis, with immediate improvement in loudness and quality noted. Because of the improved approximation of the vocal folds provided by the gel foam, he was able to begin Vocal Function Exercises. Gelfoam typically will reabsorb within 8 to 12 weeks. During this time, the patients have an improved vocal fold approximation that allows for therapy to be more effective. Exercising the voice producing system during the positive Gelfoam effect often leads to permanent improvement in voice quality, even after the Gelfoam has reabsorbed.

Patient R's voice quality did, indeed, improve perceptually to a mild dysphonia characterized by breathiness and occasional pitch breaks. He was able to continue work without major communication problems. Objective measures improved somewhat but remained abnormal. For example:

- Fundamental frequency dropped 160 to 148 Hz, still abnormally high
- Jitter measures improved for comfort level and high pitches, but remained high for low pitch

- Airflow rates dropped below 300 mL/sec, remaining well above 200 mL/sec
- Phonation times remained low for all pitch levels
- Stroboscopic observation demonstrated improvement in glottic closure with a large posterior chink noted; the vibratory pattern of both true folds was improved, again, as a result of a improved closure permitting a more stable subglottic pressure and airflow used to produce the voice.

The combination of direct voice therapy, psychological support, and surgical intervention (Gelfoam) were keys to this patient's recovery. Spontaneous recovery of the paralyzed fold was not to be Patient R's good fortune. One year following the onset of his paralysis, he underwent a vocal fold medialization. We did not have the opportunity to follow his progress through this procedure but understand that he continues to practice successfully as an orthodontist.

In the next section, Aliaa Khidr presents a tutorial on the Smith Accent Technique and its application for treating a vocal fold paralysis case 16 years postonset.

Introduction to the Smith Accent Technique

Aliaa Khidr, MD, PhD

The Smith Accent Technique (SAT) is a holistic method of voice therapy that was developed in the late 1930s by the famous Danish phoniatrician Svend Smith. It has a very clear hierarchy of exercises (Patient S Appendix A) that are designed to resolve pathologic vocal symptoms by optimizing normal vocal functions through achieving the best possible coordination between breath support, oral resonance, voice projection, articulation, body movement, and posture. The technique is widely known for its inclusive approach regarding breath support. Patients learn not only to increase and maintain sufficient air supply for speech or song, but also lhow to efficiently use this air supply to support their communicative and performance needs.

The SAT exercises drill quick, silent and deep oral air intake during inspiration; and active control of the speed and force of abdominal muscle contractions during expiration. Improving inspiratory filling as well as gaining control over shaping expiratory airflow helps patients meet their individual speech and voice demands such as utterance duration, loudness level, pitch level, and intonation contour. These skills are taught through drilling a hierarchy of tasks that gradually increase in speed of performance (slow, moderate, fast), complexity of the linguistic message (consonants, play vowels, syllables, words, phrases), complexity of vocal characters (relaxed soft low pitched voice, variety of loudness and intonation contours), and complexity of communication contexts (copying modeled stimuli, spontaneous reading, monologues, conversational dialogues, debates, vocal performance and singing).[37,38,41,42]

"Breath Support" Versus "Abdomino-Phonatory Control"

Clinicians using the "Smith Accent technique" refer to "breath support" as "abdomino-phonatory control," to indicate the "abdomino-diaphragmatic" type of breathing used throughout therapy.

This type of breathing is the most suited for voice production during speech and/or song because it allows for the greatest flow of inspiratory air into the lungs during inhalation as well as active shaping of the expiratory air flow during expiration.

During inhalation, the diaphragm contracts (lowers in position) and the abdominal muscles show brief decrements in muscle activity as well as decrease in the impedance offered by the abdominal wall, thereby allowing diaphragmatic contraction and lung expansion to resolve into a visible outward displacement of the abdominal wall. This visual observation of expansion of the abdominal wall during inspiration is used by SAT clinicians as a sign of the active contraction of the diaphragm during inspiratory filling.[43] The extent of this expansion is used as an indication of the efficiency of inspiratory filling as research shows that the amount of air breathed in and the amount of air in the lungs are strongly influenced by the length and loudness of the intended utterance.[44,45]

During exhalation for phonation, in this type of breathing, the abdominal wall actively contracts, leading to an increase in the intra-abdominal pressure and an inward as well as upward sum of force that leads to emptying the lungs.[46–48] This visual observation of inward abdominal wall displacement during the expiratory phase of speech is used by the SAT clinicians to indicate volume displacement in the expiratory direction and generation of the expiratory pressure needed to support speech or song.[49] The extent of this inward displacement is used as an indication of the efficiency of expiratory airflow shaping as research shows that the amplitude of abdominal EMG is related to the characters of the speech output.[48] Accordingly, the force and speed of abdominal wall contraction is utilized to actively control the amount of the exhaled air flow as well as the speed of its delivery for phonation.[37,42,50–53]

Two parameters have been used to record the active role of the abdominal wall muscles during phonation. The actual extent of (passive) outward abdominal wall displacement during inhalation, and (active) inward abdominal wall movement during exhalation using plethysmography,[46,54–57] as well as the extent of decrease in amplitude of abdominal muscle activity during inhalation and increase during exhalation using electromyography.[48]

Skills Needed to Acquire Abdomino-Phonatory Control

For most "Smith Accent" voice clinicians, acquiring abdomino-phonatory control means using abdomino-phonatory breathing to actively support and control speech and voice. This entails acquiring the following six basic skills:

1. Adequate inspiratory filling using quick, deep and silent oral inhalations. Oral air intake offers the least resistance compared to nasal air entry. Accordingly, it is the fastest way for entry of a sufficient amount of air to support the intended utterance and avoid repeated refilling, which can interrupt the speech flow and distract the listener.
2. Adequate force and speed of abdominal wall contractions during voicing. The adequacy of the speed and force of abdominal wall contractions within each stage and throughout each session are continuously monitored. The clinician verbally high-

lights positive productions and occasionally points out their effects on the patient's vocal output.

3. Appropriate abdomino-phonatory tuning, in which the abdominal wall contraction delivers the expiratory air pulse needed for the targeted utterance length and vocal characters. No pausing between the end of inspiration and the start of expiration is allowed and the expiratory flow is tuned with phonation.
4. Adequate air reserve after voicing thus avoiding running out of air at the end of the utterance. This is particularly critical in patients using a vocal fry due to the usage of insufficient small airflow rates during phonation.
5. Adequate production of targeted vocal characters (see Patient S Appendix B). The clinician usually selects the vocal characters that will be targeted during the exercises. Selection criteria vary from one patient to another depending on the different factors leading to the current voice problem. Clinicians usually start with one target such as the easiest to produce or the most problematic to the patient and will add others as therapy progresses. The "on target" voice productions are highlighted to the patient. As therapy progresses, the patients are expected to become good listeners to their voice and able to identify the negative and positive vocal qualities.
6. Adequate production of targeted speech characters (see Patient S Appendix C). In the last stage of therapy, the patient self-initiates performances without copying a modeled stimulus. During this stage, critical speech parameters needed to improve the client's conversation will be

selected and positively reinforced when correctly achieved.

Training these six basic skills takes place through modeling and drilling five consecutive levels of abdomino-phonatory control during phonation. These can be summarized as follows:

Although active control of inspiratory filling and active shaping of expiratory air flow for speech and song are the basis for this hierarchy; the following supportive voice production skills receive similar attention throughout each stage: general posture, tension in the face, mouth, larynx, neck, shoulder and chest muscles, articulation, oral resonance, voice projection, associated body movements, self-monitoring and self-correction, as well as turn taking and interjection during conversations.

Training the four basic skills needed to acquire abdomino-phonatory control takes place through modeling and drilling five consecutive levels of abdomino-phonatory control during phonation.

The Five Levels of Abdomino-Phonatory Control

Level 1: Abdomino/Diaphragmatic Breathing. Patients demonstrate gradual abdominal muscle contraction on a relaxed oral expiration.

Level 2: Abdomino-Phonatory Control in Largo Rhythm. Patients demonstrate visible 2 to 3 accentuated abdominal muscle contractions to produce a slow speed 2 to 3 consonant, vowel play, and syllable or word utterance. Drills start by nonphonatory voiceless stimuli and proceed to different voiced stimuli.

Level 3: Abdomino-Phonatory Control in Andante Rhythm. Patients demon-strate visible 4 to 5 accentuated abdominal muscle contractions to produce a medium speed 4 to 5 vowel play, syllable, or word utterance.

Level 4: Abdomino-Phonatory Control in Allegro Rhythm. Patients demonstrate six or more equally accentuated abdominal muscle contractions to produce a matching fast-speed vowel play, syllable, or word utterance. Discrete movements of the abdominal wall cannot be seen clearly anymore. Accentuations take place quickly, one after another, and will be seen as a continuous inward movement of the abdominal wall. The larger repertoire available for exercising drills in this stage makes it very suitable for stabilization of the acquired skills.

Level 5: Generalization. Patients demonstrate abdomino-phonatory control during spontaneous speech and song. In this level, the patient receives minimal modeling followed by no modeling from the clinician. They are expected to spontaneously adjust the speed and force of abdominal muscle contractions according to the intended utterance. This is practiced during reading, monologues, dialogues, group conversations, and debate; according to the patient's communicative needs. Performers will practice using different scripts and/or songs according to their performance and singing style.

Supportive Voice Production Skills

Within each level of abdomino-phonatory control and throughout each SAT session, the clinician constantly focuses on the development and maintenance of additional supportive skills that are critical for voice production. These include: (1)

optimum posture with no signs of physical tension in the face, mouth, articulators, larynx, neck, shoulder, and chest regions; (2) facilitation of optimum physical tension by use of associated body movements during exercises. These include such as gentle hand, arm, and whole body movements that enhance the practiced largo, andante, and allegro rhythms; (3) adequate orality (relaxed and open mouth space) needed for oral resonance and optimum voice projection; (4) adequate copying of predictable and unpredictable stimuli. The clinician models each performance and the patients follow closely the clinician's model; (5) adequate self monitoring and self correction of abdomino-phonatory control and supportive voice production parameters, as well as (6) timely turn taking during exercises and question/answer drilling and timely interjection during conversations

1. Optimum Posture and Muscle Tension.
Posture and muscle tension in the face, mouth, articulators, larynx, neck, shoulders, and chest muscles are gently modified and monitored throughout each session. The patient's self-monitoring and self-correction attempts are positively reinforced.

2. Associated Body Movements.
These subtle movements help keep the body in a nontense state. The patient usually is not instructed to copy the modeled movements, but those who start copying them receive positive feedback for the "on target" movements as well as occasional corrective feedback if needed.

3. Oral Resonance and Voice Projection.
Relaxed yet exaggerated jaw movements with adequate mouth opening are used in the SAT drilling exercises. The clinician

highlights positive productions and helps the client realize the effect of improving oral opening on vocal quality, projection and oral resonance. The patient's self-monitoring and self-correction attempts are positively reinforced.

4. Copying Modeled Stimuli.
The clinician usually starts with modeling simple predictable stimuli for the patient to copy. Later, these become more complex, and as therapy progresses, they become unpredictable in nature as well. This prepares the client for the challenges of real-life conversation.

5. Self-Monitoring and Self-Correction (see Patient S Appendix C).
Therapy is terminated when the patients are able to self-monitor and self-correct their abdomino-phonatory control skills including the targeted vocal characters, as well as self-monitor and self-correct the supportive voice production skills. These patients figure out the underlying physiologic factors that contribute to the vocal outcome through their own performances and the resulting vocal output they hear. These patients are able to carry on their newly acquired skills and self-adjust as needed.

6. Turn Taking and Interjection During Conversations.
In the first four levels of the SAT, the patient takes equal, predictable turns with the clinician in a "ping pong" game fashion with no pauses in-between. This means that the clinician models abdomino-phonatory control, then the client immediately copies the modeled performance as soon as the clinician is done. To do that, the patient has to start inspiratory filling before the clinician ends the modeled utterance, as well as adjust on the spot

the speed and strength of abdominal wall contractions to match that of the clinician. This builds up the patient's readiness to participate in regular conversations and interject as needed in a timely manner.

Progress Criteria. Although the Smith Accent technique has clear guidelines on what to do in therapy, only a few SAT clinicians have reported on progress along the hierarchy of exercises. Voice clinicians in general tend to use their own subjective impressions to judge the patients' acquisition of targeted skills and progress in therapy thus is dependent on undocumented rating scales. This has never prevented successful outcomes of therapy but it has prevented clinicians from analyzing these therapy outcomes. In this day and age, scientific replication should be ensured in order to assess efficacy of therapy, which entails clearly documented criteria for progress in therapy and termination of therapy. This requires three steps: describing the subjective criteria used, finding a functional way to rate that criteria consistently, and setting clear proficiency scores to move from one therapy level to another.

The suggested Therapy Progress Form (see Patient S Appendix C) provides a means to rate the targeted abdomino-phonatory control skills using the overall number of correct performances per therapy trial. These ratings are expressed as correct "on target" performance in 25% of the trials up to 90% of the trials. Although abdomino-phonatory control skills are not the only skills targeted in SAT, these skills were considered to be the most critical in deciding when the patient can move to the next level of therapy. This attempt is a primary step toward getting SAT clinicians to commit

to reporting their internal criteria of evaluating progress in therapy.

Smith Accent Hierarchies

The SAT moves along few hierarchies while teaching abdomino-phonatory control. Each hierarchy starts with simple drills and gradually increases in complexity.

A. *Speed of performance:* exercises start at a slow speed and gradually increase in speed. The beat/rhythm in each level usually is kept by drumming, hence, the nick name, "the drumming technique." It also can be kept by tapping by hand on a solid surface or by foot on the floor.

B. *The linguistic message:* The SAT introduces a linguistic message right from the beginning. This makes generalization of the technique to conversational speech a natural stage in therapy. Exercises start with voiceless consonants (eg, /s/, /ʃ/ used in early drills), and move up to vowel play (eg, /hoˈ, joˈ/), nonsense syllables (eg, /naˈjə, naˈjə/, /boˈjə, boˈjə/), meaningful words (eg, hey you), reading familiar then unfamiliar texts, monologues, dialogues, group conversations, group debates, and, when applicable, song performances.

C. *Vocal characters:* Drills start with a relaxed, soft, low-pitched voice and move up gradually to use a variety of loudness levels, accentuated vocalizations and intonational contours. The soft voice productions entail a softer force of abdominal contraction, whereas the loud voice productions entail more forceful contractions of the abdominal muscle. The same is true for nonaccentuated and accentuated syllables.

D. *Communication contexts:* The patient starts with conscious copying of modeled verbal exercises and moves up to spontaneous speech/song performances. And within that spectrum, they start with predictable stimuli and move up to unpredictable ones.

Types of Feedback During Therapy. The Smith Accent technique utilizes visual, tactile, kinesthetic, and auditory perceptual feedback.

A. *Visual:* In the earlier sessions, the clinician models each task in front of a full length mirror. It helps patients compare his or her performance to that of the clinician.

B. *Tactile:* In the earlier sessions, the clinician asks the patient to feel the abdominal muscle contractions of the clinician and compare them to his or her own. This is done by laying the back of one hand on the clinician's abdominal wall and the palm of the other hand on his or her abdominal wall.

C. *Kinesthetic:* The clinician occasionally adjusts and helps build the patient's awareness of inspiratory filling, abdominal muscle contractions, respiratory-phonatory tuning, and level of inspiratory reserve together with the level of tension in his or herr vocal tract, neck, face, shoulders, and upper chest. Later in therapy, the patient is expected to perceive and adjust his or her performance as needed.

D. *Auditory:* The clinician helps the patient become sensitive to selected vocal characters. Later in therapy, the patient is expected to adjust his or her performance based on kinesthetic feedback and vocal output.

Management of Unilateral Vocal Fold Paralysis 16 Years Postonset Using the Smith Accent Technique

Aliaa Khidr, MD, PhD

Case Study: Patient S

Patient History. Mr. S, a 79-year-old, healthy-looking, Caucasian male (170 lb, 5' 10") was referred to the voice lab by the otolaryngologist based on the patient's request. He suffered from left unilateral vocal fold paralysis (UVFP) of 16 years duration following a hemithyroidectomy for a benign thyroid lesion. He had a collagen injection (1 year postonset) followed by a thyroplasty (5 years postonset) and was not satisfied with his vocal outcome after either procedure. Mr. S has been a university professor for 36 years as well as the former head of several national scientific institutes during the last 16 years. He is married, has adult children and grandchildren, many close friends, and is still an active member of a professional national scientific institution. He is not a smoker nor an alcohol drinker and lives independently with his wife. Mr. S did not want to undergo any further laryngeal surgery and was very motivated to try voice therapy in order to achieve a louder voice that could help him meet his social and occupational communication needs.

Mr. S's main complaints were (1) predominant voice loss with unexpected periods of voicing, and (2) an inconsistent and weak voice that made it difficult for him to be heard by his wife when calling her from the next room or talking to her in the car. He was especially upset about the fact that 16 out of his 26 years of marriage have been without a functional voice. (3) It was also difficult for him to be heard on the phone and in small group gatherings. (4) He was unable to interject in a timely fashion in conversations, which made it difficult for him to state his point of view when needed during professional meetings and social gatherings. (5) All this made his professional meetings and social dinners very stressful for him. To compensate for his voice problem, he would try to speak quickly before losing his voice, but that would be very effortful and would cause him to run out of air, hyperventilate, become dizzy, and lose his voice altogether after 2 or 3 minutes of talking. After times such as these, he would usually be embarrassed by his voice problem and would wait until he felt better to apologize to the small crowd. (6) He also complained of his inability to interject in an ongoing conversation to state his opinion in a timely fashion. This problem made him feel left out, in both social and professional settings.

Evaluation Procedures. A detailed history and physical exam was obtained to confirm the underlying etiology of the UVFP. Voice recordings, acoustic measures, aerodynamic measures, laryngeal videostroboscopic recordings, and Vocal Handicap Index (VHI)[35] scores were collected pre- and posttherapy.

Voice samples were obtained while reading the Rainbow Passage. Recordings were obtained using a Sony DAT recorder. Acoustic measures were obtained and analyzed using the KeyPENTAX Computerized Speech Lab main acoustic analysis software. Aerodynamic measures were obtained and analyzed using the KayPENTAX Aerophone program. Laryngeal videostroboscopic recordings were recorded on a KayPENTAX videostroboscopy station. The laryngeal exam-

ination was done using a 90-degree rigid transoral endoscope. Voice recordings and laryngeal videostroboscopic recordings were independently rated by three speech pathologists, and the mean of the three ratings was used. Voice Handicap Index forms were independently filled out by the client (Table 4–11).

Speech-Language Pathology Evaluation

Auditory Perceptual Characteristics. Mr. S showed inconsistent voicing, vocal fatigue, predominant low-pitch breathy voice with intermittent periods of unnecessary vocal strain and use of falsetto register. Pitch modulation/variations during speech were normal, but pitch range was limited in both lower and upper ends. Habitual loudness level was decreased, and loudness modulation/variations during speech were poor. Patient had a soft weak voice with unpredictable bouts of relatively louder intensity levels. Voice quality reflected a consistent moderate to severe grade of dysphonia characterized by moderate to severe breathiness and asthenia, as well as mild to moderate roughness and strain.

Functional Parameters. Mr. S exhibited poor breath support and poor abdominal wall control. He ran out of air very easily and showed dominant clavicular breathing with visible chest wall movement during inhalation. He utilized noisy nasal inhalations and maintained shallow inspiratory filling during speech leading to short utterance durations.

Objective Aerodynamic and Acoustic Measures. Mr. S had an extremely short maximum phonation time (MPT) of 3.4 seconds, which explained his short utterance duration. Mean flow rates on

Table 4–11. Pre- and Post-Voice Therapy Outcome Measures for Patient S

Parameter	Client S		
	Pre	Post 1	Post 2
Auditory Perceptual Data*			
Dysphonia	4	3	1
Roughness	2	2	1
Breathiness	4	2	1
Asthenia (weakness)	4	2	1
Strain	2	1	1
Aerodynamic			
Max phonation time (sec)	3.4	3.8	4.0
Intensity /a/, dB SPL	61	68	74
Mean flow rate /a/, mL/sec	1080	550	520
Laryngeal and Vibratory Data			
Gap size*	3	2	1
Gap shape	Spindle		Longitudinal
Lateromedial supraglottal activity	2	1	1
Anteroposterior supraglottal activity	1	1	1
Strobe light triggered	No	Yes	Yes
Predominant open phase†	Not elicited	2	2
Mucosal wave on paralyzed VF	Not elicited		Mildly decreased
Mucosal wave on normal VF	Not elicited		Normal
Vocal Handicap Index (VHI) Scores			
Physical	22	18	18
Functional	18	12	12
Emotional	18	12	12
Total	58	42	42
Overall impression	Severe	Moderate	Mild

*Severity Rating, 0–5 with 0 = none, 1 = mild, 2 = mild to moderate, 3 = moderate, 4 = moderate to severe, 5 = severe.

†Severity Rating, 0–3 with 0 = none, 1 = mild, 2 = moderate, 3 = severe.

/a/ were extremely high (1080 mL/second), which explained why he ran out of air easily. His habitual intensity level was 61 dB, which did not reflect his soft voice. Mr. S's mean fundamental frequency was 102 Hz (on /a/) and 115 Hz (on /i/), his mean jitter was 1.8 (on /a/), 3.3 (on /i/), and his mean harmonic-to-noise ratio was 2.9 (on /a/), and 1.2 (on /i/).

Subjective Laryngeal and Stroboscopy Findings. Left vocal fold immobility, with the left vocal fold positioned in a paramedian position, resulting in a large size spindle shape phonatory gap. Mild to moderate latero-medial supraglottal activity with medialization of the ventricular folds, and mild anteroposterior supralaryngeal hyperfunction with medialization and advancement of the arytenoids were observed. The strobe light could not be elicited at the initial visit due to the inconsistent voicing.

Patient Self-Evaluation

Voice Handicap Index Measures:

Functional impairment score = 18/40

Physical impairment score = 22/40

Emotional impairment score = 18/40

Total vocal impairment score = 58/120

Overall Severity Rating: Severe

Patient's Self-Reported Voice Limitations.

■ His wife cannot hear him call her at home.

■ People cannot hear him on the phone.

■ People ask him to repeat himself all the time.

■ He becomes tense, dizzy, and runs out of air after talking for 2 to 3 minutes.

■ He misses his turn in talking at the dinner table because it takes him too long to prepare to speak. When ready to speak, the topic might have already changed.

■ People consistently interrupt and talk over him in meetings. He cannot state his opinions during social or professional gatherings. He can participate

only if he speaks at the beginning or is asked directly at the end.

Selection of Management Procedure. Glottal incompetence due to unilateral adductor vocal fold paralysis is encountered commonly in otolaryngology clinical practices. Patients with voice disorders due to a paralysis like Mr. S's tend to have the highest level of social and vocal disability when compared to patients with voice disorders due to other underlying etiologies.[58–61] Surgical augmentation, medialization, and re-innervation are the main surgical procedures used to manage unilateral vocal fold paralysis. In spite of the high satisfaction outcome of these surgeries, many UVFP patients prefer to enroll in voice therapy rather than undergo laryngeal surgery. These patients usually want to avoid laryngeal surgery or have already undergone surgery and are not satisfied with their vocal outcome. Mr. S was one of the latter group patients. He had already undergone two laryngeal surgical procedures and was not willing to undergo a third procedure without trying voice therapy first. He went to the otolaryngologist to obtain a referral for voice therapy.

Voice therapy, in general, has four different approaches. First, the hygienic approach that focuses on improving vocal habits. Second, the symptomatic approach that focuses on improving problematic voice characteristics. Third, the physiologic approach that focuses on directly modifying the physiology of the vocal mechanism. And fourth, the psychogenic approach that focuses on addressing the different stressors contributing to the voice problem.[62] Although Mr. S's voice therapy plan would include hygienic and psychological goals, it was obvious that his voice problem could not be addressed by either of these approaches alone. So it was either selecting a symptomatic voice therapy technique that works on improving the loudness or a physiologic voice therapy technique that works on optimizing the balance between the different elements involved in voice production such as posture, breathing, glottal closure, voicing, and resonance.

The latter was more suited for Mr. S because we needed to improve his breath support and glottal closure as well as train him to interject timely in ongoing conversations, whether social or professional. The Smith Accent technique, which is a holistic voice therapy technique, was selected as the first choice of therapy as it is designed to work on posture, breathing, glottal closure, voicing, and resonance as well as conversational turn taking and interjections. To utilize this technique for Mr. S, we had to satisfy the criteria of "evidence-based practice" (EBP), a critical theme emerging in the field of speech-language pathology that entails answering three basic clinical questions regarding (1) best current evidence, (2) clinical expertise of the clinician providing the therapy, and (3) the client's values.

A. Best Current Evidence Questions:

1. What is the effectiveness of the Smith Accent (SA) voice therapy technique in the rehabilitation of patients with UVFP?
2. How do other behavioral voice therapy techniques compare to the SAT?
3. Is there any available data regarding effective and efficient restoration of vocal functions and voice quality after administration of the technique?

Research Question: In the treatment of patients with UVFP disorders, does the SA technique effectively and efficiently restore vocal function and voice quality against the alternative of other behavioral intervention methods?

Question 1: Does the SAT have "Sound Physiologic Basis" for Voice Therapy?

Answer: Yes.

- The value of using "abdomino-diaphragmatic breathing" and "abdomino-phonatory control" to modulate inspiratory filling and expiratory air flow for phonation is documented through ample basic physiologic research.[43-49]
- The ability of the SAT to employ abdomino-phonatory control with active accentuations in the abdominal muscles that lead to changes in the vocal outcome is documented through several clinical basic research studies on normal individuals.[41,63,64]

Question 2: Does the SAT have a "Clear Treatment Protocol"?

Answer: Yes.

- The SAT treatment protocol is clearly reported in three books and several articles, as well as the recommended number, duration and frequency of therapy sessions.[37,38,42,65-71]

Question 3: Does the SAT have a "Clear Assessment Protocol"?

Answer: Yes.

- All clinical studies using the SAT have documented clear subjective and objective assessment methods including times of assessment.

Question 4: Have any of the SAT Publications Addressed Reliability of Reported Data?

Answer: Yes

- Some SAT studies have used multiple raters for subjective measures.
- None of the SAT studies used examiner/rater blinding for subjective measures.
- Some SAT studies have used objective measures derived from multiple performances.
- Some SAT studies have used objective data appropriately grouped by age, gender, and diagnosis.

Question 5: Is There "Reasonable Belief of Benefit"?

Answer: Yes

- The holistic nature of the SAT and its sound physiologic basis, besides the relevance of the SAT to the training of breath support and conversational skills provide reasonable belief of benefit.
- The overall quality of research documenting its effectiveness with other populations and the few studies that have reported on the outcomes of SAT in patients with UVFP provide reasonable belief of benefit.[65–71]
- The presence of positive general prognostics for a good outcome of therapy. He was well educated and held a healthy lifestyle. He was socially and professionally active and needed his voice to meet these needs. He was highly

motivated to do behavioral voice therapy as he did not want to undergo further laryngeal surgery. He understood the challenges presented by the long duration of his voice problem (16 years), his poor breath support, and the large size his phonatory gap leading to huge air loss during phonation. He was committed to at least two consecutive rounds of therapy (8 sessions each) to be able to deal with these challenges. He understood that the SAT would not undo his vocal fold immobility but would help him optimize his vocal output through controlling different aspects of the voice production mechanism.

B. Clinical Expertise of the Clinician Providing the Therapy. The clinician providing the SAT was trained to use this technique by students of Dr. Svend Smith, developer of the SAT. She started by spending 3 years providing SAT therapy with variable levels of supervision. After which she accumulated more than 20 years of experience using this technique with different voice disorder patients including patients with UVFP.

C. The Client's Values. Mr. S wanted to receive voice therapy and was interested in pursuing this technique as he determined it was fit to his current needs and values. As a scientific researcher, he appreciated the availability of supportive research. He also appreciated that the technique might help him produce voice on demand, improve his intensity, decrease vocal effort and fatigue as well as work on timely interjections and punctual turn-taking in conversational settings.

Probing. Mr. S was probed for ability to copy modeled abdomino-diaphragmatic breathing with emptying as much air as possible on exhalation then allowing the air to flow smoothly through a relaxed open mouth. This modeling was done with the patient lying down on his back, one leg extended and one flexed at the hip and knee, one hand on his chest and the other on his abdomen. The clinician placed one of her hands on her chest and one on her abdomen to demonstrate no chest movement during inhalation, an outward abdominal wall movement during inspiratory filling and an inward abdominal wall movement during exhalation for speech. Mr. S was able to copy the modeled performance correctly after 4 to 5 trials and was able to maintain it once it was achieved. This probing was considered successful and Mr. S was expected to do well in therapy.

Voice Therapy Goals. Both long- and short-term therapy goals were outlined for each round of the voice therapy program. (see Patient S Appendixes A and B)

The Smith Accent Technique. Mr. S received two rounds of the SAT of voice therapy with a total of 16 sessions. Each round consisted of an eight 60-minute sessions, twice per week for 4 weeks. The first round of eight voice therapy sessions was completed successfully in 4 weeks, and he achieved his goals of abdomino-phonatory control, self-monitoring and self-correction of targeted abdomino-phonatory skills, body tension, and vocal output. After a 1-month break, Mr. S returned for a second round of 4 weeks of SAT voice therapy (eight 60-minute sessions twice/week) to stabilize the newly learned technique in different conversational modes. Ther-

apy progressed along the five basic levels of abdomino-phonatory control and the newly acquired skills were independently evaluated by two speech pathologists at the end of every other voice therapy session. Ratings were compared and discussed until a consensus was reached and documented.

Progress in SAT of Therapy. A special Therapy Progress Form (see Patient S Appendix C) was developed and used to provide a functional method to identify and evaluate targeted voicing characters, speech characters and supportive voice production parameters. Each targeted parameter was rated as: (no) not being on target throughout the session, (fairly) fairly being on target when the patient shows the targeted parameter inconsistently, and (yes) when consistently on target more than 75% of the attempted trials. In this study, rating was done by consensus of two SLPs, and interrater reliability was not evaluated.

Another form (Patient S Appendix D) was developed and used to subjectively evaluate and rate the individual abdomino-phonatory skills acquired in each level of abdomino-phonatory control. Each skill was rated according to how stable the productions were that were produced throughout the session. The overall rating for each level required a subjective rounding of all the subcharacters rated. In this study, rating was done by consensus of two SLPs, and interrater reliability was not evaluated.

An abdomino-phonatory control level was considered achieved after acquiring the following five basic skills: (1) adequate inspiratory filling, (2) active (voluntary) control of speed and force of abdominal muscle contraction in a manner appropriate for the evaluated level, (3) optimum abdomino-phonatory tuning with no pause between the abdominal contraction and the produced sound, (4) sufficient inspiratory reserve where the patient does not run out of breath or produce a vocal fry at the end of the utterance, and (5) adequate performance of targeted voice quality. Each character was assigned a success rate of 0%, 25%, 50%, 75%, or 90% reflecting the stability of correct productions throughout the session.

Progress in Abdomino-Phonatory Control. Progress in abdomino-phonatory control was evaluated by monitoring the overall percentage of correct performances per therapy trial. These were expressed as correct abdomino-phonatory performance in 25% of the trials up to 90% of the trials. Although abdominophonatory control skills are not the only skills targeted in SAT, these skills were considered to be the most critical in deciding when the patient can move to the next level of therapy. Once Mr. S demonstrated correct abdomino-phonatory control in 75% of the trials, therapy moved up to the second level.

During the first round of therapy, Mr. S progressed fast in acquiring abdomino-phonatory control in the three basic tempos. He used the second round of therapy to work on generalizing his newly acquired skills to every day's vocal performances. By the end of the second round of therapy he was able to produce clear, relaxed, and full resonant voicing on demand by employing proper abdomino-phonatory control in different levels of communicative complexity such as reading, monologues, predictable dialogues, and challenging group discussions.

Progress in Targeted Voicing Characters. Breathiness and asthenia (weakness) were the main characters of Mr.

S's voice, followed by roughness and strain. Yet, the primary vocal characters targeted during the first round of therapy were: a relaxed (not strained) and effortless (not effortful) voice. This selection was intended to help Mr. S identify and avoid excessive build up of tension that not only leads to the sense of vocal effort and fatigue, but also prevents him from starting voicing and/or maintaining voicing for an appropriate period of time. Once these targeted vocal qualities were achieved, the second set of targeted qualities became a full (not breathy), and strong (not weak) voice. That was now necessary to produce a more audible and projected voice.

He was able to produce an easy effortless resonant voice on demand by the end of his 5th voice therapy session and was able to project a full and relatively loud voice on demand by the end of the 11th session of therapy.

Progress in Targeted Speech Characters. By the end of the seventh voice therapy session, Mr. S was able to employ a functional 3- to 4-word utterance length during monologues. And by the end of the last voice therapy session, he was able to consistently share in small group conversations without withdrawing or hyperventilating

Progress in Supportive Voice Production Parameters.

Physical tension. Patient was able to stop chest movement and allow oral air intake during inhalation by the end of the first voice therapy session.

Associated body movements. Patient did not feel that these movements were facilitating his skill acquisition, so they were not employed by him, although consistently modeled by the voice clinician.

Oral resonance and voice projection. Patient started demonstrating sufficient oral resonance with sufficient mouth opening during voice production by the end of his fifth voice therapy session.

Copying modeled stimuli. Patient was good in copying modeled vocal and abdomino-phonatory performances. He actually was able to copy every modeled abdomino-phonatory level by the end of the therapy session during which it was introduced

Self-Monitoring and Correction

Abdomino-phonatory control. By the end of the first round of therapy (eight sessions), Mr. S was able to monitor, self-correct and maintain a fast, silent, and deep oral inspiratory filling during speech. By the end of the second round of therapy, he was able to maximize his inspiratory filling and pace his speech rate so that he does not run out of air. He also was able to sense sufficient inspiratory filling by feeling his abdominal wall against his waist belt and utilize quick, deep, and silent inspiratory filling as soon as needed without losing concentration regarding the content of the conversation.

Voice characters. By the end of therapy, Mr. S was able to monitor his voice and correctly identify vocal performances that lead to vocal effort, fatigue, strain, breathiness, and/or asthenia as well as correctly identify vocal performances with full and projected voice productions. He also showed stable attempts of self-correction to improve his vocal outcome.

Speech characteristics. By the end of therapy, Mr. S was able to monitor

his speech rate, pause location, and duration, and adjust his inspiratory filling and abdomino-phonatory control to match the intended utterance.

Timely turn taking. By the end of the first round of therapy (session 8), Mr. S was on target with turn taking regardless of the complexity of the modeled verbal stimulus or its predictability. He commented that his practice at home with the audio recording tuned him better for timely turn taking. By the end of therapy (session 16), Mr. S reported that he was now able to prepare for speech as the current speaker is ending his phrase.

On target self-initiated performances. By the end of therapy (session 16), Mr. S was able to self initiate monologues and answer dialogues while maintaining an easy, relaxed, and resonant voice with good volume and projection in more than 75% of the trials.

Outcomes of Voice Therapy. Improvements were seen in objective aerodynamic and acoustic values, as well as subjective voice quality, vocal fold vibratory patterns, abdomino-phonatory control levels and supportive voice production parameters. The VHI scores, reported by Mr. S, also showed improvement in his physical, functional, and emotional limitations as well as his overall impressions regarding the severity of his voice problem. (see Tables 4–11 and 4–12, Fig 4–5).

1. Auditory Perceptual Outcomes. All rated auditory perceptual parameters of grade, breathiness, asthenia, and strain showed consistent progressive improvement throughout therapy in

Table 4–12. Progress Profile: Supportive Voice Production Parameters for Patient S

Supportive Parameters*	Pretherapy	Post-therapy 1	Post-therapy 2
Copying modeled performance	average	good	excellent
Monitoring targeted voice qualities	average	average	good
Monitoring abdomino phonatory control	average	good	excellent
Self-initiated verbal performances	poor	fair	good
Timely turn taking-skills	poor	fair	good

*Severity rating: poor, fair, average, good, and excellent.

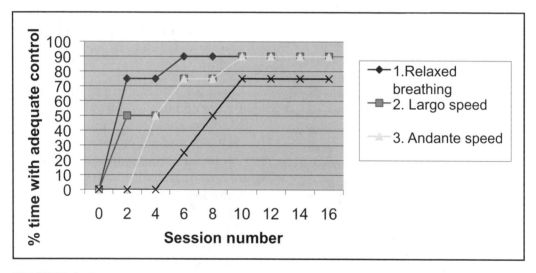

FIGURE 4–5. Progress profile: Proficiency of abdomino-phonatory control.

spite of the size of the underlying phonatory gap and the large values of the mean flow rates.

2. Aerodynamic and Acoustic Outcomes. A significant decrease in mean flow rates (MFR) was achieved by the end of the first round of therapy (from more than 1 L/second to around 500 mL/second). Although these rates are still considered very high (five times the norms) when compared with normal mean flow rates, the resultant voice was not as breathy as expected to be with such high rates. Also a 13 dB increase in intensity was achieved, which gave the voice a functional volume to carry on conversations in small groups. The maximum phonation time (MPT) showed minimum increase in duration (3.4 seconds to 4.0) seconds), but the patient was able to keep his utterances short to match his very short MPT and very high MFRs.

3. Laryngeal and Strobe Outcomes.
The size of the phonatory gap and degree of supraglottal hyperfunction decreased. In addition, there was significant improvement in the mucosal wave on both vocal folds. The normal vocal fold had normal mucosal wave and the paralyzed left showed a mucosal wave that was only mildly decreased. The presence of a mucosal wave on both vocal folds explains the vocal outcome in spite of the persistent phonatory gap and predominant open phase during vibration.

4. Voice Handicap Index Outcomes.
Although the improvement in the physical handicaps caused by the disordered voice were limited (from 22 to 18), the improvement in the functional and emotional handicaps caused by the disordered voice was more appreciated by the patient (18 to 12). The level of improvement in the handicap scores was maintained after the first round of therapy, but the overall impression regarding the severity of the voice disorder was improved. He rated it as a severe problem at the beginning, a moderate problem after the first round of therapy, and a mild problem after the second round of therapy.

5. Patient Self-Reported Outcomes.

1. I can speak on the phone without being asked to repeat myself.
2. My spouse can hear me talking across the house.
3. My spouse comments on how loud my voice has become. We were married for 10 years before I lost my voice and it has been 16 years since my vocal cord became paralyzed. She says that this voice is substantially louder and more pleasing in comparison to my paralysis voice and is more like my original normal voice.
4. I can hold long conversations with friends at dinner parties without running out of air and feeling fatigued.
5. I can break into the conversation and be listened to.
6. I can enjoy social gatherings more and no more withdraw from conversations.
7. I have learned how to voluntarily relax my shoulders, neck, and jaws, take in a good breath that fills up my "abdominal balloon," and use that air without pausing.
8. I know I've got enough air in on inspiration, when I feel my abdominal wall against my belt.
9. These exercises serve as "voice warm-ups." I feel like I am sort of tuning my vocal apparatus. I can hear the difference in my voice after these warm-ups. My voice becomes louder, clearer, more resonant, and less breathy. I am also able to keep this voice up for longer durations without fatiguing.
10. Nowadays, I find it easier to achieve a reasonably loud and resonant voice.

Patient S Appendix A
Treatment Plan: Stage I (Session 1–8)

Client Name: Mr. S, 78 years old

Duration of therapy: Four weeks: 8 voice therapy sessions, twice/week, 60-min each

Baseline/ Client's Present Level of Functioning

Complaints: Patient unable to voice on demand. Can't be heard even when in a quiet room. Not heard on the phone. Runs out of air after 2 to 3 minutes of talking and becomes dizzy. When talking to a small crowd becomes very tense and loses his voice all together.

Communicative Needs: Heard by his wife, heard on the phone, carry out social and professional conversations in an acceptable manner.

Signs: Voice characters: dominant aphonia, poor oral resonance (muffled voice), infrequent unpredictable periods of voicing characterized by an effortful voice of low intensity, occasional falsetto register, as well as severe dysphonia characterized by breathiness, asthenia, and strain.

  Breath support: None. Clavicular breathing, no inspiratory filling during speech, rushes through his utterance to avoid running out of air.

  General posture: Within normal limits.

  Excessive muscle tension: In neck and shoulder muscles during spontaneous speech.

Prognosis: Good: patient is highly educated, highly motivated, has successfully copied the modeled diaphragmatic breathing when probed, is willing to commit to behavioral therapy, and is not in hurry for immediate results.

Overall Functional Goal(s)/Rationale, Objectives, and Outcomes

Patient will be able to voice on demand, maintain longer periods of phonation without losing his voice and becoming dizzy, produce an "easy" (not strained, noneffortful) and "resonant" (not muffled) functional voice.

Patient will demonstrate timely copying of modeled performances as well as verbal interjections in simple conversations.

(Both are critical for him to meet his social and occupational demands.)

This overall goal will be achieved through the following treatment objectives:

1. **Hygiene:** Patient will adhere to a vocal hygiene program to avoid voice loss as well as promote longer periods of phonation without vocal fatigue.

2. **Physiologic:** Patient will acquire sufficient inspiratory filling using quick, deep, and silent inspiratory air fillings.

> Patient will demonstrate adequate abdomino-phonatory control to produce voicing on demand as well as targeted vocal qualities during therapy, first using predictable verbal stimuli of increasing tempo, then using unpredictable verbal stimuli with variable stress, volume, and intonation.

> Patient will demonstrate proper self-monitoring and self-correction of targeted abdomino-phonatory control.

> Patient will demonstrate proper self-monitoring and self-correction of excessive tension in laryngeal muscles, neck muscles, and mouth (decreased orality→limited mouth opening for voice projection).

> Patient will demonstrate timely inhalatory filling, abdomino-phonatory tuning, and turn taking throughout the levels of therapy.

3. **Symptomatic:**

   A. Targeted vocal characters: noneffortful, relaxed (nonstrained), resonant (nonmuffled) voice in the modal register (not falsetto)

   B. Targeted speech characters: Not yet

4. **Psychogenic:** Patient will implement suggestions offered by the clinician and generated by himself to alleviate the stress caused by his disordered voice in social gatherings and professional meetings.

Medical/Surgical: Not in consideration at this time

Breakdown of Plan I into Short-Term Treatment Objectives:

Hygiene

1. Demonstrate understanding of vocally challenging environments and situations and how to compensate for them with healthy vocal habits (eg, avoiding speaking against a noisy background, limiting talking on the phone to alerting the other about a written correspondence that will be sent, avoid talking or calling across a distance, proper use of voice magnification in conferences), by turning in weekly logs that demonstrate the times he identified potentially challenging vocal environments and highlighting how he compensated for them.

2. Increase hydration to enhance optimum laryngeal function and give himself phonatory breaks during conversations.

Physiologic

1. Demonstrate awareness of appropriate muscle tension in neck and laryngeal muscles through self-monitoring of tightness in neck and larynx as well as the resulting aphonia or strained voice quality. Patient will attempt to self-correct

body tension by relaxing neck and laryngeal muscles leading to production of a more relaxed voice.

2. Demonstrate appropriate and consistent abdomino-diaphragmatic breathing at rest in the supine, sitting, and standing positions in more than 75% of trials with no cues.

3. Demonstrate targeted vocal characters by incorporating proper and consistent abdomino-phonatory control when producing predictable and unpredictable stimuli with vowels, syllables, and words at largo speed in more than 75% of trials with no cues.

4. Demonstrate targeted vocal characters by incorporating proper and consistent abdomino-phonatory control when producing predictable and unpredictable stimuli with vowels, syllables, and words at andante speed in more than 75% of trials with no cues.

5. Demonstrate targeted vocal characters by incorporating proper and consistent abdomino-phonatory control when producing predictable and unpredictable stimuli with vowels, syllables, and words at allegro speed in more than 75% of trials with no cues.

6. Demonstrate targeted vocal characters by incorporating proper and consistent abdomino-phonatory control when producing vowels, syllables, and words at unexpected variable speeds, loudness levels, and intonation contours in more than 75% of trials with no cues.

7. Demonstrate stabilization of targeted vocal characters and abdomino-phonatory control in attempts to read, scripted dialogue, and simple question/answer exercises in more than 75% trials with no cues.

8. Demonstrate awareness of proper abdomino-phonatory control and will attempt to self-correct as needed throughout the different stages of therapy.

Symptomatic

1. Demonstrate ability to self-monitor and attempt to self-correct effortful, strained, muffled, and falsetto voice characters in his own voice during therapy.

Psychogenic

1. Patient will utilize the following alternatives to alleviate his voice-related stress:

    A. prepare written backup for professional meetings (eg, slides or handouts)

    B. limit conversations to one on one in social meetings, stay away from addressing the group

2. Patient will self-suggest other compensatory techniques that are appropriate for him.

3. Patient will keep a weekly log, highlighting the stressful situations and the techniques that proved helpful for him.

Patient S Appendix B
Treatment Plan: Stage II (Session 9–16)

Client Name: Mr. S, 78 years old

Duration of therapy: Four weeks: 8 voice therapy sessions, twice/week, 60 min each

Baseline/ Client's Present Level of Functioning

Complaints: Patient still not heard clearly on the phone, still runs out of air and fatigues toward the end of a short 10-min conversation, still becomes tense when talking to a crowd, and cannot interject easilyin the conversation.

Communicative Needs: Be heard clearly by wife, be heard clearly on the phone, carry out social and professional conversations in an acceptable manner.

Signs:

Improved voice characters: infrequent periods of aphonia, longer periods with good oral resonance (resonant voice), longer periods of voicing characterized by a noneffortful voice of low intensity and modal register.

Persistent vocal problems: moderate to severe dysphonia with moderate to severe breathiness and asthenia and occasional strain.

Improved breath support: uses diaphragmatic breathing in all basic speeds.

Persistent breath support problems: infrequent inspiratory filling during speech, still rushes through utterance.

General posture: within normal limits

Excessive muscle tension: noticed in neck and shoulder muscles at the end of utterances or speech.

Prognosis: Good. Patient is still motivated to continue, has successfully acquired diaphragmatic breathing through all first four stages of SAT.

Overall Functional Goal(s)/Rationale, Objectives, and Outcomes

Patient will be able to produce and maintain a functional voice that is louder in volume (not soft) and full (not breathy) while maintaining the previously acquired easy (not strained) and resonant and projected, (not muffled) voice. This is critical for meeting his social and occupational needs.

Patient will demonstrate timely interjection in conversations using a clear and projecting voice.

This overall goal will be achieved through the following treatment objectives:

Treatment Objective:

1. **Hygiene:** Continue to adhere to the vocal hygiene program to ensure longer periods of phonation without vocal fatigue or dizziness.

2. **Physiologic:** Patient will incorporate abdomino-diaphragmatic breathing and appropriate posture during spontaneous speech production.

3. **Symptomatic:**

   A. **Targeted vocal characters:** louder intensity (not soft) and full character (not breathy), in addition to maintaining the previous set (Treatment Plan I).

   B. **Targeted functional characters:**

      Patient will maintain relaxed, nontense, laryngeal and neck muscles and sufficient orality to optimize his voice projection during conversation.

      Patient will use larger abdominal accents to support louder voice productions, when needed, without tensing laryngeal and neck muscles.

   C. **Targeted speech characters:** Timely interjection in the conversation by starting abdominal filling as the current speaker is ending his utterance and move in right away with what he wants to say. Decrease rate of speech. Avoid running out of air.

4. **Psychogenic:** Patient will prepare himself for stressful situations such as social dinners, and professional meetings by warming up his voice using the Smith Accent Exercises for 10 minutes before the meeting/gathering. That will help tune his voice production system for the meeting.

Medical/Surgical: Not in consideration at this time.

Breakdown of Plan II into Short-Term Treatment Objectives

Hygiene

1. Demonstrate understanding of vocally challenging environments and situations and how to compensate for them with healthy vocal habits (eg, avoiding speaking against a noisy background, limiting talking on the phone to alerting the other about a written correspondence that will be sent, avoid talking or calling across a distance, proper use of voice magnification in conferences), by turning in weekly logs that demonstrates the times he identified potentially challenging vocal environments and highlighting how he compensated for them.

2. Increase hydration to enhance optimum laryngeal function and give himself phonatory breaks during conversations.

Physiologic

1. Maintain appropriate muscle tension in neck and laryngeal muscles and will successfully self-monitor and correct as needed.

2. Generalize the use of abdomino-phonatory control in everyday situations, reading unfamiliar texts, challenging dialogue and conversations more than 75% of the time with no cues.

3. Successfully self-monitor and self-correct adbomino-phonatory control during spontaneous conversations.

Symptomatic

Successfully self-monitor and self-correct targeted vocal qualities during spontaneous conversations.

Psychogenic

Warm up his voice by practicing "SAT" exercises before big social gatherings and professional meetings to provide his voice production system with the warm-up/tuning he needs to easily access his goal of a clear and projected voice.

Patient S Appendix C
Targeted Performances

Targeted Performances (check selected items) No = not on target Fairly = occasionally on target Yes = >75% on target	ON TARGET			
	Date __/__/__ (No) (Fairly) (Yes)	Date __/__/__ (No) (+/-) (yes)	Date __/__/__ (No) (+/-) (yes)	(No) (+/-) (yes)
A. Targeted Voicing Characters				
Appropriate pitch levels (lower, higher)	(No) (+/-) (yes)	(No) (+/-) (yes)	(No) (+/-) (yes)	(No) (+/-) (yes)
Appropriate loudness levels (softer, louder)	(No) (+/-) (yes)	(No) (+/-) (yes)	(No) (+/-) (yes)	(No) (+/-) (yes)
Resonant Voice (oral and not muffled)	(No) (+/-) (yes)	(No) (+/-) (yes)	(No) (+/-) (yes)	(No) (+/-) (yes)
Easy Onset Voice (no hard glottal attacks)	(No) (+/-) (yes)	(No) (+/-) (yes)	(No) (+/-) (yes)	(No) (+/-) (yes)
Clear Voice (not rough)	(No) (+/-) (yes)	(No) (+/-) (yes)	(No) (+/-) (yes)	(No) (+/-) (yes)
Full Voice (not breathy)	(No) (+/-) (yes)	(No) (+/-) (yes)	(No) (+/-) (yes)	(No) (+/-) (yes)
Strong Voice (not asthenic)	(No) (+/-) (yes)	(No) (+/-) (yes)	(No) (+/-) (yes)	(No) (+/-) (yes)
Relaxed/Easy (not strained)	(No) (+/-) (yes)	(No) (+/-) (yes)	(No) (+/-) (yes)	(No) (+/-) (yes)
Absent Vocal Fry	(No) (+/-) (yes)	(No) (+/-) (yes)	(No) (+/-) (yes)	(No) (+/-) (yes)
B. Targeted Speech Characteristics				
Appropriate speech rate	(No) (+/-) (yes)	(No) (+/-) (yes)	(No) (+/-) (yes)	(No) (+/-) (yes)
Appropriate intonation contour	(No) (+/-) (yes)	(No) (+/-) (yes)	(No) (+/-) (yes)	(No) (+/-) (yes)

Targeted Performances (check selected items)	ON TARGET		
No = not on target **Fairly = occasionally on target** **Yes = >75% on target**	*(No) (Fairly) (Yes)*	*(No) (+/–) (yes)*	*(No) (+/–) (yes)*
Appropriate pause location	(No) (+/–) (yes)	(No) (+/–) (yes)	(No) (+/–) (yes)
Appropriate pause duration	(No) (+/–) (yes)	(No) (+/–) (yes)	(No) (+/–) (yes)
Appropriate utterance duration/breath group	(No) (+/–) (yes)	(No) (+/–) (yes)	(No) (+/–) (yes)
C. Targeted Supportive Voice Production Parameters			
Optimum physical tension (posture-mouth-larynx-neck-shoulder-chest)	(No) (+/–) (yes)	(No) (+/–) (yes)	(No) (+/–) (yes)
Facilitation by associated body movements	(No) (+/–) (yes)	(No) (+/–) (yes)	(No) (+/–) (yes)
Adequate oral resonance and voice projection	(No) (+/–) (yes)	(No) (+/–) (yes)	(No) (+/–) (yes)
Adequate copying of			
Predictable stimuli:	(No) (+/–) (yes)	(No) (+/–) (yes)	(No) (+/–) (yes)
Unpredictable stimuli:	(No) (+/–) (yes)	(No) (+/–) (yes)	(No) (+/–) (yes)
Adequate self-monitoring and self-correction			
Abdomino–phonatory control	(No) (+/–) (yes)	(No) (+/–) (yes)	(No) (+/–) (yes)
Voice characteristics	(No) (+/–) (yes)	(No) (+/–) (yes)	(No) (+/–) (yes)
Speech characteristics	(No) (+/–) (yes)	(No) (+/–) (yes)	(No) (+/–) (yes)
Timely turn taking	(No) (+/–) (yes)	(No) (+/–) (yes)	(No) (+/–) (yes)
"On target" self-initiated performances	(No) (+/–) (yes)	(No) (+/–) (yes)	(No) (+/–) (yes)

Patient S Appendix D
Therapy Progress Form

Abdomino-phonatory control	Date _/_/_	Date _/_/_	Date _/_/_
1. Appropriate abdomino-diaphragmatic breathing (rest): Supine-sitting-standing	......% time		
passive outward abdominal wall movement on inspiration	0 25 50 75 90		
gradual inward abdominal wall movement on expiration	0 25 50 75 90		
2. Appropriate abdomino-phonatory control in largo (2–3 beats): consonants-vowel play-syllables-words	......% time		
adequate (quick, deep, and silent) oral inspiratory filling	0 25 50 75 90		
adequate force of abdominal wall contraction	0 25 50 75 90		
appropriate abdomino-phonatory tuning	0 25 50 75 90		
adequate inspiratory reserve	0 25 50 75 90		
adequate production of targeted vocal characters	0 25 50 75 90		
3. Appropriate abdomino-phonatory control in andante (4–5 beats): vowel play-syllables-words	......% time		
adequate (quick, deep, and silent) oral inspiratory filling	0 25 50 75 90		
adequate force of abdominal wall contraction	0 25 50 75 90		
appropriate abdomino-phonatory tuning	0 25 50 75 90		
adequate inspiratory reserve	0 25 50 75 90		
adequate production of targeted vocal characters	0 25 50 75 90		

Abdomino-phonatory control	Date _/_/_	Date _/_/_	Date _/_/_
4. Appropriate abdomino-phonatory control in allegro (6,7, . . .): vowel play-syllables-words	......% time		
adequate (quick, deep, and silent) oral inspiratory filling	0 25 50 75 90		
adequate force of abdominal wall contraction	0 25 50 75 90		
appropriate abdomino-phonatory tuning	0 25 50 75 90		
adequate inspiratory reserve	0 25 50 75 90		
adequate production of targeted vocal characters	0 25 50 75 90		
5. Generalization of abdomino-phonatory control to spontaneous speech: reading/monologue/ dialogue/. . .	Modeled/ Spontaneous		
adequate (quick, deep, and silent) oral inspiratory filling	0 25 50 75 90		
adequate force of abdominal wall contraction	0 25 50 75 90		
appropriate abdomino-phonatory tuning	0 25 50 75 90		
adequate inspiratory reserve	0 25 50 75 90		
adequate production of targeted vocal characters	0 25 50 75 90		
adequate production of targeted speech characters	0 25 50 75 90		

Balancing Vocal Function After Surgery for Unilateral Vocal Fold Paralysis

Maria Dietrich, PhD, CCC-SLP

Case Study: Patient SS

In this case study Maria Dietrich demonstrates how important it is to provide early solutions for patients with unilateral vocal fold paralysis to prevent the development of maladaptive vocal behaviors while maximizing vocal functionality in daily life.

Patient History. Patient SS is a 39-year-old woman who has been referred to a Voice Center for a voice evaluation and treatment performed by a voice care team. Patient SS underwent a thyroid surgery and has struggled with her voice since. Her surgeon observed a unilateral vocal fold paralysis of the left vocal fold, which persisted 3 months postsurgery. At that point, he decided to refer her to a specialized Voice Center for confirmation and treatment options. SS declined any voice problems prior to her thyroid surgery. Her medical history was unremarkable before the onset of her thyroid disease. She did not have any previous surgeries nor any sort of trauma to the head or neck and rarely suffered from upper respiratory infections. Patient SS lived a healthy lifestyle, exercised regularly, balanced her diet, and did not smoke. She denied issues with allergies or reflux disease. She reportedly drank about 32 ounces of water per day and two cups of either coffee or tea per day.

Patient SS was married with no children and had been working in Human Resources for a medium-sized company for 14 years. As part of her job, she would speak for most of the time during the day, be it one-on-one, on the telephone, to small groups (up to five people), or seminars with larger numbers of employees (20–30 people). She recalled instances of occasional vocal fatigue, but she denied having had any longer lasting voice problems. SS relied on her voice for work, and she became increasingly worried about her ongoing voice problem. Although she was an upbeat and optimistic person, she acknowledged that she was a worrier, and moreover, she started to feel anxious that she might lose her job in these uncertain economical times. In fact, she entered a situation where she had to take days off from work several times due to her voice problems. She was a lively person and outside of work she enjoyed an active recreational and social life including sports (tennis, hiking) and frequently meeting up with friends. However, she had to stop all her sports activities and she became increasingly frustrated that she had to limit her speaking.

History of the Problem. Patient SS noticed a hoarse voice after the thyroid surgery, which persisted at the 1-month follow-up medical visit. Her surgeon noticed that her left vocal fold was immobile and suggested to wait for spontaneous recovery and recommended a follow-up visit 3 months postsurgery. However, 3 months postsurgery, patient SS still struggled with her voice. Her physician did not see any improvement in vocal fold movement of her left vocal fold and this time suggested a visit to a Voice Center to discuss treatment options. The laryngologist at the Voice Center diagnosed SS with a unilateral vocal fold paralysis of the left vocal fold with secondary muscle tension dysphonia (MTD).

The voice disorder was deemed iatrogenic in nature and was linked to direct injury of the patient's left recurrent laryngeal nerve during thyroid surgery. Abnormalities of the cricoarytenoid joint were ruled out.

Almost 4 months had already passed since SS's thyroid surgery at the time of the visit with the laryngologist. At this point, patient SS felt that her symptoms had gradually worsened. Now her voice was not only extremely hoarse and weak but also associated with an increasing degree of vocal effort and frequent vocal fatigue, which had been present before but not as pronounced when the voice problems began. She also experienced periods of aphonia about three times per week that occurred mostly at the end of a speaking-intensive work day. On some days she did not recover well and had to take off time from work or cancel speaking engagements. Furthermore, she felt she could not be heard and ran out of air constantly during speech. She also noticed shortness of breath with exertion, which led to her quitting any sports. With regard to swallowing, patient SS observed that she had to be careful swallowing solids and especially liquids. She reported occasional choking and coughing, but she became more careful and adapted to the situation.

Based on the history of the problem and the worsening trajectory of the voice disorder, the laryngologist suggested a temporary vocal fold injection into the left vocal fold to provide instant relief to the patient. The vocal fold injection would improve vocal fold closure immediately by increasing the size of the paralyzed fold and should take care of many vocal symptoms at once. But the laryngologist coupled injection with the request that patient SS undergo a course of voice therapy postsurgery to reduce or avoid any carryover of vocal hyperfunction and to balance the vocal system postsurgery. For the long run, the patient was told she may be a candidate for a permanent medialization thyroplasty (moving the paralyzed vocal fold toward midline) if the nerve function will not recover by the time the temporary vocal fold augmentation wore off (approximately around the 7 months postsurgery mark). The patient agreed to the treatment plan. A vocal fold injection with Cymetra (acellular dermis) into the left membranous vocal fold was performed with a direct laryngoscope under general anesthesia (the patient opted against an office procedure because she was too anxious).

Evaluation Procedures. The evaluation procedures included a visual-perceptual and auditory-perceptual evaluation as well as standard vocal function testing (acoustic and aerodynamic analyses).

1. *Visual-perceptual.* A videoendoscopic and videostroboscopic examination was performed of patient SS's vocal folds with a 70-degree rigid endoscope and without a topical anesthetic. The left vocal fold was neither adducting nor abducting and was positioned in the paramedian position (slightly off midline). As a result, incomplete closure of the vocal folds was evident. The patient was able to produce a glissando pitch glide with visible bilateral vocal fold lengthening at higher pitches, which indicated normal function of the superior laryngeal nerve. The affected vocal fold had a severely reduced mucosal wave and vibrated only irregularly resulting in aperiodicity as seen on stroboscopy. A plane difference of the

vocal folds was not seen. Furthermore, supraglottic medial compression of the ventricular folds was observed during phonation consistent with secondary muscle tension dysphonia (MTD). The secondary MTD was found to be a compensatory response to the underlying glottal insufficiency. The unaffected vocal fold was free of lesions or abnormalities as was the surrounding tissue including the posterior larynx.

2. *Auditory-perceptual.* The Consensus Auditory Perceptual Evaluation of Voice (CAPE-V)[36] protocol was used to rate patient SS's voice quality. Ratings were based on conversational speech, sentence productions and sustaining the vowels /a/ and /i/. SS could sustain vowels only for a maximum of 3 seconds. The following scores of SS's voice quality refer to a visual analogue scale of 100 mm. The patient presented overall with a severe dysphonia (66 mm) consisting of severe breathiness (80 mm) mixed with moderate roughness (36 mm), severe vocal asthenia (88 mm), and severe strain (66 mm). Loudness was severely reduced and pitch appeared mildly increased. All impressions were observed consistently. Patient SS rated her vocal effort as 600 during conversational speech using direct magnitude estimation (100 normal and comfortable amount of effort in voice, 300 three times as much effort as normal and so forth). Her total score on the Voice Handicap Index (VHI) was 88/120.

3. *Acoustic analysis.* Voice fundamental frequency (F_0) as measured during the all-voiced sentence "we were away a year ago" (of which only a portion was all-voiced) was found to be increased with 285 Hz as compared to normative values matched for age and sex. A high-pitched voice can be a common compensation to improve vocal fold closure as well as a result of a chronic vocal fold paralysis with increasing fibrosis of the affected vocal fold. Her speaking intensity was reduced with 50 dB SPL. Reliable values for jitter and shimmer could not be determined due the stark presence of aperiodicity and noise in the signal (Type 3 signal).[72] Furthermore, the patient's pitch and vocal intensity ranges were reduced at the top of the range. A pitch glide on /i/ was recorded (frequency range 87 Hz), and the patient was asked to produce /a/ as quietly and as loudly as possible (intensity range 23 dB SPL).

4. *Aerodynamic measures.* Phonatory airflow and subglottic pressure as derived from intraoral pressure were measured with the Phonatory Aerodynamic System (PAS, Model 6600, KayPENTAX). The patient was asked to repeat /pi/ five times. Both values were increased in comparison to normative values matched for age and sex. Average phonatory airflow was 437.2 mL/sec, which confirmed the presence of glottal incompetence, and subglottic pressure was 11.4 cm H_2O, which provided a physiologic correlate for perceived phonatory effort.

Description and Rationale for Therapy Approach. The review of patient SS's medical history and history of the problem revealed that the source of her voice disorder at the point of her evaluation by a voice center team was twofold. First, there was a clear primary etiology for her voice problems, namely, her left vocal fold paralysis. Second, she developed secondary muscle tension dysphonia (MTD), which was a compensatory response to her glottal insufficiency that aggravated vocal symptoms. Due to her long history of vocal hyperfunction before she was offered relief, SS was at risk for a carryover of this vocal hyperfunction postsurgery. Hence, from the perspective of voice production, a primary goal was to absorb any tendencies for continued vocal hyperfunction while shaping her voice production patterns into a well-balanced, functional, and powerful voice in light of improved vocal fold closure post vocal fold injection. A secondary goal was to modify her work and private environment to optimize her functionality in the face of residually compromised vocal endurance and vocal power.

Accordingly, four treatment goals were chosen. The goals were (1) to follow a tailored vocal hygiene program; (2) to build awareness for excessive laryngeal and bodily muscle tensions and to eliminate them; (3) to start a regular vocal function exercise program; and (4) to learn resonant voice as an alternative and efficient mode of voice production. To sum up, it was necessary for the patient to fully understood her medical and vocal physiologic situation, develop awareness for daily vocal demands as well as awareness for changes in her laryngeal system and body that might affect voice, and be ready to embark on a regular vocal exercise program to optimize and fine tune vocal function.

Goal 1. First, the patient and clinician will review SS's presurgery and postsurgery vocal fold pathophysiology to build an understanding for the required modifications. Then, the clinician and SS will work out a comprehensive

vocal hygiene program tailored to her needs, which will include hydration, awareness training, and real-life adjustments. Specifically, patient SS will increase her water intake to 64 ounces throughout the day and decrease her caffeine intake to one cup per day. Further, she will scrutinize her work, family, and recreational schedules with the twofold goal of realizing the extent and type of her vocal demands and ultimately to balance speaking times and vocal resting times.

Rationale. It was crucial that patient SS understood the anatomy and physiology of her laryngeal condition and the functional extent of her chronic, although manageable, voice disorder so that it was reasonable for her to comply with adaptations that were required of her. Although patient SS's voice quality immediately improved as the result of the left vocal fold injection, her vocal endurance was likely to remain limited, thus increasing her vulnerability for experiencing vocal fatigue. Moreover, SS was a professional voice user and as such was already at a higher risk for developing a voice disorder. Fortunately, she did not have to struggle with her voice prior to the onset of her voice problem; however, with the current combination of her vocal status with her professional voice use, she definitely had to revisit her vocal load and behavior.

As a first awareness exercise, SS was asked to create a weekly chart of all vocal times starting with the moment she would wake up to the time she went to bed. The schedule was discussed in detail and peak times of heavy voicing were identified with regard to both amount and type. As a human resources employee, SS had some control over the scheduling of her one-on-one or group sessions with new or existing employees, interviews, and presentations. She was advised to avoid any back-to-back scheduling of sessions, to space out vocal demands across the week, to schedule quiet work times several times a day (eg, 30-min to 1-hour blocks), to avoid large group sessions at the end of the day, and to allow for rest and recovery before, during (10 min), and after presentations of a duration of 1 hour or longer.

This clearly was a team effort as her supervisor and colleagues had to be on board with the plan. Everyone was extremely supportive and, for example, respected SS's quiet time during which she would work on E-mails and paperwork only. Also, this was a work in progress and weekly charts would be reviewed where SS would mark times that were vocally difficult and times that were vocally successful. In the end, with the help of her chart and her notes, she figured out a work routine that was vocally feasible for her.

Finding the point of best vocal functionality in work and personal life was the foremost goal. At a private level, her husband was involved early on to create a mutual understanding of the medical situation and the functional needs that have evolved. He attended the second therapy session during which the clinician asked SS to review her weekly chart and explain positive and negative vocal events to her husband and the clinician in physiologic terms. Thus, it was ensured that SS understood her voice disorder and matured in monitoring herself independently. During outings with friends, the clinician was advised to choose a location that was conducive to her adhering to vocal hygiene. For example, if she wanted to catch up with friends, a quiet location should be preferred. If she found herself

in a noisy environment, she was advised to sit close the person she was talking to, including switching positions, and to limit the time she would speak in such an environment. Her husband and friends were extremely supportive to accommodate her needs and felt they learned from the experience too.

Finally, as an advantage, SS already led a healthy lifestyle, did not smoke, and drank water. Only a few adjustments were recommended such as to increase the water intake to 64 ounces throughout the day, and to limit caffeine on days with longer speaking engagements or larger groups. In addition, voice amplification was recommended for any large group presentations or whenever she felt like it to make the vocal experience as comfortable as possible.

Goal 2. Patient SS will create awareness for excessive muscle tension in the larynx, neck, and upper back and will learn to monitor and eliminate it to allow easy and effortless flow phonation. She will be introduced to a short routine of progressive muscle relaxation for the face and neck and a deep breathing exercise to calm down from psychologic and physiologic stress. The ultimate goal here will be to rebalance the laryngeal musculature.

Rationale. Unfortunately, patient SS had a long history of compensatory behaviors for her vocal fold paralysis. Her compensations included intralaryngeal and extralaryngeal muscular tension beyond what is usually seen in healthy voice users and which were directly linked to her experience of vocal effort and vocal fatigue. As a first step, SS had to realize that she indeed engaged in compensatory muscle behaviors and that now, postsurgery, such compensations would not be necessary and rather counterproductive. In other words, she was specifically asked to change her psychological *mindset* and attitude toward voicing. Her new visualization was supposed to be an easy and effortless voice. She liked the idea of this mindset so much that she decided to put up Post-It notes at work and at home reminding her of it.

A series of progressive muscle relaxation steps were then practiced to make the patient aware of muscle tension in the her face, neck, and upper body by increasing and releasing tension.[73] Such checks would also be performed at the beginning of each subsequent therapy session and SS was asked to use them periodically throughout the day, in particular before any speaking engagements. Also, she was asked to mark on her chart how often she found herself "tensed up" and the various triggers for it. SS learned to listen to her voice and neck and became very good at monitoring her muscular behaviors. She noticed that she would automatically increase muscular tension when in "presentation mode" or when she was excited or annoyed about something. She remembered that the psychological stress coming from her voice problems had made her feel choked up at times in the past. However, now that she was on the way to recovery, she felt a lot of pressure lifted off her shoulders, which she acknowledged, in hindsight, had made her voice problem harder than it already was. As an adjunct to progressive relaxation, SS also was introduced to a simple routine of a few deep breaths as a stress reliever to immediately calm her physiologic system (deep breathing decreases heart rate immediately by way of an increase in vagal tone).[74] Over time, she could record progress on her chart and she felt less and less bothered by muscle tension as confidence in her new voice in-

creased. Last, but not least, based on her newly acquired knowledge of laryngeal anatomy and physiology, SS was directed to focus on the interplay between airflow and voicing. Tension at the level of the vocal folds was demonstrated by negative practice involving breathholding and voicing. The patient was a quick learner and realized that there was a comfortable point of airflow in her voice that would support phonation. Flow phonation was then practiced using the hierarchical steps as described by Stone and Casteel[75] progressing from sound through words to dialogue.

Goal 3. Patient SS will master a series of vocal warm-ups and exercises to improve vocal function. SS will practice twice daily, and additionally as needed (eg, before presentations).

Rationale. Patient SS's vocal fold vibratory behavior will always be chronically affected by the underlying vocal fold paralysis despite significant surgical and behavioral improvements. Thus, a regular exercise program was essential to maintain the positive therapy outcome. The patient was introduced to a routine of exercises geared toward exercising the entire vocal range and a variety of vocal postures. The exercises included lip trills and pitch glides and sustaining of vowels at different pitches. The routine followed Stemple's Vocal Function Exercises program.[31,76] The exercises were also recorded on CD and the patient synched them on her i-Pod where she would listen to the instructions and the examples.

Goal 4. Patient SS will learn to produce resonant voice in isolation and in conversational context.

Rationale. A major problem with vocal fold paralysis is breathiness and asthenia with the perceptual result of lack of projection and vocal fatigue. Again, although the vocal fold injection provided the patient with a significant improvement in glottal closure, residual problems such as vocal fold irregularities during phonation are likely to persist. The most reasonable route of treatment for this particular problem was to train resonant voice. Resonant voice therapy is a well-known and well-researched voice therapy approach to produce a voicing pattern that is easy and efficient (ie, minimum phonatory effort to achieve a louder sound). Resonant voice was trained hierarchically starting with the experience of vibrations in the face and negative practice, the perfection of a basic training gesture (humming)[76,77] and the progressive extension to syllables, all voiced phrases, sentences, and conversational speech.

The patient did not find it difficult to produce resonant voice in isolation, but caught herself falling out of resonant voice easily during a sentence. With time, she became increasingly adept at switching back and forth between her regular conversational voice and resonant voice. Brief video- and audio recordings of the patient during therapy with time for feedback helped to hone the patient's vocal and auditory skills. A CD with resonant voice exercises was created as well, which the patient liked to use at home. SS noticed that resonant voice remarkably improved her vocal endurance and voice quality and she was very pleased with the outcome.

Results of Therapy. Patient SS participated in a total of eight 45-minute therapy sessions over an 8-week period. The therapy outcome was excellent both from the point of view of the patient as well as the speech-language patholo-

gist. Although improvement already was generated by way of the vocal fold injection, the patient's excellent compliance with therapy was critical in making the most of the situation. Her drive to improve her voice as much as possible as well as daily successes served as a strong motivation to adhere to the recommendations. This attitude especially paid off while the effects of the vocal fold injection started to wear off. During that time SS was able to maintain her level of functionality.

The follow-up visit was scheduled 1 week posttherapy (7 months postthyroid surgery). On the same day, a laryngeal needle electromyography (EMG) was scheduled to investigate the neural status of the patient's vocal fold paralysis in order to guide further treatment. As both, the visual-perceptual evaluation and the laryngeal EMG confirmed the continued presence of the left vocal fold paralysis, the laryngologist suggested a permanent laryngeal framework surgery instead of a repeat vocal fold injection to which the patient agreed. A Gore-Tex medialization thyroplasty was performed under general anesthesia. The intent of the surgery was again to improve the position and contour of the affected vocal fold by pushing the affected vocal fold medially. The surgery was performed with local anesthesia under sedation. The patient's voice was monitored during surgery to find the optimal position for the implantation material through a window in the thyroid cartilage.

One postop refresher voice therapy session was scheduled to monitor the patient's adaptation to the latest surgery. Patient SS adapted excellently to the latest surgery, continued to use what she learned in voice therapy, and was discharged without the need for further therapy. The following data refer to the treatment status at the conclusion of therapy post vocal fold injection and prior to the medialization thyroplasty.

1. *Visual-perceptual.* The videoendoscopic and videostroboscopic examination confirmed the left vocal fold paralysis as did the laryngeal needle EMG. As a result of surgery, the vocal folds, however, achieved closure during phonation. The mucosal wave of the affected vocal fold was reduced. The vocal folds vibrated, albeit periodicity was still irregular. No secondary muscle tension dysphonia was observed.
2. *Auditory-perceptual.* The CAPE-V protocol was used to rate patient SS's voice quality. SS was now able to sustain vowels for a maximum of 16 seconds. The patient presented overall with a mild dysphonia (6 mm) consisting of mild breathiness (4 mm), roughness (7 mm), asthenia (2 mm), and strain (3 mm). Loudness and pitch appeared adequate. All impressions were observed consistently. Patient SS rated her vocal effort as 150 during conversational speech using direct magnitude estimation. Her total score on the Voice Handicap Index (VHI) was 30/120. Overall, her voice quality had improved significantly and both the patient and the speech-language pathologist were extremely pleased.
3. *Acoustic analysis.* Voice fundamental frequency (F_0) was found to be at the higher end of the normal range (220 Hz). Her speaking intensity was within normal limits (68 dB SPL). Values for both jitter (1.2%) and shimmer (0.3%) were close to normative values matched for age and sex. The noise-to-harmonic ratio

was 0.112. Furthermore, the patient's frequency (160 Hz) and vocal intensity ranges (28 db SPL) improved.

4. *Aerodynamic measures.* A re-evaluation of the patient's phonatory airflow and subglottic pressure confirmed the perceptual improvements. Both values were found to be in the normal range matched for age and sex. Average phonatory airflow rate was 275.4 mL/sec and subglottic pressure was 8.0 cm H_2O.

> *In the next case presentation, Lisa Kelchner describes the evaluation and treatment of a medically challenged individual with a vocal fold paralysis causing voice loss and dysphagia.*

Management of Dysphonia and Dysphagia in Iatrogenic Vocal Fold Paralysis

Lisa Kelchner, PhD, CCC-SLP

Case Study: Patient T

Patient History. Patient T was a 75-year-old woman who was referred for voice and swallowing management following removal of a jugular glomus tumor involving the left vagus nerve in April 1998. Surgical resection of the tumor resulted in a sacrifice of a section of the vagus nerve above the carotid bifurcation at the skull base. Resulting sequelae included mild left pharyngeal hemianesthesia and paresis, left vocal fold paralysis, and hemiparesis of the left cricopharyngeal muscle, all of which resulted in severe dysphonia and dysphagia. The initial hospital course was rocky, and a G-tube was placed to provide nutritional support and avoid aspiration.

Pertinent medical history for this patient included previous (10-year) right neck surgery for removal of her parotid gland, right carotid endarterectomy (4 years prior), transient ischemic attacks (TIAs) attributable to her significant vascular disease (6 years prior), and left XIIth nerve damage. The preexisting left lingual weakness was thought to be secondary to either a mild CNS event or a XIIth nerve neuritis. Her available medical history was uncertain on this point. The patient also suffered a hiatal hernia and gastroesophageal reflux disease (GERD). Despite these other significant health events, the patient or family did not report any previous difficulties with voice, speech, or swallowing.

Patient T was a widow who lived alone prior to her surgery. She had two attentive daughters who lived close by and alternated staying with their mother during the first few months following surgery. Interests included family activities and gardening. Patient T was a delightful and cooperative woman but extremely anxious about her medical condition and concerned about the changes in sensation and function within the pharynx and larynx.

Initial Evaluation. The patient presented to the office 1 month postsurgery. Initial evaluation included videostroboscopy and clinical voice and dysphagia exams. Initial videostroboscopy revealed a spindle-shaped gap configuration to glottic closure, and supraglottic activity was significant for compression of the right ventricular fold in an attempt to compensate for the fixed left true vocal fold. Clear, thin, pooled secretions were noted in the pyriform sinuses and were worse on the left. The vertical level of the vocal folds appeared to be equal. The edge of the left TVF appeared smooth but was significantly bowed, whereas the right TVF presented as smooth and straight. Mobility of the vocal folds revealed a fixed left TVF in an intermediate position and a mobile right TVF. Because of the significant compression of the right ventricular fold, only vibratory characteristics of the left TVF could be observed. Because of the intermediate position and flaccid bowed edge of this fold, there was a mild-to-moderate increase to mucosal wave and amplitude of vibration. The open phase of the vibratory cycle dominated, and phase symmetry was at least 75% irregular. Overall laryngeal function during conversation was noted to fluctuate between hypo- and hyperfunction secondary to changes in effort with fatigue. The perceptual quality of the patient's voice during this initial evaluation was a severe dysphonia marked by a harsh breathy hoarseness. Patient T was able to sustain phonation for only 5 seconds, and these attempts resulted in harsh coughing. In fact, she felt it necessary to expectorate secretions every few minutes. Pitch range was quite limited, and intensity was judged to be reduced. Because of the apparent extreme sensitivity of the glottis and harsh dysphonic signal, formal acoustic and aerodynamic evaluation of voice was deferred.

The initial clinical dysphagia evaluation revealed oral-motor function to be within normal limits for labial and facial muscle function. Lingual function demonstrated mild persistent deviation of the tongue to the left and mildly diminished strength of velopharyngeal closure left. Sensitivity for the gag reflex was intact bilaterally. Laryngeal elevation and tilt of larynx during dry swallows were considered diminished, and secretions were continuously problematic for the patient. At the time of the initial exam, the patient was not permitted anything by mouth (NPO). Medical treatment and precautions for reflux were already in place. The patient's lungs were clear to auscultation, and there were no clinical signs of lower respiratory difficulties.

Considering the generally fragile medical condition of this patient and the multiple problems requiring therapeutic intervention, the following clinical needs were prioritized:

- airway protection and secretion management
- maintain nutritional status and hydration per G-tube
- improve strength and coordination of the pharyngeal phase of the swallow for eventual intake by mouth (PO)
- improve glottic closure with reduced ventricular effort for voicing
- ongoing patient and family education and support.

Although these are presented as separate areas of clinical focus, they were not treated in a mutually exclusive fashion.

Goal 1. Improve Airway Protection and Secretion Management. This lovely woman never went anywhere without a large box of tissues and a small disposal bag because of continuous expectoration of small amounts of thin, clear secretions. Early in her recovery, this was a necessary behavior to maintain a comfortable airway, and she often had laryngeal penetration if not aspiration of her secretions (no swallow studies were conducted while she was an inpatient). Obviously, her status was severe enough to require enteral feedings. An in-office flexible endoscopic examination of swallowing (FEES) revealed that, despite pharyngeal weakness and reduced airway pro-

tection, secretions could be cleared from the hypopharynx with multiple effortful swallows and a head turn to the left. Within the first few sessions of therapy, it became clear the harsh expectoration had become a habituated action. Having seen previous patients with the same difficulty and considering her pulmonary status, as well as the actual small amount of secretions being produced, the patient was instructed to "Hold your breath (as hard as possible) and turn your head left while pushing your tongue to the roof of your mouth while swallowing." Vocalizations following these attempts were judged to be "dry." We practiced this substitute behavior repeatedly during the first several therapy sessions and the patient was asked to do this as many times as possible during the day. Family members were enlisted to cue the patient at home regarding the frequency of her coughing and then suggest that she substitute a swallow attempt. The patient required constant cuing and reassurance to resist a cough. This harsh expectoration also contributed to the general hyperfunction of the laryngeal mechanism. Despite improvements in all areas, it was 4 to 5 months before this behavior began to diminish for good. Patient T was reluctant to travel without her tissues and bag for a few months beyond that. As successful oral intake increased, this behavior finally was extinguished.

Goal 2. Maintain Nutritional Status and Hydration. Throughout the rehabilitative process, there was close monitoring of the patient's nutritional status and hydration. Initial caloric intake was tracked through G-tube feedings that included five cans of Ensure Plus per day plus a 100-cc water flush. The patient's desired weight was approximately

132 lbs, but she lost weight immediately following surgery and remained in the low 120s. The eventual transition from G-tube feedings to oral intake was gradual and allowed a careful shift of the enteral supplements to a well-rounded oral diet, although the patient's appetite remained somewhat suppressed throughout her recovery. Even as swallowing function improved, she needed to continue with nutritional supplements by mouth to maintain her weight.

Goal 3. Improve Strength and Co-ordination of the Pharyngeal Phase of the Swallow for Eventual Oral Intake.

In addition to the effortful swallow exercises for secretion management, several direct oral-motor and pharyngeal strengthening exercises were routinely practiced within our once-to-twice per week sessions. The patient, who was always accompanied by one of her two daughters, was also instructed to do these at home on a daily basis. These exercises included:

- lingual range of motion in all directions (× 20 bid)
- lingual resistance exercises on protrusion and lateralization: hold for 5 sec relax (× 10 each alternate direction bid)
- lingual base exercises designed to work on increasing strength and laryngeal elevation.

The first exercise attempted was to keep the mouth open, hold the anterior tip of the tongue with gauze, and try to swallow. This is a challenging exercise, and many patients have a difficult time initiating the first few swallows. In this case, swallowing while pushing against a tongue blade had to be the first step. Patient T was instructed to do these five times daily. Eventually, the tongue hold

maneuver was possible in a sequence of two or three.

The initial FEES exam had been conducted to observe the patient's management of secretions and airway protection during the swallow. Blue food coloring and ice chips were the only items introduced during that exam. Results indicated management of both was possible with the strategies of head turn left and multiple swallows. Initially, this approach using small trials of ice chips was fatiguing for the patient. Nonetheless, the patient progressed and small therapeutic trials of pureed consistencies were offered successfully. At that point, a modified barium swallow (MBS) was conducted to thoroughly evaluate all stages of the swallow.

During the initial MBS, thin, honey-thickened liquids and pureed consistencies were offered. This study revealed a severe pharyngeal phase dysphagia marked by:

- reduced laryngeal elevation
- decreased tongue base strength
- residue in the valleculae
- a significant amount of pooled contrast in the left piriform sinus postswallow
- significantly reduced cricopharyngeal relaxation on the left
- a moderate degree of laryngeal penetration for all trials with thin liquids more likely to be poorly controlled. (Using a head turn left-lean right and multiple swallows, airway protection and hypopharyngeal clearance improved.)

Goals in therapy now included a more aggressive trial feed schedule that used pureed and honey-thickened liquid consistencies. Initial bolus sizes offered were less than 5 cc. Close clinical monitoring of pulmonary activity was instituted, and the family was compliant and reliable with all those recommendations. As therapy progressed, the patient was instructed to attempt small trials at home under the supervision of family. Still uncomfortable with the altered pharyngeal and laryngeal sensations, Patient T progressed slowly at home.

A second modified barium swallow study conducted shortly after a vocal fold medialization (3 months postsurgery) revealed significant improvements in the pharyngeal phase of the swallow with only trace residues remaining in the valleculae and left piriform sinus. Reduced cricopharyngeal opening on the left remained and continued use of aforementioned strategies was a must for safe oral intake. With improved airway protection, increased pharyngeal strength, and continued recovery, the patient was able to tolerate more aggressive diet advancement. Once the majority of intake was oral, exercises were discontinued. The transition to total oral feeds for all consistencies without nutritional compromise or pulmonary excitement was complete by December. The G-tube was removed the following month. The pace of this part of treatment was slowed somewhat by the patient's constant need for reassurance and strict guidance.

Goal 4. Improve Glottic Closure and Reduce Ventricular Effort During Voicing. From the start of therapy, it was apparent that Patient T was engaging in an excessive use of supraglottic laryngeal area tension during voicing. This was evidenced by observation of effort during conversation and patient complaints of fatigue, as well as the endoscopic views previously described. Results of the first videostroboscopic examination revealed a significant bow

to the paralyzed left vocal fold, and the continuous harsh coughing and general hypersensitivity to the alterations in hypopharyngeal and laryngeal sensations only added to this problem. Trials involving sustaining the tense vowel /i/ almost always resulted in coughing. Sustaining lax vowels /o/ and /u/ actually resulted in clearer tones and longer times because she was able to reduce some of the ventricular compression while maintaining appropriate tension of the mobile vocal fold. The patient was asked to sustain the vowels /o/ and /u/ for as long as possible, using a forward focus technique of exaggerated lip rounding and attempt to buzz the lips. This gesture had to be trained over time with much reinforcement and visual feedback. Helping this patient identify supraglottic versus glottic tension was a challenge. The therapeutic nuances of gestures to reduce tension and enhance forward focus were difficult for this patient to appreciate. Emphasis was also placed on proper breath support through attention to abdominal breathing technique. Within-therapy, success was achieved in reducing supraglottic tension during these sample tasks, but carryover to conversation was extremely difficult.

The patient was inconsistent with this part of her home-program routine. Frankly, she had many tasks to perform, and although the tasks complemented each other, there were too many of them at once. Several weeks into the recovery and therapy process, the surgeon was approached to consider a Gelfoam injection to assist in relieving the significant glottic gap of the paralyzed vocal fold. Because of the nature and extent of the original surgery, the surgeon decided immediately to proceed with performing a type I thyroplasty.

Type I Thyroplasty. The surgical procedure was carried out in the typical fashion with the patient under general sedation and local anesthetic. When the Silastic stent was ready to be placed, a fiber-optic endoscope was passed transnasally to allow for visualization of the vocal folds. Silastic stent placement immediately resulted in straightening the edge of the left vocal fold and improving medialization of the mid-anterior segment of the vocal fold edge. Perceptual quality of the patient's voice was stronger with less harsh breathy hoarseness. The surgery was completed without complication, and the patient was advised to remain NPO and on voice rest for 7 days. Previously described strategies to reduce coughing also were encouraged.

Postoperative laryngeal videostroboscopy confirmed complete elimination of the left true vocal fold bow, improved medialization, and less lateromedial compression of the right ventricular fold. In the weeks after surgery, exercises designed to encourage vocal fold approximation were resumed. These included a modified version of Vocal Function Exercises sustaining the lax vowels /o/ and /u/ on only three pitch levels (low, mid, high). Pitch variability remained restricted (3–4 note range A–D). The patient eventually was successful in sustaining these for up to 10 seconds.

A modification of the Resonant Voice Therapy protocol also was introduced to address goals of achieving efficient glottic tension while discouraging ventricular compression. The patient was asked to hum at comfortable pitch levels and with variable (as possible) melodic contours. Tasks progressed to chanting words and short phrases. These techniques resulted in a moderate improvement and "fine tuning" of the medialization results for conversational voice quality. Patient T had to be cued continually to attend to levels of laryngeal tension and effort. Toward the end of therapy, voice quality variations were secondary to the patient's general feeling of well-being and how much energy she had to attend to the subtleties of the therapeutic techniques she had acquired.

Goal 5. Ongoing Patient and Family Education and Support. The complex nature of this patient's physiologic and emotional needs made for a long and intensive therapy process. All the voice and swallowing goals required direct physiologic treatment. Clearly, the turning point in airway protection and voice improvement was the result of the vocal fold medialization. Progress experienced with the early intervention exercises for pharyngeal strengthening and secretion management improved her basic distress and allowed her to be ready physically and mentally to proceed with the thyroplasty. During the course of therapy, the patient often would become excessively anxious about her health and various sensations in the neck region. One time, she called the office to report having swallowed the Silastic stent and was afraid she would soon be "passing it." It took an interim videostroboscopy to convince her that her stent had not dislodged and that she was fine.

There was no rushing this fine elderly woman. Explanations were provided and provided again to reassure and educate. Her daughters were most helpful, and once the acute phase of her medical care was over, they were supportive in reacting to only true medical concerns. All therapeutic goals were met, and the patient was seen only for periodic rechecks.

> *Superior laryngeal nerve paralysis can leave patients with notable voice concerns. However, the subtlety of the condition's auditory and laryngeal presentation often results in the problem being overlooked or misdiagnosed. In the section that follows, Bruce Poburka offers an overview of superior laryngeal nerve paralysis and shares the case study of a 20-year-old music major confronting this diagnosis.*

A Brief Discussion and Case Presentation of Superior Laryngeal Nerve Paralysis

Bruce J. Poburka, PhD

Compared to recurrent laryngeal nerve (RLN) paralysis, considerably less attention has been paid to cases involving the superior laryngeal nerve (SLN). This is likely due to the fact that clinical manifestations of SLN paralysis are more subtle than RLN paralysis; often causing it to be overlooked.[78] The SLN is a branch of the vagus (Xth) nerve, and its external branch innervates the circothyroid (CT) muscle. When contracted, the CT exerts tension on the vocal folds and increases the fundamental frequency.[79] The SLN may incur damage from trauma, viruses, high vagus nerve lesions, and iatrogenic causes.[80] The following discussion summarizes diagnostic findings and treatment strategies for SLN paralysis.

Diagnostic Findings

Auditory perceptual signs and patient complaints associated with SLN paralysis have been reported to be mild to moderate in severity. They include mild breathiness, mild dysphonia, volume disturbance, fatigue, reduction of fundamental frequency range, and loss of upper register.[79-83] Some studies reported that patients exhibited signs of strain and muscle tension, which were thought to be compensatory in nature.[81]

Studies using acoustic assessment to evaluate the effects of SLN paralysis yielded mixed results. Robinson et al[84] reported increases in jitter, shimmer, and noise-to-harmonic ratio (NHR). Roy et al[82] found modest increases in jitter only, but no significant changes in NHR or shimmer. Both studies reported reductions in fundamental frequency range. Interestingly, Roy[82] found fundamental frequency "compression," meaning that range was reduced on both the high and low ends of the range.

A variety of endoscopic findings have been reported for SLN paralysis, but history reveals a long-standing lack of agreement over which laryngeal signs are most useful for identifying SLN paralysis.[85] Among the reported findings are amplitude and phase asymmetry, a shift or rotation of the posterior glottis toward the paralyzed side, vertical level differences, mild vocal fold bowing, hypomobility or lack of brisk adduction/abduction, and rotation of the larynx.[80,81,86] These observations were reported from a variety of clinical settings involving patients who varied with regard to time postonset and use of compensatory behaviors. In a study designed to identify specific voice tasks and laryngeal signs that may reveal CT dysfunction in its acute phase, Roy et al[85] induced SLN paralysis in 10 otherwise vocally healthy subjects using lidocaine block. Their findings showed no consistent evidence of hypomobility or axial rotation of the larynx. The most robust finding was for deviation of the petiole of the epiglottis toward the weak side. Not surprisingly, high-pitched vocal tasks were found to be most helpful in revealing laryngeal dysfunction associated with CT denervation.

Treatment

Treatment options for SLN paralysis include pharmacological, surgical, and behavioral methods. Corticosteroids and antiviral medications have been used in the first 2 to 3 weeks postonset.[81] Beyond that time, observation and behavioral intervention are most commonly used. However, Nasseri and Maragos[80] reported a surgical solution in which Isshiki type IV thyroplasty (cricothyroid approximation) is combined with type I (medialization) thyroplasty. After using this approach on nine patients, the authors concluded that the cricothyroid approximation surgery corrects differences in vocal fold height and cover tension, whereas the medialization procedure improves acoustic power which was reduced when the type IV procedure was used alone.

Behavioral intervention strategies offer an important element in the management of SLN paralysis. A review of the literature revealed that most therapeutic approaches involved patient education, improvement of vocal function, elimination or prevention of vocally abusive compensatory behaviors, and exercises to increase the fundamental frequency range. These exercises included gentle upward and downward glissandos.[81,86] It was stressed that, in performing these exercises care should be taken to avoid strain or other hyperfunctional behaviors. Finally, in cases where the patient is a singer, collaboration with a singing teacher was recommended.[87]

In the following case, a singer diagnosed with superior laryngeal nerve paresis is discussed. This case involves many factors that were discussed above in relation to diagnosis and treatment of SLN paralysis.

Superior Laryngeal Nerve Paralysis

Bruce Poburka, PhD

Case Study: Patient U

Patient History. Patient U, a 20-year-old female college student majoring in vocal music education, was referred to the clinic following a visit to an otolaryngologist who made a diagnosis of left superior laryngeal nerve (SLN) paresis. She began experiencing vocal difficulties several months earlier after a virus caused an extended period of laryngitis. After a slow return of her voice, her residual complaints included mild to moderate hoarseness, a reduction in her fundamental frequency range, a tense throat on extended speaking or singing, and pain in the laryngeal area; especially when attempting to sing high notes. Her vocal music education major required a considerable amount of singing, which amounted to approximately 2 to 3 hours per day on average. Patient U was working with a vocal instructor who also noted changes in vocal quality and a reduction in vocal range.

With the exception of the severe viral infection, Patient U's medical history was otherwise unremarkable. She was careful to maintain hydration by drinking 1 to 2 liters of noncaffeinated beverages per day. She exercised regularly and did not talk during exercise activities.

Evaluation Procedures. U's evaluation involved two separate clinics, and she was seen by Otolaryngology and Speech-

Language Pathology services. Evaluation procedures included laryngeal videostroboscopy, auditory perceptual assessment, an abbreviated oral mechanism exam, hearing screening, and selected maximum phonatory performance tasks.

Videostroboscopy. The videostroboscopic examination revealed mild asymmetry of vibration with the right vocal fold slightly leading the left. Furthermore, muscle imbalance was observed that indicated SLN paresis. Specifically, the larynx was noted to rotate toward the left side. Vocal fold mobility and mucosal wave were excellent, and there was no evidence of vocal fold lesions, infections, edema, or erythema.

Auditory Perceptual. Patient U's vocal quality was judged to be somewhat breathy with mild hoarseness. Vocal fry was observed frequently and appeared related to reduced breath support. Other observations included reduced jaw opening and a lack of oral resonance. This diminished her ability to project the voice across larger spaces. There was no evidence of nasal resonance problems.

Vocal Performance Tasks. Maximum phonation time averaged 13.5 seconds across two trials. She was able to sing notes across 1.5 octaves, which was reduced compared to her normal vocal range. Patient U was asked to sing a choral piece as part of the voice evaluation. During singing, she demonstrated improvements in breath support, vocal quality, loudness, and projection. This revealed a discrepancy when compared to the vocal technique she used during her conversational speech.

Oral Mechanism/Hearing Screens. An abbreviated oral mechanism examina-

tion revealed normal structure and function. Range of motion, strength, speed, and coordination were normal. Glottal adduction on voluntary cough was excellent. Connected speech was normal with regard to articulation and prosody. Speech intelligibility was judged to be 100%. A pure-tone hearing screening was passed in both ears at 500, 1000, 2000, and 4000 Hz.

Impressions. The clinician's impression was that Patient U developed several compensatory behaviors in the wake of her long bout with laryngitis and the vocal changes that resulted from SLN paresis. These behaviors may have developed as a result of trying to "make the voice work" despite its impaired condition. Additionally, after observing her vocal behaviors, it also was thought that U assumed that her voice needed "protection" and that she was "scaling back" her normal approach to voice production. This impression was compatible with the observations of reduced breath support, fry, and restricted oral cavity opening. Furthermore, the compensatory use of muscles may also explain the sensation of tension and pain in the laryngeal area during extended speaking and singing situations. Although SLN paresis certainly could account for some of her complaints, the clinician felt that maladaptive compensatory behaviors could explain several of her symptoms and complaints. Finally, it appeared that U was more likely to use these undesirable compensatory behaviors during conversational speech compared to singing.

Description and Rationale for Therapy Approach. It was felt that the compensatory behaviors that U used were compounding any residual dysfunction associated with her SLN paresis and possibly creating new problems such as vocal fry, reduced projection, and the sensations of tension and pain. Accordingly, a treatment plan was developed to: (1) provide patient education about SLN paresis and laryngeal function in general; (2) restore more normal use of breath support; (3) increase oral cavity opening and anterior oral focus; and (4) promote relaxation in the laryngeal area. It was felt that these changes would promote more stable vocal fold vibration, enhance resonance and projection, and reduce uncomfortable sensations.

Goal 1. Patient U will demonstrate a basic understanding of normal laryngeal function as well as how SLN paresis may impact voice production. This will be measured informally in conversations with U.

Rationale. Basic education about laryngeal function and SLN paresis was provided for two main reasons. First, because U was a vocal music major, it was thought that she could benefit from having this information as part of her academic preparation for a career in singing. Second, because U seemed to be compensating and "protecting" her voice, it was thought that she might better understand the nature of SLN paralysis, and that protecting the voice was not necessarily needed for continued recovery and that the compensations may even be counterproductive.

Goal 2. Patient U will use optimal breath support during spontaneous conversations outside the clinical setting with 90% success as judged by the clinician and/or client report. Optimal breath support was defined as a moder-

ate-sized breath, abdominally focused, and sustained through the end of the utterance.

Rationale. This goal was established to eliminate vocal fry, improve loudness control, and to help eliminate muscle strain associated with talking beyond a normal breath supply.

Goal 3. Patient U will use optimal phonatory technique during spontaneous conversation outside the clinical setting with 90% success as judged by the clinician and/or client report. Optimal phonation technique was defined as using a coordinated onset, relaxed phonation, and a relaxed laryngeal area during speech production.

Rationale. This goal was intended to eliminate muscle fatigue and/or strain associated with patient U's use of compensatory techniques such as "scaling back" or "holding back" her voice. It is important to note that in this case, muscle strain was not associated with pressed voice or hyperadduction, but rather with holding the larynx in a "posture" or inhibiting normal function.

Goal 4. Patient U will use optimal oral resonance during spontaneous conversation outside the clinical setting with 90% success as judged by the clinician and/or client report. Optimal oral resonance was defined as using moderate mandibular movement and anterior oral focus of resonance during speech.

Rationale. This goal was developed to increase oral cavity opening and to promote optimal tuning of the oral cavity as a resonator. Secondarily, it was felt that this goal might promote laryngeal relaxation by directing the patient's mental focus away from the larynx.

Following completion of goal 1 (patient education), the remaining goals were addressed simultaneously. Thus, Patient U was taught "optimal vocal technique" using the optimal speech breathing, phonation, and resonance strategies outlined in goals 2 through 4. Tasks and treatment environments were arranged into a hierarchy ranging from single syllable words through spontaneous conversation outside the clinical setting. Therapy focused exclusively on speaking and did not address singing technique. This was due to the fact that U did not exhibit many undesirable behaviors during singing compared to speaking, and because she was already seeing a vocal singing instructor.

Results of Therapy. Patient U was seen for six voice therapy sessions over a 4-week period. She returned to her otolaryngologist for a follow-up evaluation several months after finishing therapy. U was an excellent client who demonstrated a high level of motivation and quick learning ability. At the conclusion of therapy, she had achieved all of the therapeutic goals with excellent overall results, which are detailed below.

Auditory Perceptual. At the time of discharge from therapy, U used appropriate breath support in conversational speech. This had a positive effect on phonation, which was clear with no evidence of vocal fry. Resonance and projection were improved, and U reported far less fatigue during extended speaking and singing. Additionally, her complaint of pain diminished considerably, and she only experienced this when she sang without warming up.

Videostroboscopy. Follow-up videostroboscopy was completed on her return to otolaryngology several months after discharge from voice therapy. The examination revealed normal symmetry of vibration and none of the laryngeal rotation that was observed at the time of initial diagnosis. All other aspects of phonation remained normal.

Improvement of Vocal Fold Closure in a Patient with Voice Fatigue

Joseph C. Stemple, PhD

Case Study: Patient V

> *Glottal incompetence also may be seen as a result of functional, or muscular, concerns. In the following case, Joe Stemple, describes the management of a middle-aged male with an anterior glottal gap and vocal fatigue.*

Patient V was a 36-year-old systems analyst for a large computer networking company with no previous history of voice difficulty. Eight months prior to the voice evaluation, he had experienced bronchitis with associated harsh coughing and hoarseness. Within 2 weeks, all symptoms had resolved. Since that time, however, the patient had noticed that his voice was not quite as "strong" and that it seemed to get "tired" easily. At first, the voice fatigue occurred only occasionally and was usually associated with a busy workday or a normal social gathering. In the previous 2 to 3 months, however, the "tired" voice had become a daily occurrence and, according to the patient, was getting worse.

On a daily basis, the patient's voice quality was slightly hoarse when he awakened at 6 AM, cleared to nearly normal by 8 AM, but then began fatiguing, often by 11 AM. The fatigue was accelerated if he was required to talk on the telephone or make a presentation to a small group. The patient described his voice quality, when the voice was fatigued, as being "breathy and muffled . . . almost like talking out of a barrel." He described an increased effort to talk and complained that the harder he tried to talk, the worse the quality became.

Except for persistent throat clearing, Patient V was not a voice abuser. By his own admission he was a "couch potato." When not working at his computer at work, he was working on his home computer, watching television, or reading. Social activities were limited to family gatherings, movies, and quiet dinners with friends. He had been married for 10 years and had no children. His wife was an accountant.

The patient's medical history was unremarkable; no surgeries, hospitalizations, or chronic disorders were reported. The patient took no medications; had never smoked, although he grew up in a smoking environment; and drank alcohol only occasionally. His liquid intake was not adequate, consisting mostly of morning coffee and evening iced tea; both were caffeinated. The bronchitis, experienced 8 months ago, was an unusual occurrence for this normally healthy man.

Examination. Laryngeal videostroboscopic examination revealed grossly normal-appearing vocal folds bilaterally. Glottic closure demonstrated a moderate-sized anterior glottal gap with a slight ventricular fold compression. The bilateral amplitude of vibration and mucosal wave were moderately decreased and slightly decreased, respectively. The open phase of the vibratory cycle was slightly dominant, whereas the symmetry of vibration was irregular during extremes of pitch and loudness. No mass lesions, paresis, or paralysis were evident.

This vocal fold condition left Patient V with a mild dysphonia characterized by a dry, breathy hoarseness, high pitch, and intermittent pitch and phonation breaks. The patient was visibly pushing to produce voice in conversation and was using a forced back focus, often speaking at the end of expiration as a result. This subjective judgment of voice quality was confirmed by objective measures including the following:

- High fundamental frequency (142 Hz)
- Limited frequency range (115 to 380 Hz)
- High jitter measure for sustained vowels
- High airflow rates (comfort, 205 mL/second H_2O; high pitch, 216 mL/second H_2O; low pitch, 320 mL/second H_2O)
- Low phonation times at all voice conditions.

Patient V was evaluated in the late afternoon, when he was most symptomatic, of a typical workday. Because he had never experienced vocal difficulties prior to suffering bronchitis, it was speculated that the persistent harsh coughing had strained the laryngeal musculature. Presence of the anterior glottal gap, the unusually high pitch, and his inability to produce a more normal lower pitch range suggested the possibility of a laryngeal muscle imbalance. Indeed, Patient V's attempts to sustain lower tones during the stroboscopic examination yielded a larger anterior glottal gap. The presence of this gap during low-pitch production was confirmed by the unusually high airflow rate of 320 mL/H_2O/sec. Continued effort to produce voice by force was causing the symptoms not only to persist, but to worsen.

Management. The management approach developed for Patient V included the following:

- education
- relaxation of laryngeal area musculature during phonation
- direct training in respiratory support and frontal focus
- vocal function exercises
- evaluation-modification of telephone voice
- elimination of throat clearing
- hydration program.

Education. The video recording of the stroboscopic examination was used to demonstrate the relationship between the glottal gap, high airflow rate, and increased effort to produce voice. Patient V was made to understand that even with the increased effort, the voice remained weak and breathy; therefore, the effort was useless and indeed harmful to the laryngeal mechanism. The patient's understanding of why his voice was failing was a key to his becoming a willing participant in the therapeutic process. The patient had seen two laryngologists who had reported that his vocal folds were normal. He was frustrated because he knew he had a problem, but no one could "find" it. The relationship between his symptoms and his physiology "made sense," and he was ready to proceed to eliminate the bothersome problem.

Relaxation. As patient V's voice began to fatigue, his response was to tense his neck and shoulders in an effort to help force a more normal sounding voice. This effort, of course, had the opposite effect causing more laryngeal tension and fatigue. The education process was a major step in modifying this tensing behavior. The patient needed a cue for when he was too tense, however. Once cued, he needed a simple technique for reducing unwanted tension.

The cue established for the patient was to set the alarm on his watch to sound every hour. When the alarm sounded, his task physically was to relax his neck and shoulders by rolling his head and by stretching his arms back and forth, up and down. This task took less than 1 minute but was quite effective for this patient in reducing physical tension.

The patient had found that neck and shoulder tensing often occurred while he sat at his computer, even when he was not talking. He noticed that on occasion, he would not speak for 2 to 3 hours while working at the computer. Then, when he did speak, his voice was weak. The relaxation exercise was helpful in eliminating this problem.

Respiratory Support and Frontal Focus. Because of the increased airflow necessary to drive the vocal folds, Patient V often felt breathless while talking. One reason for this breathless feeling was his inability to complete a phrase on a normal expiration without pushing and using his maximal air reserve. Using his air reserve added to laryngeal tension, which contributed to a backward tone focus. In his attempt to compensate for lack of glottic closure, the patient began elevating his larynx and contracting his tongue to improve laryngeal constriction. A symptomatic therapy was therefore utilized to modify these behaviors.

The following is a description of the four-step Frontal Focus Exercise used by Patient V:

1. *Patient education.* We began by teaching the patient about the concept of resonance by demonstrating how one sentence may be said with various resonance characteristics. Patients are made aware of how celebrity impersonators change the resonance of the voice to sound like other people. The concepts of frontal, back, and midfocus are introduced by first demonstrating a tight, constricted, back-focused phrase that the patient is asked to imitate. Because this type of tone placement is most often implicated as the problem, most patients, although somewhat embarrassed, are able to produce this voice. Second, a breathy, poorly focused tone is imitated followed by an exaggerated, almost nasal forward-focus. It is explained to the patient that, although the ultimate goal was not to talk in a nasal quality, practicing this placement would help to approximate the desired focus. Practice of this exaggerated forward placement would be one step toward learning the desired placement.

2. *Nasalized phrase production.* The patient was instructed to slowly and softly chant the following phrases on a comfortable pitch level slightly above his fundamental frequency:

   OH MY OH MY OH MY OH MY . . .

   OH ME OH ME OH ME OH ME . . .

   OH NO OH NO OH NO OH NO . . .

   OH MY NO OH MY NO OH MY NO . . .

   OH ME OH MY OH ME OH MY . . .

The forward resonance of each phrase is exaggerated to the extreme, and the patient is instructed to feel and sense the energy of the tone in the nose, on the lips, in the front of the face, and so on. Audio recordings of the phrases are made for both the clinician and the patient, and ear training is accomplished as needed.

Once the phrases are produced to the satisfaction of voice pathologist, negative practice is used. The patient is asked to alternate between forward and back focuses to demonstrate the mastery of the focus technique on these simple phrases.

3. *Introduce intensity and rate variations.* Using the same phrases, Patient V was asked to repeat each phrase multiple times using the following routine:

   - Very slow and very soft
   - Faster and louder
   - Fast and loud
   - Slower and softer
   - Very slow and very soft.

All steps of the routine are accomplished in one breath.

Changing the rate and loudness of the chanted phrases adds a new dimension to the exercise that forces the patient to concentrate on maintaining the forward placement even as the intensity and rate are increased. The pitch remains the same.

4. *Introduce inflected phrase and normal speech.* When Patient V succeeded in mastering the first three steps, the

same practice phrases were modified from the single pitch chant to a more "sing-song" or overinflected vocal presentation and then directly into a normally spoken phrase:

- Soft and slow
- Louder and faster
- Exaggerated inflection
- Normal speech.

Again, all steps of this routine are accomplished in one breath.

The proper focus of the tone is closely monitored during each one of the steps utilizing the phrases. Negative practice is used throughout each session. Some patients move quickly through each of these steps and master a forward focus with ease. Others require many therapy sessions to master the appropriate focus. The final step is to expand the ability to produce a forward focus from these phrases into expanded phrases and sentences, paragraph reading, and conversational speech.

Patient V was gradually able to expand into longer phrases. Negative practice was used judiciously throughout the therapy process to confirm the patient's understanding and control of the concepts of frontal and back focus.

Vocal Function Exercises. Concurrent with the other therapeutic tasks, Patient V was instructed in Vocal Function Exercises (VFE; see Chapter 3). In our clinical practice, these exercises have proved extremely effective in dealing with obvious hypofunctional voice disorders. This patient had an airflow volume of approximately 4000 mL H_2O. He should have been able to sustain a tone for at least 35 to 40 seconds. His baseline VFE measures were:

Note	Seconds
E/F	22
C	15
D	16
E	24
F	26
G	30

The patient was instructed to do the Vocal Function Exercises two times each, twice daily, in the morning and evening.

Evaluation and Modification of Telephone Voice. During the evaluation, Patient V indicated that his voice fatigued more quickly when he was required to talk on the telephone at work. To determine why this occurred, a telephone scenario was utilized. The patient was instructed to call the therapist during the morning, before the onset of typical voice fatigue.

The phone call revealed that the patient artificially lowered his pitch, spoke in a back focus, and talked louder than normal on the telephone. Many of us have "telephone voices" that differ from our normal speaking voices. Patient V created more tension and strain, and thus fatigue, by talking with his "telephone voice."

To modify this behavior, the patient was instructed to imagine that the person with whom he was talking was sitting directly in front of him. In addition, he was instructed to hold the receiver to his ear only when listening and to move it 3 to 4 inches away when he was talking. By holding the receiver away from his ear, he would be monitoring his voice in the same manner as if the listener were present. The telephone receiver would not distort his auditory feedback system.

Eliminate Throat Clearing. Throat clearing became more and more evident as the patient's voice fatigued. Behavior modification and the forceful swallow (see Chapter 3) were utilized to eliminate this behavior.

Hydration Program. Patient V's liquid intake was inadequate for promotion of laryngeal lubrication. He was instructed to drink six to eight 8-oz glasses of noncaffeinated, nonalcoholic liquids per day. Water and fruit juices were the preferred liquids.

Results of Therapy. Three months of therapy were required to complete this program successfully. During this time, the combined therapy approaches were practiced, monitored, and modified as needed. Patient V first began to notice that his voice fatigue began later and later in the day. He then began to develop more of a downward extent of pitch in his VFE and more timbre in his speaking voice. By the middle of the month, he proclaimed his voice to be normal.

Posttherapy stroboscopy demonstrated a tiny anterior glottal chink only at low pitches. All other observations were within normal limits. Perceptually, his voice quality was judged to be normal. Objective measures were as follows:

- Fundamental frequency (128 Hz)
- Frequency range (98 to 560 Hz)
- Jitter measures (normal)
- Airflow rates (all less than 200 mL H_2O/sec)
- Phonation times for Vocal Function Exercises (averaged 36.5 seconds)

The original complaints of voice that lacked strength and tired easily were resolved. Patient V was placed on a maintenance program of modified VFE and discharged from therapy. A 3-month recheck revealed that the patient had successfully discontinued the maintenance program and maintained normal voicing. Combining direct symptom modification with laryngeal exercises and vocal hygiene training proved successful in resolving voice fatigue.

References

1. Bless D, Glaze L, Biever-Lowery D, Campos G, Peppard R. Stroboscopic, acoustic, aerodynamic, and perceptual attributes of voice production in normal speaking adults. In: Titze I, ed. *Progress Report 4.* Iowa City: University of Iowa, National Center for Voice and Speech; 1993:121–134.
2. Titze I. *Principles of Voice Production.* Englewood Cliffs, NJ: Prentice-Hall; 1994.
3. Stemple JC, Stanley J, Lee L. Objective measures of voice production in normal subjects following prolonged voice use. *J Voice.* 1995;9(2):127–133.
4. Eustace CS, Stemple JC, Lee L. Objective measures of voice production in patients complaining of laryngeal fatigue. *J Voice.* 1996;10(2):146–154.
5. Stemple J. *Voice Therapy: Clinical Studies.* St. Louis, MO: Mosby Yearbook; 1993.
6. Case J. *Clinical Management of Voice Disorders.* 3rd ed. Austin, TX: Pro-Ed; 1996.
7. Hirano M, Bless D. *Videostroboscopic Examination of the Larynx.* San Diego, CA: Singular Publishing Group; 1993.
8. McFarlane S, Holt-Romeo T, Lavorato A, Warner L. Unilateral vocal fold paralysis: Perceived vocal quality following three months of treatment. *Am J Speech Lang Pathol.* 1991;1:45–48.
9. McFarlane S, Watterson T, Lewis K, Boone D. Effect of voice therapy facilitation techniques on airflow in unilateral

paralysis patients. *Phonoscope*. 1998;1: 187–191.

10. Colton R, Casper J. *Understanding Voice Problems: A Physiological Perspective for Diagnosis and Treatment*. 2nd ed. Baltimore, MD: Williams & Wilkins; 1996.

11. Boone D, McFarlane S. *The Voice and Voice Therapy*. 5th ed. Englewood Cliffs, NJ: Prentice-Hall; 1994.

12. Boone D, McFarlane S. *The Voice and Voice Therapy*. Needham, MA: Allyn & Bacon; 2000.

13. Sanabria A, Carvalho AL, Silver CE, et al. Routine drainage after thyroid surgery —a meta-analysis. *J Surg Oncol*. 2007; 96(3):273–280.

14. Shandilya M, Kieran S, Walshe P, Timon C. Cervical haematoma after thyroid surgery: management and prevention. *Irish Med J*. 2006;99(9):266–268.

15. Isshiki N, Morita H, Okamura H, Hiramoto M. Thyroplasty as a new phonosurgical technique. *Acta Otolaryngol*. 1974;78(5–6):451–457.

16. Behlau M. Consensus Auditory-Perceptual Evaluation of Voice (CAPE-V), ASHA 2003. *Rev Soc Bras Fonoaudiol*. 2004;9: 187–189.

17. Hogikyan ND, Sethuraman G. Validation of an instrument to measure voice-related quality of life (V-RQOL). *J Voice*. 1999;13(4):557–569.

18. Verdolini K, Rosen C, Branski R. *Classification Manual of Voice Disorders-I*: Mahwah, NJ: Lawrence Erlbaum Associates; 2006.

19. Harries ML, Morrison M. The role of stroboscopy in the management of a patient with a unilateral vocal fold paralysis. *J Laryngol Otol*. 1996;110(2): 141–143.

20. Behlau M, Hogikyan ND, Gasparini G. Quality of life and voice: study of a Brazilian population using the voice-related quality of life measure. *Folia Phoniatr Logop*. 2007;59(6):286–296.

21. Frohlich M, Michaelis D, Strube HW, Kruse E. Acoustic voice analysis by means of the hoarseness diagram. *J Speech Lang Hear Res*. 2000;43(3):706–720.

22. Sataloff RT, Mandel S, Mañon-Espaillat R, et al. Laryngeal electromyography. In: Sataloff RT, ed. *Professional Voice. The Science and Art of Clinical Care*. 3rd ed. San Diego, CA: Plural; 2005.

23. Chan WF, Lang BH, Lo CY. The role of intraoperative neuromonitoring of recurrent laryngeal nerve during thyroidectomy: a comparative study on 1000 nerves at risk. *Surgery*. 2006;140(6):866–872; discussion 872–863.

24. Steurer M, Passler C, Denk DM, Schneider B, Niederle B, Bigenzahn W. Advantages of recurrent laryngeal nerve identification in thyroidectomy and parathyroidectomy and the importance of preoperative and postoperative laryngoscopic examination in more than 1000 nerves at risk. *Laryngoscope*. 2002;112(1):124–133.

25. Witt RL. Comparing the long-term outcome of immediate postoperative facial nerve dysfunction and vocal fold immobility after parotid and thyroid surgery. *J Voice*. 2006;20(3):461–465.

26. Zambudio AR, Rodriguez J, Riquelme J, Soria T, Canteras M, Parrilla P. Prospective study of postoperative complications after total thyroidectomy for multinodular goiters by surgeons with experience in endocrine surgery. *Ann Surg*. 2004;240(1):18–25.

27. Behrman A. Evidence-based treatment of paralytic dysphonia: making sense of outcomes and efficacy data. *Otolaryngol Clin North Am*. 2004;37(1):75–104, vi.

28. D'Alatri L, Galla S, Rigante M, Antonelli O, Buldrini S, Marchese MR. Role of early voice therapy in patients affected by unilateral vocal fold paralysis. *J Laryngol Otol*. 2008;122(9):936–941.

29. Miller S. Voice therapy for vocal fold paralysis. *Otolaryngol Clin North Am*. 2004;37(1):105–119.

30. Schindler A, Bottero A, Capaccio P, Ginocchio D, Adorni F, Ottaviani F. Vocal improvement after voice therapy in unilateral vocal fold paralysis. *J Voice*. 2008; 22(1):113–118.

31. Stemple JC, Lee L, D'Amico B, Pickup B. Efficacy of vocal function exercises as a

method of improving voice production. *J Voice.* 1994;8(3):271–278.

32. Ramig LO, Countryman S, O'Brien C, Hoehn M, Thompson L. Intensive speech treatment for patients with Parkinson's disease: short-and long-term comparison of two techniques. *Neurology.* 1996;47(6): 1496–1504.

33. Isshiki N. Mechanical and dynamic aspects of voice production as related to voice therapy and phonosurgery. *J Voice.* 1998;12(2):125–137.

34. Bridge PM, Ball DJ, Mackinnon SE, et al. Nerve crush injuries—a model for axonotmesis. *Exp Neurol.* 1994;127(2):284–290.

35. Jacobson BJ, Johnson A, Grywalski S, et al. The Voice Handicap Index (VHI): Development and validation. *Am J Speech Lang Pathol.* 1997;6:66–70.

36. Kempster GB, Gerratt BR, Verdolini Abbott K, Barkmeier-Kraemer J, Hillman RE. Consensus auditory-perceptual evaluation of voice: development of a standardized clinical protocol. *Am J Speech Lang Pathol.* 2009;18(2):124–132.

37. Kotby MN. *The Accent Method of Voice Therapy.* San Diego, CA: Singular Publishing Group; 1995.

38. Smith S, Thyme K. *Accent Metoden: Special Paedogogisk.* Herning, Denmark: Forlag Herning; 1978.

39. Aronson A. *Clinical Voice Disorders.* New York, NY: Thieme Medical Publishers; 1990.

40. Ballanger J. *Disease of the Nose, Throat, Ears, Head, and Neck.* 3rd ed. Philadelphia, PA: Lea & Febiger; 1985.

41. Smith S, Thyme K. Statistic research on changes in speech due to pedagogic treatment (the accent method). *Folia Phoniatr (Basel).* 1976;28(2):98–103.

42. Thyme-Frokjaer K, Frokjaer-Jensen B. The Accent Method: a rational voice therapy in theory and practice. *Speech Mark.* 2001:2–11.

43. Iwarsson J. Effects of inhalatory abdominal wall movement on vertical laryngeal position during phonation. *J Voice.* 2001;15(3):384–394.

44. Winkworth AL, Davis PJ, Adams RD, Ellis E. Breathing patterns during spontaneous speech. *J Speech Hear Res.* 1995; 38(1):124–144.

45. Winkworth AL, Davis PJ, Ellis E, Adams RD. Variability and consistency in speech breathing during reading: lung volumes, speech intensity, and linguistic factors. *J Speech Hear Res.* 1994;37(3): 535–556.

46. Hixon TJ, Mead J, Goldman MD. Dynamics of the chest wall during speech production: function of the thorax, rib cage, diaphragm, and abdomen. *J Speech Hear Res.* 1976;19(2):297–356.

47. Hoit JD, Hixon TJ, Watson PJ, Morgan WJ. Speech breathing in children and adolescents. *J Speech Hear Res.* 1990; 33(1):51–69.

48. Hoit JD, Plassman BL, Lansing RW, Hixon TJ. Abdominal muscle activity during speech production. *J Appl Physiol.* 1988;65(6):2656–2664.

49. Watson PJ, Hixon TJ. Effects of abdominal trussing on breathing and speech in men with cervical spinal cord injury. *J Speech Lang Hear Res.* 2001;44(4): 751–762.

50. Awan SH. *The Voice Diagnostic Protocol: A Practical Guide to the Diagnosis of Voice Disorders.* Gaithersburg, MD: Aspen Publishers; 2001.

51. Gregg JW. From song to speech: how do we breathe for speech and song? *J Singing.* 1998;55(2):57–58.

52. Ingram DB, Lehmen JJ. Management of high-risk performers in clinical practice. *Curr Opin Otolaryngol Head Neck Surg.* 2000;8(3):143–152.

53. Irving RM, Epstein R, Harries ML. Care of the professional voice. *Clin Otolaryngol Allied Sci.* 1997;22(3):202–205.

54. Hixon TJ. Kinematics of the chest wall during speech production: volume displacements of the rib cage, abdomen, and lung. *J Speech Hear Res.* 1973;16(1): 78–115.

55. Hoit JD, Banzett RB, Brown R. Binding the abdomen can improve speech in

men with phrenic nerve pacers. *Am J Speech Lang Pathol.* 2002;11:71–76.

56. Iwarsson J, Sundberg J. Effects of lung volume on vertical larynx position during phonation. *J Voice.* 1998;12(2):159–165.

57. Iwarsson J, Thomasson M, Sundberg J. Effects of lung volume on the glottal voice source. *J Voice.* 1998;12(4):424–433.

58. Benninger MS, Ahuja AS, Gardner G, Grywalski C. Assessing outcomes for dysphonic patients. *J Voice.* 1998;12(4):540–550.

59. Benninger MS, Crumley RL, Ford CN, et al. Evaluation and treatment of the unilateral paralyzed vocal fold. *Otolaryngol Head Neck Surg.* 1994;111(4):497–508.

60. Benninger MS, Gillen JB, Altman JS. Changing etiology of vocal fold immobility. *Laryngoscope.* 1998;108(9):1346–1350.

61. Fitzpatrick PC, Miller RH. Vocal cord paralysis. *J La State Med Soc.* 1998;150(8):340–343.

62. Stemple JC. Principles of voice therapy. In: Stemple JC, ed. *Voice Therapy: Clinical Studies.* 2nd ed. San Diego, CA: Singular Publishing; 2000:1–15.

63. Kotby MN, Shiromoto O, Hirano M. The accent method of voice therapy: effect of accentuations on F$_0$, SPL, and airflow. *J Voice.* 1993;7(4):319–325.

64. Thyme K, Frokjaer-Jenson B. *Results of one week's intensive voice therapy (the Accent method).* Paper presented at: XIX IALP Congress, 1983; Edinburg, Scotland.

65. Bassiouny S. Efficacy of the accent method of voice therapy. *Folia Phoniatr Logop.* 1998;50(3):146–164.

66. Dalhoff K, Kitzing P. Voice therapy according to Smith comments on the accent-method to treat disorders of voice and speech. *J Res Singing Appl Vocal Pedagog.* 1987;11(1):15–27.

67. Fex B, Fex S, Shiromoto O, Hirano M. Acoustic analysis of functional dysphonia: before and after voice therapy (accent method). *J Voice.* 1994;8(2):163–167.

68. Harris S. The accent method in clinical practice. In: Stemple JC, ed. *Voice Therapy: Clinical Studies.* San Diego, CA: Singular Publishing Group; 2000.

69. Khidr AA. Effects of the "Smith Accent Technique" of voice therapy on the laryngeal functions and voice quality of patients with unilateral vocal fold paralysis. In: Series IC, ed. *17th World Congress of the International Federation of Oto-Rhino-Laryngological Societies (IFOS).* Vol 1240. Cairo, Egypt: Elsevier Press; 2003:1235–1241.

70. Koschkee D. Accent method. In: Stemple JC, ed. *Voice Therapy: Clinical Studies.* 1st ed. St. Louis, MO: Mosby Year Book; 1993.

71. Kotby MN, El-Sady S, Bassiouny S, Gadallah M, Abou Ross Y, Hegazi M. Efficacy of the Accent Method of voice therapy. *J Voice.* 1991;5(4):316–320.

72. Titze I. Workshop on acoustic voice analysis: summary statement. Iowa City, IA: National Center for Voice and Speech; 1995.

73. Jacobson E. *Progressive Relaxation.* Chicago: University of Chicago Press; 1938.

74. Benson H. The relaxation response: history, physiological basis and clinical usefulness. *Acta Medica Scandinavica, Suppl.* 1982;606:231–237.

75. Stone R, Casteel R. *Restoration of Voice in Non-organically Based Dysphonia.* Springfield, IL: Charles C. Thomas; 1982.

76. Stemple J. *Vocal Function Exercises.* San Diego. CA: Plural Publishing; 2006.

77. Verdolini Abbott K. *Lessac-Madsen Resonant Voice Therapy.* San Diego, CA: Plural Publishing; 2008.

78. Ward P, Berci G, Calcaterra T. Superior laryngeal nerve paralysis: An often overlooked entity. *Am Acad Ophthalmol Otolaryngol.* 1977;84:78–89.

79. Sanders I, Wu BL, Mu L, Li Y, Biller HF. The innervation of the human larynx. *Arch Otolaryngol Head Neck Surg.* 1993;119(9):934–939.

80. Nasseri SS, Maragos NE. Combination thyroplasty and the "twisted larynx:"

combined type IV and type I thyroplasty for superior laryngeal nerve weakness. *J Voice.* 2000;14(1):104–111.

81. Dursun G, Sataloff RT, Spiegel JR, Mandel S, Heuer RJ, Rosen DC. Superior laryngeal nerve paresis and paralysis. *J Voice.* 1996;10(2):206–211.

82. Roy N, Smith ME, Dromey C, Redd J, Neff S, Grennan D. Exploring the phonatory effects of external superior laryngeal nerve paralysis: an in vivo model. *Laryngoscope.* 2009;119(4):816–826.

83. Thorson C. *The singer's voice and superior laryngeal nerve dysfunction: An introduction, guide, and personal account.* MFA Thesis, Minnesota State University-Mankato; 2006.

84. Robinson JL, Mandel S, Sataloff RT. Objective voice measures in nonsinging patients with unilateral superior laryngeal nerve paresis. *J Voice.* 2005;19(4):665–667.

85. Roy N, Barton ME, Smith ME, Dromey C, Merrill RM, Sauder C. An in vivo model of external superior laryngeal nerve paralysis: laryngoscopic findings. *Laryngoscope.* 2009;119(5):1017–1032.

86. Eckley CA, Sataloff RT, Hawkshaw M, Spiegel JR, Mandel S. Voice range in superior laryngeal nerve paresis and paralysis. *J Voice.* 1998;12(3):340–348.

87. Sataloff R, Brandfonbrener A, Lederman R, eds. *Textbook of Performing Arts Medicine.* New York, NY: Raven Press; 1991.

5

Management of Functional Voice Disorders

Introduction

When viewed from a strict physiologic point of view, hyperfunction and hypofunction of the laryngeal mechanism are not difficult to understand. All the management approaches outlined seek equilibrium of the respiratory, laryngeal, and resonatory systems. Nonetheless, when personality, emotions, psychosocial behaviors, and relationships are thrown into the mix, these factors often complicate the therapeutic process. It is well known that a person's physical condition and emotional status may be directly reflected in the quality of voice. With this in mind, presentation of the following group of disorders focuses on management techniques for functional voice problems.

The term "functional" has been cho-sen to describe voice disorders that present with perceptual voice changes, often in the presence of normal-appearing vocal folds. Various texts have classified these disorders as psychosocial, psychogenic, conversion, personality-related, psychosexual, and so on. Because of disagreement concerning the causes of these disorders, the somewhat benign term "functional" is used here. Agreement does exist, however, for the premise that the person cannot be separated from the voice disorder. With this premise in mind, case studies focusing on voice change and personal awareness are presented for disorders related to:

■ Environmental stress
■ Severe muscle tension dysphonia
■ Functional aphonia
■ Functional dysphonia
■ Functional falsetto

Management of Muscle Tension Dysphonia Resulting from Environmental Stress

Joseph C. Stemple, PhD

Case Study: Patient W

Many events in life can lead to emotional and physical stresses that may provoke vocal disorders in some individuals. Unknown by the individual, these stresses often lead to extreme musculoskeletal tension. Laryngeal area tension, whether caused by hyperfunctional behaviors as previously discussed (Chapter 3) or emotional stress, is a primary cause of functional vocal disturbances. The following case study describes the management approach utilized for Patient W, who suddenly found herself in the middle of an unpleasant life experience.

Patient History

Patient W was a 45-year-old nurse, wife, and mother of two sons, ages 16 and 20 years. She was referred from the laryngologist with a moderate-to-severe dysphonia characterized by a strained, raspy phonation. Videolaryngoscopy yielded grossly normal-appearing vocal folds bilaterally. Stroboscopic examination of the vocal folds demonstrated significantly decreased amplitude of vibration and a strongly dominant closed phase of the vibratory cycle.

Visually, Patient W presented with a well-groomed, pleasant appearance. Her smile, however, was rather fixed and forced. It was one of those smiles where the mouth went up at the corners, but the eyes were hollow. Her breathing was shallow, with occasional deep sighs. Her neck and shoulders appeared stiff, with the larynx elevated and the tongue retracted.

The patient became symptomatic with hoarseness approximately 3 months prior to the voice examination. She reported that she thought she must have had a cold when the symptoms first started, but she wasn't quite sure. Over the past 3 months, the voice quality had worsened. Not only was she hoarse, but she also had the laryngeal sensations of extreme dryness, a "lump-in-the-throat" feeling, and an actual aching that occasionally ran from her larynx, up her neck, and to her ears. When the pain was greatest, the patient experienced what she described as "blocked hearing."

Patient W's medical history involved a complete hysterectomy at age 40, frequent D & Cs prior to the hysterectomy, and a tonsillectomy as a child. Chronic disorders included frequent headaches (daily), sinusitis, and stomach pain. In addition, she had begun to experience a "shortness of breath" when speaking. Medications included estrogen (Premarin) for hormonal balance, acetaminophen (Tylenol) for headaches, antihistamine (Zyrtec) for sinusitis, and antacid preparation (Mylanta) for stomach pain. Patient W had recently begun smoking again after not smoking for 5 years. Her liquid intake was adequate. She reported that on a day-to-day basis she felt only "fair" because she was "always tired."

Obviously, this patient was demonstrating many signs of emotional tension and stress. During the interview section of the voice evaluation, our patients are always asked, "On a day-to-day basis, how do you feel?" Medical history may tell physical condition, but this question explores the patient's emotional condition. When Patient Y answered "fair," this was the therapist's opportunity to explore the emotional side of the problem. Patient W was asked, "Why only fair?" Her response was that she was so busy, she always felt tired. She couldn't seem to get enough sleep. This issue was then explored while probing the patient's social history.

The patient had been married for 21 years. Her husband was a manufacturer's representative and was on the road 50% of the time covering a multistate territory. Her 20-year-old son was an honor student attending an out-of-state university. The 16-year-old son attended a local high school. Patient W was a licensed practical nurse who worked part-time at a nursing home.

When speaking of her 20-year-old son, the patient's entire demeanor changed. Her voice quality improved somewhat, and her tension visibly diminished. However, the opposite response was noted when questions focused on her younger son. Noting this response, the patient was encouraged to talk about his schooling and his outside activities such as sports, clubs, and so on. The patient became visibly agitated and finally, in tears, told of the problems this son was having.

Three months before the examination, not coincidentally at the same time as the onset of her voice problems, Patient W's son had been arrested at the high school with two other boys for selling and using various drugs. He was presently in a residential rehabilitation program as required by the juvenile court. The stress of this problem had caused marital problems that had "always been there" to surface. Instead of being able to rally support for their son and each other, the patient and her husband were discussing divorce. The husband was now constantly working, and the patient felt alone in her efforts to deal with these problems.

After releasing this extreme tension by verbalizing the problem and crying, the patient's voice quality actually was much improved. This was pointed out

to the patient. The relationship of stress and tension to voice strain was described and discussed in detail. Understanding the problem was the first step in remediating the symptoms.

Although Patient W now understood why she was hoarse, she could not automatically decrease the musculoskeletal tension in the manner that her catharsis had permitted. Subsequent therapy sessions introduced a means of decreasing tension known as digital massage.[1] (This method is described in detail in a case by Nelson Roy later in this chapter.) Several other methods of laryngeal tension reduction have been suggested. Some of these include progressive relaxation,[2] chewing exercises,[3] and electromyographic and thermal biofeedback.[4]

Patient W responded well to digital massage, and her voice quality improved to normal within 3 weeks of the evaluation. A recommendation was made for family counseling, which was begun automatically as part of her son's rehabilitation program. Environmental stress led to extreme tension in the patient's laryngeal area, causing functional voice strain. A management program involving education, tension reduction, and counseling was successful in remediating the voice component of this stress-related disorder.

Comments on Functional Aphonia and Dysphonia

Joseph C. Stemple, PhD

At times, environmental tension and stress may become so severe that, in the attempt to draw attention away from the real problem, people develop various avoidance behaviors. These behaviors may be functional reactions that permit individuals to deny awareness of the stress or emotional conflict. The behaviors are unconscious methods of avoiding strong interpersonal conflicts that cause stress, depression, or anxiety. Two such behaviors are functional whispering and functional dysphonia, again in the presence of normal vocal folds.

By the time patients seek help from the laryngologist or voice pathologist, the need for the functional reaction often has passed, and they are ready to have the voice problem resolved. It must be stressed, however, that these patients are not malingering. They do not know that they have the capability of producing normal voice. Some patients may continue to receive secondary gains from the disorder and resist all therapy modifications, but the majority will respond quickly to direct voice therapy.

Functional dysphonias, may be more difficult to diagnose. The voice pathologist will recognize unusual vocal presentations as functional when:

- the medical examination yields normal vocal folds
- the history of the problem yields no strong evidence for the occurrence of a hyperfunctional voice disorder
- the voice quality produced is not typical of "normal" dysphonia
- when the patient demonstrates the ability to produce normal phonation during nonspeech voicing behaviors such as coughing, throat clearing, or laughing or when the patient has evidenced brief, unexpected periods of normal voicing during the course of the disorder.

The majority of functional voice disorders occur in women[5]; however, we have treated men, women, and children with this diagnosis. The following case study will present some general principles of therapy used with both functional aphonia and dysphonia.

> *In the following cases, Joe Stemple, Nelson Roy, and R. E. (Ed) Stone share treatment methods for functional dysphonia and aphonia and the nuances of treating this segment of the voice-disordered population.*

Management of Functional Dysphonia and Aphonia in a 13-Year-Old

Joseph C. Stemple, PhD

Case Study: Patient X

Patient History

Patient X, a 13-year-old, eighth-grade student, was referred with a 4-week history of "voice loss." The patient and her mother were interviewed together, and then the interview was continued when the mother was asked to leave the examination room. As is the case with many functional voice problems, the onset of whispering was associated with a cold. The patient's mother reported that her daughter had developed "laryngitis" 4 weeks prior to this examination and then "lost her voice totally" 2 days later. The cold quickly resolved, but the patient's voice had not yet returned.

The patient was reported to be a rather shy child who succeeded reasonably well in her academic activities. Socially, she had two "best" friends and participated in the school choir, library club, and 4-H activities. Her medical history was unremarkable as related to this problem. Although she had never experienced vocal difficulties before, her mother reported that the girl had experienced a "chronic cough" 1 year earlier for which no diagnosis could be found. Following several weeks of excessive coughing, the behavior suddenly stopped. The child's mother was hoping the voice would come back in the same manner.

Laryngeal videostroboscopy was performed at this point of the evaluation as a means of educating the patient about the anatomy and physiology of the laryngeal mechanism and vocal folds. Patient X presented with normal-appearing vocal folds. The whisper, of course, did not permit slow motion observation of fold vibration, but the folds were shown to adduct toward the midline, only to stop in an incomplete closure. The lack of approximation of the folds was pointed out to the patient with an explanation similar to the following:

> *Your vocal folds look very good and healthy. For some reason, the muscles that pull them together are simply not pulling the way that they should. Therefore, the vocal folds are not closing all the way. When they do not close all the way, they do not vibrate, and we hear whispered speech. Our goal in therapy, therefore, is to do whatever is necessary to encourage those muscles to pull hard enough to make the vocal folds come together.*

With this approach, the voice pathologist has given the patient a nonthreatening explanation as to why phonation is not occurring. No comment is yet made regarding the patient's inherent ability to phonate. In fact, the "blame" for lack of phonation has been removed from the patient and placed squarely on the faulty mechanism.

Traditional management approaches then might examine the patient's ability to phonate during nonspeech phonatory behaviors such as coughing, throat clearing, laughing, crying, or sighing. When clear phonation is identified during one of these behaviors, it is then shaped into vowel sounds, nonsense syllables, words, and short phrases. The voice pathologist must demonstrate patience at this time. Most patients have not phonated for several weeks. The possibility of proceeding too quickly and frightening the patient away from phonation is present. Once good, consistent phonation is established under practice conditions, the voice pathologist begins to insist gently that it be used during the therapy conversations. Some claim that, when voice is regained in this manner, it is seldom lost again, and patients do not substitute other symptoms. [6] Long-term studies are needed to substantiate this claim.

Another technique that we have found useful is the use of direct visual feedback using laryngeal videoendoscopy. While the patient is being scoped, with either a rigid or flexible endoscope, an explanation is given related to the positioning of the vocal folds and how that positioning relates to the present vocal problem. The patient is able to monitor the video over the voice pathologist's shoulder. The patient is then instructed in various manipulations of the vocal folds, such as deep breathing, light throat clearing, laughing, and attempts to produce tones of various loudness levels and pitches. We have had surprising success in the quick return of normal voicing using these visual biofeedback procedures.

A different management strategy was used with Patient X, that is, the use of falsetto voice as a facilitator of normal voicing. It was explained to the patient that we were going to manipulate her vocal folds in a manner that would encourage her muscles to pull the folds together. The therapist then produced a high-pitched falsetto tone on the vowel /ai/. The patient was told, in a matter-of-fact manner, that, by stretching the vocal folds for this high pitch, the folds are more closely approximated. Everyone, even those with vocal problems, can produce this tone. The falsetto again was demonstrated, and the patient was told to produce the same sound.

Following several unsuccessful attempts, the patient produced a high-pitched squeak. This was promptly reinforced with praise and repeated several times. As the falsetto voice strengthened and the sound became clearer, other vowel sounds were introduced and stabilized at this pitch level.

It was explained to Patient X that we were going to use the muscle tension created by producing the falsetto tone to encourage the vocal folds to pull together normally. The patient was given a list of 150 two-syllable phrases and asked to read them in the falsetto voice. During this exercise, she was constantly encouraged to read swiftly and loudly. After the voice stabilized in a relatively strong falsetto, the patient was halted and asked to match the clinician when singing down the scale about three to four notes from the original falsetto tone. The patient was then asked to continue reading the phrases at this new pitch level. The same procedure was repeated two to three more times until the young woman's pitch closely approximated a normal pitch level. She was continually encouraged to produce these phrases louder and faster until her voice eventually "broke" into normal phonation.

Occasionally, the patient will approximate normal phonation but then hesitate as if somewhat reluctant to produce normal voice. When this occurs, the patient is asked to "drop way down" and produce a guttural voice quality while reading the phrases. This will "produce more appropriate muscle pull." After a few minutes, the patient is taken back to the falsetto voice with the break into normal phonation usually occurring soon after.

It is extremely important for the voice pathologist to be patient when utilizing this technique. The normal time frame from aphonia to normal voice is approximately 30 to 45 minutes. The voice pathologist must not only be patient but also must present a very matter of fact, confident manner. Voice pathologists are not cheerleaders. They are simply presenting a technique that they know will work.

Why do these techniques work?

- The patient is ready for change.
- The voice pathologist has given a reasonable explanation for what the vocal folds are doing.
- The voice pathologist has demonstrated confidence in the therapeutic techniques.

Following return of voice, it is necessary to explore the actual cause for the voice disorder. It is desirable to do this in a direct manner. For example the voice pathologist could say:

I'm very pleased that the muscles are all functioning well now and that your voice has returned to normal. It sounds really good. The thing that still puzzles me somewhat is why the muscles stopped closing the folds in the first place. I can tell you quite frankly that with a lot of other patients that we have seen with the same problem, the cause has been something that has happened that was very upsetting or emotionally draining. Can you think of anything that has been going on lately that has been upsetting to you?

By this time, it is hoped that the patient has developed strong confidence in the voice pathologist and will "open up a floodgate" of information about deaths, family problems, work problems, and the like. In discussing these problems, the voice pathologist attempts to accomplish two major objectives: (1) Give the patient total and final control over the laryngeal mechanism and (2) determine the patient's general emotional state to decide the need for further professional counseling.

Up to this point, the voice pathologist has been manipulating the voice. The patient now must understand that despite the ultimate cause of the aphonia, he or she is in total control of the voice and does not need to permit the problem to recur. If it does, the patient knows how to regain control of the voice.

Finally, just because the need for the functional reaction no longer may be present, this does not mean that formal family, psychiatric, or psychological counseling would not be helpful. If the voice pathologist feels the problem is not resolved and further counseling is in order, the suggestion should be discussed with the patient, and appropriate referrals should be made.

In discussing the problem with the patient's mother, it became evident that Patient X had experienced other episodes of possible functional behaviors, most notably several long-term coughing spells. Patient X was shy and she lacked confidence. Physically, she was overweight and had, in the past year, become sensitive about her appearance. Her mother reported that around the onset of this voice problem, her daugh-

ter had come home from school very upset about being teased by some classmates about her weight. Like many children in this age group, she was sensitive to comment by her peers and was struggling to find her own identity. Suggestions were made for further counseling.

In a follow-up voice therapy session, Patient X had maintained normal voicing. As a matter of fact, she was looking forward to singing with her school choir in a concert that week. Her ability to control her voice production was reinforced. She was told that if she felt the whisper returning, all she needed to do was produce the falsetto tone and most likely her voice would return to normal. That was our last contact with this patient.

Manual Circumlaryngeal Techniques in the Assessment and Treatment of Muscle Tension Dysphonia (MTD)

Nelson Roy, PhD

Case Study: Patient XX

Without exception, contemporary voice texts cite excessive or poorly regulated activity of the intrinsic and extrinsic laryngeal muscles as important causal considerations in a variety of voice disorders.[1,7–11] This "imbalanced" laryngeal and paralaryngeal muscle activity seems to be the common denominator behind a class of voice disorders referred to as hyperfunctional or musculoskeletal tension voice disorders. [12] In this regard, manual circumlaryngeal techniques recently have received attention in the clinical voice literature as potentially valuable diagnostic and treatment tools. This case study illustrates the use of these manual laryngeal techniques and highlights important procedural considerations.

Voice and Medical History

Patient XX, a 55-year-old "paralegal," presented with a 6-month history of chronic mild-to-moderate dysphonia with sporadic acute exacerbations. These acute episodes, which bordered on aphonia, persisted for less than a week and resolved gradually. The patient indicated that she seemed to be gradually "losing the full force of her voice." She reported a persistent ache and tightness of the anterior neck, larynx, and shoulder regions. She had also noticed episodic neck swellings that she labeled as "swollen glands." According to the patient, these "lumps" would worsen according to her amount of voice use, and the degree of perceived laryngeal tension, fatigue, and effort. She added that the swellings coincided with the acute dysphonic exacerbations and that their appearance was not accompanied or preceded by symptoms of an upper respiratory infection (URI). The patient reported no change in health status and occupational or social voice use preceding the onset of vocal symptoms. Her recent medical history included treatment for asthma, allergies, hypertension, depression, tension headaches, gastroesophageal reflux disease (GERD), and temporomandibular joint dysfunction. Her current medications included: Altace (antihypertensive), Prozac (antidepressant), Cimetidine (antacid), and Premarin (estrogen replacement). She had received psychological treatment for clinical depression 4 years previously, but she was not currently consulting a mental health professional.

Psychosocial Interview

During the psychosocial interview, Patient XX reported numerous work-related stresses. She indicated that just prior to the onset of her voice difficulties "her workload at the firm had become horrendous and had doubled following a company takeover." Patient XX explained, "I found every single day stressful at work, and that's when some of this started . . . Every day I went into work to put out the fires, rather than doing something fresh—it was constant pressure." She admitted feeling overwhelmed and exhausted. Patient XX indicated that 2 months earlier, she had missed work for 1 week with "chronic fatigue" accompanied by complete voice loss. Although she was frustrated by the increased workload and the limited support offered by her superiors, she had not expressed this dissatisfaction to her manager and was reluctant to do so. Her employer had hired additional office help recently, but she was solely responsible for training that individual. Consequently, she was forced to neglect some of her own duties in the process, only adding to the burden. In addition to the work-related stresses, the patient admitted to a long-standing communication breakdown with her only daughter. She had not communicated with her daughter over the past several years. Despite probing by the clinician, Patient XX denied knowing the precise cause of the communication breakdown, but she confessed to thinking about the unresolved conflict on a daily basis.

Voice Evaluation

Perceptually, her connected speech was characterized by a mildly pressed, tight vocal quality, which worsened over the course of the assessment period. By the end of the interview, Patient XX was in glottal fry 80% of the time. Repeated readings of a standard passage produced further deterioration in voice. Sustained vowel production was somewhat superior in quality when compared with connected speech. She displayed reduced pitch range and experienced noticeable phonatory disintegration early during upward pitch glides. She seemed to be functioning toward the bottom of phonatory frequency range.

Rigid videolaryngostroboscopy revealed no evidence of structural or neurological pathology. Both vocal folds moved symmetrically and were free of mucosal disease. Mild mediolateral supraglottic compression was noted. Vocal fold vibratory characteristics, including mucosal wave and amplitude of vibration, were essentially within normal limits; however, the closed phase dominated the vibratory cycle.

Focal Laryngeal Palpation. At rest, musculoskeletal tension was appraised manually by palpation of the laryngeal area to assess the degree, nature, and location of focal tenderness or muscle nodularity or pain. Care was taken to avoid sustained carotid artery compression during these maneuvers. With the occiput gently supported in a neutral position, pressure was directed (1) over the major horns of the hyoid bone, (2) over the superior cornu of the thyroid cartilage, (3) within the thyrohyoid space, and (4) along the anterior border of the sternocleidomastoid muscle. During palpation, the degree of compression applied was roughly equal to the pressure required to cause the thumbnail tip to blanch when pressed against a firm surface. When this amount of pressure was used, focal sites of tension evoked dis-

comfort and pain. The patient winced, withdrew, and vocalized her discomfort when tender points were specifically identified. These sites of tenderness were over the major horns of the hyoid and the superior cornu of the thyroid cartilage. The patient confirmed that these sites were the location of her episodic laryngeal swellings. The discomfort was more pronounced on the left than on the right and radiated to both ears. This severe tenderness in response to pressure in the laryngeal region was considered abnormal and highly suggestive of excess laryngeal musculoskeletal tension.

The extent of laryngeal elevation was examined by palpating within the thyrohyoid space from the posterior border of the hyoid bone to the thyroid notch. The patient demonstrated a narrowed thyrohyoid space that caused the larynx to be suspended high in the neck. This finding was also highly suggestive of excess muscle tension. Attempting to maneuver the larynx from side to side along the horizontal plane tested its mobility. Ample resistance to lateral movement indicated generalized extralaryngeal hypertonicity.

Voice Stimulability Testing Using Manual Techniques. With the index finger and thumb situated within the thyrohyoid space, the clinician applied gentle downward traction over the superior border of the thyroid lamina while the patient vocalized a sustained "ah" vowel. The voice improvement associated with such laryngeal lowering (reposturing) was immediate and audible to both the patient and the clinician. Such a positive response to laryngeal reposturing and stimulability testing was informative regarding the patient's potential for normal voice and was suggestive of muscular tension and laryngeal elevation as possible causal mechanisms. (Other manual reposturing techniques, including pressure in a posterior direction over the inferior aspect of the hyoid bone, did not produce noticeable improvement in voice quality.) Before proceeding with manual circumlaryngeal therapy, the diagnosis of muscle tension dysphonia was explained to the patient, and she was educated regarding the negative effects of excessive musculoskeletal tension on voice and the possibility that such tensions may be responsible, solely or in part, for her voice disorder. In addition, the results of the laryngoscopic examination were reviewed, emphasizing the absence of vocal fold pathology sufficient to account for the severity and fluctuating nature of her voice symptoms. Once she appeared to understand the relationship between muscle dysregulation, stress, and voice, the manual therapy procedure was outlined, and the positive outlook for recovery was explained. She was warned that the technique may produce some initial discomfort but that with continued kneading of the musculature, the pain gradually would remit. She was also encouraged to attend carefully to any voice improvement and the laryngeal sensation accompanying such improvement.

Circumlaryngeal Massage

Rationale. Once the assessment procedures were completed and the results were explained to the patient, the manual tension reduction technique (ie, circumlaryngeal massage) was undertaken according to the description of Aronson.[1] Skillfully applied, systematic kneading of the extralaryngeal region is postulated to stretch muscle tissue and fascia, promote local circulation with removal of metabolic wastes, relax tense muscles, and relieve pain and discomfort associated with muscle spasms.[13] The putative physical effect of such massage is reduced laryngeal height and stiffness and increased mobility.[14] Once the larynx is "released" and range of motion is normalized, an improvement in vocal effort, quality, and dynamic range should follow. Focal palpation and massage helps patients become more aware of where they are holding tension. By being conscious of these laryngeal "trouble spots" the patient can begin to focus on relaxing them during self-massage, which can be undertaken on a daily basis. In a series of articles, Roy and colleagues have evaluated the clinical utility of manual techniques with a variety of functional voice disorders.[15–18] The results of these investigations suggest that the majority of patients studied derived noticeable voice improvement within a single treatment session using manual circumlaryngeal therapy.

Description of the Technique. The hyoid bone was encircled with the thumb and index finger, which were then worked posteriorly into the tips of the major horns of the hyoid bone. Pressure was applied in a circular motion over the tips of the hyoid bone. The procedure was repeated within the thyrohyoid space, beginning from the thyroid notch and working posteriorly. The posterior borders of the thyroid cartilage medial to the sternocleidomastoid muscles were located, and the procedure was repeated there. With the fingers over the superior border of the thyroid cartilage, the larynx was stretched downward and, at times, moved laterally. Sites of focal tenderness, nodularity, or tautness were deliberately given more attention. Gentle kneading or sustained pressure was focused over these sites and then released. The procedure began superficially, and the depth of massage was increased according to the degree of tension encountered and the tolerance of the patient. The clinician extended the technique into the medial and lateral suprahyoid musculature, because excess tension and pain was encountered over those sites. The patient was encouraged by the clinician to "unhinge her jaw and assume a more relaxed jaw position." The immediate effects of massage were noticeable on the skin. A slight reddening and warming of the skin accompanied friction and circular stroking movements.

During the above procedures, Patient XX was asked to sustain vowels while both the clinician and the patient noted changes in vocal quality. The patient, as an active participant in the therapy process, was encouraged to continually self-monitor the type and manner of voice produced. Given her marked sensitivity to pressure in the laryngeal region, some discomfort during the procedure was unavoidable. Nonetheless, the clinician's goal was to achieve sufficient tension reduction without inducing reactive-reflexive muscle tensing because of pain. Improvement in voice was noted almost immediately and was combined with reductions in pain and laryngeal height. Such changes were suggestive of a relief of tension. The patient commented, "Even though it hurts, it still feels good." Over the course of approximately 20 minutes, the improved voice was extended from vowels to words (automatic serial speech, ie, counting, days of the week), to short phrases loaded with nasals (eg, "many men in the Moon," "one Monday morning"), to sentences and paragraph recitations, and then to conversation. Once sufficient tension was released

and the patient assumed a more normal laryngeal posture, progress was swift, with complete amelioration of the dysphonia. Following the procedure, Patient XX commented that the voice felt free of tension and effort.

On repeated laryngeal palpation, the sites of most severe tenderness were no longer apparent. Pain no longer radiated to the ears. The patient was warned that she could experience some mild laryngeal discomfort over the next 24 to 48 hours as a consequence of the intense massage, but that this should resolve.

Patient XX was instructed in self-laryngeal massage techniques and encouraged to perform them twice daily and whenever she experienced any tightness or fatigue in the laryngeal region. She was scheduled for a follow-up visit in 1 month to assess progress and determine future management. Patient XX was instructed to contact the clinician should she experience any acute exacerbations. In the interim, the patient was encouraged to make modifications to her work schedule to alleviate some of the situational stresses and to explore psychological counseling to acquire relaxation skills.

Recurrence and Relapse

Patient XX contacted the clinician 2 weeks later with a severe strained dysphonia (with frequent aphonic breaks) that had suddenly begun a day earlier, which was Sunday. Until this exacerbation, the patient reported symptom-free voice for the 2-week posttreatment period. She indicated that her recent attempts at self-laryngeal massage were completely unsuccessful in modifying the voice. She denied any new situational conflicts, stresses, or voice-use patterns that may have contributed to the onset but had not pursued counseling.

Rigid and flexible videolaryngostroboscopy revealed an extraordinary sequence of laryngeal movements, most obvious during laryngeal ddks (rapid abduction and adduction of vocal folds). The laryngeal movement pattern was characterized by prephonatory supraglottic compression with complete obliteration of the view of true vocal folds by the hyperadducted ventricular folds. Phonatory initiation was preceded by abduction of the left arytenoid complex while the right arytenoid remained adducted, producing an irregular shaped posterior glottic and supraglottic chink (Fig 5–1). This paradoxical movement of the left arytenoid during phonatory initiation appeared to represent a decoupling of conjugate vocal fold movements.

The dysphonia was interpreted by the clinician to be a more severe manifestation of the original muscle tension disorder. Manual circumlaryngeal therapy again was undertaken according to the previous description. In spite of paralaryngeal tension and pain that was judged to be more severe than the original visit, normal voice quality was again rapidly reestablished within a single treatment session. This time, the patient transitioned through several stages of decreasing vocal severity until normal voice was restored. One intermediate stage of dysphonia was quite reminiscent of her original dysphonia. Posttreatment rigid videolaryngostroboscopy (same session) showed no evidence of the atypical and asymmetric arytenoid movement pattern and confirmed normal vibratory characteristics (Fig 5–2).

The pre- and posttreatment sustained vowel acoustic analyses are shown in Figures 5–3A and 5–3B, respectively.

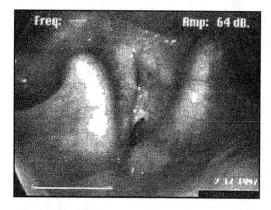

FIGURE 5–1. Pretreatment rigid videolaryngoscopy obtained during sustained phonation illustrates the asymmetric appearance of the arytenoids, combined with mediolateral and anteroposterior supraglottic constriction that was sufficient to obscure the view of the true vocal folds. An irregular-shaped, posterior glottic and supraglottic chink was created by the partially abducted left arytenoid complex.

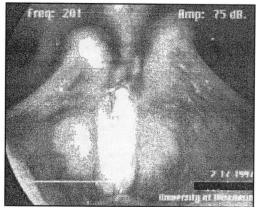

FIGURE 5–2. Videolaryngoscopy completed immediately following successful manual circumlaryngeal therapy (same session) confirmed normal glottic and supraglottic symmetry and function. All vibratory parameters, as assessed by stroboscopy, returned to within normal limits.

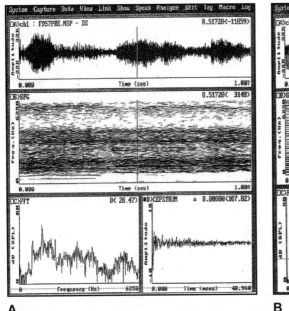
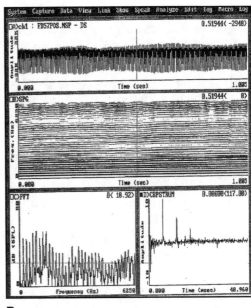

A   B

FIGURE 5–3. Acoustic analysis before (**A**) and after (**B**) manual circumlaryngeal therapy for the acute exacerbation (ie, recurrence). Each figure illustrates the middle 1-second segment extracted from the pre- and posttreatment sustained vowel /a/ productions, sampled at 25 kHz, and acoustically analyzed using the Computerized Speech Lab (CSL Model 4300B. Kay Elemetrics Corp., Lincoln Park, NJ). (a) sound pressure waveform; (b) narrowband spectrogram of the preemphasized downsampled (12.5 kHz) waveform generated using a 36 Hz analyzing filter; (c) FFT (power spectrum) at the cursor location; (d) cepstrum power spectrum. The time axis is frequency and shows the dominant energy corresponding to the harmonic peaks in the spectrum. A prominent peak in the cepstrum is called the dominant harmonic, and its amplitude reflects the harmonic structure of the voice signal. Visual inspection of the pre- and posttreatment acoustic analyses confirms substantial improvement in spectral and cepstral characteristics following manual circumlaryngeal therapy. Improvement in harmonic intensity and structure following treatment is apparent in the posttreatment narrowband spectrogram (b) and power spectrum (c). The presence and amplitude of the dominant harmonic in the posttreatment cepstrum (d) substantiates these improvements.

Her severely disturbed voice in the pretreatment analysis is replaced by a normal posttreatment voice. All results are based on samples obtained within the same assessment and treatment session.

Once the voice was restored, a frank discussion ensued regarding the complex interplay of laryngeal muscle tension, life stresses, situational conflicts, and her apparently ineffectual coping strategies. She agreed that she needed to develop more pragmatic coping skills and that long-term maintenance of voice improvement probably would require supportive psychological counseling. Arrangements were made for her to return to her counselor.

Short- and Long-Term Follow-Up

The patient was reevaluated in the voice clinic at 3 and 6 months posttreatment.

On each occasion, she reported no further relapse. Initially posttreatment, Patient XX completed self-laryngeal massage on a daily basis, then weekly, and eventually as needed. She returned to her psychologist for relaxation training and short-term cognitive-behavioral therapy. By 6 months posttreatment, she had discontinued counseling, self-laryngeal massage, and had made many positive life and work adjustments. Contact by telephone approximately 2 years posttreatment confirmed maintenance of therapy gains without any evidence of partial or complete relapse.

Comparisons with Existing Research

Patient XX's positive response to manual circumlaryngeal therapy and her subsequent relapse and exacerbation is compatible with the results of an investigation of 25 patients with functional dysphonia (FD) conducted by Roy and colleagues.[16] All functional dysphonia patients received a single treatment session of manual circumlaryngeal massage. Although the majority of patients improved across perceptual and acoustic indices of vocal function, interviews during the follow-up phase revealed that over two thirds of the patients who had initially responded favorably reported infrequent, partial, and self-limiting recurrences early in the follow-up phase (ie, less than 2 months posttreatment). It appears, then, that the case presented here is not exceptional from a treatment-and-relapse perspective. Roy et al [16] advised that, for some patients, superior long-term results might be found when manual laryngeal techniques are combined with supportive counseling, more frequent clinical support, or both. Certainly, Patient XX's eventual sustained voice improvement following manual circumlaryngeal ther-

apy and short-term psychological counseling seems to support this contention.

During the second treatment, Patient XX progressed through stages of decreasing dysphonia and laryngeal discomfort until voice symptoms gradually remitted. These findings are also consistent with Aronson's[1(p315)] accounts and the reports of Roy, Bless, et al[16] Whether this gradual remission of dysphonia and laryngeal pain during treatment represents a steady reduction in laryngeal tension, as Aronson maintained, remains open for debate.

It is apparent from this case study that voice and musculoskeletal symptoms can be consequences of specific environmental triggers and stressors combined with individual differences in coping style.[19,20] Understanding the contribution of laryngeal and extralaryngeal muscle dysregulation to these disorders , therefore, is critical to proper diagnosis and selection of appropriate treatments. Manual techniques, including focal palpation, laryngeal reposturing maneuvers, and circumlaryngeal massage are valuable tools that augment the voice practitioner's diagnostic and treatment armamentarium.

Management of Functional Dysphonia in a Child

R. E. (Ed) Stone Jr, PhD

Case Study: Patient Y

In the next case study, R. E. (Ed) Stone, Jr., demonstrates the advantages of imagination and clinical experience in developing and implementing a "speaking situations hierarchy" for functional dysphonia in a 10-year-old child.

Patient History

Patient Y was only 10 years old but represented one of the greatest intervention challenges I have encountered in nearly 30 years of clinical practice. At the mother's telephone contact for an appointment, I learned that Patient Y came home from school one day with extreme dysphonia after attending a soccer game. She thought that he had developed laryngitis. When supper was over, he produced no voice and indicated that he couldn't talk. Professional help from various disciplines over a 7-week period was unproductive in restoring normal voice and communication.

When we met, Patient Y's only vocalizations were utterances of vocal fry but with no accompanying lip, jaw, or tongue movements needed for word formation. These movements were not elicited even when the boy was asked to whisper. If it weren't for the vocal fry productions, he might have been thought to show elective mutism. One got the impression that his talking was reduced to a series of vocal-fry grunts that may have showed syllabification, thought pauses, and interphrase silences. Additionally, the pitch and loudness of the grunts varied within restricted limits but seemed to suggest his attempts at prosody.

Patient Y was adopted during infancy into a home of two older female siblings. The family life seemed healthy. The parents were well educated, and the father was a vice president of a large company in a large metropolitan Midwestern city. Both parents were energetic and had outgoing personalities. They did not give the impression of being overbearing or unreasonably demanding of their children.

A history provided to the clinician (C) by the mother (M) follows:

C: "Tell us a little bit about when Patient Y started talking with a really tight voice."

M: "OK. He came home from school hoarse. They had a soccer game; he had some voice, but it sounded like he had been screaming a lot. Within maybe 2 hours, the voice was completely gone."

C: "All he could do, then, was produce this sound?"

M: "He did not even do that; there was just nothing."

C: "Did he mouth his words, or did he stop talking altogether?"

M: "He stopped talking, and when I would ask him to try, he would just make indications that there was nothing there."

C: "How long after that was it before he started pushing air through the larynx a little bit" (strained sounding voice-making that vocal-fry kind of voice)?

M: "I would say it was like a week. He went to a pediatrician the following day, and he thought it was laryngitis, so he told him not to try to talk. So he made no attempt of any kind to talk for a week until he went to a throat specialist who then got him to make that vocal-fry noise. That was when he started with . . . "

C: "So he kind of learned to produce the sound then, huh?"

M: "Yes, I think so, yes."

C: "What other things has he done in trying to get voice back again? You have been to the pediatrician and to an ear, nose, and throat specialist."

M: "And he was hospitalized for a week and was treated then by a psychologist, a throat specialist, and a physical therapist. All who were trying to make him relax enough to be able to make his vocal cords work. They said they were too tight."

C: "What kinds of things did they do for relaxation?"

M: "They did hypnotic suggestion, they put him in whirlpool baths, they played games with him, and they just talked to him about other things, anything that was unrelated to his being unable to talk."

C: "You spent a great deal of money pursuing this then, haven't you?"

M: "Yes, about $7,000."

During the intake interview with Patient Y's parents, a colleague met with the patient in another room. They unproductively probed the child's potential for voice production using a variety of facilitative techniques, [21] including inspiratory voice, yawn-sigh, humming, throat clearing, coughing, and chewing.

My involvement with Patient Y was governed by a model I have called "erg." In physics, an erg is a unit for measuring work. It involves moving a mass through a certain distance in a given unit of time. Applied to the therapeutic setting, one might consider taking a patient (mass) from one point of behavior to another (distance) within an individual therapy session (or segment of it) divided into three parts:

1. **Evaluation** of behavior or skill that is needed or (needs to be aban-

doned) to bring the person closer to normal
2. **Recommendation** of desirable behavior through verbal instruction and modeling
3. **Getting** on with developing the use of the desired skill (or absence of the undesired behavior) in a hierarchy of speaking situations

After the patient achieves success criterion at one level of the hierarchy, the erg is repeated at another level. Each recycling would involve a new bit of behavior. The bits are designed to shape the individual's eventual performance into the use of normal physiology for phonation, finally in normal proposition communication.

Evaluating Patient Y, initially, I sought to recognize those behaviors he brought to the task of communication that obviated normal voice production. Hollien[22] has reviewed the characteristics of vocal fry (pulse register) productions, suggesting there is increased glottal resistance and decreased airflow. Patient Y consequently needed to reduce muscle effort and increase airflow to the task of voice production. Teaching muscular relaxation[23] of the interarytenoid, lateral cricoarytenoid, and thyroarytenoid muscles to a 10-year-old child within 1 or 2 days (before he and his parents returned home several hundreds of miles away) seemed an unrealistic clinical undertaking.

Recommendation, therefore, deemphasized formal relaxation training and focused on increasing airflow. I learned quickly that asking Patient Y to change behavior during speechlike activities led to failure. When a patient fails at a task that I recommend, I am obligated to assume the responsibility for the error in asking something that is too difficult or in not adequately communicating what I want of the person. Because failure tends to foster undesirable thoughts in a patient and unproductive consequences of my guidance, I must present requests that the individual can understand and accomplish.

Teaching increased airflow, at what task could I expect Patient Y to succeed? Finally, I merely asked him to blow against his upheld index finger as if he were blowing out a match. This was nonpropositional use of airflow and was a request of a behavior with which he had previous experience. It was behavior that easily could be molded by later instruction and was a task with a simplicity that anyone with normal anatomy could do. The component or partial behaviors to which Patient Y's attention was drawn through verbal instruction included unimpeded inspiration, no holding of the breath between inspiration and expiration, and lack of work (muscular action) in the neck area (and consequently in the larynx) on exhalation. These partial behaviors were adopted, then, as the recommended behaviors to be employed repetitively (that is, practiced, which constitutes "getting on with the behavior") in a variety of tasks one might consider as constituting a speaking-situations hierarchy.

Lowest on the hierarchical ladder was purposeful flow of air through the untensed speech mechanism. Next, Patient Y practiced flow of air while his mouth and lips were placed in various static positions. This was done by asking that he produce a relaxed flow of air with his mouth open, then somewhat closed with the corners of the lips pulled back, then with lips rounded, and so forth. (These positions resulted in the production of different whispered vowels; however, this fact was not pointed

out to Patient Y because of the need to avoid the chance of failure that might have accompanied a request to "whisper /i/, whisper /a/," for example.)

After the boy successfully produced multiple events, meeting at least 80% success in the desired partial behaviors while instruction (discriminative stimulus) and positive feedback were withheld, it was pointed out that he indeed produced many tokens of various vowels. He then was asked to practice production of airflow (no voice) on vowels that he read from flash cards. (This represented another level of the hierarchy: purposeful vowel production with flow of air through an untensed mechanism.)

The use of unvoiced flow of air through a relatively relaxed speech mechanism was eventually shaped through carefully graded increments of a speaking hierarchy into employment for propositional speech. At this point, after approximately 1 hour of intervention, Patient Y was whispering normally. Mouth, lip, and tongue movements had become reestablished communication behaviors along with unimpeded flow of air. Not only had an erg been accomplished, but the idea of elective mutism as a diagnostic label no longer was an appropriate consideration.

The second session began with an evaluation of what behavior was needed to bring Patient Y a step closer to normal communication. Even the uninitiated clinician would recognize the patient's need for vocal fold activity superimposed on the flow of air through a relatively relaxed speech mechanism. But how could vocal fold activity be recommended without a statement such as, "OK, now produce the airflow like you did last hour, but this time with voice?" The reader also may ask, "What's wrong with asking for voice?" Maybe nothing would be wrong, but I submit that it would have risked the patient adopting behaviors similar to those he demonstrated when he first entered therapy (which was vocal fry). Guarding against this possibility, I was compelled not to refer to "voicing." Also, I did not want to ask the patient to do any of the activities my colleague requested earlier because he failed at them. What could I do that might rely on referents that the child knew, that were not requests "to produce voice" (because he 'knew" he couldn't produce voice), and that would ensure success?

I decided to approach voice production by recommending gargling. Unvoiced gargling really wasn't much different from the activity Patient Y had engaged in during the previous hour. The recommendation proceeded as follows, where C is the clinician and P is the patient.

C: "I know you can let air flow out of your mouth. This time I'd like you to do so while gargling a small mouthful of water." (Clinician models, tilting the head backward and gargling with voice.) "Now you do it."

P: The patient tried. He produced the bubbling sound, but no voice.

C: "Okay, you kept the air flowing out all the time. That's a good thing, too! If you hadn't, you'd have done a lot of choking. Keeping the air going is pretty important. Now, this time let's have you gargle like your Dad might do—with a lot of sound." (Clinician models vocalized gargling.) "Now, you do it."

P: The patient tried. He produced the bubbling sound louder than before, but still no voice. After he swallowed the mouthful of water, he gave a little laugh with one short period in which the voice was produced in a high-pitched squeal sound.

C: Immediately, the clinician remarked, "Hey, did you notice that part of your laugh had some voice to it? Here, gargle another sip of water and make that little squeak sound as you gargle."

P: Patient Y succeeded.

C: "Do that again, but this time make the sound longer."

P: Again, Patient Y succeeded.

C: This time, make your gargle sound bigger, like your Dad might sound."

P: Again, Patient Y succeeded.

C: "Okay, this time make that sound, but without using a sip of water."

P: Again, the patient succeeded. Voice was produced, and the gurgling sound probably resulted from interruption of the voice airstream by repetitive action of the uvula against and away from the base of the tongue.

Practice followed until the patient and the clinician both felt assured that this behavior could be repeated any time the patient wished. The next evaluation established the need to alter the boy's head position to an upright posture.

Accomplishing this was done in three trials in which gradual increments of head position change minimized the potential for failure that might have accompanied moving the head in a single trial to a position more suitable for communication.

Next, the evaluation established the need to alter the gurgling of sound to a continuous voice production by eliminating the tongue-uvula vibration. The recommendation to the patient was a simple instruction to open the mouth widely (separating the tongue from the uvula) accompanied by providing a mode of sustained /a/. Five trials were done before the patient indicated that he felt able to do this consistently whenever he wanted.

The next intervention step needed to establish Patient Y's ability to maintain continuous voice while moving parts of the speech mechanism without triggering his dysphonic behaviors conditioned to the act of speaking. The recommendations involved leading the boy, by modeling, through a sequence of behaviors starting with opening and closing the mouth (vowel productions) with continuous voice. Next, vowel-like utterances were made individually rather than the continuous vowel series. Following this, individual vowel productions each were terminated with an articulatory valving; then, vowels were initiated and terminated with consonants. Even though Patient Y was producing nonsense and finally meaningful syllables at this time, the fact that he merely was copying the model set by the clinician seemed to keep him from recognizing that he was using voice in speechlike units. Finally, after the boy had produced several CVC units that would have resulted in meaningful words if

they had been uttered in reverse, it was pointed out that the patient had been saying words backward. For example, "tube" said backward would be "boot." "You have been speaking backward, let's now say some words forward," was the recommendation used to elicit meaningful words.

Use of words to form phrases and sentences was based on increasing the length of utterance, word for word, and then finally uttering the entire unit. For example:

C: "Say 'I'."

P: "I."

C: "Say, 'I want'."

P: "I want."

C: "Say, 'I want some'."

P: "I want some." (etc, etc)

P: "I want some eggs for breakfast."

By the end of this session (2 hours), Patient Y was able to engage in dialogue, maintaining voice that was different from that with which he presented initially and was closer to normal. The voice still had a falsettolike quality and was produced with guarded participation. I decided to accompany Patient Y and his parents to lunch and observe the degree to which the boy maintained his present skill outside the clinical setting. He did admirably. Not once did he lapse into vocal fry, and during lunch he even seemed to modify voice production to be more normal. After lunch, intervention resumed and constituted a review of the processes the boy had used in reacquiring use of voice. With a trend during lunch for him to improve voice toward normal, formal activities focusing on voice normalization were deferred until the next day.

Patient Y returned the next day, and his parents vouched for the accuracy of his contention that he had maintained use of the improved vocal function established during the previous afternoon and evening. Although he presented this morning with normal voice, I was uncertain of his awareness of the clinical processes and goals. To test this, I asked the boy to demonstrate the way he talked before we started intervention. He did. Then, he successfully switched at will between normal voice and that which he used previously.

One last evaluation seemed necessary. Because Patient Y lived nearly 300 miles away, and he could not conveniently return to the clinic, I needed satisfaction that he knew what to do to reestablish normal voice if he ever began speaking with his pre-intervention behaviors. Notice the absence of the term "remission." Within a behavioral model of intervention, the use of medical terms such as "remission," "exacerbation," and "cure" tend to be used in ways that do not foster a patient's development of the awareness that the behavior brought to the task of speaking is the responsibility of the patient. I was seeking indication that this patient had become his own clinician and that he had an appropriate plan of approach to solving future problems of voice of a similar nature should he exhibit them. Patient Y reiterated and successfully demonstrated the intervention steps he used to re-establish normal voice.

Because his parents participated in the therapy sessions, it seemed important to sample the parents' understanding of how their son implemented a change to normal and the implications of this change. This was assessed on the second morning through an interview at the end of the patient's hour-long session.

C: "What thoughts went through your mind as you and the family were experiencing this?"

M: "Well, we were told that our son's problem was purely psychological, that until he could learn to cope with a lot of the fears and things that were going on inside of him he would not be able to produce a voice that his subconscious would not allow him to speak. So we went through a whole lot of guilt and embarrassment. I think that each one of us wondered . . . were we the ones who caused that kind of trauma and what have we done when we thought that we had a typical normal family. You know there was a lot of self-doubt and wondering if he would ever get over this."

C: "Pretty spooky!"

M: "Yes, it was very scary, yup."

C: "Do you have any concerns or questions now that you know he is producing voice again?"

M: "No, I don't think so; I guess, if he comes down with laryngitis I will be very nervous. I think I am really satisfied with the psychological end of it and . . ."

C: "Explain what you mean."

M: "Well, I guess I worried about a lot of deep-seated problems and, you know, I don't think I am worried about that anymore. In the beginning, I would have said if he had gotten his voice back maybe there would be another time when if a traumatic experience occurred, he would lose it again. I see it now more as a physical thing that he can deal with and we can help him if he, you know, if it would come to a point where there was a problem with voice, I think we would know how to handle it."

Management of a Functional Dysphonia Initially Masquerading as a Paralytic Dysphonia

Claudio Milstein, PhD

Case Study: Patient Z

Voice disorders often are complex in nature and challenging to fully define at the time of the initial evaluation. Consequently, clinicians may find themselves reconsidering their initial impressions as they walk with patients through the therapeutic process and observe the patients' response to various methods. The following case of functional dysphonia by Claudio Milstein highlights the importance of approaching clients with an open mind and a flexible treatment plan.

The patient is a 39-year-old woman who was referred by her ENT for a 3-month history of hoarseness and change in voice quality following a total thyroidectomy. She is a trained singer, and has worked as an elementary school music teacher (K through 6) for the last 10 years. She had a 4-year history of formal classical voice training in college, and over

the years has continued to take short periods of individual voice lessons to "tune-up" her voice. Her teaching technique consists of demonstrating the songs to her students, and then singing with them throughout the entire class. Therefore, over the course of an 8-hour working day, she estimates that she sings for about 4 to 5 hours. She has not had a voice problem in the past and was able to complete her working days with no vocal fatigue.

Her past medical history is significant for occasional sinus problems. Otherwise, she is a healthy woman. Her history was negative for smoking. She rarely consumes alcohol, consumes one serving of caffeine daily, and reportedly drinks "lots of water." Medications include thyroid hormone replacement therapy and birth control pills. She states that she is very protective of her voice, is well aware of vocal hygiene guidelines, and does not do any vocal behaviors that "would put my voice at risk."

Prior to undergoing a total thyroidectomy, her surgeon explained the potential risks of damage to laryngeal nerves, and stated that she would probably experience some hoarseness after the procedure. She had a noneventful postoperative period and was sent home the same day. She experienced minimal pain during the following 2 days. She noticed a change in her voice quality and some hoarseness immediately following the surgery but was not concerned about it initially, as she expected to have some temporary voice changes. However, after a month of hoarseness, she consulted with her surgeon, who indicated that the laryngeal nerves were monitored during the operation, and that, as far as he could tell, there had been no nerve trauma as a result of the procedure. She was referred to her local ENT, who confirmed that both vocal folds were mobile. He found generalized laryngeal edema and erythema and prescribed antireflux medication. The patient discontinued this medication after 3 weeks because of lack of improvement. On her next ENT follow-up visit, she was urged to comply with the reflux management recommendations. After 3 months of medical treatment with no improvement, the ENT referred the patient to our clinic for what he described as a "frustrating lack of progress."

During her first evaluation, the patient reported that she had returned to work full time but was having significant difficulties performing her job. She was unable to sing and was experiencing extreme vocal fatigue at end of the day. She had started using a microphone at school when teaching, but this was not helping much. She appeared quite anxious about the future of her voice and indicated that this was catastrophic for her career both as a music teacher and a singer. She described her symptoms as follows:

1. Consistent hoarseness
2. Straining to speak
3. A significant drop in her speaking voice, with a "very deep voice"
4. A significant drop in her singing pitch range with a 1½ octave loss in the upper range
5. Inability to increase loudness beyond a quiet voice
6. Pain described as "cramping" localized to the lateral aspect of the larynx, hyoid, and submandibular area bilaterally when high pitches were attempted
7. Voice fatigue that increased with voice use
8. Increased shoulder/neck tension with voice use

9. Globus sensation with difficulty swallowing.

She indicated that her thyroid hormone levels were balanced, as per her endocrinologist. On the weekends, when she did no talking at all, her energy levels were good. She attributed the fatigue to the constant effort required for speaking.

Initial Evaluation

Trauma to the laryngeal branches of the vagus nerve following thyroid surgery is a known potential risk of this procedure. The nerves may be stretched, bruised or severed, resulting in unilateral neuropathy, and more rarely in bilateral involvement.[24] In some patients, the damage is permanent, whereas others experience spontaneous recovery up to 9 months after the nerve insult. Trauma to the recurrent laryngeal nerve may result in unilateral vocal fold paralysis or paresis, causing hoarseness and sometimes dysphagia. Superior laryngeal nerve (SLN) transient or permanent injuries are relatively frequent and are often underestimated.[25,26] Deeper voices and a loss of the upper part of the register are not infrequent in these cases. Based on this patient's case history and symptomatology, trauma to the SLN was considered.

On initial evaluation, her voice quality was judged to be consistently mildly hoarse and low pitched, with a consistently low loudness level. Her average speaking F_0 was 165 Hz, which was considered low for her age and gender. She had an inability to increase either pitch or loudness. When asked to perform a pitch glide toward higher pitch levels, the patient reported throat pain starting consistently at around 250 Hz. She was unable to go any higher than

260 Hz. Palpation of the neck musculature during this voice task revealed sudden and severe tightening of the laryngeal and paralaryngeal musculature. When prompted to increase volume, her voice remained soft and weak.

Videostroboscopic evaluation revealed essentially a normal larynx. There were no lesions, tumor, masses, ulcerations or areas of leukoplakia identified. Mobility of the vocal folds was within normal limits bilaterally. There was no edema or erythema. The vocal folds appeared with good color, and straight edges. During phonation at a comfortable pitch level, the pattern of glottal closure was complete. Phase symmetry was regular. Amplitude of vibration and mucosal waves were within normal limits bilaterally.

The only significant finding was an odd laryngeal posturing when the patient attempted to phonate above 250 Hz. There was noticeable narrowing of the posterior pharyngeal wall, and supraglottic constriction, with significant tilting forward of the arytenoids. In other words, laryngeal posturing was normal below 250 Hz, and a severe constriction with an odd posturing was observed as soon as that pitch level was reached. This was confirmed with multiple pitch glide repetitions, in which constriction was elicited exactly at the same pitch level every trial. When the patient was asked to produce a louder voice, she simply could not do it, despite perception of a legitimate attempt to do so.

After the initial evaluation, several therapeutic probes, which included digital laryngeal manipulation and neck stretching, were implemented. Following this brief treatment, the patient was able to raise pitch up to 300 Hz with relative ease, but not any higher. She could not increase loudness level.

Based on the results of this evaluation, nerve trauma was suspected. The deepening of her conversational voice, together with the inability to produce higher pitches, and the odd laryngeal posturing seen during endoscopy were thought to be secondary to insult to the superior laryngeal nerve. In addition, musculoskeletal tension was observed. Although the decrease in pitch range could be attributed to SLN neuropathy, there was no physiological explanation for the inability to go beyond a soft voice. The comprehensive evaluation did not reveal any physiological impediment for increasing loudness, as her respiratory system, ability to produce large subglottic pressures, and laryngeal mechanism and valving appeared to be intact.

Treatment recommendations included an electromyographic study (EMG) to evaluate status of laryngeal nerves and the initiation of an individual course of voice therapy to address musculoskeletal tension. The patient refused to undergo a diagnostic EMG examination for fear of needles and the invasive nature of the procedure. She agreed to initiate voice therapy.

Therapy Approach

The goals of therapy were established toward increasing pitch range and loudness levels while decreasing muscular tension and achieving effortless and relaxed sound. Even if a neuropathy was confirmed at a later time, it was believed that a therapeutic approach would be beneficial to decrease the hyperfunctional component. Prognosis for voice improvement was deemed good based on the initial positive response to therapeutic intervention during her evaluation.

The patient initially presented for two therapy sessions where several therapeutic techniques were tried. These included:

- laryngeal massage
- digital laryngeal manipulation
- head-neck-shoulders relaxation
- coordination of respiratory and phonatory behaviors
- breath support for increased loudness
- pitch glides with lip and tongue trills
- voice placement with forward focus.

All of these techniques failed to improve pitch or loudness ranges. Even though she had responded well to digital laryngeal manipulation during her evaluation, further improvement was not achieved with therapy. It appeared as if there was a threshold for both pitch and loudness above which the patient could not operate. Phonation below that threshold could be achieved in a relaxed manner, with no hoarseness or discomfort, but above it, severe tension was elicited.

By mutual agreement, a third session was scheduled to focus exclusively on vocal loudness, based on the clinician's belief that there was no physiologic impediment for producing louder voice. An overview of the therapeutic approach follows. The process occurred within a 30-minute time frame:

C: "Okay, I want you to look out of the window (office located on 7th floor). See that person there about to cross the street? Try to yell "Hey you!" loud enough to get that person's attention."

P: "I don't think I can do that."

C: "Just try."

P: *Patient initiates a series of "Hey You!" productions, trying to increase loudness after each trial as*

prompted by the clinician. Her willingness to do the required task was evident; however, the more she tried to get loud, her voice would become breathier and more strained, but not any louder.

C: *As the patient would stop and "think" between trials, the clinician prompted her to: "Just do it—don't think—just do!" The more the patient tries, the more frustrated she gets by her inability to get louder, and becomes emotional and tearful. The emotional display did not stop the unrelenting prompts by the clinician to continue to try to yell.*

P: "I'm exhausted, I can't do anymore, this is not going to work."

C: "Keep trying, as loud as you can!" "Yell now!" "One more time!"

After approximately 15 more trials, the patient was able to produce a very loud voice. Encouraged, she tried a couple more times, actually yelling, and this elicited an emotional catharsis. Evaluation of her voice quality after this sequence of events revealed a normal voice, with normal loudness level, and ability to voluntarily increase volume as desired. Moreover, and this was surprising to both the patient and the clinician, once loudness range was re-established, her average fundamental frequency during conversational speech was noticeably higher. Immediate evaluation of her pitch range revealed complete recovery of her pitch range without further intervention. The patient was able to produce pitch glides up to 1050 Hz without effort or discomfort. This appeared to be a simultaneous benefit of the breakthrough with loudness.

A 1-week over-the-phone follow-up revealed that she had maintained a normal voice quality, with an increase in her overall fundamental frequency for speech, ability to phonate at normal and loud voice levels, and recovery of her normal pitch range. She was able to stop using a microphone at work and was able to teach all day without discomfort. She also reported a significant improvement in her singing voice. Post-therapy videostroboscopic examination was deemed unnecessary.

Discussion

This case demonstrates the use of an enabling voice therapy technique in a patient who had developed an inability to phonate above a specific threshold. It appeared that the patient had acquired maladaptive strategies in an attempt to "protect" her voice after surgery, as if she was "holding back" for fear of further damage.

Even though some of the symptoms appeared consistent with postoperative SLN injury, this was a unique manifestation of what turned out to be a case of functional dysphonia, or musculoskeletal tension. Muscle tension disrupted two parameters of vocal function, creating a "ceiling-effect" beyond which the patient could not operate. Below those levels, physiologic parameters of voice production were intact. Once the patient regained access to volume control, it appeared to recalibrate the entire system, with immediate restoration of full pitch range.

The clinical relevance of this case lies in the therapeutic approach. As demonstrated, coaching of this patient required gentle guidance, at times, and at other times to be more assertive and harsh. The approach was met with resistance, in terms of the patient believing she could not perform the required tasks. The actual dialogue was neither sophisticated nor particularly varied. It was a relentless, continued urging of the patient to get louder, louder, louder, followed by additional prompts such as: "You can do this," "You need to push yourself," "It doesn't matter how it feels, just do it," and so on. This focused around only one goal, to force the patient to overcome her limitation. Not surprisingly, there was significant emotional catharsis manifested in crying, not only during the process, but after the breakthrough. The patient's reflection was that it was really hard, and she was convinced she could not do it. She genuinely believed she was physically unable to get louder. She was grateful that the clinician pushed her beyond levels that she did not think possible. The reader should understand that sometimes "tough love" is required in therapy. We cannot use the patient's words, or emotional reaction of resistance, to be the indicators of the end point of the therapeutic approach. In order to allow the patient to push through an emotional and physiologic limit, sometimes the guidance has to be done in an encouraging but strict manner.

Voice improvement in this case was not a slow, gradual response to therapy to obtain a normal voice. In the treatment of patients with functional dysphonia, often there is little or no evidence of success during the therapeutic process, until the patient reaches a breakthrough moment, after which recovery is achieved quite rapidly. In these cases, the clinician's persistence is paramount to success. It appears as if, once the patient reaches a level of exhaustion (mental or physical) during the therapeutic process, his or her physical or mental blocks go down, and patients are not able to continue to hold on to the maladaptive pattern of vocal function that results in dysphonic voice.

> At times, individuals present with pitch concerns that are functional in nature. Although these issues most frequently arise in pubescent males, they may be seen in other populations. The cases that follow discuss treatment for functional pitch concerns in a postpubescent teenage male, a hearing-impaired teen, and an adult female.

The size and general positioning of the male larynx undergo marked changes in a relatively short period of time during puberty. These anatomical changes dramatically alter the physiology of phonation and require a new mechanism of laryngeal neuromuscular control. At the same time, anatomic changes bring about a significant reduction in fundamental frequency and, consequently, present a challenge to the individual's auditory feedback system. Most pubescent males proceed through the above changes without difficulty, making the necessary motor and sensory adjustments without thought or effort. However, in some males, the system does not adjust to the changing anatomy, and the individual persists in the higher range.

Physiologically, the mutational voice is produced when the suprahyoid and cricothyroid muscles are contracted, and the thyroarytenoid muscle is disengaged. The result is a tense laryngeal mechanism that is positioned high in the neck. The vocal folds themselves are elongated and tense and exhibiit decreased vibration and inadequate closure. This posture results in a high-pitched, weak, breathy voice, often accompanied by roughness and pitch breaks. Therapies

aimed at engaging the thyroarytenoid muscle and moving the larynx into an improved posture have proven quite helpful in remediating this voice concern.

The use of an inappropriately high-pitched voice beyond puberty in males has been commonly presented in voice literature[1,6,7] and has taken on a number of names, including: mutational voice, mutational falsetto, persistent falsetto, and puberphonia. The problem is most commonly observed in adolescent males in the months immediately following puberty when hormonal shifts bring about dramatic changes in the size and function of the vocal mechanism as described above. Although rare, some cases have been reported to extend beyond puberty into adulthood.

The presence of the mutational voice can be confirmed clinically in several ways. For example, throat clearing, coughing, laughing, and production of the hard glottal attack should engage the thyroarytenoid muscle and result in a dramatic lowering of pitch into the modal register. Furthermore, digital manipulation of the larynx initially will reveal an elevated larynx that can be gently manipulated to a lower position with systematic, digital manipulation of the thyroid cartilage.[1,7]

Mutational Voice in a 16-Year-Old Male

Lisa Fry, PhD

Case Study: Patient AA

Patient History

Background and Referral Information. Patient AA was a 16-year-old male referred to the university voice center by a local otolaryngologist for evaluation and treatment of mutational voice. In a telephone conversation with the patient's mother prior to the evaluation, she expressed deep concern over her son's abnormal voice and its impact on his interaction with peers and teachers at school.

The patient was brought to the evaluation session by his mother. The mother was present during the interview portion of the evaluation session and left the room after historical information had been obtained. The patient provided the majority of the background and historical information related to his voice condition. AA was reserved throughout the evaluation session, speaking only briefly when asked direct questions by the clinician and offering only limited detail in his comments.

History of the Problem

The client presented with the primary complaints of a "high voice" and intermittent vocal fatigue at the close of the day. He could not recall the exact time of onset or any circumstances surrounding the onset but believed that the problem had been in existence for about 2 years. AA reported that his voice did not really bother him and that he did not pay much attention to it. He stated that his mother was much more concerned about the problem than he was and that she was the primary instigator of the otolaryngology and voice therapy appointments.

During the history-taking portion of the evaluation, AA was asked about his voice behaviors and if/when he had ever heard himself produce "another" voice. (Some young men with this condition experience brief periods where the new, lower pitched voice is heard; however, they find themselves unable to sustain this mode of phonation for

functional use.) AA indicated that he had heard this "other" voice from time to time. He recalled that this generally happened first thing in the morning, just upon waking. He stated that he generally makes only a few statements in this other voice before the high-pitched voice returns and remains for the course of the day.

Medical History

AA's medical history was significant for mild nasal allergies and acne. Current medications included an oral antibiotic for treatment of acne and an over-the-counter pain medication as needed for sports-related orthopedic pain/soreness.

Social/Educational History

AA was a sophomore at the local high school where he participated in the school's junior varsity basketball team. As part of the team requirements, he attended practice 4 to 5 times per week and engaged in weightlifting 2 to 3 times per week. He reported great enthusiasm for the sport and indicated that most of his close friends at school were his fellow members of the basketball team. When questioned about his behavior and general performance at school, AA indicated that he was "an OK student." He reported that he rarely spoke up in class and rarely talked with teachers apart from his basketball coaches. AA did converse with close friends in the hallway before and after school and during breaks, but he suggested that these hallway conversations were, at times, difficult, as he could not project his voice over the surrounding noise. AA stated that his friends did not comment on his voice but indicated that when people met him for the first time they often asked if he had a cold.

AA lived at home with his father, mother, and younger sister. He described the home as typically "quiet" and uneventful. There were no smokers living in the home. The family had one small indoor dog. AA reportedly filled his spare time with basketball, hanging out with friends, and attending church-related youth activities.

Vocal Hygiene History

AA described his amount of voice use as "average." He reported occasional allergy-related coughing and throat clearing and occasional yelling at sporting events. He sang in a church youth choir twice weekly. AA denied smoking and alcohol use. He drank 64 ounces of water and approximately 32 ounces of caffeinated soda per day.

Brief Summary of the Perceptual Voice Evaluation

AA spoke in a falsetto voice throughout the evaluation session. His voice quality was moderately harsh, and loudness was reduced. He displayed intermittent pitch breaks into the modal register during conversation. A mild degree of strain was present during voicing. Specific parameters of AA's voice were rated using the Consensus Auditory Perceptual Evaluation—Voice (CAPE-V).[27] Specific results are outlined Table 5–1. In brief, AA presented with moderate to severe dysphonia, characterized by a severe deviation of pitch, moderate breathiness, moderate roughness, and a mild to moderate reduction in loudness. Intermittent pitch breaks were noted.

Acoustic Measures. Key acoustic measures were taken with the Computerized Speech Lab (KayPentax). Results are shown in Table 5–2. In brief, fundamental frequency of sustained phonation and conversational speech were increased at 236.37 Hz and 229.97 Hz, respectively. Conversational dB was mildly decreased. Harmonics-to-noise ratio as well as jitter and shimmer calculations indicated an increased degree of noise and aperiodicity in the voice signal.

Videostroboscopic Examination. AA's vocal folds were easily visualized with a 70-degree rigid scope. Vocal fold edges were smooth and straight bilater-

Table 5–1. CAPE-V Scores for Client AA

Parameter	Score	Consistency
Roughness	40	Consistent
Breathiness	39	Consistent
Strain	20	Consistent
Pitch (increased, falsetto)	85	Consistent
Loudness (reduced)	31	Consistent
Voice breaks (downward)	25	Inconsistent
Overall Severity	74	

Table 5–2. Pre and Posttreatment Acoustic Measures for Case AA

	Pretreatment	Posttreatment
F_0—sustained phonation	236.37 Hz	110.6 Hz
F_0—conversation	229.97 Hz	105.7 Hz
dB—conversation	74.90 dB	82.60 dB
Harmonics-to-noise ratio	10.3	14.6
Jitter (in %)	.67	.55
Shimmer (in dB)	.26	.14

ally, and vocal fold coloration was normal. Arytenoid movement was normal bilaterally. Glottic closure pattern was incomplete, characterized by a slight gap running the length of the vocal folds. Amplitude of vibration and mucosal wave were mildly reduced bilaterally. The open phase of vibration was moderately longer than the closed phase. The vocal folds were elongated and tense during phonation.

Impressions and Recommendations

The client presented with mutational voice characterized by an abnormally high pitch, roughness, breathiness, voice breaks, and reduced loudness. It was recommended that AA participate in 1 to 2 intensive voice therapy sessions to lower pitch to an appropriate level and generalize its use to all speaking situations.

Therapy

Background. Most cases of functional falsetto in the pubescent male can be successfully managed in only 1 to 2 treatment sessions. In many cases, the initial treatment session can, in fact, be conducted at the time of the diagnostic voice evaluation, saving the client pre-cious time and offering tremendous support and encouragement to the client and family. In some cases in which the functional use of the falsetto register has been maintained over the course of many years, a few additional treatment sessions may be necessary.

Because the mutational voice is generally amenable to modification and can be managed efficiently, a few guidelines regarding scheduling are generally followed. First, when clinic scheduling permits, it is helpful to arrange an extended block of time for the initial evaluation/treatment session. I generally schedule a 2- to 3-hour session for these cases. When more than one session is required, every attempt should be made to avoid long period between sessions, as this may permit the client to revert back to previous vocal behaviors; arranging sessions on consecutive days is quite helpful.

Goals for AA

- AA will consistently achieve the targeted lower pitched voice after facilitating techniques.
- AA will extend use of the new pitch to increasingly complex linguistic contexts (syllables through conversation).

- AA will develop a plan for generalizing the new voice to new listeners and situations.
- AA will use the lower pitched voice in all speaking contexts.
- AA will express satisfaction and comfort with his new speaking voice.

Management of AA

Education. Treatment began with a thorough description of the anatomy and physiology of voice production and a discussion of how these features change at puberty. Line drawings by the clinician and a laryngeal model supported the explanation. The clinician reminded the client that his laryngeal structures were normal on exam and that his voice concerns were related to muscle use issues. The physiology of the mutational voice (ie, disengaged thyroarytenoid muscle amid tense suprahyoid and cricothyroid muscles) was presented. The client was reassured that changes in laryngeal anatomy at puberty create challenges for the system and that he was not alone in his experience. Finally, methods of facilitating proper muscle activity were reviewed; the rationale for each method and its ability to restore normal physiology was explained.

Facilitating and Stabilizing the Lower Pitch. After the above discussion, the clinician spoke with AA about the "other voice" that he reported hearing upon waking some mornings. The clinician asked if AA could produce that voice on command. AA made several attempts to produce the lower pitch without success. (*Note:* In some instances, this simple technique is sufficient to prompt the lower pitched phonation, which can then be shaped into conversational speech.)

As AA was unable to produce the lower pitch on command, a simple facilitating technique—the hard glottal attack—was used. Production of the hard glottal attack requires engagement of the thyroarytenoid muscle and moves the larynx away from the falsetto posture into an appropriate posture for the lower pitch. In keeping with this line of thought, AA was asked to produce a hard, abrupt "ah." His initial attempts yielded only breathy, high-pitched "ahs." The clinician continued to request a harder, louder tone, eventually asking the client to press hard against her hands while attempting the abrupt "ah." With this maneuver, the glottal attack was produced, immediately triggering a lower pitched, frylike phonation. The client was instructed to repeatedly produce the glottal attack until the lower pitched tone was stable. Once consistent hard glottal attacks were heard and the client was able to hear/identify the targeted pitch, the abrupt "ah" was sustained for longer periods of time. Eventually, the hard onset was faded, and AA was able to sustain the "ah" for several seconds on command.

After the target tone had been stabilized, the tone was slowly extended into other speech contexts. First, the client was asked to generalize the tone to other sustained vowels. Once that step was mastered, the clinician trained the client in chanting, all-voiced nonsense syllables (eg, mamama, momomo, minimini). Chanting syllables such as these permitted AA to extend the low-pitched voice to a variety of articulatory contexts without altering the newly acquired laryngeal posture for inflection or for production of a voiceless consonant. Consequently, the new voice became more stable, and the client was less likely to return to the high pitch as a result of laryngeal maneuvering that would have been required of voiced-voiceless syllables.

AA continued chanting all-voiced productions through word, phrase, and sentence levels. Once mastered, AA progressed to producing voiced-voiceless syllables, words, phrases, and sentences in the context of a chanting style. Eventually, the chanting style was faded, and the client was able to gradually produce the new pitch with longer utterances with normal prosody. The client was advanced through various readings and conversational topics.

Generalizing the Lower Pitch. Because of the dramatic nature of voice changes during treatment for mutational voice, transition of the voice outside of the therapy context can be challenging. Consequently, it is recommended that the clinician and client openly discuss this challenge and develop a structured plan for generalizing the new voice.

In the case of AA, the clinician posed the question "What do you think others will say about your new voice?" to which AA replied "They will be shocked. I don't know if they will like it." The clinician reassured the client that, although the new voice was notably different, it was also quite pleasing and appropriate. To confirm this for the patient, digital recordings of the new voice were made and played back for the client. After hearing only a few brief statements, the client expressed his pleasure with the new voice, stating that it made him sound stronger and more confident.

At this point, the speech pathologist suggested that the client develop a hierarchy of persons and situations where the voice could be gradually introduced. The client agreed to use the new voice with his immediate family and two close friends on the day of the session; he would be free to use his

higher pitched voice if he so desired with other individuals on that day. On the first day following therapy, AA would expand use of his new voice to include the coaches and members of his basketball team and members of his extended family. By the second day posttherapy, AA would use the voice with all teachers and with friends and acquaintances in the school hallway. Finally, by the third day following therapy, AA expected to use his lower pitched voice in all situations.

With the above plan in place, the session drew to a close. The speech pathologist asked that the client remain in the treatment area while she went to get his mother. Prior to taking the mother into the treatment area, the clinician took a few moments to prepare the mother for AA's new voice. The results of the session were discussed, and the speech pathologist asked that the mother not respond too dramatically or emotionally to the new voice but that she simply make a few brief comments about the appeal of the new voice. It was believed that preparing the mother for the new voice and practicing her response would reduce the likelihood of that she would overreact to the new voice and, thereby, cause the client to be fearful of future interactions where he used the new voice with friends and family.

Refining the Lower Pitched Voice. At the close of the initial session, AA's lower pitched voice possessed an element of glottal fry, suggesting that AA had lowered the pitch a bit beyond the target and that a degree of muscle imbalance was still present. To deal with this situation, an additional therapy session was recommended to refine the lower pitched tone and to promote a proper tone focus. AA followed up for the second session 1 week following the initial visit. He had been using the lower pitched voice in all contexts for several days. Consistent use of the voice and an increasing comfort with the voice had resulted in a lessening of the fry and a more appealing voice quality. Nonetheless, an abbreviated program of resonant therapy was introduced, and AA was given a program of daily resonance exercises to complete over the next 2 weeks.

A follow-up call was placed to the client 2 weeks following the last session. AA indicated that he was doing well with the lower pitched voice and that the gravelly quality had dissipated. He expressed pleasure with the new voice and an increasing social confidence as well.

Functional Falsetto in a Young Male with Hearing Impairment

Robert C. Peppard, PhD

Case Study: Patient BB

Although functional falsetto is most often described in postpubescent males, it can be identified in other populations as well. One group at increased risk for functional pitch concerns is the hearing-impaired population. In the next case, Robert Peppard presents principles of managing functional falsetto in a young man with a hearing impairment.

High Risk in the Hearing-Impaired Population

My clinical experience suggests that hearing impairment may be a risk factor that makes persistent high-pitched voice use more likely in adolescent males. It has been reported that children who have deafness and lack normal auditory feedback mechanisms may not develop the lower pitched voice of typical postadolescents.[28,29] Thus, the incidence of puberphonia, fairly rare in hearing male adolescents, may be more prevalent in the hearing-impaired population. Children with hearing impairments, having only tactile and kinesthetic feedback to direct them, may attempt to stabilize the variable function of the mutating larynx by consistently using the falsetto mode. Although such use is less efficient than a lower pitched register, it may at least provide some measure of vocal stability. Furthermore, the focus of speech treatment for the hearing-impaired population often is perfecting articulation to ensure intelligible speech, and the speech clinician may not feel comfortable addressing the voice needs of these children.

Patient History

At the time of the evaluation, Patient BB was a 15-year-old boy with hearing impairment. His height was 68 in, and his weight was 135 lb. He had a bilateral, symmetrical, moderate-profound sensorineural hearing loss (pure-tone average, 95 dB HL), which was acquired postlingually following meningitis at age 3 years. He wore binaural, ear-level aids at volume levels of 2 for both ears. He had an aided speech reception threshold of 42 dB. Patient BB was mainstreamed and doing well in a ninth-grade public school classroom. His expressive and receptive language skills were excellent, and he communicated primarily through good oral speech, aided hearing, and lip reading. He also used American Sign Language with his nonspeaking deaf peers.

With the exception of a few phonetic distortions, his speech was intelligible and he had not been enrolled in speech therapy since fourth grade. During a recent hearing reevaluation, his audiologist noted that Patient BB's voice was high pitched and had a strained quality. She recommended that he be seen for a voice evaluation.

Voice Evaluation

Patient BB was seen in a university hospital voice clinic by a laryngologist and a speech-language pathologist specializing in voice disorders. A complete medical evaluation, including otolaryngologic examination and voice evaluation, was performed. He was accompanied to the evaluation by his mother, who reported that she was pleased with her son's academic and communication abilities. The family was aware of their son's high-pitched voice, but assumed that it was a consequence of the hearing loss, and they had come to accept this pitch level as normal for their son.

Vocal Symptoms. Patient BB's only voice complaints were occasional voice fatigue and periodic voice breaks. He reported that classmates sometimes teased him about his high-pitched voice. He was aware that his voice varied from his peers, but did not believe anything could be done about it. He was unaware of being capable of producing any other voice.

Medical and Laryngeal Examinations. Medical examination revealed a normal, healthy, postpubescent male with no hormonal abnormalities. Indirect laryngeal examination was normal, with the larynx appearing normal in size for a boy of his age, with no abnormalities in structure or function. Larynx height

was noted as elevated with a good deal of tension in the neck muscles.

Videostroboscopic Examination. Patient BB's vocal folds were difficult to visualize as a result of tension and high laryngeal position. A topical anesthetic was used to reduce the gag reflex, which then permitted the following observations. Glottic closure pattern was incomplete. The vocal folds appeared stretched and tense, with reduced mucosal wave. The vocal folds exhibited light contact with thin edges. Vibration was characterized by long open phases and very short closed phases. Reduced amplitude of vibration was also noted.

Auditory Perceptual Signs. Patient BB's voice was high pitched with occasional downward pitch breaks. He sounded strained, breathy, weak, and low in intensity, with little range in either intensity or pitch.

Acoustic Signs. The patient's fundamental frequency averaged 260 Hz in both sustained vowels and contextual production. His frequency range was restricted to less than one octave. Intensity was reduced, averaging 60 dB sound pressure level (SPL) in both sustained and contextual situations. SPL range was also limited, with maximum voluntary production being 75 dB SPL.

Diagnostic Therapy

Some young men with puberphonia are aware of their ability to produce another voice. With assurances that this second, lower pitched voice is desirable, they are able to quickly shift to the new voice in all situations. Because Patient BB reported no knowledge of a second voice, several nonspeech vocalizations were used to test for the presence of puberphonia. These included coughing, throat clearing, and hard glottal attack.

These vocalizations all demonstrated the dramatic downward shift of pitch characteristic of puberphonia. Similar descents in pitch were obtained with shouted productions because falsetto cannot be sustained at maximum volume levels. When questioned, the patient reported that he could feel differences in his habitual mode of voice and these new, lower pitched productions, although he felt the lowered productions were not appropriate.

Somewhat reluctantly, the patient agreed to begin an intensive schedule of voice therapy to determine if the lower pitched voice was more efficient. His reluctance was in part due to concerns that therapy would interfere with his other school and social activities and in part to his doubt that the new lowered voice was appropriate.

Therapy

In some cases of puberphonia, the more appropriate pitch levels discovered during diagnostic activities can be quickly carried over into conversational speech, and a permanent change in pitch level may be possible after one session.

Because hearing impairment limits the person's ability to monitor the changed pitch level, a longer period of therapy is usually required in which non-auditory methods, such as visual feedback, are used to achieve consistent use of the new voice. To account for these additional needs, multiple therapy sessions were scheduled for Patient BB to establish use of the new, lower pitched voice.

Caution. If too little time is allotted for each session or if the sessions are too far apart, the patient may revert to the habitual falsetto pattern, which, although less efficient than the mutational voice, may be more comfortable because of its familiarity, especially for the hearing impaired. Goals for treatment included teaching Patient BB

- the method of producing the lower pitched voice, including the ability to move voluntarily between rnodal and falsetto registers
- consistent use of a more optimal vocal register in all speaking situations
- acceptance of the new voice mode as appropriate.

Session 1. The initial therapy session was scheduled for a 3-hour block with two rest breaks, 2 days after the initial diagnostic visit. It was during this session that the clinician began the process of persuading the patient that a mode of vibration that felt quite different from his habitual mode was actually optimal.

The first goal of this session was for Patient BB to consistently use the lower pitched voice in sustained vowels, in reading of single words and short phrases, and in spontaneous speech consisting of short replies to simple questions. These limited contexts gave the patient many opportunities to practice the new voice register. Occasionally, he would revert to his habitual pitch level, especially in spontaneous utterances. At those times, the clinician would signal the patient to produce the utterance again, using a lower pitch. If the higher voice persisted, the patient was asked to initiate voice with hard glottal attack or louder volume, which almost always resulted in an appropriate downward pitch shift.

A Visi-Pitch (KayPentax, Lincoln Park, NJ) that displayed real-time measures of pitch levels on a monitor occasionally was used as visual feedback to show the patient his ability to achieve target pitch levels. Although such feedback was seldom needed for Patient BB, this visual feedback may be a highly desirable method for other persons with hearing impairment who are in treatment for falsetto.

During this first session the patient occasionally exhibited some behavioral problems. At times, he would refuse to try a task. He avoided looking at the clinician and he would say, "What's the point?" Such resistance to change should be expected even by patients with no psychogenic component, because— especially for the hearing-impaired population—the new register may feel uncomfortable.

An analogy proved useful in helping the patient accept the discomfort he was experiencing in shifting to his new voice. It was suggested that shifting to his new voice was "like learning to use a stick shift on a car after having driven an automatic transmission." He was told that "with the new voice system you will occasionally 'stall out,' but, with practice, you'll soon learn to use your new voice system and that as with a stick shift, your now voice will be a very efficient method of voice production, requiring less effort and vocal fatigue than your old voice."

Toward the end of the first session, the patient used negative practice in which he voluntarily shifted between the optimal and falsetto registers. This shift demonstrated the control that he had over the two voices and prepared him for any involuntary upward shifts he might have outside the therapy room.

By the end of the first session, the patient was successfully producing a more optimal pitch level, averaging 140 Hz at the 90% level. He had also begun self-monitoring and correcting inappropriate pitch productions without clinician prompting.

In planning for the next session, Patient BB chose his mother and younger brother as two people with whom he would begin using the new voice during the next therapy session, which was scheduled for a 2-hour block on the following day.

Session 2. The goal of this session was to stabilize and expand the number of situations in which the new voice was used. At the beginning of the session, Patient BB consistently was using the lower pitched register with the clinician. The new voice was also noted to be louder than the pretreatment voice. Some slight dysphonia and glottal fry quality were noted in the lower pitched voice, as was some slight decrease in Patient BB's overall speech intelligibility, due to an increase in phonetic errors.

Such decreases in intelligibility have been noted in other young men with hearing impairment who dramatically lower their pitch. This articulatory change may be related to posterior tongue position that often accompanies the lowering of the larynx necessary for production of the modal register. Additional speech therapy may be needed to decrease these errors and increase intelligibility.

Patient BB selected from a number of practice options for carryover of the new voice. He used the new voice in telephone calls to other university departments and to an airline. Important was his use of the new register outside the therapy room in a conversation with the clinic receptionist and while ordering lunch in the hospital cafeteria. The clinician provided positive feedback at Patient BB's consistent success in using the new voice in these situations. At no time did the patient revert to the pretreatment voice, and after completing these assignments, he reported that, although he was still self-conscious about using the new voice, he was feeling increasingly comfortable with the new register.

The patient's mother and brother then joined the session for a short conversation about family vacation plans, in which Patient BB consistently used the new register. Finally, the patient agreed to utilize the new voice as much as possible outside the therapy room until the next therapy session.

It should be noted that following this session, Patient BB's mother reported some unease with her son's new voice quality. She said that her son's lower pitched voice sounded unfamiliar and asked was it really appropriate for his age. She accepted assurances that indeed this was an appropriate mode for her son. The next session was scheduled 2 days later to give Patient BB time to practice the new voice.

Session 3. The goal of the third session was to evaluate the progress Patient BB had made in the consistent use of his new voice. The patient was much more relaxed at the start of this session than at any previous meeting. His pitch had descended even further and averaged 130 Hz. His voice was less dysphonic and displayed little glottal fry quality.

The patient reported that he was using the new mode in all situations and that only twice had he reverted to the high-pitched voice, both times when he had become excited while playing tennis. He had immediately known that the pitch was too high and quickly shifted to the optimal level. He further reported that he was becoming much more comfortable with the new voice

and that friends and family seldom commented about the pitch change as he had feared they might.

The patient tried some additional negative practice and laughed when he found it difficult to shift back into the higher register. With some effort, he succeeded in doing so and reported that the higher voice now was more uncomfortable to produce than his new voice. The patient agreed with the clinician that the new pitch level was appropriate. He further agreed that additional speech therapy to improve his intelligibility would be desirable.

Therapy was terminated with an agreement that the patient would continue to use his new voice in all situations and that he would be contacted for follow-up evaluation in 3 months.

Follow-up

A phone contact was made with Patient BB's mother 3 months following termination of voice therapy. She reported that her son had continued to use the lowered pitch voice in all situations. He also had been seen by the public school speech pathologist, who helped him reduce phonetic errors, and it was reported that the patient's intelligibility was again at the excellent pre-voice-change levels.

Conclusions

It has been suggested that puberphonia may have a higher incidence in the hearing-impaired population because of altered feedback mechanism. It is strongly recommended that adolescent male speakers with hearing impairment be carefully monitored and screened for the presence of this voice disorder by communications disorders specialists.

As the preceding case study demonstrates, with some additional time, some variation in treatment, and the use of feedback, puberphonia in individuals with hearing impairment is highly treatable. Successful treatment results in a more efficient voice, which also more closely compares with the speech of hearing peers.

Functional Falsetto in the Adult Woman

Joseph C. Stemple, PhD

Case Study: Patient CC

As previously mentioned, functional falsetto is associated most often with the postpubescent male. This author, however, has treated several adult women with this disorder. In the most recent case, Patient CC was a 52-year-old, third-grade teacher who was referred by a friend with the complaint of having a "weak voice." The weakness was something that she had noticed all her life, but she never thought that it could be modified.

Stroboscopic examination of her vocal folds revealed normal-appearing folds that approximated in a near-parallel relationship. Glottic closure was complete, but the amplitude of vibration was severely decreased with just the medial edge of the folds vibrating. The open phase of the vibratory cycle was dominant; however, the symmetry of vibrations was regular.

Perceptually, Patient CC's voice quality was mildly dysphonic, characterized by a high-pitched, weak phonation. Objectively, she presented with a fundamental frequency of 220 Hz. Her pitch range was 205 to 860 Hz. Most interesting was the fact that she could not shout without overdriving the vocal folds into a high-pitched explosion of sound. Even with young men, one diagnostic sign of this disorder is the inability to shout. The positioning of the vocal folds for falsetto will not permit an appropriate buildup of subglottic air pressure to support a shouting behavior. The tenseness of the folds will not permit the greater amplitude of vibration required for the louder phonation.

How does one tell a 52-year-old woman who has always used this voice that it is not her real voice? First, you explore her knowledge of other voices. Patient CC was asked if she could produce voice in any other manner. Her only response was a puzzling look that, without words, questioned the sanity of the therapist.

The next attempt to describe the problem was the intellectual approach. Through the use of the stroboscopic videotape and line diagrams, functional falsetto was explained in some detail to the patient. Patient CC showed an intellectual understanding of the disorder but was still somewhat skeptical of the diagnosis as related to her weak voice.

The clincher turned out to be the direct approach. Patient CC was instructed in how to produce a hard glottal attack on the vowel /ae/. Her first attempt resulted in the deepest, loudest tone that she had ever heard emanate from her mouth. The sound also shocked and puzzled her. The therapist explained, "That was normal vibration of the vocal folds."

Once the shock diminished, Patient CC was most interested in pursuing this form of voice production. Because of the deep sound, she was not yet interested in permitting anyone else—office staff, family, or friends—to hear her speak in this manner. Indeed, desensitization is an important step in dealing with functional falsetto. This patient had a lifetime of using her "old" voice. Her auditory feedback system kept repeating, "That's not me, that's not me." Systematic practice from words (at first using the hard glottal attack), through phrases, paragraph readings, and directed conversations were necessary to stabilize the "new" voice. Audio recordings were used liberally to demonstrate the normalcy of the "new" voice.

Once stabilized in therapy, Patient CC had to begin using the new voice with others. She started with a most sympathetic ear, my secretary, who had learned long ago when to positively reinforce. We then developed a hierarchy of situations to be tackled with the new voice, including

- ordering food at a drive-through restaurant
- ordering food in a restaurant
- calling for information about a store product
- talking directly to her daughter
- talking to her husband
- talking to her class (who she was sure would laugh and giggle).

At the following session, which was 2 weeks later, Patient CC returned to report on her progress. Her new voice was stable and demonstrated remarkably improved inflection and flexibility. Now it was my turn to be puzzled. Patient CC reported that the day after our last session, she developed a bad cold. In the past, she reported becoming aphonic during the initial stages of a cold, and so it was this time. Using her falsetto voice, she "lost" her voice. "So, I decided, what have I got to lose? I tried to talk the new way and my voice came out fine. So, I've been using it

everywhere ever since. I just tell people my cold changed my voice."

So much for brilliant hierarchies and desensitization plans. Final stroboscopic observation yielded normal wide amplitude of vibration and phase closure. The patient's fundamental frequency stabilized at 196 Hz. Her pitch range expanded to 159 to 880 Hz. Most important, her voice was strong, easily produced without effort or fatigue, and was heard in all situations.

References

1. Aronson A. *Clinical Voice Disorders: An Interdisciplinary Approach.* 3rd ed. New York, NY: Thieme Medical Publishers; 1990.
2. Jacobson E. *Progressive Relaxation.* 2nd ed. Chicago, IL: University of Chicago Press; 1938.
3. Froeschels E. Chewing method as therapy; a discussion with some philosophical conclusions. *AMA Arch Otolaryngol.* 1952;56(4):427–434.
4. Stemple JC, Weiler E, Whitehead W, Komray R. Electromyographic biofeedback training with patients exhibiting a hyperfunctional voice disorder. *Laryngoscope.* 1980;90(3):471–476.
5. Herrington-Hall BL, Lee L, Stemple JC, Niemi KR, McHone MM. Description of laryngeal pathologies by age, sex, and occupation in a treatment-seeking sample. *J Speech Hear Disord.* 1988;53(1): 57–64.
6. Stemple J. *Clinical Voice Pathology: Theory and Management.* Columbus, OH: Merrill; 1984.
7. Boone D, McFarlane S. *The Voice and Voice Therapy.* 5th ed. Englewood Cliffs, NJ: Prentice-Hall; 1994.
8. Case J. *Clinical Management of Voice Disorders.* Austin, TX: Pro-Ed; 1996.

9. Colton R, Casper J. *Understanding Voice Problems: A Physiological Perspective for Diagnosis and Treatment.* 2nd ed. Baltimore, MD: Williams & Wilkins; 1996.

10. Morrison M, Rammage L. *The Management of Voice Disorders.* San Diego, CA: Singular Publishing Group; 1994.

11. Stemple J. *Voice Therapy: Clinical Studies.* St. Louis, MO: Mosby-Year Book; 1993.

12. Hillman RE, Holmberg EB, Perkell JS, Walsh M, Vaughan C. Objective assessment of vocal hyperfunction: an experimental framework and initial results. *J Speech Hear Res.* 1989;32(2): 373–392.

13. Peifang C. Massage for the treatment of voice ailments. *J Trad Chinese Med.* 1991; 11:209–215.

14. Roy N, Bless D. Assessment and treatment of voice disorders using manual circumlaryngeal techniques. *Curr Opin Otolaryngol Head Neck Surg.* 1998;6: 151–155.

15. Roy N. Ventricular dysphonia following long-term endotracheal intubation: a case study. *J Otolaryngol.* 1994;23(3): 189–193.

16. Roy N, Bless DM, Heisey D, Ford CN. Manual circumlaryngeal therapy for functional dysphonia: an evaluation of short- and long-term treatment outcomes. *J Voice.* 1997;11(3):321–331.

17. Roy N, Ford CN, Bless DM. Muscle tension dysphonia and spasmodic dysphonia: the role of manual laryngeal tension reduction in diagnosis and management. *Ann Otol Rhinol Laryngol.* 1996;105(11): 851–856.

18. Roy N, Leeper HA. Effects of the manual laryngeal musculoskeletal tension reduction technique as a treatment for functional voice disorders: perceptual and acoustic measures. *J Voice.* 1993; 7(3):242–249.

19. Roy N, Bless D. Toward a theory of the dispositional bases of functional dysphonia and vocal nodules: exploring the role of personality and emotional adjustment. In: Kent R, Ball M, eds. *The Handbook of Voice Quality Measurement.* San Diego, CA: Singular Publishing Group; 1999.

20. Roy N, McGrory JJ, Tasko SM, Bless DM, Heisey D, Ford CN. Psychological correlates of functional dysphonia: an investigation using the Minnesota Multiphasic Personality Inventory. *J Voice.* 1997;11(4):443–451.

21. Boone D, McFarlane S. *The Voice and Voice Therapy.* 4th ed. Englewood Cliffs, NY: Prentice-Hall; 1988.

22. Hollien H. On vocal registers. *J Phonetics.* 1982;2:25–43.

23. Jacobson E. *Modern Treatment of Tense Patients.* Springfield, IL: Charles C Thomas; 1970.

24. Crumley RL. Unilateral recurrent laryngeal nerve paralysis. *J Voice.* 1994;8(1): 79–83.

25. Dursun G, Sataloff RT, Spiegel JR, Mandel S, Heuer RJ, Rosen DC. Superior laryngeal nerve paresis and paralysis. *J Voice.* 1996;10(2):206–211.

26. Rosato L, Avenia N, Bernante P, et al. Complications of thyroid surgery: analysis of a multicentric study on 14,934 patients operated on in Italy over 5 years. *World J Surg.* 2004;28(3):271–276.

27. Kempster GB, Gerratt BR, Verdolini Abbott K, Barkmeier-Kraemer J, Hillman RE. Consensus auditory-perceptual evaluation of voice: development of a standardized clinical protocol. *Am J Speech Lang Pathol.* 2009;18(2):124–132.

28. Boone D. Modifications of the voices of deaf children *Volta Rev.* 1966;68:686–694.

29. Zaliouk A. Falsetto voice in deaf children. *Aktuel Probl Phoniatr Logop.* 1960;1: 217–226.

6

Irritable Larynx Syndrome and Respiratory Disorders

Introduction

Since the first edition of this text was published in 1993, the field has gained a greater understanding of the larynx's role in a variety of nonphonatory disorders. Because of our knowledge of the upper airway and our unique abilities to affect behavioral change, speech-language pathologists have increasingly become the medical providers of choice for the management of these interesting sensory and respiratory-based disorders.

Exciting developments in this area of the field have led us to incorporate two comprehensive tutorials into the chapter. The first tutorial by Linda Rammage and Murray Morrison looks at irritable larynx syndrome (ILS) and the spectrum of concerns that fall under that diagnostic classification. Later in the chapter, Michael Trudeau and Jennifer Thompson discuss in more detail the spe-

cific condition of paradoxical vocal fold dysfunction. Case studies illustrating various presentations of ILS are presented throughout the chapter.

Overview of Irritable Larynx Syndrome

Linda Rammage, PhD, CCC-SLP and Murray Morrison, MD, FRCSC

Introduction

Irritable larynx syndrome (ILS) is a term that was proposed in 1999 to identify and hypothesize an etiologic explanation for a commonly observed clinical symptom complex. The original definition proposed that ILS represents "hyperkinetic laryngeal dysfunction resulting from a variety of specific causes in response to a definitive triggering stimulus."[1] The hyperkinetic laryngeal dysfunction, more specifically laryngeal muscle spasm, can produce symptoms of airway obstruction, often labeled "vocal cord dysfunction (VCD)," "laryngospasm," or "paradoxical vocal fold motion (PVFM);" episodes of cough when a specific cause is not evident; globus pharyngeus; and/or dysphonia.

Proposed Physiologic Mechanisms

The proposed mechanism by which these symptoms develop is complex, but much of the etiologic theory can be inferred from research and theory in chronic pain and a number of other chronic conditions.[2–7] This body of literature provides a foundation for the hypothesis that, in ILS, brainstem control of laryngeal sensory-motor processes has been altered so that abnormal muscle tension or spasm occur in response to normal levels of sensory stimuli. In the larynx, a number of central nervous system (CNS) pathologic processes may lead to chronic laryngeal motor stimulation and heightened sensory irritability.

Neural plasticity may affect the way that laryngeal motor and related systems react to sensations or thoughts. Literature on chronic pain is a helpful source of information and understanding about plasticity and its possible role in development of ILS.[3] Central neurons may undergo plastic adaptation in one or several ways:

- Afferent inputs may be withdrawn from the central neuron in response to peripheral nerve or tissue injury. New connections are then made by resprouting dendrites or reactivating "silent" synapses. In this situation, an afferent stimulus that used to result in one response now may elicit a different one.

- Viral illnesses may attack the CNS and effect a change in the central sensory-motor control of laryngeal muscle systems. Central nervous system viral infections, such as herpes zoster, can result in genome changes that alter laryngeal motor control. Specifically, viruses may affect reactions in the periaqueductal gray (PAG) area of the brainstem, known to be involved in vocalization, and make it more reactive to sensory stimulus from the larynx and adjacent structures. This is assumed on the basis of known responses to stimulation or damage of the dorsal and lateral regions of the PAG. Stimulation of the PAG has evoked vocalization in some animals,[8] and lesions produced in the PAG will result in mutism.[9] Supramaximal stimulation of the internal branch of the superior laryngeal nerve in the cat has been shown to increase fos labeling in dorsomedial and dorsolateral regions of the PAG.[10] This type of genome change can be associated with hyperreactivity to sensory stimuli from the larynx and pharynx.

- Emotional states and defense reactions, known to be related to PAG activity, may result in hypersensitivity when the larynx is, or should be, involved in the expression of the emotion.[11,12] Jurgens has proposed that the PAG serves as a link between sensory and motivation-controlling structures and the periambigual reticular formation, allowing it to coordinate the activity of muscles involved in phonation.[13] Through the PAG, then, there is potential to mediate muscle spasm in the larynx under situations of psychological arousal and repressed emotional expression.

■ Asthmalike reactions may be elicited in the upper airway in the same way that bronchial muscles react to irritants in lower airway disease. Specifically, parasympathetic branches of the laryngeal muscle systems may be involved in hyperreactivity to a variety of stimuli introduced through sensory channels, including the olfactory channel. A suspected common stimulus is refluxate. The laryngeal effect may produce muscle misuse voice problems, chronic cough, and/or paradoxic vocal fold respiratory reactions. A direct reflex relationship between stimulation of the lower esophagus and thyroarytenoid muscle activity has been demonstrated in a porcine model.[14] It is possible that chronic laryngeal reflux irritation affects the PAG, where neural plastic change results in long-term effects on laryngeal function.

The original ILS theory describes how these factors and combinations of them affect the laryngeal CNS control network to produce a hyperirritable "spasm-ready" state in the peripheral laryngopharyngeal muscles that is thought of as the "untriggered" state. The transition from the "spasm-ready" state to ILS symptom manifestation requires a trigger, typically in the form of some sensory input, and possibly heightened by muscle tone modulators, such as psychological stressors or postural factors that make the laryngopharynx more susceptible to spasm triggered by a sensory irritant. The trigger usually is an episodic sensory irritant, such as acid refluxate, airborne particles, or odors.

Differential Diagnostic Criteria

The original description of the ILS included three categories of inclusion criteria:

1. Symptom(s) that can be attributed to tension in the larynx and related muscle systems. These include dysphonia and/or airway obstruction (respiratory laryngospasm, VCD, PVFM), cough, and/or globus pharyngeus. Episodes of airway obstruction due to laryngospasm, when they exist, may be identified by patients as the dominant symptom, as they tend to be sudden and fairly distinct occurrences and may cause both physical and emotional distress. These are characterized by partial to total adductory activity of the true vocal folds during inspiration. Often previously assumed to be asthmatic episodes, clinical observations of inspiratory rather than expiratory obstruction, with the inspiratory restriction at the laryngeal, rather than chest level, can help differentiate the hyperkinetic laryngeal dysfunction typical of laryngospasm from asthma. Laryngeal stridor, either voiced or unvoiced, is the sound typically observed with laryngeal adductor breathing problems, as opposed to the characteristic respiratory wheezing noted during asthma attacks. Muscle tension dysphonia associated with ILS often is a more persistent accompanying symptom, although it also may be exacerbated by triggering stimuli, and when it is reported as the dominant symptom, it arises and abates with the triggers.

2. Evidence of laryngeal and paralaryngeal muscle misuse, identified during

visual examination and/or palpation of paralaryngeal muscles. Although the larynx usually looks structurally normal, physical findings include abnormal laryngeal posture and palpable muscle tension in and around the larynx, as originally described by Lieberman.[15] The specific muscle misuses can be delineated and scored using a previously described clinical technique.[16]

3. Identification of specific trigger(s) that may include airborne particulates (often first identified by accompanying odors); reflux, and/or other esophageal activity—eating certain foods or drinking certain liquids, sometimes with temperature as a contributor, postural changes (typically positions that might increase reflux episodes); voice use; exercise; and/or recognized psychologic stressors.

The ILS diagnosis is withheld under certain definitive exclusion criteria, including:

1. Organic laryngeal/pharyngeal/esophageal pathologies that could account for peripheral hypersensitivity and/or laryngeal symptoms of dysphonia, laryngospasm, chronic cough and/or globus.
2. Definitive neurologic diseases known to cause any of these symptoms.
3. Pre-existing psychiatric diagnosis. This does not preclude consideration of psychologic symptoms such as anxiety and/or depression that may arise as a result of ILS symptoms, or recognized psychologic stressors, such as repressed expression of negative emotions, that may act as symptom triggers.

Demographic and Descriptive Data

The original demographic study reported demographic and clinical data for 39 patients. An expanded data base of 218 patients collected from 2000 to 2008, using the same diagnostic and exclusion criteria, strengthens the trends noted in 1999.

1. Over 85% of the patients with ILS were female, with an average age of 50.
2. 21% of the patients were on disability leave or pension due to their symptoms.
3. The dominant ILS symptom was laryngospasm in over 50% of the patients; chronic cough in approximately 13%; and dysphonia in approximately 9%. Almost 50% of the patients with laryngospasm as their dominant symptom also experienced chronic muscle tension dysphonia, 42% complained of cough, and 11% experienced globus sensation.
4. For those patients dominant ILS symptom was cough, most also experienced episodic dysphonia and a small percentage experienced chronic globus pharyngeus.
5. Approximately 45% of patients for whom dysphonia was the dominant ILS symptom also experienced episodic cough, and a few experienced globus pharyngeus.
6. High scores of palpable muscle tension were assigned to over 75% of all ILS patients for all four paralaryngeal muscle groups normally assessed during clinical evaluation.[16]
7. The most common trigger for ILS symptoms was airborne, specifically odors such as perfume.

8. Reflux was diagnosed by 24-hour pH test or diagnosis by drug therapy in over 90% of patients with ILS.

ILS as a Central Nervous System Hypersensitivity Disorder

The original sample of 39 patients to which the diagnostic criteria were applied revealed several common reported patterns of symptom onset, the most prevalent of which were viral illness and acute episodes of gastroesophageal reflux, fueling the foundation for a theory of neuroplastic change mediating a hyperirritable larynx. Scrutiny of the subsequent larger sample reveals compelling evidence of comorbidities with a number of other syndromes associated with CNS hypersensitivity triggered by neuroplastic change, suggesting that ILS may be encompassed in a much broader etiologic group of syndromes known as central nervous system hypersensitivity disorders (CHD).[17]

Using the diagnostic criteria established in 1999, records were examined of 219 patients seen from 2000 to 2008 who were assigned a diagnosis of ILS. This suggested frequent comorbidity for ILS and other symptom complexes such as irritable bowel syndrome (IBS), fibromyalgia (FM), chronic fatigue syndrome (CFS), irritable bladder syndrome (IBL), chronic headache (HD), and temporomandibular joint dysfunction (TMJ). Patients reported that many of these other symptom complexes were triggered by environmental irritants or other sensory stimuli, and many had been assigned a diagnosis of multiple chemical sensitivity disorder (MCS).

The literature on these syndromes that appear frequently in patients with ILS suggests a common pathophysiology, specifically central nervous system mediation of peripheral symptoms that can be attributed to hyperreactivity to internal or external stimuli. Although no definitive cause has been identified in the other syndromes in this proposed group of CHD, theories of neural plastic change following virus and chronic systemic irritation abound in the literature, and the literature on chronic pain is referenced frequently to explain symptom formation and perpetuation. Proposed causes of the various forms of CHD include a predisposed personality, life traumas, burnout, neurochemistry, genetic factors, immune disorder, viruses, and infections. The presence of significant GER seems to play a major role in development of throat (ILS) symptoms in patients with CHD.

Among the compelling findings in the larger ILS study are comorbidities of ILS with IBS (>50%); HD (45%); CFS (37%); and FM (25%). Most ILS patients complained of more than one of these associated diagnoses. The prevalence of comorbidity for other CNS hypersensitivity disorders was proportional for personal and clinical demographics, suggesting comorbidity was not proportionally higher in patients grouped by dominant symptoms or demographic characteristics.

ILS Treatment

Treatment for patients with ILS typically involves a team approach. The first step in helping patients reduce symptoms is ensuring they have an understanding of the nature of their disorder and the need to approach treatment at multiple levels. Reassuring patients that we, the professionals, have an understanding of their problem goes a long way toward motivating them to play a role in improving their status. (This is highlighted because many patients with ILS and other CHDs have sought explanations and treatment from many professionals before consulting the voice clinic; they may have previously received several conflicting explanations, or declarations that the consultants cannot explain the symptoms.) Once the voice care team has confirmed the patient understands and trusts our explanation of the problem, a three-level treatment strategy is used to help patients reduce hypersensitive reactions to normal sensory stimuli:

Level 1: Minimize Sensory Stimuli (Reflux, Odors)

Initially, patients are instructed to minimize exposure to known irritants. Reflux is assumed to play a major role as a sensory trigger of ILS symptoms, and maximal lifestyle and pharmaceutical treatment regimens generally are prescribed, including daily use of proton pump inhibitors, sometimes supplemented with gastrointestinal motility drugs. A small proportion of ILS patients may be candidates for surgical treatment such as fundoplication of the lower esophageal sphincter.

By being more attentive to specific airborne triggers such as perfume or car exhaust, patients can minimize exposure in environments under their control, such as making their homes and workplace "scent-free."

Level 2: Reprogram the Maladaptive CNS Response

A review of the brain's role in precipitating and perpetuating ILS symptoms sets the foundation for use of motor learning principles to alter inappropriate muscle response patterns to stimuli, thereby reducing symptoms. Changing the laryngeal sensory-motor control patterns may involve a combination of approaches:

- reducing overall postural muscle tension around the laryngopharynx using postural, behavioral and/or manual therapy techniques[18,19];
- learning specific exercises, such as sniffing, pursed lips breathing, openthroat breathing, and sustaining fricative phonemes, that inhibit the maladaptive muscle patterns of adductory laryngospasm, cough, and hyperadducting phonation, and re-direct awareness to anatomically distant regions, more appropriate sensations and muscle activity[20,21];
- undergoing cognitive behavioral therapy with a skilled psychotherapist to help recognize and reduce anticipatory anxiety or repressed vocal expression of emotions that may trigger and/or exacerbate symptoms, and to help patients eliminate other psychologic factors, such as depression or primary or secondary gain, that may affect their motivation to help themselves.

Level 3: Neuropsychotropic Medication

Some patients with ILS and other CHD syndromes benefit from centrally active prescription medications. To help patients understand the potential benefit of this approach, we explain that the nerve cells involved in their sensory-motor disorder use chemicals to communicate with each other and that modifying brain chemistry might make it possible for them to communicate more effectively. Selective serotonin reuptake inhibitors and combined serotonin and norepinephrine reuptake inhibitors, such as venlaxitine, are the most frequently used preparations. Tricyclic antidepressants, more frequently used in chronic pain and fibromyalgia, have a mouth and throat drying side effect that is sometimes a problem for those with throat symptoms. Baclofen, a centrally acting spasmolytic drug, and gabapentin, an antiepileptic, also may be effective. In instances where significant psychological factors are suspected in playing a role in symptom formation, complete psychiatric evaluation is recommended, and medication selection and dosage should be determined and monitored by the psychiatrist.

BOTOX injection into the thyroarytenoid muscles is employed in selected cases of paroxysmal coughing and adductory laryngospasm.

A regular exercise program is known to improve mental health and is frequently recommended as part of the treatment program. The benefits of regular production of endorphins, through aerobic activity, probably exceed exogenous medication in the long term.

Summary

Although ILS remains a theoretical concept, it can help the voice care team explain a central mechanism that mediates a symptom complex, and plan intervention accordingly. According to theory, ILS arises when brainstem laryngeal controlling neuronal networks undergo neuroplastic change so they are held in a perpetually hyperexcitable state, which lowers the threshold for muscle reactions to sensory stimulation. The common ILS

symptoms of laryngospasm, muscle tension dysphonia, chronic cough, and globus pharyngeus are triggered by sensory stimuli (irritants) that, in the absence of ILS, would be tolerated as minor or transient irritants and not result in chronic symptoms. The presence of significant gastroesophageal reflux seems to play a role in development of ILS and frequently also is a symptom trigger. Symptom triggers typically are predictable for each patient.

ILS appears to fall into a broad syndrome group that includes IBS, CFS, FM, and other clinical conditions generally are assumed to comprise disorders of central hypersensitivity, and for which specific etiologies are yet indefinite.

The goal of treatment is to minimize disability, reduce distress, improve general health, and reduce the use of medical resources.

Management of Irritable Larynx Syndrome

Linda Rammage, PhD, S-LP(C)

Case Study DD

Patient History. When we first met her, DD was a 54-year-old woman, married with three adult children, one of whom still lived with her and her husband in a metro suburb. Her daughter who was living at home accompanied DD to the first voice clinic appointment, and DD described this girl as her "angel." Her husband of 30 years was a heavy smoker, but had been smoking outdoors exclusively for the past 10 years. She claimed she was happily married, but worried about her husband, due to his smoking.

DD had worked in customer service in an indoor shopping mall for 5 years until 3 months previously, when her doctor advised her to discontinue her work. She enjoyed her job immensely, as she is very sociable and enjoys meeting and talking to customers, many of whom friends and neighbors. DD's compliance with her doctor's order to stop working had negative economic and psychologic impacts. She explained that, in addition to missing the social contact, her husband's business was experiencing some slowdown, which increased the financial burden on the family.

DD had undergone multiple abdominal surgeries, including spleenectomy, inguinal hernia repair, appendectomy, hysterectomy, and multiple laparoscopies, and she sustained back injuries during a motor vehicle accident. Her mother died of colon cancer. Her father was still alive and suffered some cardiovascular problems. On her voice clinic intake form, she declared the following problems: anxiety; asthma; arthritis; breathing problem; chronic fatigue syndrome (CFS); chronic coughing and choking; depressed mood; fibromyalgia (FM); chronic headaches (HD); heartburn; hoarseness; irritable bladder syndrome (IBL); irritable bowel syndrome (IBS); lump in throat sensation; multiple chemical sensitivity (MCS); neck or back injury; postnasal drip (PND); severe snoring; swallowing problem; and chronic throat-clearing. She stated she had been moderately overweight all her life, but since going on sick leave and reducing her physical activity, she had gained an additional 25 pounds, which frustrated her. She did not eat regular meals during the day but enjoyed a large meal in the evening with her husband and daughter. She drank 8 cups of water daily, and several cups of herbal tea. She was a lifelong abstainer of alcohol and tobacco. She stopped drinking caffeinated tea and

coffee a few months previously, after consulting a naturopathic practitioner, who advised her that these agents would aggravate her irritable bowel and bladder.

DD suffered daily headaches, limb pain, back pain, chronic fatigue, heartburn, need for frequent urination, unpredictable bowel patterns, sleep disturbance, and breathing and throat problems (as described below). Consultation with an allergist revealed allergies to various antibiotic medications and nuts, but no airborne allergies. DD previously had consulted a respiratory specialist, who performed a battery of tests and concluded she had "borderline asthma," exacerbated by exercise and allergies. Her family doctor had prescribed a number of drugs to reduce anxiety and improve her ability to sleep, and steroid inhalers to reduce her "asthma" attacks.

History of the Problem. Over the previous 18 months, DD had experienced progressive difficulty with voice quality, breathing, and swallowing. She did not recall any acute illnesses that might have coincided with the onset of the symptoms. She first noticed this when she started working in a department store, adjacent to the perfume department. Initially, she noticed that her voice became increasingly hoarse, which she described as "squeaky," and it took greater effort to talk as the working day progressed. Initially, the hoarseness abated overnight, but eventually it persisted even after a full night's sleep. After a few weeks of chronic hoarseness, DD noticed her breathing also was affected when she was in the store. She described a wheezing sensation in her throat when she was trying to take a breath in, and the effort of breathing increased the longer she spoke. She also described struggling to inhale, as though she were breathing from only the top half of her lungs. Her dysphonia worsened with the onset of the breathing problem. Aware that she was straining her voice, DD asked the manager to turn down the background music in her department, and he complied. A few months after the onset of her throat symptoms, when she took her breaks at work, DD began to experience difficulty swallowing. She described increasing effort to swallow solid food, and a feeling of panic when preparing to go on her breaks. She typically took her break with a long-time friend, who regularly expressed great concern about DD's symptoms, and hoped that she didn't have throat cancer from her husband's secondhand smoke or from the chemicals coming from the perfume department, which seemed to aggravate DD's symptoms. Based on these comments, DD asked her manager for a transfer to another department, and he complied. She was transferred to a clothing section and initially felt relieved until she noticed a peculiar scent as she opened some new garment packages. These odors triggered the same throat symptoms: increased dysphonia followed by difficulty breathing in. It was in describing these symptoms to her doctor that the diagnosis of multiple chemical sensitivity was ascribed and he recommended that she stop working. As DD had been experiencing increasing symptoms of IBS, IBL, CFS, HD, and FM, she agreed that taking some time from work was necessary. She was finding it increasingly difficult to get up for work, and fatigue and anxiety were worsening. Her doctor referred her to a number of specialists after she stopped working, and although some queried the contribution of psychological stress, asthma, allergies, and fibromyalgia, she was not aware of a definitive diagnosis.

As her symptoms persisted, her concern about throat or lung cancer increased, despite a clear chest X-ray and declaration from an otolaryngologist that he could not "see anything to be concerned about."

Evaluation Procedures. DD underwent detailed evaluation of her problem by a multidisciplinary team comprised of a laryngologist, speech-language pathologist, and psychiatrist. Adjunctive consultations also were sought. The evaluation procedures undertaken in the voice clinic included a detailed interdisciplinary history, evaluation of general posture and laryngeal and paralaryngeal muscle use; laryngeal examination and visual perceptual scoring of laryngeal postures and vibratory characteristics; acoustic and perceptual-acoustic evaluation; and trial of therapy techniques.

Detailed, Interdisciplinary History. The information obtained from the interdisciplinary interview allowed the voice clinic team to identify a number of physiologic and psychologic factors that may have contributed to the development of irritable larynx syndrome and/or acted as symptom triggers. Asked how her problems have impacted her life, DD stated: "My throat problems took my life away, and I just want to get my life back!"

Predisposing Factors

Abdominal Tension: DD's history of multiple abdominal surgeries over a span of 40 years may have contributed to an observed tendency to hold her abdominal muscles hypertonic, which represents the "splinting" behavior that inhibits painful abdominal muscle stretching on inspiration during recovery from abdominal surgery. Her lower back injury also may have contributed to muscle hypertonicity in the abdominal muscles. Furthermore, she was aware that her abdomen and back became very tense when she recalled her mother's pain during her fight with colon cancer.

Gastroesophageal Reflux: DD's chronic heartburn, globus pharyngeus, sensation of postnasal drip, chronic throat-clearing, and choking when supine are common symptoms of reflux. These symptoms had existed as long as she remembered, but had increased as she had become more sedentary, started going to bed immediately after meals, and subsequently gained weight. Her tendency to hold her abdominal muscles hypertonic may have compounded the propensity for reflux.

Psychological Factors: DD's pre-occupation with the possibility she had cancer caused growing anxiety and was fueled by the unabated throat and breathing symptoms. In discussion with the voice clinic team, it was evident that DD was burdened by unexpressed fear that she would inherit her mother's colon cancer (the memories of which may have contributed to abdominal tension, as discussed above), or alternatively that her long-term exposure to her husband's second-hand smoke might have induced cancer. This cancer fear may have been inadvertently reinforced by her close friend. Furthermore, it was clear that DD had developed anticipatory anxiety about her throat, specifically her difficulty breathing in certain environments. Her anxiety may have been borne of previous

inconclusive or inadequately explained diagnoses of "borderline asthma" and "multiple chemical sensitivities," particularly as she was cautioned against exposing herself to environmental agents that seemed to cause these symptoms and had already been exposed to triggering irritants for prolonged periods. A symbolic olfactory association also may have existed during the onset of symptoms. On reflection and discussion with the psychiatrist, DD stated that she had never appreciated perfumes since she was a child and a relative who she disliked and distrusted always wore perfume when she visited.

Central Nervous System Hypersensitivity Disorder (CHD): DD had been suffering a number of symptoms that had led to diagnoses of multiple CHDs: IBS, IBL, CFS, HD, and FM. If, as has been proposed, ILS represents a CHD, DD may have been predisposed to neuroplastic changes that affect the sensory-motor system, with other physiologic and psychological factors contributing the laryngopharyngeal focus for symptom formation.[22]

Evaluation of General Posture and Laryngeal and Paralaryngeal Muscle Use General Body Alignment. Visual observation and manual techniques were used to assess general body alignment in sitting and standing postures. Misalignment patterns in both positions suggested spinal lordosis, and head retraction and jaw jutting posture were noted in sitting position. DD's scapulae were moderately adducted and tender to touch. Her head was held rigidly on her neck, due to general neck muscle hypertonicity, and her suboccipital muscles were extremely tender to palpation. The general postural muscle tension and tenderness noted are consistent with symptoms of FM and HD.

Abdominal Muscles. Circumferential palpation of DD's abdomen and lumbar spine regions revealed minimal palpable displacement on inhalation during speech and at rest in upright positions. In supine position, following a brief relaxation exercise, appropriate abdominal displacement was noted.

Facial Postures. Visual observation and palpation were used to evaluate facial muscle use. DD's eyebrows were held in adducted position for the duration of our interview. Her jaw was clenched, and when asked to release her jaw, she pushed it forward rather than relaxing it down. No TMJ crepitus or asymmetry were noted on palpation during normal-range movements and speech. Her face was tender on palpation between the maxilla and mandible, due to hypertonic jaw muscles. DD's tongue periphery was scalloped, imprinted from her bottom teeth against which she chronically pressed her tongue.

Paralaryngeal Muscle Evaluation. Using the grading criteria set out previously, four paralaryngeal muscle groups were evaluated at rest and during vocal activities.[16] The suprahyoid, thyrohyoid, and cricothyroid muscles all were maximally tense and her cricoid cartilage was displaced anteriorly. The cricopharyngeal muscle region was moderately hypertonic.

Laryngeal Examination and Visual Perceptual Scoring of Laryngeal Postures and Vibratory Characteristics. Transnasal fiberoptic laryngoscopy was conducted and digitally recorded with continuous and stroboscopic light during sustained vowels, connected speech, pitch and loudness dynamics, diadochokinetics, rest breathing, maximal inhalation and exhalation, and a trial of therapy techniques. Use of the transnasal scope with camera "chip-in-the-tip" technology allowed the team to view DD's pharyngeal and laryngeal postures and afforded them an excellent tool for obtaining stroboscopic images.

DD's breathing pattern changed initially in response to the sensory stimulus of the transnasal scope fueled by her apprehension about the procedure; some lightly voiced laryngeal inspiratory stridor was viewed and recorded. This provided excellent visual and auditory feedback for a demonstration of the laryngeal muscle misuse pattern and afforded an opportunity for initial training in extinguishing the behavior. Using the sniffing technique, DD was able to reverse her adduction laryngospasms while watching the video monitor. She continued to use the technique throughout the examination.

In addition to the adduction laryngospasm noted at the true vocal fold level, muscle misuse patterns observed in the laryngopharynx included larynx elevation for speech and pitch ascension (due to suprahyoid and thyrohyoid muscle misuse), elongated vocal fold posture during speech, and absence of vocal fold shortening during pitch descent (due to maximal contraction of the cricothyroid muscles). DD also was observed to clear her throat multiple times during the evaluation and the muscle and tissue misuse intrinsic in this behavior was explained to her as she viewed it on the monitor.

During evaluation of vocal fold vibratory patterns with stroboscopic light, notable features included reduced amplitude of vibration bilaterally for all vocal tasks, incomplete closure during high-pitched phonation and speech, and reduced mucosal wave bilaterally. Amplitude, mucosal wave, and closure patterns were normal when a voice onset technique "M Hm"; "M Hmmm-mmm . . . " was used to help DD initiate and sustain phonation in modal register.

Laryngeal evaluation with continuous light revealed moderate erythema in the posterior glottis, including arytenoid surfaces and vocal processes and interarytenoid areas of the true vocal folds. The arytenoid bodies were edematous, as was the interarytenoid area. Pseudosulci were noted inferior to the vocal fold margins. These signs all were interpreted by the laryngologist as representing effects of reflux on the larynx. No other structural or movement abnormalities were noted.

Acoustic and Perceptual-Acoustic Evaluation.

Software provided by KayPEN-TAX was used to evaluate DD's mean fundamental frequency (F_0) and physiologic range; mean intensity and dynamic range; laryngeal diadochokinetics, perturbation, and interharmonic noise. DD's mean F_0 during speech was 278 Hz, with a low and high range from 270 to 314 Hz. She demonstrated a physiologic F_0 range from 125 Hz to 857 Hz, produced during a glissando exercise simulating a "siren" noise, which allowed her to explore her vocal range in the absence of her typical misuses.

DD's average vocal intensity during speech was 50 dB, but with encouragement she was able to demonstrate a dynamic range of 42 dB, by imagining she was yelling at someone who had annoyed her, to a maximum intensity level of 92 dB.

Perturbation values on sustained vowel productions were outside the normal range for measures of pitch perturbation (jitter), amplitude perturbation (shimmer), and harmonics-to-noise ratio.

Perceptually, DD's voice during speech was characterized by moderately strained, breathy and aesthenic quality. Her breath groups tended to be short and phrasing periodically inappropriate, due to the tendency to run out of air during speech.

Trial of Therapy Techniques.

The therapy trials were initiated during the laryngeal examination, using the transnasal fiberoptic technology for visual feedback as exercises were introduced to reduce adductory laryngospasm (sniffing); and cricothyroid spasm ("M Hm"; "Hm!"; humming; glottal fry). DD responded very positively to immediate auditory, sensory, and visual feedback provided during successful use of these techniques. Her daughter provided additional reinforcement and immediately initiated a "game" of having her mother respond to questions or comments, using the spontaneous utterances that helped DD restore her normal modal voice.

Adjunctive Consults.

Adjunctive consultations were sought from colleagues in respiratory medicine, gastroenterology, physical therapy, and dietetics.

Description and Rationale for Treatment Approach.

The interprofessional voice clinic team concluded that DD was suffering ILS, which followed similar onset patterns to her other CNS hypersensitivity disorders. Reports from the respiratory consultant confirmed that DD did not meet criteria for an asthma diagnosis and recommended discontinuing steroid inhalers. He suspected gastroesophageal reflux was a significant contributor to her respiratory symptoms, which was reinforced by the report from the gastroenterologist, who found that DD was experiencing significant amounts of reflux daily, due primarily to poor closure in the lower esophageal sphincter and a hiatal hernia. He recommended lifestyle changes, weight loss, and 40 mg of a proton pump inhibitor twice daily. The dietician's consult concluded that DD's high-carbohydrate diet and eating schedule contributed to her weight gain as well as reflux and provided guidelines for more appropriate diet and eating routine. The physical therapist identified multiple areas of postural misuse and initiated treatment for postural adjustment and muscle relaxation.

A multidisciplinary approach to treatment was deemed necessary to address the various physiologic, lifestyle, and psychologic factors contributing to DD's ILS symptoms.

Goals set were as follows:

Goal 1. DD will demonstrate an understanding and acceptance of the multifactorial nature of her breathing and voice problems.

Rationale. DD will need to "buy into" the concept of ILS as a CNS hypersensitivity disorder with multiple interacting causes, so she can commit to making major life-style changes that will be required to reduce her symptoms. Following detailed description of her laryngeal status, the voice care team will provide reassurance that DD does *not* have laryngeal cancer and, in fact, is not at risk for either laryngeal or lung cancer, and that the symptoms she suffers can be fully accounted for by ILS. This reassurance will be reinforced regularly throughout treatment.

Goal 2. DD will minimize sensory stimuli that are acting as triggers for her ILS symptoms of adductor laryngospasm, dysphonia, and globus pharyngeus. Reflux treatment will be a major part of this goal, and pharmaceutical intervention as recommended by the GI specialist will be initiated immediately. The voice care team and dietician will continue to reinforce and monitor DD's efforts at changing her diet and eating schedule, with special focus on eating frequent small meals, increasing her protein intake, remaining upright for a minimum of 3 hours after meals or snacks, and sleeping with the head of her bed tilted.

DD also will be instructed to minimize exposure to known airborne irritants, although this exposure has been largely eliminated since she stopped working. She will be seen with her husband, so the irritation caused by his second-hand cigarette smoke can be discussed.

Rationale. DD's medical history, as well as her ILS history, suggest that reflux has played a major role in predisposing her to laryngeal muscle spasm. Her reflux symptoms have increased since she has gained weight, become more sedentary, and spent more time resting in supine position.

Goal 3. DD will reprogram the maladaptive CNS response causing her ILS symptoms. This will include gaining an understanding of how negative thought processes, repression of vocal expression of fears/emotions, and olfactory stimuli can serve as triggers for ILS symptoms. The psychiatrist will play a leading role in helping DD recognize how her fears about cancer and her general health, other potential unexpressed negative emotions, olfactory memories, and sensory stimuli from reflux or airborne irritants can become inappropriately paired to cause abnormal muscle responses to common sensory stimuli.

In conjunction with cognitive psychotherapy, DD will engage in physical and speech therapy to improve her general posture, increase her exercise tolerance, and reduce specific muscle misuses in the abdomen, head, face, and neck. Selective manual therapy will be used to give DD an opportunity to experience sensations associated with relaxed muscles in the paralaryngeal muscles that have been chronically hypertonic. Voice therapy will be incorporated into the physical program and used in conjunction with manual therapy to re-establish modal register phonation, using simple voice onset techniques that were successful during trial therapy.

DD will be instructed to use the sniffing technique many times daily, to reprogram her larynx to abduct during inhalation.

A desensitization program will be included in later stages of the physical and cognitive therapies to allow DD to incorporate her therapy strategies while exposed to odors that previously served as ILS symptom triggers.

Rationale. DD uses muscle tension throughout her body as a defense reaction, and the consequent pain and fatigue are recognized as hallmark symptoms of FM, HD, and CFS. The pain sensation tends to reinforce itself through fear of what it represents. If this cycle is broken, using a general to specific muscle relaxation process, her chronic symptoms associated with CHD should subside.

The desensitization program will allow DD to learn to extinguish the maladaptive responses to normal sensory stimuli and will give her the confidence to return to environments that previously were problematic, including her work-

place. This will "give her her life back."

Goal 4. Explore use of neuropsychotropic medication. In consultation with DD, her general practitioner and the laryngologist, the psychiatrist will take responsibility for determining which, if any, prescription medications, such as selective serotonin reuptake inhibitors and combined serotonin and norepinephrine re-uptake inhibitors, might assist DD in reducing ILS symptoms. He also will consider DD's current medication regimen to determine whether it is achieving maximum benefit or if it should be altered. If progress is being demonstrated early in the physical and speech therapy program, he will hold off on prescription of antispasmolytic medications. The psychiatrist will also help DD evaluate and monitor psychological effects of her physical exercise program.

Rationale. Some patients with ILS and other CHD syndromes benefit from centrally active prescription medications. The neurons involved in the sensory-motor disorder of ILS and other CHDs use chemicals to communicate with each other, and modifying brain chemistry might make it possible for them to communicate more effectively.

A regular aerobic exercise program is known to improve mental health due to production of endorphins, and the long-term benefit to DD will probably exceed effects of neuron-psychotropic medication.

Results of Treatment

Symptom Abatement. Within 3 weeks of BID proton-pump inhibitor (PPI) therapy and reflux-control lifestyle measures, DD noticed swallowing was easier and she was sleeping better, despite reducing her sleeping medication.

She lost 5 pounds on the new eating regime, without reducing calorie intake. An additional benefit of her reflux treatment was absence of heartburn for the first time since she was pregnant with her eldest child. The recognition of her symptom reduction encouraged DD, and she demonstrated a dogged determination to continue with her success. Within 6 weeks of commencing physical therapy, she was walking 60 minutes daily with friends whom she had not seen for a long while. She recognized a significant reduction in her general body pain and fatigue. At her 3-month voice clinic reassessment she reported she had not experienced breathing problems (except for being short of breath when she increased her exercise) for 6 weeks, that swallowing was normal most of the time, that she rarely cleared her throat, and that her voice was normal most of the time. She also stated that she was "getting her life back."

General Posture and Laryngeal and Paralaryngeal Muscle Use. The physical therapist and speech-language pathologist both observed progressive improvement in body alignment and reduced sensitivity to palpation of specific muscle areas. DD herself stated she was "taller" since she started therapy. She monitored tension in her neck, face, jaw, tongue, and suprahyoid muscles several times daily, and was able to accurately report improvement as she observed it visually, proprioceptively, or by palpation. At 3-month reassessment, scores for four target paralaryngeal muscle regions indicated only mild residual hypertonicity.

Laryngeal Examination and Visual Perceptual Scoring of Laryngeal Postures and Vibratory Characteristics. Three-month reassessment with the transnasal scope confirmed lowered larynx position during phonation, appropriate laryngeal posture for modal register phonation, normal vocal fold closure pattern, vocal fold vibratory amplitude, and mucosal wave bilaterally. DD initially did demonstrate some adductory spasm when the flexible scope was inserted, but she was able to control the symptoms quickly by sniffing repeatedly and performing what she called her "body meditation" (her term for tuning into positive sensations in her body). The laryngeal exam revealed reduced erythema and edema in the larynx, but a mild pseudosulcus was still evident.

Acoustic and Perceptual-Acoustic Evaluation. At 3-month reassessment, measures of vocal perturbation and interharmonic noise were within normal limits for sustained vowels. Her physiologic ranges for F_0 and intensity remained within normal limits. DD's speaking voice was predominantly clear and produced in modal register. However, when she spoke of issues that caused anxiety, such as being able to return to work and financial pressures, she tended to revert to her "squeaky voice," which was high pitched and breathy, but less strained than previously. She recognized the voice change, and, with the assistance of the speech-language pathologist, was able to recover clear modal register phonation.

The rapid abatement of DD's ILS symptoms can be attributed largely to her motivation to improve her health and return to a normal lifestyle. An intelligent and insightful woman, she was able to recognize and evaluate her physical and emotional responses to various situations and employ appropriate techniques to reduce or extinguish inappropriate muscle responses to symptom triggers. The multiprofessional collaboration provided her with consistent messages about the causes and appropriate treatments for her symptoms. Although it was almost a year after her first visit to the voice clinic that she claimed to be "symptom-free," DD accepted the gradual improvement as a predictable response and gave herself due credit for the amount of time and effort she contributed to the changes she made.

> As noted in Rammage and Morrison's tutorial at the opening of the chapter, chronic cough may be one manifestation of ILS. In the following case, Susan Shulman, describes her behavioral approach to treating chronic cough and associated voice concerns in an adolescent female.

Symptom Modification for Chronic Cough Syndrome

Susan Shulman, MS

Case Study: Patient EE

Patient History. Patient EE, a 13-year-old junior high school student, reported a 10-month history of chronic cough precipitated by a 5-day exposure to smoke odors from the forest fires during "El Nino." At the time of the exposure, she was participating in a highly competitive soccer tournament. The daily temperatures reached more than 100°F. She remembers having difficulty breathing, especially when running, and relates the onset of her cough to that time. She was utilizing an inhaler for asthma without benefit. Approximately 8 months ago, she began wearing braces and felt that this increased the severity of her cough. Laryngeal examination indicated moderate laryngeal edema.

Voice Evaluation Results

Acoustic Analysis (as determined by the Visi-Pitch II)

- appropriate habitual modal pitch of 201 Hz
- reduced range of inflection for conversational speech of 37 Hz
- reduced pitch range of 134 Hz to 435 Hz
- slightly elevated jitter of .87%
- normal shimmer of 2.9%.

Loudness Measurement and Breath Support

- reduced volume for conversation of 61 dB
- reduced range of volume of 53 dB to 75 dB
- rate of speech was normal to slow
- sustained phonation times were /a/ 15 seconds, /s/ 20 seconds, and /z/ 11 seconds
- breath support was shallow, clavicular
- breathing characteristics including speaking on residual air, mouth breathing, breath holding
- poor airflow control.

Physical Analysis

- marked laryngeal and jaw musculature tension
- elevated laryngeal posture during phonation
- restricted jaw movement with jaw clenching
- retracted, elevated tongue posture
- body tension: locked head and neck position, elevated shoulder posture
- screening oral peripheral examination: elevated, tense velum during /a/
- digital laryngeal massage: marked sensitivity and pain to light touch of

the jaw, the superior cornu of the hyoid cartilage, and the thyroid cartilage

■ approximate number of coughs per hour: 30 to 40.

The overall voice quality was consistent with a mild-to-moderate dysphonia with glottal fry and low, back-tone focus. Hydration was poor. Although speaking seemed to trigger a cough at the end of a phrase or sentence, she frequently coughed even when she was not speaking. In response to a question concerning tongue placement at rest, she indicated that the tongue was "tight and against the roof of the mouth."

The following goals were established for therapy:

1. Focus patient's attention on exhalation and release of breath
2. Reduce jaw and laryngeal tension with digital laryngeal massage
3. Increase mandibular opening during phonation
4. Reduce or eliminate coughing
5. Eliminate clavicular breath support
6. Diminish glottal fry
7. Increase hydration.

Therapeutic Procedures. The procedures employed to reach the above goals included the use of videotapes for visual feedback and audiotapes for voice practice. Charting behaviors including number of coughs per hour were essential to the success of the program.

First Session. It is always important that patients understand the function of the vocal folds and the rationale and procedure for the digital jaw and laryngeal massage technique. This information helps educate patients and enlist their participation in the therapy process. Using a mirror for visual feedback, Patient EE was instructed in the massage technique. It was recommended that she use the massage technique at least 4 to 6 times per day for approximately 1 minute at a time. It was also advocated that she use a small massager to release tension in the jaw and the neck. A simple exercise of counting from 1 to 10 with slightly increased downward movement of the lower jaw released jaw tension. The patient was instructed to exhale frequently throughout the day (eg, each time she walked outside, each time she picked up the phone, etc).

Second Session. At the beginning of each session, auditory and sensory symptoms were reviewed. Patient EE reported that she had "significantly" reduced her coughing and that she increasingly was aware of jaw tension. She also had tried to exhale frequently throughout the day, especially when running. Her throat felt less closed and she could talk for longer periods of time without coughing.

Therapy techniques to be practiced frequently throughout the day were twofold:

1. Relaxed tongue posturing:
   ■ Tongue relaxed on the floor of the mouth
   ■ Speak from the "tip" of the tongue
   ■ Speak in a yawn position and not a swallow position

2. Breathing technique:
   ■ Inhalation through the nose
   ■ Lips lightly together
   ■ Abdominal expansion
   ■ Exhalation of voiceless /s/
   ■ Easy release of breath
   ■ Gentle abdominal contraction

Third Session. Patient EE noted that she was able to run for 15 minutes without coughing. She was also able to talk for longer periods without feeling the need to cough. She had increased her water intake and was consistent with the voice exercises. She was able to use the breathing technique to interrupt a cough. Her overall voice quality was freer with improved oral and nasal tone focus. Her jaw was more relaxed, and she was not holding on to the breath as much as she had in prior sessions.

Therapy recommendations were to continue with the previous exercises, to increase flexibility and awareness of tongue placement and to encourage slight upward inflection at the end of a phrase or sentence.

1. Tongue placement exercises:
   - Increasing tongue tip control and flexibility
   - Repetition of single sounds with anterior tongue placement (eg, /t/, /f/).

2. Repetition of lists of words with anterior tongue placement, emphasizing easy onset of sound.

3. Short sentences in the form of a question with slight upward inflection.

Fourth Session. Patient EE reported that the jaw tension was minimal, coughing was essentially eliminated, and it was "easier to speak." Jaw clenching was reduced. The presenting voice quality was essentially clear with balanced tone focus. Breath support was improved, and overall body tension was significantly lessened. She reported increased awareness when she felt tense and held onto the breath or started to speak without first inhaling. She did not cough during the 45-minute session.

Therapy recommendations were to begin voice strengthening exercises, which included humming and prolongation of sustained tones. Singing exercises that included sustained final /ŋ/ were introduced. Patient EE was instructed to continue with the audio CD of voice exercises on a daily basis for 2 months and return as needed.

Outcome of the Voice Therapy Program

- Quality of the voice and ease of speaking essentially within normal limits
- Overall body tension significantly reduced
- Coughing essentially eliminated
- Sensitivity to digital jaw and laryngeal manipulation minimal
- Pitch range increased from 191 Hz to 877 Hz
- Volume range increased by more than 30 dB, 50 dB to 85 dB
- Inflection increased to 86 Hz
- Volume for conversation speech increased to 70 dB.

Comments and Summary. The chronic coughing that the patient exhibited initially was triggered by exposure to noxious fumes. The problem most likely was complicated by exposure to heat, intense physical exercise in a dry environment, reduced hydration, reduced mouth opening during phonation, and laryngeal-pharyngeal tone focus. The persistent and frequent coughing resulted in a mild dysphonia with reduced pitch range, poor airflow control, glottal fry, and reduced inflection for normal conversation. Follow-up laryngeal examination was within normal limits. A telephone recheck 1 month following the final session indicated that she continues to progress and had not experienced a return of symptoms.

Patient EE responded well to voice therapy techniques that included increased hydration, more relaxed tongue posturing, reduced jaw and laryngeal hyperfunction, and improved breath support. At the end of the fourth session, she coughed only infrequently and breath support was abdominal-thoracic with less pronounced breath holding. The reduction of coughing resulted in elimination of the initial auditory and sensory symptoms and of the vibratory trauma to the vocal folds. Individuals with chronic cough syndrome should be referred for voice therapy so that coughing behaviors can not only be investigated, but also understood and eliminated.

As indicated above, the irritable larynx syndrome manifests itself in a variety of ways. One common presentation is characterized by paradoxic movement of the vocal folds during respiration. Michael Trudeau and Jennifer Thompson offer additional insights into this specific manifestation of ILS. Their tutorial is followed by a series of case studies showing how paradoxical vocal fold dysfunction is managed in a variety of patient populations.

Overview of Paradoxical Vocal Fold Dysfunction

Michael Trudeau, PhD, CCC-SLP, and Jennifer Thompson, MA

The serious student of voice disorders can attest to the dynamic growth in this area of practice. Paradoxical vocal fold dysfunction (PVFD) typifies this growth. Twenty years ago speech-language pathologists (SLP) rarely participated in the care of persons with PVFD. Textbooks failed to mention the disorder. Now the SLP is an intrinsic member of the team treating these patients. Professionals quibble about the proper terminology: paradoxical vocal fold dysfunction, paradoxical vocal fold motion, vocal cord dysfunction, psychogenic stridor,[23] and so on. Google did not exist in 1989; but had it existed, a Google Scholar search in 1989 would have identified only 21 references touching on this subject. A similar search in 2009 returned approximately 3863 references (search terms "paradoxical vocal" and "vocal cord dysfunction"). For the serious student of voice disorders, this is an exciting topic and time.

By way of introduction, paradoxical vocal fold dysfunction (PVFD), as with many "voice disorders," requires the clinician to bear certain important caveats in mind. The first of these is that it is not a voice disorder. PVFD does not alter the acoustics of the human voice. There is no dysphonia, although PVFD may coexist with dysphonia. PVFD also is not typified by some identifiable laryngeal lesion. It is typified by an action typical of a sphincteric valve, namely constriction.

The second caveat is that PVFD is a descriptive label more than a diagnosis. A person with PVFD constricts the laryngeal airway at inappropriate times, thereby interfering with respiration. Assigning a label of PVFD, therefore, does not delineate the etiology of the respiratory problem.

Related to the preceding caveat, a third introductory caveat is that the nature of PVFD is not well understood. There are several possible etiologies. It is almost certain that not all persons with PVFD share the same underlying cause. It also is possible that the laryngeal behaviors that define PVFD in a given person arise from more than one etiology. The simple determination that a person does have PVFD does not, of itself, lead to an appropriate focus for treatment.

Returning to the Google search, a final caveat is that there is still much to know about PVFD, particularly in the realm of evidence-based practice. Refining the search by using a search tool such as Mednar and eliminating redundant entries reduces the likely scholarly contributions from 3863 to 154. Of these, over half (80) were case studies. Another 40 articles were summaries of knowledge in the area (eg, reviews, tutorials, editorials, etc). Of the remaining 34 citations, only 21 posed testable positions (ie, experimental in nature), only 14 were prospective in design, and only 7 dealt specifically with treatment. The scholarly clinician will recognize in these figures that there appears to be a large body of intuitive or experiential knowledge of PVFD, but very little empirically based, scientific knowledge with which to guide assessment and intervention.

Paradoxical vocal fold dysfunction occurs with mistimed laryngeal valving disrupting respiration. Simply put, the affected individual experiences intermittent interruptions in inspiration, expiration, or both. These interruptions are sufficient in duration or frequency or both to produce shortness of breath or dyspnea. Persons with this disorder typically report sudden onsets of dyspnea, sometimes with no known trigger, but often with the onset associated with mild exertion or increased stress. In contrast, the episodes frequently occur while the patient is sleeping, producing a startled arousal with a sensation of strangling or choking (night chokes).

Although clinicians find it convenient to use the term PVFD as if it were itself the cause of the dyspnea, this useful shorthand does not convey the true nature of the problem in terms of etiology, diagnosis, and treatment. In studying PVFD, it is useful to view the larynx as a valve in the respiratory system, rather than as the organ of phonation. The basic reflexive action of the larynx in this system is to protect the lower airway by closing. A second function of the larynx in the respiratory system is to regulate pulmonary airflow and, indirectly, thoracic pressure.

In terms of diagnosis and treatment, PVFD represents a condition in much the same way as dysphonia represents a condition produced by a variety of disorders and diseases. If the view is held that PVFD is more a symptom than a disorder, then questions about the etiology of PVFD must address the underlying cause. Similar to our understanding of aphasia, more than one taxonomy has been proposed for PVFD. One approach to classifying PVFD yields at least five possibilities:

First, laryngospasm is the larynx's response to noxious stimuli. It is an abrupt, reflexive laryngeal constriction of such strength as to obstruct respiration. One such stimulus is gastroesophageal reflux (GER), or, more appropriately for PVFD, gastrolaryngopharyngeal reflux (GLPR).[24,25] The patient who awakes with "night chokes" is probably experiencing GLPR. GLPR is more likely to occur during sleep because the individual is supine or prone, eliminating gravity's effect in containing gastric contents to the stomach.

After examining more than 1000 patients with PVFD, this clinician's impression is that many of these individuals produce chronic GLPR and are completely unaware that they are doing so. When observed by nasendoscopy, they appear to be airway protective in the sense that they maintain a constricted laryngeal posture (vocal folds and ventricular folds medialized, epiglottis positioned posteriorly, and arytenoid cartilages drawn anteriorly, hooding over the glottis) as if in anticipation of refluxed material penetrating the airway. There also are the typical signs of reflux irritation: interarytenoid pachyderma, edema of the arytenoid cartilages, postcricoid edema, diffuse erythema, and so forth.

At rest, this partially constricted posture has little effect. Respiration is not forceful enough to create audible turbulence (stridor), and the person exchanges sufficient air in each respiratory cycle to remain comfortable. With exertion, however, such constriction produces an inefficient, effortful respiratory pattern and dyspnea. This may explain why many patients with PVFD report onset of shortness of breath coinciding with mild exertion (carrying laundry, vacuuming, raking leaves, etc) and a primary control strategy of just sitting still for 5 or 10 minutes.

GLPR may serve as a primary cause of episodic dyspnea (ie, laryngospasm) and as a predisposing condition. Patients with this form of GLPR often have a long history of misdiagnosis, typically of asthma. In addition to the typical inhalers, they also take a steroid (usually prednisone) and frequently are dependent on it. GLPR-related PVFD might be the single most common form of PVFD. Control of the reflux, however, may not eliminate the patient's habituated protective laryngeal posture. Additionally, although this position appears to explain the development of PVFD in a person, it does not explain why, in other persons for whom GLPR appears to be chronic, PVFD does not develop.

Second, some patients with observed laryngeal constriction or complete closure during respiration unconsciously use the laryngeal valve to maintain positive thoracic pressure throughout the respiratory cycle. Such a pattern has been reported for asthmatic patients[26–29] and for patients with cystic fibrosis.[30] In this clinic, it also has been observed in patients with lung cancer and patients who have experienced severe pulmonary irritation (eg, ammonia inhalation). These persons appear to be maintaining some degree of lung inflation in compensation for pulmonary injury or disease.

Third, the consistent profile of adolescents with PVFD strongly suggests that PVFD among adolescents represents a distinct form of the condition. The 10- to 20-year-old patient with PVFD often is a good student who is heavily involved and successful in extracurricular activities.[31] These activities usually are sports related but may simply be strenuous in and of themselves (eg, marching band). The shortness-of-breath episodes typically occur during such activities, interrupting, but not eliminating, the student's participation. These adolescents are displaying an immature strategy for dealing with unacceptable levels of stress in their lives. They are not necessarily unhappy individuals. They (and their parents) frequently object to a stress-oriented explanation by expressing how much they enjoy all their activities and successes. It may be that an individual activity is the locus of the stress, but it also may be that an individual activity was simply the final straw to cause a "stress" fracture of the camel's back.

Fourth, the paradoxical motion of the vocal folds (and possibly other laryngeal structures) may represent a form of conversion reaction similar to functional aphonia. The dyspnea, therefore, is a subconscious mechanism for avoiding some deep-seated emotional conflict.[32,33] Recent work by Husein et al[34] supported this view with approximately three out of four persons with PVFD exhibiting a personality type prone to conversion reaction. This etiology may account for the reportedly high incidence of sexual abuse among women with PVFD.[35] Typically, these individuals are women in their fourth or fifth decades who report increasingly severe and frequent episodes of shortness of breath. The episodes cause them sufficient discomfort that they resort to local emergency rooms for treatment. They generally report that they have asthma but note that they do not respond well to asthma medications.

A reasonable practice is to interview patients with PVFD by themselves without family or friends present. This permits greater privacy and sensitivity when broaching a topic as difficult as a history of abuse. The clinician should bear in mind that, if the patient were aware of the connection between abuse and laryngeal problems, she probably would not have the problem. It is likely that the patient's denial of the abuse will extend to answering questions about its potential occurrence. The clinician must be circumspect, sensitive, and patient in obtaining information about this matter. Frequently, the patient will deny any involvement in abuse, only to raise the issue for clarification later in the session or during therapy.

Finally, inappropriate laryngeal constriction during respiration may indicate a level of incoordination typical of a focal dyskinesia.[36] In these cases, the paradoxical motion is similar to the abrupt adduction of the vocal folds characteristic of adductor spasmodic dysphonia. Although some patients exhibit a degree of vocal instability (unstable zero-phase during stroboscopy, elevated jitter in sustained phonation), dysphonia is not a typical concern of the patients. Neurogenic voice disorders are not cited in the literature as common among patients with PVFD.

From the foregoing, it should be apparent that PVFD is a complex issue and that management of the condition may involve numerous disciplines. For many patients the first step in management is a visit with their family physicians. Here, an initial diagnosis of asthma frequently is made. The family physician becomes concerned, however, when the patient responds poorly to asthma medications. This prompts a referral to a pulmonologist and a comprehensive evaluation of the patient's pulmonary function. When these results fail to support a diagnosis of asthma or the severity of the asthma is inadequate to explain the patient's severity of complaints, the pulmonologist looks for other explanations. Increasingly, they are referring patients to speech-language pathologists (SLPs).

The role of SLPs in treating the patient with PVFD parallels their role in treating dysphagia. Neither disorder directly affects communication. Just as SLPs' education and training in the motor aspects of the speech system prepare them for the specialized perspective needed to assess and treat swallowing disorders, so also do their education and training in respiratory and laryngeal physiology and in modifying laryngeal behavior for voice disorders prepare them for the assessment and treatment of PVFD. This is accomplished by modifying the patient's laryngeal valving during respiration using laryngeal control therapy (LCT).

Laryngeal endoscopy is a crucial tool in the diagnosis of PVFD because it can confirm the presence of the paradoxical motion.[29,37] The results also may implicate the role of GLPR and aid in focusing treatment. Although laryngeal endoscopy via the oral cavity can detect the inappropriate laryngeal constriction, this method also is susceptible to the confounding effects associated with stimulating a gag reflex. Therefore, nasendoscopy is preferable, but even this method has limitations, the most important of which is that the examiner cannot observe the glottis for extended periods. The examination generally is limited to 10 minutes or less and paradoxic motion may or may not occur during this time.

An equally crucial tool in diagnosing PVFD is the patient interview. The interview cannot confirm the diagnosis with the same confidence of a direct observation of paradoxical motion. It does permit the gathering of other very important information, however.

- How long has the patient had breathing difficulties?
- How frequently do the episodes of dyspnea occur?
- What does the patient do when they occur?
- What other assistance (professional or otherwise) has the patient sought?
- Is the severity or frequency of the episodes increasing?
- How long do episodes persist?
- What impact have the episodes had on the patient's life?
- When do they occur in terms of both time of day and preceding activities?
- What approaches has the patient used to control respiration?

- What signs of gastrolaryngopharyngeal reflux problems are present?
- What are the stressors and what are the levels of stress in the patient's life?
- How do these relate to both the onset of the symptoms and present occurrences of the dyspnea?
- Has the patient been a victim of verbal, emotional, physical, or sexual abuse?
- If so, has there been any counseling to aid in recovery from that trauma? When did counseling take place?

A basic assumption in treating persons with PVFD is that the underlying etiologies must be addressed. GLPR must be brought in check where it is contributory. Psychologic and emotional issues (eg, a history of abuse or inefficient stress management strategies) must be addressed for the patient to progress to safe, normal respiration. Clearly, a major role for the SLP is to recommend appropriate referrals to other professionals. A second role is to provide support and encouragement to increase patient compliance with the treatment programs initiated by other professionals.

A second basic assumption is that these individuals are unaware that the larynx is the source of their respiratory difficulties. For a significant minority of these persons, simply becoming aware of the laryngeal nature of their dyspnea resolves the problem or at least gives them sufficient direction so that they do not require further professional assistance in its management.

Another basic assumption is that these individuals can bring laryngeal behaviors under volitional control. Respiration is essentially a visceral function subject to autonomic, brainstem control, however.[38] Phonation as a component of speech is subject to cortical control. Particularly for persons who have habituated a constricted laryngeal posture during respiration, the major goal of therapy is to establish awareness of and conscious control over respiratory functions. These are the basic assumptions of laryngeal control therapy.

Useful tools for therapy promote an open laryngeal posture in the patient. Viewed during nasendoscopy, nasal inspiration typically stimulates a maximally open glottis. Pairing nasal inspiration with diaphragmatic breathing tends to produce a relaxed inspiratory pattern. To gain control over expiration, an audible but relaxed exhalation (such as with a sustained, breathy /s/) is useful. Sometimes simply asking the patient to blow gently produces a relaxed, effortless pattern; it is essential to emphasize this pattern. Many persons with PVFD have grown accustomed to labored, effortful breathing, whereas others have adopted a rapid, "panting" pattern as a compensation for the laryngeal constriction. Conversely, some clients will significantly improve respiratory control and limit dyspnea when coached in panting as a compensatory strategy. Still others will force an open airway by coughing, which quickly becomes chronic and frequent. The SLP's goal, therefore, is to establish a new pattern, supportive of efficient respiration. Just as the SLP probes client performance in evaluating articulation, so does the SLP probe respiratory behaviors during assessment and early treatment for PVFD in order to find useful strategies for improving breathing.

Although unconscious breath holding is central to PVFD, conscious breath holding can be a valuable clinical tool for creating increased awareness of and control over respiration and in aiding the patient in identifying when paradoxical vocal fold motion is occurring. This tactic is not useful in every case. In fact, some patients seem to respond poorly to increased laryngeal awareness. Persons with PVFD are not a homogeneous clinical group. Part of the clinical challenge is to find the right tool for the particular patient. One group where breath holding does seem to improve function is athletes. The student athlete typically complains of shortness of breath only during practice or competition (ie, during periods of vigorous exertion). Apparently, they either are constricting the airway at these times or the degree of constriction that they typically produce becomes an impediment at these times.

Increased awareness of breath holding allows athletes to monitor their respiratory patterns during training and competition and to identify inadvertent breath holding. One added challenge in this scenario is educating the athletes' coaches or trainers. They may view alterations in training regimen as intrusions into their programs.

Management of PVCD: A Case of Physical and Emotional Abuse

Michael Trudeau, PhD, and Jennifer Thompson, MS

Case Study: Patient FF

Patient FF was a 48-year-old woman with a 2-year history of episodic shortness of breath. She reported that these episodes occurred approximately four times daily and typically were associated with activities requiring mild exertion (eg, walking up stairs, carrying heavy objects, etc). The episodes typically lasted for approximately 10 minutes but had, on occasion, persisted for upward of 2 hours. In general, she avoided activities that demanded more than mild exertion because she felt they would produce too much difficulty breathing.

Patient FF had been employed as a sales associate in a department store since graduating from high school. She had been married for 20 years and had two children (18 and 15 years old) with her present husband and a child (28 years old) from her first marriage, which ended when she was 21 years old.

Patient FF had never used tobacco products and was a self-described "health nut." She was careful about her and her family's diet. She was exercising regularly until the breathing difficulties began 2 years before.

The patient stated that she had had asthma "for years." On closer questioning, she revealed that she first experienced breathing problems 29 years ago. She did not recall any particular health issues or stressful events at that time. She did note that the episodes were increasing in severity over the past 2 years.

Initially her dyspnea responded well to the use of inhalers (eg, Ventolin), but the effectiveness of these medications had declined. Her apprehension about her breathing had increased simultaneously. In the past year, she had sought treatment four times in her local hospital's emergency room because her medication failed to restore normal breathing. On these occasions, she was "given a breathing treatment." She was never admitted to the hospital. The ER staff would observe her for 2 to 3 hours, during which time her breathing stabilized, and she then would return to her home.

Following her most recent ER treatment, the attending physician arranged for Patient FF to see a pulmonologist. This physician completed pulmonary function testing (PFT). The results, particularly a flat inspiratory loop, were inconsistent with asthma.[29,33] Based on these findings and the patient's repeated use of the emergency room, the pulmonologist performed a methacholine challenge test. When this test failed to produce an asthmatic response, the pulmonologist determined that a diagnosis of asthma was inappropriate and began seeking another diagnosis for her.

The next step was referral to an SLP experienced with PVFD and accomplished in videonasendoscopy. The intake interview with the SLP was organized to aid Patient FF and the SLP in detailing her breathing difficulties.

From the intake information, the SLP discerned that the dyspnea began in the year prior to the birth of the patient's first child. Although Patient FF reported no health problems associated with the onset of her difficulties, the SLP asked how long before the birth of her child the dyspnea began. The patient recalled that she first experienced breathing problems during her pregnancy, which was also marked by severe morning sickness.

During this part of the interview, Patient FF volunteered that she probably experienced that severity of morning sickness because she was "too young." When asked to expand on this, she explained that at age 16 she had started to see an older boy. Because he wanted to start a family when she finished high school, she gave up her plans for college and married.

When asked whether she had been a victim of emotional, verbal, physical, or sexual abuse, she denied any such history. Later in the evaluation, however, she asked if her first husband yelling at her constituted verbal abuse. Further inquiry and clarification by the SLP revealed that her first husband had emotionally abused Patient FF for years beginning before their marriage. The patient next asked if striking her would be physical abuse. The pattern that emerged was that her first husband was an alcoholic who emotionally and physically abused his wife to the point of stabbing her.

Fortunately, fear for her infant impelled Patient FF to leave her husband shortly after the child's birth. She had never had any form of support or counseling for the emotional or physical trauma experienced during her first marriage.

The videonasendoscopic examination revealed a narrowing of the glottis, particularly during inspiration and following loud, sustained phonation. There was no evidence of laryngeal lesion, and vocal fold movement was symmetrical and rapid. In contrast with many individuals with PVFD, the examination did not reveal any signs of GLPR.

Based on the interview and examination, the SLP informed Patient FF that she felt that PVFD was present and that there was a possibility that it was related to her past history of abuse. The SLP had two recommendations. First, the patient should enroll in laryngeal control therapy. The nature of the program was outlined for her. Second, she should seek some form of counseling, at least to determine whether the abuse issue was relevant to her breathing problems.

Patient FF was willing to enroll in LCT but unwilling to seek any form of counseling. After consulting with the referring pulmonologist and presenting her findings, the SLP accepted the patient's decision and enrolled her in treatment. During the first session, which focused on diaphragmatic breathing, the patient repeatedly commented on her apprehension about her daughter dating and on how she had not been sleeping well for the past 2 years, waiting up for her daughter to return from a date. The SLP pointed out that the daughter's dating, Patient FF's apprehension, and her respiratory symptoms appeared to have arisen at the same time and that she had experienced emotional trauma at approximately the same age in her own life.

Again, Patient FF was reluctant to accept the connection between past trauma and present breathing problems. Her husband, who had attended therapy at the patient's request, encouraged her to "follow-up on this idea," however. He volunteered to accompany her if it would make her more comfortable. The SLP provided the couple with a list of mental health resources in the area.

At the beginning of the second session Patient FF, informed the SLP that she was feeling more comfortable about her breathing and that the exercises were helping her. She asked if it was correct to begin using the diaphragmatic breathing even if she were not practicing. The SLP informed her that diaphragmatic breathing was simply an efficient method of breathing, and she could use it whenever she wished.

Patient FF had been asked to keep a log of the occurrences of her shortness-of-breath episodes and of what activities she was engaged in at the time. The SLP and Patient FF reviewed this and found that at the beginning of the week she was having approximately four episodes daily. These typically occurred during times of mild exertion, such as carrying the laundry, running up stairs from the basement to answer the phone, and so forth. They also occurred whenever she spoke to her daughter's boyfriend. This latter observation was not lost on the patient, who informed the

SLP that she had scheduled an appointment with one of the counselors on the SLP's list.

In the third session, a review of the log revealed that in the last week Patient FF had had only five shortness-of-breath episodes. These were always associated with exertion. Per her report, these episodes were less severe than in the past and provoked less apprehension. Patient FF expressed greater confidence in her skills in managing her breathing. She also informed the SLP that her first session with a psychologist had been informative and not a bit painful.

Use of diaphragmatic breathing was extended to mild exertion (stair climbing). No dyspnea occurred. The next session was delayed for 2 weeks to allow the patient to practice her breathing and to continue in counseling. At that session, her log indicated that no episodes of dyspnea had occurred. Patient FF expressed satisfaction with her progress. The final session was scheduled for 4 weeks later to ensure stability of results. At that time, she continued to be free from the shortness-of-breath episodes. She was completing her counseling and was extremely pleased at how rapidly she had progressed.

In ending laryngeal control therapy, the SLP emphasized that all the progress in the past 2 months had been the result of Patient FF's efforts. She was reminded that she had learned the skills to maintain her present pattern of efficient respiration, but that if she needed assistance, the SLP would be happy to provide her with "booster" sessions.

Patient FF's case depicts several important points in dealing with persons with PVFD. First, patients can be vague about the onset of their symptoms. The vast majority will not mislead the SLP or physician purposefully, but

they make no direct connections between stressful or traumatic times in their lives and problems with breathing. The case history is a useful tool for "teasing out" possible connections. In this case, clues were a broken marriage, ages of children, young age of the patient at the time of symptom onset, and the change in her life plans.

Second, even when it is appropriate, a referral or recommendation for psychiatric or psychologic counseling often is met by resistance or outright rejection by the patient or patient's parents (in childhood PVFD). The topic keeps resurfacing during interactions with the patient because the patient returns to issues germane to the clinician's suspicions of emotional trauma or stress.

The approach in this clinic is to be direct in suggesting an appropriate referral and to be sensitive and careful in explaining the reasons for this suggestion but not to be insistent. If the matter is pertinent, there will be additional opportunities to discuss it and to provide direction. Additionally, the progress (if there is any) in therapy is likely to be sporadic and slow. This lack of progress often is critical in convincing the patient that seeking the assistance of a competent mental health professional is necessary. Having a list of local mental health resources is helpful.

Asking patients to keep a log of their breathing difficulties aids both patient and SLP in defining the extent of the problem. Many patients initially provide few useful details about the actual episodes of shortness of breath. Maintaining a daily log can fill in details. It also allows the patient to chart progress in regaining control over respiration.

The role of family members in therapy can be vital for both adolescents and adults. They often serve as coaches and cheerleaders, providing feedback and motivation. They also may have a better sense of the nature of the problem than does the patient.

Treatment of PVCD: A Case of GERD

Michael Trudeau, PhD, and Jennifer Thompson, MA

Case Study: Patient GG

Patient GG was a 54-year-old woman with a 6-year history of episodic shortness of breath. She also had a very low-pitched, gravely voice, but this did not concern her. She was 5 feet, 4 inches tall and weighed 200 pounds. She had been a two-pack-a-day cigarette smoker for 36 years but had ceased all tobacco use 1 year ago. She drank "at least two pots" of coffee daily and consumed essentially no beverages or fluid without caffeine. She reported a steady use of over-the-counter antacids because she experienced heartburn or indigestion on a daily basis.

When asked if she had discussed this discomfort with her physician, she responded that the problem ran in her family. She simply had learned to live with it. This prompted a question about her diet. Patient GG replied with amusement that she preferred "seafood. When I see food, I eat it." She consumed three large meals and several snacks daily. The final snack was a bowl of ice cream just before bed.

She recently had begun experiencing night chokes and was concerned about this change. Having read a magazine article about sleep apnea, she had self-diagnosed this disorder based on the night chokes. She also had cut out an

article from her local paper on gastroesophageal reflux, Barrett's esophagus, and esophageal cancer. Her long history of cigarette use coupled with her reading sufficiently concerned her that she went for her first "annual" physical in several years.

Her physician diagnosed Patient GG with hypertension, chronic gastroesophageal reflux, obesity, and emphysema. He also observed that the patient had a low-pitched, dysphonic voice. He placed her on a diet, prescribed omeprazole for control of the reflux, and arranged for her to see a pulmonologist and an otolaryngologist. When the patient bent over to tie her shoes following the examination, she became short of breath and began coughing violently.

Her physician had attended an in-service presentation conducted by a local SLP on PVFD. Based on the information he received, he called the SLP to discuss the case and eventually referred Patient GG for evaluation for possible PVFD and dysphonia. The evaluation, including videonasendoscopy, was conducted jointly by the SLP and the otolaryngologist.

Her breathing complaints were of episodic shortness of breath during mild exertion, a chronic cough, and night chokes. The shortness of breath occurred repeatedly throughout the day as Patient GG provided day care in her home for between four and six preschool-age children. During the interview, the patient reported that the night chokes occurred five to six times weekly. She asserted that she was "always" short of breath, but the SLP gained better definition by asking her to describe when she had been short of breath on the day of the examination. It became apparent that Patient GG became short of breath with any attempt at mild exertion but that she experienced shortness of breath and severe coughing whenever she bent over to lift something (eg, picking up toddlers, retrieving objects from under furniture, etc). The exertion-induced dyspnea typically persisted for 3 to 5 minutes. Patient GG considered these occurrences as inconvenient. She considered coughing to be severely limiting because it interfered with her care of the children in her charge.

Patient GG reported a happy marriage of 34 years producing three children and five grandchildren. She denied any history of abuse. She expressed general satisfaction with her life and could not identify any particular stress or event associated with her breathing difficulties.

Videonasendoscopy revealed a chronic narrowing, but not complete closure, of the glottis during resting inspiration and expiration. Patient GG was asked to count to 10 loudly. Following this, she was observed to adduct the vocal folds completely and to maintain this posture for 3 seconds before inhaling. The SLP asked her if she was having any difficulty breathing or tolerating the examination. She said she was fine. This task was repeated later in the endoscopy with the same results.

Additional findings were of leukoplakia and diffuse edema and erythema of the endolarynx, but these were more severe posteriorly than anteriorly. There was pachyderma in the interarytenoid area. The edema and vibratory pattern of the vocal folds led the otolaryngologist to diagnose polypoid corditis. In adduction and abduction, the vocal folds moved rapidly and symmetrically with maximum abduction observed during nasal inspiration.

The SLP and otolaryngologist concluded that Patient GG in fact did have PVFD and that laryngeal control therapy

(LCT) was appropriate. Both also felt that the problem was closely related to GLPR. The otolaryngologist was concerned enough about the leukoplakia to consider biopsy but opted to delay the decision for biopsy until the patient had been on GLPR management for at least 8 weeks. Both concurred that Patient GG was moderately dysphonic with a voice characterized by abnormally low pitch and consistent use of glottal fry. The patient was unconcerned about her voice, "just as long as you didn't find any cancer."

Patient GG enrolled in LCT. The primary goals of the first session were to establish diaphragmatic breathing and to promote GLPR management. Both goals proved challenging.

The patient was extremely resistant to altering her diet in terms of content or timing. The main obstacles were the following: (1) her view that this was just something that happened in her family, a resignation to reflux inevitability; (2) she liked to cook and to eat what she cooked; (3) she felt she shouldn't change the diet she always had offered the children in her care; (4) her family, especially her husband, "would be disappointed if I change my kitchen;" and (5) she felt better after taking omeprazole for 2 weeks. The night chokes had ceased and the "fullness" in her throat was better. She preferred to continue taking a pill to altering her diet.

Over the course of 10 sessions, the SLP diplomatically revisited the GLPR issue and the desirability of using diet management; but Patient GG simply was not interested in this method. The SLP explained that diet management was important not only for GLPR management, but also for weight management given the family physician's diagnosis of obesity and hypertension with the concurrent recommendation for weight reduction. The patient acknowledged that this was good advice; however, she was "not going to live on rabbit food." The SLP also offered to arrange for a session with the institution's dietitian. Patient GG declined the opportunity.

Over the time period, the patient initially reported reduced frequency of episodes of dyspnea. Per the clinic's recommendation, her husband constructed a platform to elevate the head of their bed 6 inches. For her part, Patient GG substituted decaffeinated coffee for her second pot of the day. She also continued with 15 mg of omeprazole daily.

The daytime occurrences of shortness of breath and frequent coughing appeared to be improving. The progress was essentially associated with Patient GG identifying, altering, or eliminating those activities that tended to precede the episodes. She understood from the diagnostic session that her posture was a significant contributor to the severity of the episodes. With this in mind, she taught her children to pick up their toys. She stopped bending from the hips to pick up the children and began bending from the knees and keeping her back straight. She made no changes in diet.

Developing diaphragmatic breathing was a difficult task for Patient GG. She seemed anxious about the exercise and maintained clavicular breathing throughout the first therapy session. In the second session, she began to produce diaphragmatic breathing but not to the proficiency that the SLP felt home practice was appropriate. By the end of the third session, the SLP felt that Patient GG could perform this task adequately to assign this for home practice. This was assigned in cycles of 10 breaths (requiring about 2 minutes) for five sequences daily.

A review of Patient GG's home practice log at the start of the sixth session indicated that she seldom practiced even once daily. She felt she simply did not have the time, and she was uncomfortable practicing in front of the children. The log also revealed that her episodes were occurring 14 times daily with half of these also affected by the severe coughing. The coughing episodes were lasting approximately 10 minutes and producing nausea. The other episodes continued to be approximately 5 minutes long and had no lasting physical effects. The SLP suggested trying to make time before and after the children came for two practice sessions and to make a game of breathing in which she would teach the children to use the appropriate pattern. The SLP assured Patient GG that using relaxed diaphragmatic breathing would be healthy, not harmful, for the children.

A review of her log at the eighth session indicated that Patient GG had improved home practice to once daily, typically in the evening. At this point, she noted that the exertion-induced episodes had declined in duration to typically 2 to 3 minutes, but the frequency continued to be seven times daily on average. The episodes related to laryngospasm had not declined.

The 10th LCT session occurred just after the patient met with the otolaryngologist to determine the need for biopsy. By mirror examination, the leukoplakia and polypoid corditis had not improved. The otolaryngologist felt that biopsy was needed but offered to delay the procedure for another 8 weeks if Patient GG's attempts to control the GLPR would include modification of her diet. He also indicated that following the biopsy, the patient would be on voice rest for 5 days and would not be able to provide child care during this time.

Fear of surgery and concern over lost income induced Patient GG to accept the recommended changes in her diet. She asked the SLP to arrange for a meeting with a dietitian, and she implemented the dietary recommendations. She also began practicing her LCT exercises three times daily.

Based on these changes, the SLP scheduled therapy to occur once every 2 weeks. By the 12th session, the patient reported a dramatic decline in the frequency of laryngospasm to once or twice a day. The exertion-induced episodes remained at seven daily, but she continued to manage them well. She continued to demonstrate appropriate performance of the breathing exercises. The SLP scheduled the next session for 4 weeks later and emphasized to the patient the need to keep a good log over that period.

At the 13th session, Patient GG and the SLP reviewed the log. The exertion-induced episodes continued to occur, but the patient generally was unconcerned about them. The laryngospasms had declined to once daily, and she expressed that she could recover from these rapidly; the severe cough was gone. The SLP noted in the log a period of 3 days where the episodes increased to 4 to 5 daily. Patient GG was a little embarrassed to relate that her sister had come to town for a 3-day weekend and the family had "partied." She had gone off her diet, and, as she put it, "I had to pay the price."

A final session was conducted in conjunction with the otolaryngologist. Patient GG had been controlling her diet for more than 2 months and had been using omeprazole for more than 4 months. She was 15 pounds slimmer

and volunteered that her husband had also lost weight. She continued to experience dyspnea associated with exertion and continued to view this as unavoidable and simply bothersome. The dyspnea associated with laryngospasm and severe coughing was reduced to one brief occurrence daily.

The laryngeal examination revealed decrease in the erythema; however, the polypoid corditis and leukoplakia were still present, but not worse. Because Patient GG's laryngeal symptoms had improved, the otolaryngologist selected a strategy of watchful waiting with the patient visiting the office every 3 months over the next year to ensure early diagnosis of malignant change, should any occur.

Patient GG's case demonstrated several helpful lessons concerning PVFD treatment. The first is that many of these patients are not so much motivated to treat what they have as by what they do not have. Patient GG sought treatment because she was afraid she had some form of serious disease. She did have several serious health problems (obesity, emphysema, GLPR, PVFD), but not the ones she was most worried about (cancer and sleep apnea).

A second issue is that patients often are unwilling to change their lifestyles or to change their lifestyles further. Patient GG already had made some significant changes in her life: She ceased tobacco use, she sought medical treatment, and she enrolled in LCT. She was not motivated to make additional changes, especially in the area of diet.

A third issue is that many patients will have partial improvement in their symptoms after partial treatment of their problem. Use of omeprazole had a positive effect on this patient's breathing difficulties. Her physicians and the SLP knew that additional gains were possible, but from the patient's perspective, taking a pill once daily had already accomplished a great deal.

These three issues all conspire against progress in therapy. The patients are noncompliant in applying therapy techniques outside of the clinical settings. Their primary motivation for consulting was fear of a specific problem; once that has been relieved, they perceive that their health actually is better than they imagined. They also have the feeling that they have complied with the demands and suggestions of their health care providers. Because of their partial compliance, their main symptoms have, in fact, improved. In all this, the clinicians are challenged to find new motivation for the patient.

This new motivation may arise from educating the patients about their current health (eg, hypertension and emphysema are serious medical conditions). The SLP may challenge the patient's work ethic: "You've sacrificed and worked hard to get the improvement you've made. Let's finish the job by _____." The daily logs may prove helpful in documenting to the patient just how intrusive the breathing problem remains. For Patient GG, the resurrected fear of cancer (need for biopsy) and the possible loss of income stimulated her to greater efforts in controlling her health.

This case study also demonstrated a conundrum. Many of these patients have coexisting additional respiratory diseases or other health issues affecting respiration. For Patient GG, hypertension, emphysema, and obesity limited her respiratory function. With diet, exercise, and medication the hypertension and obesity could be controlled or elim-

inated. The emphysema or chronic obstructive pulmonary disease born of too many cigarettes over too many years is unlikely to improve, even with smoking cessation. As a result, LCT holds the promise of improving the patient's respiration, but not of restoring it to normal.

Neither PVFD nor the model of treatment for it is complex. By education and inclination, the SLP is prepared to contribute substantially to the management of this problem. The patients with PVFD are the sources of complexity. They challenge the SLP with the vagaries, strengths, weaknesses, habits, and injuries of their personalities and lifestyles. The adept clinician confronts these factors in any caseload and finds the greatest personal and professional rewards in aiding the most complex patients to improve.

> *In the next case, Michael Trudeau and Jennifer Thompson discuss the treatment of a PVCD case with multiple etiologic factors.*

Management of PVCD with Functional Aphonia: Considering a Psychogenic Factor in Treatment

Michael Trudeau, PhD, and Jennifer Thompson, MA

Case Study: Patient HH

HH was a 46-year-old Caucasian female with a 4-year history of severe, chronic breathing difficulties and intermittent aphonia. At the time of HH's visit, she had been whispering for the past 10 weeks, and stridor was present with both phases of the respiratory cycle. Dyspnea was chronically present, but increased with even slight physical activity. Although she stated that she truly enjoyed her occupation as a respiratory therapist, her present respiratory and phonatory difficulties made it hard for her to carry out duties and so she had been away from work for several weeks.

The patient was a smoker of more than 20 years and currently was at 2.5 packs per day. Likewise, her caffeine habit was significant at six colas per day and several cups of coffee; but with limited water intake (2–3 cups/day). Otherwise, HH would be classified as an average-sized, middle class woman. She reported a generally good marriage with a supportive husband.

At the onset of HH's complaints 4 years prior, paradoxical vocal fold dysfunction was diagnosed via videonasendoscopy at a different facility. Per her report, findings at that time were also consistent with chronic gastrolaryngopharyngeal reflux. Symptoms including dyspnea, dysphonia, globus, and throat clearing had emerged 7 years before the initial assessment.

When HH lost her 17-year-old son unexpectedly in a motor vehicle accident, the shortness of breath and voice loss both increased in severity and began to interfere with the patient's abilities to functional professionally and socially. Per her account, her son had an argument with his girlfriend. On the way home, he lost control of the car and hit a telephone pole just hundreds of yards from their home. The telephone pole crushed the vehicle. HH and her son, her only child, were "buddies." She did not share much information about the whereabouts of her husband at the time but she was careful during the interview process to mention that he was supportive.

Because there was such a strong stress and anxiety component to HH's symptoms, psychologic counseling was suggested as the primary treatment strategy at her initial assessment. Prior to that time, the patient had never sought treatment for her complaints. Over the next 4 years, HH proceeded to see several psychiatrists who, per HH's report, simply prescribed anxiolytics to assist with the anxiety and antidepressants. The patient expressed frustration that none of the counselors helped her "work through" her grief and suffering from losing her son. HH eventually overdosed on the medications because the pain of her son's death was too much to bear. She decided to completely stop taking antidepressants after surviving the overdose.

HH had never been to the emergency room for her complaints; however, she visited several clinics for assistance and tracheotomy was suggested on several occasions. HH was a respiratory therapist and refused this mode of treatment each time.

Pulmonary testing was completed but it was unremarkable much to HH's and her family's surprise. Her family members and friends were growing more and more concerned about her condition. To accommodate them, she decided to pursue possible treatment of her complaints once again.

Following consultation with an ENT close to her home, primarily for voice loss, she was referred to the clinic (an hour drive from her residence) for a videolaryngoscopy with stroboscopy (VLS) examination to potentially identify the nature of her voice loss. As previously mentioned, when HH arrived for her appointment, she was whispering and had audible stridor with both phases of respiration.

VLS revealed near total glottic closure during both phases of respiration at rest. There was full ventricular fold compression during phonation of sustained pitches and also during laryngeal valving tasks. In an attempt to assess vocal fold mobility and to probe for effectiveness of laryngeal control therapy, the clinician coached HH through nasal inhalation and blowing exhalation. One long nasal inspiration yielded little to no improvement in glottic opening. Short multiple sniffs through the nose showed that the vocal folds were mobile bilaterally and glottic opening did improve with application of this technique. Likewise, pulsing air through pursed lips for exhalation gave way to glottic opening. These findings suggested (1) severe PVFD and (2) mobile vocal folds with no signs of paresis or paralysis.

Given HH's occupational background, she was already familiar with laryngeal landmarks and the desired positioning of the vocal folds during respiration. It was with this in mind that HH was encouraged to look at the video monitor and observe her own vocal fold activity on the screen throughout the remainder of the VLS. The clinician encouraged HH to maintain continuous airflow by applying the effective techniques. She was very encouraged to see that vocal fold abduction was achieved and that she could maintain an open airway with concentration on the technique.

Once glottic opening was continuous during respiration, the clinician continued using the VLS as biofeedback to attempt production of voice. HH was coached to hum. Humming provided false vocal fold retraction and allowed for free vibratory movement of the vocal folds and therefore voice production. Resonant voice exercises were applied

during this portion of the examination to establish phonation. The vocal folds had a full and erythemic appearance consistent with HH's deep pitched voice. There was interarytenoid pachyderma and severe edema of the postcricoid area and bilateral arytenoid complexes. This portion of the examination and biofeedback suggested that (1) HH had polypoid corditis that was likely from smoking and (2) her report of being "unable to talk" was functional in nature as there was no paralysis or paresis and phonation was achieved.

The speech-language pathologist staffed the case with the otolaryngologist following the examination. The two concluded that HH's conditions were primarily functional in nature, but that HH's smoking and gastrolaryngopharyngeal reflux contributed to the heightened sensitivity and her facile airway protection response. Both also surmised that the laryngeal irritants probably served as physiologic triggers for the functional aphonia and PVFD. The otolaryngologist suggested regular sessions of biofeedback for both PVFD and voice. He concurred with the recommendation for grief counseling. He requested consistent updates on the laryngeal health of HH because the speech-language pathologist would have frequent opportunities to view the patient's phonatory mechanism. The otolaryngologist also offered to review pharmacologic options for aiding in smoking cessation; however, HH declined the offer, indicating a preference for "going cold turkey."

HH was encouraged to enroll simultaneously in laryngeal control and voice therapies with biofeedback using the flexible nasendoscope. Otherwise, she was advised to work toward smoking cessation and to observe a diet low in acid-inducing foods. Grief counseling was strongly suggested because it appeared that her laryngeal findings likely were functional and tied to the death of her son. HH agreed to seek counseling with the speech pathologist's assistance to find an appropriate match. Likewise, she agreed to enroll in regular weekly sessions of biofeedback despite the 60-minute drive to the clinic.

Several sessions of biofeedback were conducted following the initial VLS. Sessions concentrated primarily on PVFD as HH felt the resonant voice exercises always assisted with return of normal voicing. During the biofeedback sessions for PVFD, HH concentrated on establishing laryngeal abduction using the practiced breathing techniques when several triggers were applied: physical activity including lifting, pushing and pulling, and exposure to strong scents. Each situation was replicated in the clinic while the patient observed her vocal fold activity on the screen. Activity was completed using a stationary bike. HH was also exposed to several strong scents to manage dyspnea triggered by noxious agents. Perhaps her greatest trigger was lifting and moving patients while at work. To simulate this situation, HH lifted a graduate student from the examination chair while watching her vocal fold movement on the video monitor. With each situation, HH's goal was to maintain abducted vocal folds throughout each activity.

HH showed greater management as she progressed through biofeedback sessions. Her voice was more stable than it had been for months by performing resonant voice exercises each morning. She returned to work soon after the initial session, and she maintained her typical work load even though it required heavy lifting and moving of patients. In effort to relieve her symptoms, HH

even reduced her smoking habit from 2.5 packs per day down to 1 pack. Hydration was still poor in terms of water intake versus coffee and soda consumption. She felt this was a "good compromise" for the reduction in smoking. Her PPI regimen, prescribed after the initial videoendoscopy 4 years ago, was already at maximal dosage so she simply continued the regimen. She also continued to see her counselor on a weekly basis (again despite the long drive), and she felt she made more progress emotionally in those few short weeks than she had since her son passed away several years prior.

After some time, HH's symptoms worsened at the same time of year that her son died. Although the otolaryngologist was regularly updated on HH's case, she was encouraged to continue seeing her ENT at home. When her complaints, including dyspnea and near aphonia, returned and worsened, the otolaryngologists suggested BOTOX as a treatment strategy. When the day for the injection came, the otolaryngologist decided against the procedure considering the strong emotional nature of her conditions, especially the PVFD. As is the case with initial trials of BOTOX, there is the risk that one's voice will become breathy. The otolaryngologist felt there was potential that HH would respond to this functionally and experience a setback with her vocal progress. Instead of the injection, the physician suggested re-enrollment in biofeedback and continued consultation with the psychologist.

HH's case highlights many important applications for improvement or resolution of PVFD. Commonly, the cause of PVFD is not solitary. Several patients' contributors are multifactorial just as HH's were. Many patients with PVFD can benefit from laryngeal control therapy alone; however, treatment of the root cause of their condition is of primary importance whether it is emotionally/psychologically based, medically based, or environmentally based.

It is clear in HH's case that the death of her son was the strongest trigger for symptoms. The stress produced behaviors (ie, smoking and poor diet decisions) that led to increased laryngeal irritation and, in turn, worsened PVFD. This cycle demanded an extensive treatment process that required a determination to change on HH's part, both psychologically and behaviorally. Pharmacologic and medical management also were required for the duration of her treatment. HH's case demonstrated the complexity of PVFD, the complexity of the treatment of PVFD for all professionals involved, and the need for interdisciplinary management.

When treating clients with PVFD, it is important for the speech-language pathologist to be creative in developing an effective and customized behavioral plan with various modes of feedback for each patient to identify with and benefit from. The speech-language pathologist also needs to recognize that a multidisciplinary approach is required for a patient. Often, PVFD is a secondary condition and it does not resolve until other medical or emotional conditions are treated. The speech-language pathologist often finds that the greatest contribution to a patient's care lies in encouraging and making appropriate referrals.

In the following series of cases, Mary Sandage, Edie Swift, and Mary Andrianopoulos discuss the treatment of PVCD in young athletes. The cases demonstrate how treatment is tailored not only to the individual, but also to the specific sport in question.

Treatment of PVCD in a Collegiate Swimmer

Mary J. Sandage, MA, CCC-SLP

Case Study: Patient II

For treatment of an 18-year-old college freshman swimmer, Mary Sandage uses information gathered from the behavioral and medical interview and the dynamic endoscopic laryngeal assessment to develop a patient-specific breathing modification program to help this patient overcome the paradoxical vocal fold motion (PVFM) events experienced while swimming competitively. Counseling for behavioral and diet changes to reduce laryngopharyngeal reflux (LPR) was also a component of the treatment plan.

Patient History. Patient II, an 18-year-old college freshman on a swim scholarship, was referred to the speech-language pathologist by her pulmonologist and sports medicine physician for an assessment to rule out paradoxical vocal fold motion (PVFM). The pulmonologist's assessment had resulted in a negative methacholine challenge, negative chest X-ray, and spirometry that indicated a flat inspiratory flow volume loop consistent with extrathoracic obstruction during inhalation. The swim team physician had referred Patient II to the pulmonologist for a thorough pulmonary assessment to better manage asthma, diagnosed 2 years earlier by the patient's pediatrician. When it was determined that Patient II did not have asthma, the treating physicians determined that the patient might have PVFM.

Patient II attended the initial speech-language pathology evaluation by herself and served as the sole reporter for her behavioral and medical history. She described some confusion about the referral to a speech-language pathologist (SLP), as she did not believe that she had any difficulty with her speech or language. It was explained that the evaluating SLP specialized in breathing disorders in athletes and worked closely with pulmnologist and sports medicine physicians.

Patient II described a successful high school swimming career with subsequent recruitment to an excellent collegiate swimming program. During high school, she typically competed in the 200- and 400-meter freestyle. During her first season of collegiate swimming, her new coach targeted her training and competition for the 200-meter freestyle. Patient II reported intermittent breathing problems during swimming for about 3 years with a diagnosis of asthma 2 years prior to her referral to the Voice Clinic. The patient described her first year on a collegiate swim team as challenging and stressful and described anxiety about losing her scholarship if her breathing problem was not resolved quickly. Patient II indicated that she set high personal goals for herself, both academically and athletically, and her ultimate goal was to make the USA Olympic Swim Team.

The patient's medical history was remarkable for diagnosed allergies to pollen, mold, and dust mites, the primary symptoms of which included nasal congestion and sneezing. The patient had no other diagnosed medical conditions. She denied any surgical history and indicated that she did not smoke or drink alcohol. When asked about symptoms of laryngopharyngeal reflux (LPR), Patient II indicated that she experienced a persistent globus sensation and often cleared her throat secondary to a perception of phlegm in her throat. She attributed the throat irritation to her history of allergies. Patient II described some nausea and acidy burps before and during swim meets, for which she took over-the-counter antacids. The patient reported that she took birth control pills and over-the-counter allergy medication when her allergies were bothering her. Albuterol, a rescue inhaler, had been prescribed for her to take when she experienced asthma attacks.

When asked about her eating habits, Patient II indicated that she frequently ate a high protein snack before practice (eg, peanut butter sandwich), and she also snacked before bed. She described drinking about four to five carbonated, caffeinated beverages per day as well as sports drinks during and after practice.

Socially, Patient II described an atypical college experience secondary to swim team practices both before and after classes. She reported that she didn't have much of a social life; however, she indicated that she had close friends on the swim team. She also described missing her family, who lived about 11 hours away.

History of the Problem. The client was first asked to describe the nature of the breathing difficulty with as much detail as possible. To avoid leading the patient in a particular direction, open-ended questions were asked with the goal of discerning the exact nature of her unique breathing difficulties. Examples of the questions asked with a summary of each response are as follows:

> *Tell me about your breathing attacks in as much detail as possible.*
>
> The breathing difficulty generally occurred during timed trials in practice and in competition when she was swimming the 200-meter freestyle. She reported that the first 100 meters of the race went well; however, she noticed more difficulty breathing during the last

100 meters. She described that she wasn't able to get enough air and, as a result, her times were slower than those that she had achieved in practice.

How often do these attacks happen?

At first, they happened occasionally; however, by the time of the evaluation, they were occurring every time she was being timed in practice and in competition.

Are your breathing attacks during swimming like asthma attacks?

The patient thought that the breathing difficulties were asthma attacks that were not getting better with medicine.

When you are having a breathing attack, do you have trouble breathing in, breathing out, or both?

Patient II reported that she always had trouble inhaling and no trouble exhaling.

Do you make a noise when you are having trouble breathing?

The patient indicated that she didn't think she made any noise, but she wasn't sure.

Do you notice any tightness in your body when you are having trouble breathing?

Patient II described that she noticed some tightness in her upper torso, but mainly in her throat.

When the race is over, what happens with your breathing?

She indicated that she took her rescue inhaler as soon as she got out of the pool and her breathing seemed better within a couple of minutes.

Does anything help your breathing get better?

Patient II indicated that the only thing that really made the breathing problem better was to stop swimming and take her inhaler.

Is your breathing difficulty getting worse, getting better, or staying the same?

The patient reported that it slowly worsened over the course of the season and that, at the time of the evaluation, she had trouble every time she was being timed or in competition.

Do you ever get short of breath with other forms of physical exertion, such as climbing a flight of stairs?

The patient indicated that her breathing difficulties were confined to the contexts already described. She also denied any difficulty breathing at night.

Can you describe how you generally breathe during the 200 meter freestyle when you are not having any trouble?

She reported that she took a breath about two strokes before a turn and then again when she resurfaced after a turn. She also indicated that her coach didn't care how many strokes she put between each breath as long as she continued to improve her times. Her coach encouraged her to try to avoid taking a breath during the last 50 meters of the race. This latter direction was new, per client report, and she described feeling a lot of pressure to achieve this benchmark.

When you are swimming as fast as you can in the 200-meter freestyle, do you hold your breath until you need another breath or do you let the air out while swimming?

The patient reported that she generally held her breath and then let it out as fast as she could before turning her head to take another breath.

Evaluation Procedures. Patient II received a standard assessment for suspected PVFM. The assessments included:

1. *Auditory-perceptual assessment.* The patient's voice quality was judged as clear by the evaluating clinician using both informal and formal methods. During conversation, the evaluating SLP did not discern any voice disturbances. The Consensus Auditory-Perceptual Evaluation of Voice (CAPE-V)[39] was used as a formal voice quality assessment, the findings of which were consistent with the informal assessment described.
2. *Visual-perceptual assessment.* The structure and function of the patient's upper airway were assessed using a flexible nasal endoscope, which was carefully advanced through the patient's nostril after application of topical nasal anesthetic. The flexible endoscope was advanced through the nasopharynx, and the tip of the endoscope was positioned with complete view of the laryngeal structure during resting breathing and breathing maneuvers. Initially, the patient's larynx was observed during several cycles of rest breathing to allow the patient to get used to the endoscope and to allow the evaluating SLP to observe the behavior of the upper airway during unstressed rest breathing. Frequent "twitching" of the arytenoids cartilages during resting breathing was observed with a patent airway during both inspiration and expiration. The tissue of the membranous vocal folds appeared smooth but somewhat edematous bilaterally, characterized by infraglottic edema bilaterally, which was observed during maximum abduction. Additionally, posterior laryn-geal edema and interarytenoid tissue changes were observed, consistent with clinical signs for laryngopharyngeal reflux.

The patient then was asked to quickly take a maximum inhalation then exhale quickly and completely through the mouth, during which the patient was observed to narrow the vocal folds about 50% to 60% of the width of the glottis during inhalation. Given that the referring pulmonologist had ruled out asthma (asthma is a contraindication for panting, which can trigger an asthma attack), the patient was asked to pant, during which the arytenoids cartilages were also observed to "twitch."

At this point in the endoscopic assessment, the patient was asked to view the screen and the patient was oriented to the anatomical structures of her larynx. While watching the screen, the patient was asked if she could imitate what a breathing attack felt like. Her reproduction of the feeling of throat tightness during inhalation resulted in near complete vocal fold adduction, with no production of stridor but obvious glottal narrowing. The patient was able to match the perception of throat tightness with the image of glottal narrowing. The patient was then asked to sniff in deeply through her nose and then exhale out of her mouth. Patient II was able to observe her larynx rapidly lower and widely abduct during the sniff and then remain open during exhalation. Again, the patient was able to match the physical sensation of the open throat with the visual image of the open glottis. Finally, the patient was asked to sip air in through a narrow mouth opening, as if sipping through a straw, with subsequent wide abduction of the glottis during inspiration.

For purposes of visual feedback and to strengthen the subsequent training of the breathing recovery exercises, the patient was asked to imitate what a breathing attack felt like and then perform the sip inhale on the following breath to simulate application of the breathing recovery method.

The dynamic endoscopic laryngeal assessment was reviewed with an otolaryngologist who concurred with the observation of clinical signs of laryngopharyngeal reflux disease and ruled out other laryngeal obstruction or disease.

Description and Rationale for Therapy Approach. The patient's pulmonary and otolaryngology assessments ruled out medical diagnoses that are part of the differential diagnosis for PVFM (eg, pulmonary disease [including asthma], subglottic stenosis, bilateral vocal fold paralysis, laryngeal mass lesion, unresolved laryngomalacia, etc). Key medical assessment information supporting the diagnosis of PVFM included the negative methacholine challenge and the flow-volume loop showing a truncated inspiratory loop only with no expiratory obstruction. Additionally, the account that her breathing difficulties resolved only a couple of minutes after taking her rescue inhaler signaled that her difficulty was not asthma—the rescue inhaler would not have worked that quickly per the pulmonologist report. The medical information in combination with the patient's description and imitation of the breathing "attacks" as well as the information gleaned from the dynamic endoscopic assessment assured the evaluating clinician that the

patient likely had PVFM and it would be safe to proceed with counseling and behavioral intervention.

The treatment program designed for Patient II consisted of the following: counseling the patient about the differences between asthma and PVFM and offering a theoretic framework to understand why these breathing attacks may have occurred; counseling regarding dietary and behavioral changes that may improve symptoms of LPR; training of breathing recovery exercises adapted for swimming; and implementation of a step-by-step application of the recovery exercises to swimming with the ultimate goal of total elimination of the breathing attacks.

Goal 1. Counsel the patient about the differential diagnosis of PFVM and describe a theoretical framework to understand the physiologic triggers for the events.

Rationale. Many patients who carry the diagnosis of asthma and then are suddenly told that they never had asthma in the first place are reluctant to drop the asthma mantle. Detailed descriptions of the physiological differences between the two diagnoses, differences between triggers, and, finally, differences in treatment approaches are important components to include. Counseling also can help patients understand that the breathing attack is not their fault and they have control over the difficulty. For this patient, stress may have played a role, but it was clear that there was a probable physiologic trigger from untreated LPR. Understanding the role that LPR as a trigger helped focus the patient on a systemic approach to recovery.

Counseling for Patient II started with the visual feedback provided during the endoscopic assessment, empowering her to see that she had at least two strategies for getting her throat open during inhalation, either via a deep, quick nasal sniff or during a sip inhale through her lips. The visual feedback also assisted the patient in pairing the physical perception of throat tightness with narrowed vocal folds, demonstrating how the breathing recovery exercises would reverse the glottal narrowing that characterized her PFVM events. Finally, the whole process of describing PVFM, the typical triggers for it, and treatment approaches, helped the patient overcome her initial confusion about the role of the SLP.

Goal 2. The patient will make dietary and behavioral changes to reduce the symptoms of laryngopharyngeal reflux (LPR).

Rationale. Given that the patient described symptoms of LPR and the endoscopic assessment indicated clinical signs of the same, counseling Patient II about behavioral and dietary changes to reduce LPR was appropriate. Given that she was an elite athlete with a rigorous training regime to follow, the guidelines established to reduce LPR needed to extend beyond the type of counseling that the average voice patient received. A list of foods that can exacerbate reflux was reviewed, and the patient was asked to avoid the following foods until her breathing attacks were well controlled: chocolate, nuts/peanut butter, carbonated and caffeinated drinks, fried food, onions, spicy foods, and high fat foods. Because the patient required a lot of calories to sustain her physical activity, the patient was asked to refrain from high fat foods only prior to practice and bedtime. The patient's medical team

prescribed medication for LPR, and the evaluating SLP worked with the physicians to make sure that Patient II timed her medication delivery to get maximum coverage while swimming.

Goal 3. Train a breathing recovery program with special adaptations for the elite swimmer.

Rationale. With all other obstructive conditions ruled out, counseling regarding the condition completed, and medical/behavioral management of LPR initiated, it was safe to train a breathing recovery program with a measure of confidence that the breathing strategies would be successful in remediating Patient II's breathing difficulties in the pool.

The breathing recovery program typically used by the evaluating clinician included three basic steps: body awareness, establishment of lower torso/belly breathing, and training of a quick, deep nasal sniff followed by complete exhale through the mouth. The first of these three steps, training body awareness, was appropriate for this patient without much adaptation. The progressive awareness tasks, a combination of progressive relaxation and mindfulness were trained, and the patient was directed to complete the exercise at least twice daily when not at swim practice.

The second step of the program, establishment of lower torso/belly breathing, was not appropriate for the patient to use in the pool. Most swimmers are coached to maintain a "streamlined" position in the pool, which translates to a perfectly straight spine with limited chest excursion during inhalation and tight abdominal muscles. The goal of the streamlined position is to create a body silhouette whereby the shoulders cut through the water first with little or no drag created by chest or abdominal excursion. To train belly breathing with a swimmer might actually slow her down instead of speeding her up in the pool. Additionally, counseling the patient to pursue a physical profile that was in direct disagreement with her coach's training may have undermined the SLP's ability to successfully engage the coach in the generalization process.

The third goal of the breathing recovery program (the quick, deep nasal sniff in, followed by the slow, complete exhale) required significant adaptation for this patient. Although many swimmers are able to learn to do the deep nasal sniff while swimming competitively, the ability to learn and apply this depends on the distance and stroke performed. It also requires patent nasal passages while swimming. Patient II competes at the middle distance 200-meter freestyle, a stroke that requires her face to be in the water most of the time while taking as few breaths as possible for the fastest time. Given that she described nasal congestion as a symptom of her intermittent allergies, it was more appropriate to train the quick "straw" sip method of inhalation. The patient was trained to purse her lips, as if sipping through a straw, draw air in quickly and completely, and then follow the inhalation with a complete exhalation out of her mouth. Complete exhalation during practice breathing while out of the pool was critical to avoid hyperventilation and the sensation of light-headedness.

During swimming, the patient described that after taking a breath, she held it and then rapidly exhaled just before taking another breath. The tension in her throat from this breath holding habit may have contributed to extraneous neck tension; therefore, she was asked to

stop holding her breath and exhale over a period of time leading up to her next breath to allow for greater inhalation. This last direction was discussed with the patient's coach, and he concurred that this change should translate into improved swim performance.

Patient II was asked to perform an appropriate repeat demonstration of the two exercises trained during the initial evaluation. She was asked to practice both steps two to three times per day, when not at swim practice, so that she could focus on the recovery exercise and make it automatic. Patient II was asked to focus on the sensation in her throat to discern when it felt tight and when it felt open. She also was asked to avoid breath holding between the inhalation and the exhalation. The exercises were assigned and the patient was scheduled to return in 1 week, at which time a plan would be established to generalize the new behaviors to the pool.

Goal 4. The patient will apply the recovery exercises in the pool, gradually working up to race speed, timed trials and, finally, competition.

Rationale. The application of the recovery exercise to elite sport required a structured step-by-step approach to support the athlete in generalizing to the pool what was relatively easy to do while sitting in a chair in the therapy room or at home. The cardiopulmonary requirements of swimming the 200-meter freestyle far exceeded those required for the therapy room. Finally, the specificity requirement for training a new physical skill required that the exercises be generalized to a pool environment while employing the freestyle stroke.

For Patient II, the generalization program started on land, using a treadmill to increase the cardiopulmonary load and require Patient II to coordinate the breathing recovery exercise at increasingly higher oxygen requirements. After the patient experienced success applying the recovery exercise in a greater oxygen demand context, the generalization process quickly moved to the pool environment in the third therapy session. Using a lane away from the swim team, Patient II was instructed to swim slowly, incorporating the recovery exercise with her stroke. Some time was spent at this stage while Patient II learned to coordinate the extended exhale before the head turn and "straw" sip for inhalation. Patient II quickly adapted the inhalation pattern but had more difficulty stopping the breath-holding, a practice that she had started when she was a young swimmer. Given that the straw-sip inhalation would not provide enough oxygen for a middle distance elite swimmer, Patient II was directed to reserve the straw-sip inhalation for the point in the race when she typically would experience throat tightness. Because Patient II knew the distance in the race at which the breathing attack typically occurred, she could start the recovery exercise before this and completely avoid the attack. After two therapy sessions at poolside, a baseline of success was established with the new breathing strategies and the patient's coach and trainer completed the remainder of the generalization.

Results of Therapy. Patient II received four sessions of therapy over the course of 1 month and attended one follow-up session 1 month following discharge from treatment. At the final clinic visit, approximately 8 weeks after her initial diagnosis, Patient II reported that she no longer experienced any breathing difficulty when competing at the 200-meter freestyle. She also described that she was gradually able to avoid the throat tightness completely and had recently started swimming successfully without the straw-sip inhalation. She was most excited to report she had steadily improved her race time. Her disposition during the clinic visit was optimistic, and she no longer reported anxiety about keeping her athletic scholarship.

The outcome of therapy was attributed to the patient's high level of motivation and compliance with the combination of medical management for LPR, the presumed physiologic trigger for the events, as well as the breathing training. The support of the patient's family and the coaching staff were also key contributors to her rapid recovery.

Management of PVCD: A Collegiate Basketball Player

Edie Swift, MA

Case Study: Patient JJ

The number of patients referred for treatment of paradoxical vocal fold motion (PVFM) has increased dramatically since publication of the classic article by Christopher, Wood, Eckert, Blager, Raney, and Souhrada.[27] This group used endoscopy and pulmonary function testing to describe paradoxical closure of the larynx during periods of respiratory distress. Inspection of the literature also suggests numerous etiologic possibilities. These include reflux,[40,41] sexual abuse,[42] laryngospasm,[40] exercise-induced asthma,[43] a sequela to laryngomalacia,[44] midbrain malformation,[45] somatization,[46] and malingering.[45] This diversity of etiologic possibilities supports the concept that this may be a multifactorial condition with a spectrum of severity and complexity.

An interesting and rewarding subgroup of patients with PVFM is the young athlete. Patient JJ is a recent example. The pediatrician/sports medicine specialist referred the patient to the voice clinic. The specialist was questioning whether part of her difficulty was PVFM. Patient JJ came on scholarship as a highly recruited basketball player. She obviously had been very successful in high school and had no problem breathing at that level of competition. Since entering the university, however, she had been dealing with shortness of breath that had escalated in severity. Her first episode was during a one-on-one practice observed by the varsity coach. The patient described this particular aspect of the practice routine as the most strenuous and stressful because she was evaluated by and against her peers. As this initial episode progressed, she simply left the court for a few minutes and felt better. When she returned, however, she again had trouble breathing. Subsequently she began experiencing difficulty with every practice and was beginning to dread practice. The basketball season was only 1 month away.

Patient JJ had received no formal allergy testing and no pulmonary function testing at the time of her initial visit. This made the diagnostic session difficult because her medical baseline was unclear, and she was in no respiratory distress. A careful history revealed that the only episodes of shortness of breath she had experienced outside of practice were at night when she had awakened gasping for air. This was becoming a weekly occurrence. Patient JJ described frequent stomach aches that she thought were secondary to anxiety about her breathing. It also became

clear, however, that she had a chaotic eating schedule. She indicated that dorm food was a significant dietary change and that she was now eating late in the evening after she finished studying. She noted that her general level of anxiety was increasing. As mentioned, she was beginning to dread practice but also was afraid of a possible major illness and concerned that the coaches would limit her playing time. She was aware that the associated anxiety was worsening the problem.

The initial diagnostic session concluded by asking Patient JJ to begin a log describing the first symptoms she experienced and exactly what she did in response. Observations were structured by suggesting she note any throat tightness, air hunger, light-headedness, or premonitory sensation. This information was used both to structure her practice and to improve her awareness. The panic associated with shortness of breath often makes self-assessment difficult, and it is necessary to train patient perceptions to help initiate alternative breathing patterns.

A flexible fiberoptic endoscopy was deferred until it could be combined with pulmonary function testing. Rigid endoscopy revealed an erythemic area on the superior surface of both arytenoids and on the posterior folds inferior to the arytenoids. There were vascular markings running the length of the superior surface of both vocal folds and considerable thick tenacious mucus throughout the glottis. Otherwise, nothing remarkable was observed. The film was reviewed with an otolaryngologist who felt there was evidence of gastroesophageal reflux disease (GERD), which was consistent with the patient's history. During his examination, the otolaryngologist also observed evidence of allergic rhinitis. The follow-up conference with the referring physician resulted in a trial treatment for GERD (Prilosec 20 mg bid), and referrals to the allergy clinic and to a pulmonologist who could perform pulmonary function testing in combination with exercise. Testing was arranged so that Patient JJ's larynx could be observed with the flexible fiberoptic endoscope immediately following exercise. It was agreed that this exercise would be extended until she reported feeling typical symptoms. With athletes, this can be a long test, and she was no exception. All pulmonary function tests, with the exception of a flat inspiratory flow-volume curve, fell within the expected range. The flexible fiberoptic observation showed clear evidence of PVFM. The aberrant movements were videotaped, and she was able to observe the behavior. Allergy testing and the initiation of therapy were scheduled within the following week.

Therapy Program. The initial session began with a review of the diagnostic videotape and the mechanics of the larynx. Instruction regarding behavioral changes was divided into three modules. The first was to teach relaxation exercises. The intent was not to maintain the relaxation of muscles because she would certainly not be relaxed during competition. The goal was to make her as aware as possible of any relative increase in tension of various muscle groups, particularly those in her chest and neck. It is important to be able to identify the first signs of trouble because intervention is more effective if initiated as early as possible. Classic progressive relaxation lends itself well to this program because it provides an opportunity to perceive both maximum tension and maximum relaxation.

The second module involved teaching "abdominal" breathing. During this first session, the goal was to teach the fundamental concept of breathing while relaxing the upper body. During the inspiratory phase, the patient is directed to first expand the abdomen and then the rib cage. The shoulders and neck stay relaxed. This adaptation is founded, in part, on breath management techniques described in the Italianate school of classical singing voice described by Miller.[47] Tactile feedback supplied by the placement of hands or use of thin rubber sheeting at the targeted levels of expansion seemed to make this easier for her. She was started in a reclining position but asked to practice at home while both standing and sitting. Practice was done using only oral (not nasal) inhalation and exhalation. There were two considerations that contributed to the therapy decisions made with respect to respiration: Patient JJ used oral breathing during maximum exercise, and competition often required her to bend from the waist, making the more traditional approach to "abdominal breathing" impractical.

The third component of the initial session was to teach firm nasal inhalation, or "sniffing," as her release mechanism. "Release" here refers to a situation in which the larynx is consciously moved toward controlled abduction. A sniff is an excellent example of the fine coordination of the various parts of the respiratory apparatus. It can be viewed as an exaggerated inspiration. The velum drops as the larynx lowers and opens widely as air is sucked into the lungs. The mechanism is easily explained by a basic principle of physics: Air flows from areas of positive pressure to areas of negative pressure. For air to be sniffed through the nasal passage where it is warmed and humidified (therefore less irritating), the larynx rapidly lowers while simultaneously opening to its maximum position. The rapid downward deflection causes a Bernoulli effect, pulling the air left in its wake into the lungs. Thus, in one swift movement, air moves from outside the body into the lungs. Sniffing is one of the easiest of maneuvers to teach as a method of inhalation that overcomes the abnormal movement patterns. Other techniques that have proved helpful include manually lowering the larynx, which mirrors the motion associated with inhalation and sniffing, albeit much slower. Laryngeal reposturing sometimes act as a trigger for inhalation, much as opening the mouth widely can trigger a yawn. Finally, for Patient JJ, shallow panting for a few cycles was effective but had to be carefully monitored to prevent her from beginning to hyperventilate. The technique could not have been used if she had asthma because panting in asthmatics may cause the airway to narrow. With Patient JJ, as with most athletes, the most successful technique was sniffing combined with three firm inhalations or one extended inhalation.

The allergy testing had indicated increased responsively to both dust and mold. The otolaryngologist and allergist agreed that a steroid nasal spray was appropriate for her. Patient JJ had begun using this, but at the end of the first week, she was still somewhat congested, making nasal inhalation more difficult. She therefore was given a SinuCleanse nasal irrigation system that used buffered hypertonic saline solution to help clear congestion from the nose. It was suggested that she continue to use this prior to using the nasal spray. She was asked to be sure that nasal inhalation duplicated oral inhalation so that the air easily inflated the lung visibly, expanding the abdominal area without concomitant tightening at the neck and shoulders. Patient JJ was encouraged to monitor the neck and abdominal movements in a mirror during home practice. The exhalation following either oral or nasal inhalation had to be oral and slow. Six seconds was her typical goal for home practice even though it obviously would be faster during play. She was told not to try to use this breathing pattern during basketball practice until it was clear both to the clinician and patient that she had all three areas of practice under control.

Treatment Session 2. Patient JJ's practice routine appeared to be going well. Generally, a wonderful thing about working with athletes is that they have great faith in their ability to control their bodies, as well as remarkable discipline. Discussion about how to carry home practice over into basketball was initiated. Basketball presents special challenges because the player often is not only bent at the waist but also has multiple cognitive demands. Additionally, unlike running or swimming, it is not a "rhythmic" sport. In home practice, relaxation is a foundation for perception of relaxed and effective respiration, and oral "abdominal" breathing is a foundation for nasal inhalation. In an actual episode of shortness of breath, the patient begins with nasal inhalation, monitors any muscle tension of the neck, and then switches to deep oral breathing. The patient then mentally scans his or her body for the need to relax or adjust and continues with oral breathing and the game.

Patient JJ was asked to work alone in the gym with her trainer and one teammate. They were instructed to begin playing slowly, and the patient was to focus more on her respiration than on her basketball skills. They continued to escalate physical demands until she noticed some tightening and then used three or four cycles of nasal inhalation with slow oral exhalation to gain control of her breathing. She was instructed to slow her play as much as needed to accomplish control but not to stop play unless she could not achieve respiratory control. Because this first gym session went well, she pushed herself harder in a second session but waited for two successful trials before rejoining the team.

Treatment Session 3. Patient JJ returned 2 weeks later, feeling very optimistic about her progress. She reported that she now realized she had been tolerating a low-grade nausea during practice that had now stopped. She attributed her lack of nausea to her change in diet and to the Prilosec. It is common for athletes to disregard negative feedback from their bodies as something to be "dealt with" because injuries are, in fact, common. Patient JJ also felt that learning to use a "deeper" breathing pattern was helping as much as "sniffing," which she used only if she felt she was losing control. Confidence in the effectiveness of any release mechanism is always a component of success. She had experienced success during her gym session and had not needed to use sniffing in over a week. Her evaluation of its reduced importance was viewed as a positive indicator of her progress.

Treatment Sessions 4 and 5. Patient JJ was seen in the clinic only twice more. Unfortunately, there is a tendency among many patients to stop therapy too soon, sometimes in response to HMO pressures and sometimes because

progress seems to come so easily. Although Patient JJ appeared to reach success by the end of the third session, prior experience with other patients with PVFM suggested additional sessions were needed to reinforce the improved respiratory control. As with other athletes, Patient JJ was advised to continue to home practice of respiratory control throughout her competitive season.

This patient's story is a common one. Effective, interdisciplinary diagnosis and the cooperation of a variety of professionals were needed for successful treatment. Although Patient JJ did not require psychological counseling to deal with her anxiety, a number of other athletes have found this an invaluable part of their treatment. It was a pleasure to follow her athletic career in the newspaper. During her sophomore year, she was a regular contributor to the team. Although risking the violation of the athletes' first rule, "never call a shutout," we are aware of only one high-level performing athlete who has been unable to return to the previous level of competition after treatment for PVFM.

Treatment of PVCD: A Young Athlete with Associated Psychosocial Contributions

Mary V. Andrianopoulos, PhD

Case Study: Patient KK

Patient History. Patient KK was a 16-year-old young woman referred by her primary care physician for evaluation and treatment of chronic, progressive "respiratory attacks" and possible "laryngeal dysfunction" of indeterminate origin. The mother of the patient requested that her daughter be seen by a voice pathologist as soon as possible, given the urgency of the matter. Apparently, the patient and family were in a state of despair because of the disabling effects of her condition on her general function and quality of life. Because of the chronicity of the respiratory "attacks," which the family presumed to be asthma related, the patient had been absent from school for a 6-week period and had yet to return to school. Moreover, medical interventions administered to date composed of multiple asthma pharmacotherapies were reported to be unsuccessful in managing her condition.

Accompanied by her mother to the voice pathology clinic on the day of the evaluation, the 16-year-old patient arrived carrying a shopping bag full of numerous pharmacologic products, such as bronchodilators, oral inhalers, nasal drops, antihistamines, muscle relaxants, steroids, anti-allergens, cough medications, and acid reflux protocols. In addition, she came prepared with 45 pages of medical reports, several emergency room and hospital records, lab results, and chest and neck radiographs from several medical specialists whom she consulted in an attempt to establish a differential diagnosis regarding her condition. According to the patient, the "asthma-related laryngeal dysfunction" began approximately 2 years prior, marked by infrequent, transient, isolated episodic periods of acute wheezing or inspiratory stridor, respiratory distress, and aphonia only during the acute attack. The acute respiratory distress and associated aphonic episodes were reported to subsequently resolve on their own in a matter of seconds without any direct intervention or administration of prescription medications.

The patient indicated that her condition was diagnosed as asthma by the attending physicians on call during one of her visits to the emergency room at a local hospital. She was emotionally labile during the diagnostic interview and intermittently stopped to administer a dose of an oral inhaler as a prophylactic measure given that she was trying to avoid the onset of an "attack." She expressed frustration and concern because the respiratory-laryngeal attacks or asthma symptoms were occurring more frequently over the past month, and the beneficial effects of the asthma medications prescribed were limited. Although she experienced some relief from some of the asthma protocols, recently it had taken much larger doses to achieve the same effects.

History of the Problem. The patient reported that she first experienced an isolated, acute episode of the asthma-related laryngeal dysfunction problem during field hockey practice at age 14 years. She was running vigorously and noticed the sudden onset of wheezing and stridor during inspiration, accompanied by upper airway obstruction at the level of the larynx that subsided after a few seconds. At the request of the field hockey coach, she pursued a general medical evaluation through her primary care physician, who reported normal findings and prescribed an oral inhaler as needed. The transient stridor and respiratory-laryngeal obstruction did not recur until approximately 2 years following the isolated episode. During March of that year, she recalled sitting on the floor reading a book one evening and suddenly developing an episode of chest and neck pain, coughing, wheezing, difficulty breathing on inhalation, and aphonia during the "attack." This precipitated a trip to the emergency room via ambulance where she was diagnosed with asthma by the attending physician on call and placed on a battery of asthma medications.

In May, she experienced a similar isolated episode of acute chest and neck pain, coughing, stridor, and aphonia as she was doing homework in the evening at home. Again, the mother transported her to the emergency room by ambulance because she was emotional, in a panicked state, and her breathing difficulties alarmed the family. The attending physician placed her on a different combination of asthma medications, and she subsequently was released. The constellation of symptoms and respiratory attacks did not recur until the following month when one day she was at her friend's house socializing during the morning hours. This incident precipitated another visit to the emergency room, and, once again, a series of asthma protocols were prescribed, as well as a Pulmo-Aide machine for home use given that the attending physician suspected her symptoms were consistent with an exacerbation of asthma. Pulmonary function tests (PFTs) were performed the following week, which revealed better than normal forced vital capacity (FVC) and forced expiratory volume at one second (FEV1) values and "borderline obstruction" findings; however, the results of flow volume loops were not reported. She indicated that an allergy screening revealed negative findings to various allergens.

She was free of any symptoms and respiratory "attacks" during the following two summer months of July and August, as well as during the month of September upon returning to school. In early October, however, she experienced another acute attack during field hockey practice just prior to the first "big" game of the season. She did not attend the game because she was taken to the emergency room for medical attention by one of her friends. She reported the same constellation of symptoms marked by acute, transient inspiratory stridor, coughing, respiratory distress, and aphonia. In the emergency room, she was administered oxygen with a mask and prednisone intravenously; an unknown type of pill medication was placed under her tongue. As she calmed down, she was released from the emergency room under her mother's care, and a different host of asthma medications were prescribed.

Following the most recent episode in early October, the patient's general condition and quality of life began to decline rapidly in that she was transported out of school at the request of the mother because the acute "asthma attacks" increased in frequency to approximately six to eight isolated episodes per day. The patient felt that her medical problem disrupted the classroom, and she could not function in school under these circumstances. Moreover, she began vomiting following the consumption of food and liquids for unknown reasons that contributed to a rapid 13-pound weight loss.

As of October, the following coexisting symptoms also were reported by the patient:

■ tightness in the neck and some chest tightness
■ throat and ear pain
■ tickling sensations in the throat
■ throat irritation
■ chronic cough and throat clearing
■ frequent bifrontal migraine headaches
■ mouth and throat dryness
■ jaw pain and tension
■ skin dryness and irritation mainly on the palms of the hands that she

attributed to possible side effects of the prescribed medications
- difficulty swallowing
- dizziness that she attributed to her recent weight loss and poor nutrition.

The exacerbation of asthma-related symptoms and coexisting problems perpetuated a comprehensive multidisciplinary medical work-up because her respiratory distress was not accompanied by much of any objective symptoms of respiratory difficulty. Her primary care physician requested consultations from the following specialties to establish a definitive diagnosis:

- Pulmonology-respiratory medicine
- Otolaryngology
- Gastroenterology
- Allergy
- Voice pathology

Differential Diagnosis. A differential diagnosis utilizing a multidisciplinary team evaluation protocol was utilized to establish a definitive diagnosis regarding the nature of her problem. Medical evaluations revealed that neuromuscular, gastrointestinal, gynecological, cardiorespiratory, and lymphatic systems all were within normal limits. The gastroenterologist reported that subjective and objective clinical findings did not support an etiology of GERD, and as a result, pH monitoring was not performed. Pulmonary function tests (PFTs) reported a normal flow volume loop during asymptomatic periods and attenuation of the inspiratory component of the flow volume loop suggestive of partial upper airway obstruction during an attack. The lungs were noted to be clear bilaterally with no signs of asthma or bronchitis. Lateral soft tissue radiographs of the neck depicted normal glottic,

supraglottic, and cervical airways. In addition, sinus, posterior-anterior (PA), and lateral chest films were normal. Allergy and skin testing were negative to foods and inhalants. Hemograms and electrolyte levels were normal. The patient's history was negative for smoking, alcohol consumption, and use of recreational drugs. She consumed approximately three to five caffeine beverages per day.

Transnasal fiberoptic laryngoscopy (TFL) performed by the otolaryngologist revealed the classic pathognomonic pattern paradoxical vocal fold movement (PVFM) marked by inspiratory adduction of the anterior two thirds of the vocal folds with a posterior diamond-shaped gap during symptomatic episodes.[27,29,40] Moreover, a normal laryngoscopic exam was immediately achieved with simple vocal reassurance by the otolaryngologist without use of any medication. Possible anterior-posterior or ventricular fold muscle tension patterns were not noted during TFL. Mucous stranding was noted along the junction of the posterior middle third of the vocal folds bilaterally. Mucosal waves were symmetric.

Voice Pathology Evaluation

Audiologic Screening. The patient passed an audiologic screening conducted bilaterally in a sound-proof booth at 20 dB for all frequencies between 250 Hz and 8000 Hz.

Oral Peripheral-Neuromotor Speech Examination. The procedures outlined in the Mayo Clinic Neurological Motor Speech Examination[48–50] were followed. The speech mechanism was observed at rest, during sustained posturing, and during movement. The following cranial nerves were assessed: V, VII, IX, X, and

XII. Facial, orolingual, velopharyngeal, and dental structures were within normal limits during all sets of tasks. A sucking reflex was not elicited. During cheek inflation, no leakage of air was noted via oral or nasal passages. No nasal emission was observed during vowel prolongation of /i/ or production of utterances devoid of nasal sounds. Speech alternate motion rates (AMRs) and sequential motor rates (SMRs) were within normal limits. Multisyllabic words were repeated with good precision. There was no evidence to support a dysarthria, apraxia of speech, or nonverbal oral apraxia.

Using Aronson's digital manipulation technique,[51] palpation of the superior and inferior neck regions revealed marked tightness, subjectively. Tightness in the temporomandibular and shoulder region was also noted subjectively. The patient complained of pain during palpation of the neck, jaw, mandible, and shoulder-clavicular regions. Chronic coughing and throat clearing were noted. On one occasion, the patient stopped responding to the examiner's questions, and she exhibited an acute onset of inhalatory stridor and respiratory distress. At this moment, the patient began to gasp for air and an audible wheezing sound accompanied the inspiratory phase. The patient exhibited what resembled a single spasm of the laryngeal area lasting approximately 10 to 15 seconds in duration. Elevation of the hyoid bone and a significant degree of muscle tension was observed visually in the neck, shoulder-clavicular, and jaw regions during the stridorous, laryngospastic, respiratory attack. The patient was temporarily aphonic only during this isolated moment.

The examiner instructed the patient to breathe in through her nose and then inhale through the oral passages with a pursed lip posturing. Following several seconds of verbal and visual feedback provided by the examiner, the patient's breathing returned to normal. She indicated that this transient "attack" exemplified the nature of her problem and associated constellation of symptoms. She denied the presence of any sensory, mechanical, or physiologic triggers that precipitate or perpetuate the nature of her problem with the exception of emotional and stress-related factors.

Auditory-Perceptual Vocal Quality. The examiner's judgment of voice quality was that the patient's voice was mildly hoarse. Pitch range was not perceived to be restricted. Habitual pitch was deemed to be appropriate for age and gender. Using a 5-point rating scale for severity of the voice disorder (0 being normal and 4 being severe), the examiner subjectively judged the patient's voice quality to be a score of 1, mild in severity.

Objective Acoustic Analysis of Vocal Quality. The Multi-Dimensional Voice Program (MDVP-4305, Kay Elemetrics, Lincoln Park, NJ) and Computerized Speech Lab (CSL-4300B, 5. X version, Kay Elemetrics) were used for objective voice analyses. Following guidelines outlined by the National Center for Voice and Speech,[52] voice samples were recorded in a sound-proof booth using a digital audiotape (DAT) recorder (Tascam, DA-P1) and a head-mounted condenser microphone (AKG, C410) placed in a 45° off-axis position to the mouth. Voice samples were fed into the CSL and MDVP programs via DAT recorder for analyses.

Although 10 tokens for vowel prolongation tasks were obtained, only the first three tokens were analyzed because of time constraints for diagnostic purposes. Voice samples were obtained for the following three tasks:

- vowel /a/ prolongation (6-second samples)
- 1-minute monologue
- 1-minute reading aloud of a standard passage.

The patient was instructed to perform each task at a comfortable pitch and loudness level. Approximately 30 seconds or 2000 pitch periods of the monologue and reading samples were analyzed to determine average speaking fundamental frequency (SFF), jitter, and shimmer, and a host of other parameters provided by the MDVP software. Results obtained and normative thresholds used for comparisons are noted in Table 6–1.

Compared with normative thresholds, the patient's jitter and shimmer values exceeded normal thresholds for conversation and reading tasks. The patient's average fundamental frequency (average pitch level) fell within the normal range for age and gender compared with norms.[53] Nonetheless, the patient's average fundamental frequency of /a/ vowel prolongation was assessed at a habitual pitch level that fell in the high average range compared with normative data for age and gender. Conversational speech was assessed to be at an average fundamental frequency level in the low-

average range. Average fundamental frequency for reading fell just above the mean level for age and gender compared with norms. Noise-to-harmonic ratio for /a/ vowel prolongation was within normal limits or below normal threshold.

Maximum Phonation Time. The following tasks were performed to calculate estimates for maximum phonation time (MPT) or maximum phonation duration (MPD): /a/ vowel prolongation and s/z ratio. Three tokens per task were obtained, and an average score was calculated. Results were noted as: /a/ vowel prolongation, MPT = 22 seconds, s/z ratio = 0.80. Compared with normative data, MPT for /a/ vowel prolongation was within normal limits.[53,54] The s/z ratio of 0.80, however, was below 1.0 and normative data for children of comparable age. This finding was suggestive of hoarseness in the presence of normal vocal folds.[55]

Psychosocial History. Because the patient's history was positive for emotional and stress-related triggers that were noted to precipitate or perpetuate her breathing difficulties, a comprehensive psychosocial history was obtained. The patient responded candidly to questions presented. She was enrolled as a junior in high school, but she had not returned to school for at least 6 weeks because of her respiratory problems.

Table 6–1. Results of Quantitative Voice Analysis Pretreatment for Client KK

Voice Task	Average F_0	SD of F_0	F_0 Semitone	Jitter	Shimmer
/a/ vowel	249.0 Hz	5.5 Hz	7	2.3%	3.52%
Conversation	196.1 Hz	29.3 Hz	19	2.9%	8.63%
Rainbow	210.4 Hz	44.1 Hz	24	5.1%	9.61%

Although she was in jeopardy of repeating her junior year as a result of the high absentee rate, she did not express concern about this possibility. She did express considerable disappointment, however, that her field hockey team had not contacted her to date regarding her health and abrupt departure to the local hospital emergency room preceding the "big game" 6 weeks prior.

In terms of varsity sports, she participated in track and field in the past and decided to quit 2 years prior for no apparent reason. Field hockey was the only sport in which she annually participated during the autumn season. She stated that she "likes getting good grades" and her grade point average was a solid "A." With respect to peer relationships, she reported two close friendships. She also indicated having a close and rewarding relationship with her mother. She suggested that her peers perceived her as belonging to a social group comprised of "cool kids." The family dynamics were noted to be tumultuous for most of her life with the exception of a 1-year period when she and her mother resided alone following her parent's divorce 2 years prior. The patient is the product of a union between her biologic parents who did not marry but cohabitated until she was 11 years old at which time her parents were married. The marriage lasted 3 years and her parents divorced at the patient's request. There were no other siblings in the family.

The patient also stated that her current living situation was intolerable because she and her mother were forced to move in with her maternal grandfather following the death of the maternal grandmother 1 year prior. The grandfather was unable to care for himself because of his poor health and frequent hospitalizations secondary to chronic seizures, multiple strokes, and emphysema attributed to a chronic smoking history. She expressed much emotional distress and sadness residing in the grandparent's home since her grandmother's death. A maternal aunt, whom she referred to as the "general," resided next door. The current living situation was described as not conducive for studying because of noise and other factors. She reported that her mother had missed a significant amount of work transporting both the patient and the grandfather to medical appointments. There was no history of voice remediation, family counseling, or formal psychotherapy to date.

Clinical Impression. Based on subjective and objective exam findings, a differential diagnosis includes the following:

- PVFM believed to be secondary to multiple etiologic factors marked by: probable emotional, stress-related, functional, or psychogenic phenomena and probable musculoskeletal laryngeal tension factors.
- Hyperfunctional voice disorder marked by mild hoarseness secondary to: phonotraumatic vocal behaviors, including chronic throat clearing and coughing, and palpable musculoskeletal tension of the larynx and perilaryngeal regions.
- Possible medically related etiologic factors, such as GERD.
- Possible irritable larynx syndrome (ILS)[1] phenomena.

Treatment Recommendations. Diagnostic therapy was recommended using a multifactorial treatment program[56,57] composed of an eclectic approach: symptomatic-behavioral, psychogenic, etiologic, and physiologic voice therapy.[58] The management program developed by this author utilizes a three-phase program. In Phase 1, a differential diagnosis and inventory of baseline data are established to address etiologic and precipitating factors underlying syndromes associated with PVFM. Medical management also should be addressed by the medical team in Phase 1. Phase 2 emphasizes behavioral management of this symptom complex utilizing principles of motor learning to ensure acquisition and carryover of target behaviors. The need for formal psychotherapy should be justified based on the presence of precipitating or perpetuating emotional, stress-related, or psychogenic phenomena and a referral to a psychologist with expertise in treating voice disorders should be made accordingly. In Phase 3, self-awareness and independence in controlling aberrant respiratory and phonatory behaviors are encouraged to facilitate sensorimotor changes in the patient by adapting behaviors that restore optimal function.

Phase 1: Differential Diagnosis-Baseline Data. Critical information and data obtained from the voice pathology evaluation session were utilized to establish specific baseline data regarding the constellation of symptoms, the presence of precipitating and triggering stimuli along with the frequency, duration, and estimated severity of each presenting variable. For example, an inventory of the following variables was determined:

■ psychologic-emotional issues
■ phonotraumatic behaviors
■ medical factors
■ muscle tension patterns
■ triggers and exacerbating stimuli
■ degree of respiratory and phonatory system involvement.

The relative importance and magnitude that each etiologic variable contributed to the presenting problem were enumerated. The use of a daily journal was implemented to help identify emotional factors, situations, and triggering stimuli that elicit aberrant respiratory and phonatory behaviors.[57] Baseline data should be substantiated with subjective and objective evidence obtained by the patient's history, diagnostic interview, medical history and reports, and laboratory reports.

Examples of psychological, emotional, and stress-related factors include: conversion reaction phenomena; functional disorders resulting from learned, maladaptive physiologic compensatory behaviors and resulting psychoemotional sequelae; and natural fears, anxiety, and stress resulting from acute respiratory distress. Medical etiologic variables, such as gastrointestinal problems, GERD, sinusitis, rhinitis, organic laryngeal problems, asthma, and bronchitis, should be ruled out and managed by the medical team. Examples of phonotraumatic behaviors include chronic throat clearing, chronic coughing, and voice misuse or overuse. In this patient, the following five variables were present:

1. PVFM or laryngospastic symptoms: six to eight episodes per day, marked to severe

2. Emotional, stress-related, or psychogenic factors precipitating or perpetuating the problem:
   ■ high rate of school absences because of the problem
   ■ chronic bifrontal migraine headaches
   ■ possible dysfunctional home environment
   ■ possible issues surrounding grandmother's death

- probable emotional, stress-related issues surrounding above factors and PVFM etiology
- referral for formal psychotherapy warranted.

3. Laryngeal and perilaryngeal muscle tension:
   - neck and perilaryngeal tightness
   - pain on palpation of above regions
   - radiating pain per patient report.

4. Phonotraumatic behaviors present:
   - chronic cough and throat clearing
   - mucus stranding noted during laryngoscopy
   - dysphonia, mild hoarseness
   - increased jitter and shimmer perturbation parameters
   - s/z ratio of 0.80
   - possible effects of chronic vomiting on laryngeal health

5. Medically related issues:
   - consumption of multiple pharmacotherapies for asthma
   - caffeine consumption and possible GERD etiology
   - etiology of throat tickle, indeterminate
   - rule out sinusitis and rhinitis etiologies
   - chronic vomiting and possible nutritional issues
   - referral to primary care physician and diagnostic team for medical treatment and follow-up
   - possible referral to dysphagia specialist for differential diagnosis of chronic vomiting.

Based on the above symptoms, the following treatment goals were addressed with the patient:

1. To manage PVFM or laryngospastic symptoms:

- Patient education and counseling regarding the nature of the problem
- Implementation of daily home journal to note food habits, situational and psychosocial phenomena, medical factors, sleep habits, and other variables that precipitate, perpetuate, maintain, or alleviate the PVFM problem
- Early intervention of voice pathology remediation, frequency of sessions, home practice of tasks, estimated duration of treatment
- Patient responsibility regarding success of treatment, carryover of intervention target behaviors, increased self-awareness, and independence in managing PVFM.

2. To manage emotional, stress-related, or psychogenic factors precipitating or perpetuating the problem:
   - The need for formal psychotherapy in conjunction with voice pathology therapy regarding management of PVFM and possible coexisting psychologic manifestations
   - Increased self-awareness of emotional, psychosocial, and stress reduction coping repertoire to restore optimal function.

3. To manage laryngeal and perilaryngeal muscle tension:
   - Suggestions for general or whole body relaxation techniques
   - Manual laryngeal musculoskeletal tension reduction techniques to treat functional laryngeal muscle tension[51,59] to be provided via voice pathology department.

4. To manage phonotraumatic behaviors:
   - Hydration therapy to alleviate cough and throat clearing

■ Elimination of laryngeal, perilaryngeal, and whole-body stress patterns.

5. To manage medically related issues:
   ■ Referral to primary care physician for medical management, follow-up, and additional medical referrals as needed.

Phase 2: Modification. In Phase 2, modification of inappropriate residual respiratory and phonatory behaviors that have not resolved in Phase 1 were addressed, and an individualized treatment program for this patient was developed. Treatment goals and objectives were organized to restore lost function and promote optimal function by utilizing purposeful activity; performance was improved with instruction, and various forms of feedback were successful for this patient. Optimal achievement and carryover of desired behaviors were restored by using motor learning principles that address cognitive, associative, and autonomous or automatic stages.[60]

To restore sensorimotor function of respiratory and phonatory systems, the cognitive phase of treatment emphasized patient education and achievement of specific target behaviors to achieve the desired effect. For example, to alleviate the laryngospastic or PVFM behaviors the following nonspeech tasks were utilized:

■ blowing
■ sniffing
■ panting
■ pursed-lip inhalation
■ nasal inhalation

The pursed-lip inhalation and nasal inhalation techniques were most successful in restoring a wide-open airway in this patient. The associative stage consisted of transitioning the patient from conscious, repetitive drills and practices to more automatic control of her breathing and laryngeal dysfunction through trial-and-error paradigms. The use of visual, auditory, and proprioceptive feedback was essential in this stage. The examiner instructed the patient to visualize or "feel" the difference between a wide-open airway sensation from a PVFM state. During the autonomous stage, the patient was able to anticipate and control or alleviate the onset and duration of each attack on a more automatic level with minimal auditory feedback from the examiner.

Laryngeal muscle tension coping repertoires were also incorporated into practice sessions, such as digital, manual laryngeal massage; head, neck, and shoulder range of motion exercises; and body-posturing techniques. Initially, the examiner physically provided the laryngeal massage to the patient and auditory and proprioceptive feedback was provided. The patient then developed this skill and provided manual laryngeal massage to herself as she sensed the laryngeal musculature tense up. In the automatic stage, the patient utilized this technique as a prophylactic measure or muscle tension coping repertoire to restore optimal function and a relaxed wide-open airway. The patient also chose to incorporate relaxation and breathing techniques she had learned in yoga classes into her daily paradigm to alleviate focal and generalized muscle tension factors.

Respiratory Retraining Tasks. Respiratory retraining was also part of Phase 2. This retraining was employed through abdominal breathing focus by encouraging the patient to distend the abdominal region during inhalation and maximizing use of the abdominal muscles during exhalation. The patient monitored her performance proprioceptively by placing her hand on the abdominal region as the examiner provided auditory feedback in the cognitive stage. She was able to perform this task automatically for nonspeech and speech tasks in a relatively short period of time. The following respiratory-phonatory synchronization tasks were employed to promote optimal function utilizing purposeful activity:

■ sibilant prolongation with and without crescendo-diminuendo tasks
■ upward and downward glides of sibilant sounds
■ lip trills
■ humming
■ nasal sound prolongations with nasal-vowel syllabic combinations
■ counting aloud
■ reading aloud
■ singing
■ spontaneous speech.

Because the patient was an athlete engaged in field hockey, variable practices using respiratory retraining tasks were incorporated into physical activities, such as walking, slow jogging, and laps up and down stairs, with good success.

Aberrant respiratory and laryngeal behaviors were best modified when symptomatic-behavioral intervention was administered early following an accurate diagnosis of PVFM. Drills or brief periods of practice were distributed over time in lieu of lengthy practices. Consistent or repeated practice on a single task was combined with variable practice involving a range of related tasks once the target behavior is achieved with at least some consistency in the associative stage. Moreover, treatment sessions were organized strategically in that the patient was seen more frequently

for shorter periods in early stages of therapy to manage the existing PVFM and coexisting clinical manifestations.

Stimulus Control. Another aspect of Phase 2 involved stimulus control. Phonotraumatic behaviors, such as chronic coughing and throat clearing, were eliminated with the use of hydration therapy techniques. The patient was instructed to take a sip of water when the need to cough or clear her throat arose. She also was instructed to drink at least eight 8-oz glasses of water daily as a prophylactic measure. Her primary care physician referred her to a nutritionist to address optimal nutritional intake because she had lost a considerable amount of weight due to chronic vomiting. Swallow was deemed to be intact by the otolaryngologist via TFL, and therefore, a formal dysphagia evaluation was deemed to be unwarranted by the primary care physician. The patient was instructed to eliminate caffeinated beverages as a prophylactic measure to eliminate possible GERD side effects.

Formal Psychotherapy. Psychotherapy was the final component of Phase 2. The patient sought the help of a psychologist with expertise in treating functional and psychogenic voice disorders. Formal psychotherapy consisted of use of the neurolinguistic programming (NLP) model,[61] which incorporated use of hypnosis and psycho-educational techniques, such as pacing, mirroring, modeling, self-awareness, guided visualization, systematic desensitization, and stress-coping repertoires, in achieving optimal laryngeal and respiratory function.

Phase 3: Generalization and Carryover. Phase 3 of treatment addressed carryover of target behaviors utilizing behavioral paradigms noted to facilitate optimal function. Although carryover strategies began in Phase 1 and Phase 2, the focus of this phase emphasized self-awareness, patient independence, and patient control in alleviating and eliminating aberrant respiratory, laryngeal, and phonatory behaviors. The use of "preparatory sets" was organized to achieve optimal function. For example, target behaviors, techniques, and established protocols to restore lost function were emphasized including:

- stimulus control (GERD, sinusitis, and rhinitis protocols, hydration therapy to control chronic cough and throat clearing, diet control, etc)
- control of musculoskeletal laryngeal and whole-body tension factors using physical methods (manual laryngeal massage) and other established tension reducing paradigms
- emotional and psychological coping repertoires to eliminate the onset or exacerbation of the aberrant respiratory-laryngeal problem.

Use of the daily home journal assisted the examiner and patient in determining the efficacy of treatment and the beneficial effects of each treatment paradigm.

Conclusion. The patient attended 12 treatment sessions and two follow-up voice pathology treatment sessions before she was discharged from therapy. She gained control of the PVFM problem and the frequency of an "attack" decreased to approximately one episode over a 3-month period. Hyperfunctional vocal behaviors were eliminated, and her vocal quality returned to normal baseline levels. At discharge, objective MDVP findings revealed that jitter and shimmer perturbation measures were below thresholds. With the help of formal psychotherapy, the patient was transitioned back to school as coping repertoires were implemented to address psychogenic and emotional manifestations underlying her problem. The patient was followed by her primary care physician for adjustment and elimination of oral medications prescribed to treat her respiratory distress. On a follow-up evaluation in otolaryngology, there was no evidence of PVFM during transnasal flexible laryngoscopy.

References

1. Morrison M, Rammage L, Emami AJ. The irritable larynx syndrome. *J Voice.* 1999;13(3):447–455.
2. Clauw DJ, Taylor-Moon D. Information about fibromyalgia. http://www.rheu matology.org/public/factsheets/fibro mya_new.asp. Retrieved May 2006.
3. Coderre TJ, Katz J, Vaccarino AL, Melzack R. Contribution of central neuroplasticity to pathological pain: review of clinical and experimental evidence. *Pain.* 1993;52:259–285.
4. Fuller NS, Morrison RE. Chronic fatigue syndrome. *Postgrad Med.* 1998;103(1): 175–176, 179–184.
5. Mihrshahi R, Beirman R. Aetiology and pathogenesis of chronic fatigue syndrome: a review. *NZ Med J.* 2005;118 (1227):U1780.
6. Mulak A, Paradowski L. Migraine and irritable bowel syndrome. *Neurol Neurochil Pol.* 2005;39(4 suppl):S55–S60.
7. Vandvik PO, Lydersen S, Farup PG. Prevalence, comorbidity and impact of irritable bowel syndrome in Norway. *Scand J Gastroenterol.* 2006;41(6):650–656.
8. Bandler R, Keay KA, Vaugh CW, Shipley MT. Columnar organization of the PAG neurons regulating emotional and vocal expression. In: Davis PJ, Fletcher NH, eds. *Vocal Fold Physiology: Controlling Complexity and Chaos.* San Diego, CA: Singular Publishing Group; 1996.

9. Davis PJ, Zhang SP. What is the role of the midbrain periaqueductal gray in respiration and vocalization? In: Depaulis A, Bandler R, eds. *The Midbrain Periaqueductal Gray Matter*. New York, NY: Plenum Press; 1991:57–66.

10. Ambalavanar R, Tanaka Y, Damirjian M, Ludlow CL. Laryngeal afferent stimulation enhances Fos immunoreactivity in periaqueductal gray in the cat. *J Compar Neurol*. 1999;409(3):411–423.

11. Behbehani MM. Functional characteristics in the midbrain periaqueductal gray in respiration and vocalization? *Progr Neurol*. 1995;46:575–605.

12. Carrive P. The periaqueductal gray and defensive behavior: functional representation and neuronal organization. *Behavl Brain Res*. 1993;58:27–47.

13. Jurgens U. The role of the periaqueductal gray in vocal behavior. *Behav Brain Res*. 1994;62:107–117.

14. Gill C, Morrison M. The esophagolaryngeal reflex in a porcine model of GERD. *J Otolaryngol*. 1997;27(2):76–80.

15. Lieberman J. Principles and techniques of manual therapy: Application in the management of dysphonia. In: Harris T, Harris S, Rubin JS, Howard DM, eds. *The Voice Clinic Handbook*. London: Whurr Publishers Ltd; 1998:91–138.

16. Angsuwaransee T, Morrison MD. Extrinsic laryngeal muscular tension in patients with voice disorders. *J Voice*. 2002;16(3): 333–343.

17. Morrison M, Rammage L, Mallett V. *Irritable larynx syndrome as a central nervous system hypersensitivity disorder*. In preparation.

18. Blager F. *Breathing Exercises for Cough; Relaxed Throat Breath with Exercise; Patient Handouts*. Denver, CO: National Jewish Medical and Research Center; 2005.

19. Rammage L, Morrison M, Nichol H. *Management of the Voice and Its Disorders*. 2nd ed. San Diego, CA: Singular Publishing Group; 2001.

20. Mathers-Schmidt B. Paradoxical vocal fold motion: a tutorial on a complex disorder and the speech-language patholo-gist's role. *Am J Speech Lang Pathol*. 2001;10:111–125.

21. Sandage M. Sniffs, gasps, and coughs irritable larynx syndrome across the lifespan. *ASHA Leader*. 2006;11(9):16–21.

22. Rammage L, Morrison M. ILS as a central nervous system hypersensitivity. Presentation at the 10th Biennial Phonosurgery Symposium. Madison, WI; 2008.

23. Wareing MJ, Mitchell D. Psychogenic stridor: diagnosis and management. *J Accid Emerg Med*. 1997;14(5):330–332.

24. Heatley DG, Swift E. Paradoxical vocal cord dysfunction in an infant with stridor and gastroesophageal reflux. *Int J Pediatr Otorhinolaryngol*. 1996;34(1–2): 149–151.

25. Koufman J. The differential diagnosis of paradoxical vocal cord movement. *The Visible Voice*. 1994. http://www.bgsm .edu/voice/paradoxical.html.

26. Barnes SD, Grob CS, Lachman BS, Marsh BR, Loughlin GM. Psychogenic upper airway obstruction presenting as refractory wheezing. *J Pediatr*. 1986; 109(6):1067–1070.

27. Christopher KL, Wood RP, 2nd, Eckert RC, Blager FB, Raney RA, Souhrada JF. Vocal-cord dysfunction presenting as asthma. *N Engl J Med*. 1983;308(26): 1566–1570.

28. Goldman J, Muers M. Vocal cord dysfunction and wheezing. *Thorax*. 1991; 46(6):401–404.

29. Martin R, Blager F, Gay M, Wood R. Paradoxic vocal cord motion in presumed asthmatics. *Semin Respir Med*. 1987;8: 332–337.

30. Rusakow LS, Blager FB, Barkin RC, White CW. Acute respiratory distress due to vocal cord dysfunction in cystic fibrosis. *J Asthma*. 1991;28(6):443–446.

31. Trudeau MD. Paradoxical vocal cord dysfunction among juveniles. *American Speech-Language-Hearing Association Voice Special Interest Division (SID 3) Newsletter*, April, 1998:11–13.

32. Craig T, Sitz K, Squire E, Smith L, Carpenter G. Vocal cord dysfunction during wartime. *Mil Med*. 1992;157(11):614–616.

33. Mobeireek A, Alhamad A, Al-Subaei A, Alzeer A. Psychogenic vocal cord dysfunction simulating bronchial asthma. *Eur Respir J.* 1995;8(11):1978–1981.

34. Husein OF, Husein TN, Gardner R, et al. Formal psychological testing in patients with paradoxical vocal fold dysfunction. *Laryngoscope.* 2008;118(4):740–747.

35. Freedman MR, Rosenberg SJ, Schmaling KB. Childhood sexual abuse in patients with paradoxical vocal cord dysfunction. *J Nerv Ment Disord.* 1991;179(5):295–298.

36. Nahmias J, Tansey M, Karetzky MS. Asthmatic extrathoracic upper airway obstruction: laryngeal dyskinesis. *N J Med.* 1994;91(9):616–620.

37. Treole K, Trudeau MD, Forrest LA. Endoscopic and stroboscopic description of adults with paradoxical vocal fold dysfunction. *J Voice.* 1999;13(1):143–152.

38. Seikel J, King D, Drumright D. *Anatomy and Physiology for Speech, Language, and Hearing.* San Diego, CA: Singular Publishing Group; 1997.

39. Kempster GB, Gerratt BR, Verdolini Abbott K, Barkmeier-Kraemer J, Hillman RE. Consensus auditory-perceptual evaluation of voice: development of a standardized clinical protocol. *Am J Speech Lang Pathol.* 2009;18(2):124–132.

40. Gallivan GJ, Hoffman L, Gallivan KH. Episodic paroxysmal laryngospasm: voice and pulmonary function assessment and management. *J Voice.* 1996; 10(1):93–105.

41. Harding S, Schan C, Guzzo R, Alexander R, Bradley L, Richter J. Gastroesophageal reflux-induced bronchoconstriction, is microaspiration a factor? *Chest.* 1995;108:1220–1227.

42. Tajchman UW, Gitterman B. Vocal cord dysfunction associated with sexual abuse. *Clin Pediatr (Phila).* 1996;35(2):105–108.

43. McQuaid EL, Spieth LE, Spirito A. The pediatric psychologist's role in differential diagnosis: vocal-cord dysfunction presenting as asthma. *J Pediatr Psychol.* 1997;22(5):739–748.

44. Smith R, Bauman N, Bent J, Kramern M, Smits W, Ahrens R. Exercise-induced laryngomalacia. *Ann Otol Rhinol Laryngol.* 1995;104:537–541.

45. Maschka D, Bauman N, McCray P, Hoffman H, Karnell M, Smith R. A classification scheme for paradoxical vocal cord motion. *Laryngoscope.* 1997;107: 1429–1435.

46. Sim T, McClean S, Lee J, Naranjo M, Grant A. Functional laryngeal obstruction: a somatization disorder. *Am J Med.* 1990;88:293–295.

47. Miller R. *The Structure of Singing.* New York, NY: Schirmer Books; 1986.

48. Darley FL, Aronson AE, Brown JR. Clusters of deviant speech dimensions in the dysarthrias. *J Speech Hear Res.* 1969; 12(3):462–496.

49. Darley FL, Aronson AE, Brown JR. Differential diagnostic patterns of dysarthria. *J Speech Hear Res.* 1969;12(2):246–269.

50. Duffy J. *Motor Speech Disorders: Substrates, Differential Diagnosis, and Management.* St. Louis, MO: Mosby; 1995.

51. Aronson A. *Clinical Voice Disorders.* New York, NY: Thieme Medical Publishers; 1990.

52. Titze I. *Workshop on acoustic voice analysis.* Iowa City, IA: National Center for Voice and Speech, University of Iowa; 1995.

53. Wilson D. *Voice Problems of Children.* 2nd ed. Baltimore, MD: Williams & Wilkins; 1987.

54. Andrews M. *Manual of Voice Treatment: Pediatrics Through Geriatrics.* San Diego, CA: Singular Publishing Group; 1995.

55. Eckel FC, Boone DR. The S/Z ratio as an indicator of laryngeal pathology. *J Speech Hear Disord.* 1981;46(2):147–149.

56. Andrianopoulos M. *Management of paradoxical vocal fold movement: How I do it?* Presentation at the 27th Annual Symposium: Care of the Professional Voice. Philadelphia, PA; June, 998.

57. Andrianopoulos M. *Irritable larynx syndrome: What are we talking about and how do we treat it?* Presentation at the 28th Annual Symposium: Care of the Professional Voice. Philadelphia, PA; June, 1999.

58. Stemple J. Pseudo-asthma. In: Stemple J, ed. *Voice Therapy: Clinical Studies.* San Diego, CA: Singular Publishing Group; 1993.

59. Roy N, Leeper HA. Effects of the manual laryngeal musculoskeletal tension reduction technique as a treatment for functional voice disorders: perceptual and acoustic measures. *J Voice.* 1993; 7(3):242–249.

60. Rosenbaum DA, ed. *Human Motor Control.* San Diego, CA: Academic Press; 1991.

61. Rosen D, Sataloff R. *Psychology of Voice Disorders.* San Diego, CA: Singular Publishing Group; 1997.

7

Management of the Professional Voice

Introduction

The young pitcher came set, paused, kicked, and released the ball. As he followed through, he felt a twinge in his pitching arm and shoulder. It was a feeling he never had felt before. It was not really pain, but a burning sensation that ran from the back of his bicep, up his arm, and through his shoulder to his neck. The pitch was low and outside, and the catcher returned the ball. The pitcher walked behind the mound, windmilled his arm in both directions, and stretched it across his body. Knowing that this was not the pitcher's normal routine, the manager became alert and stepped to the top step of the dugout for a better look. The pitcher returned to the mound. The catcher put one finger down and tapped the inside of his left leg, signaling an inside fastball. The pitcher fired the ball, which sailed high

over the batter's head. As he released the ball, he grabbed his arm, wincing in pain. The manager and trainer rushed to the mound. The relief pitcher was called into the game, and the starter was immediately sent to the hospital for preliminary X-rays. After the game, the manager told reporters that he did not think the injury was serious. Nevertheless, even though the team was in a tight pennant race, he would not rush the pitcher back into a game until it was certain he was 100% sound. The pitcher was much too valuable to the team to risk permanent damage.

The tenor was singing in the second of three acts, in the third performance of a four-performance run. The opera featured his role, and the music was extremely demanding, especially for his young voice. He had felt a little under the weather that day and was physically and vocally fatigued. While singing a strenuous duet with the female lead, he reached for the climactic note, which he reached and then suddenly released. The soprano knew something was wrong. The conductor raised his eyes to the stage. The tenor suppressed a cough caused by a severe tickle and dry feeling in his throat. He was alarmed, but knew that he must continue. Between the second and third acts, the tenor drank some warm water, which relieved the tickle. The dry feeling persisted, and his speaking voice was slightly husky. The soprano quietly asked of his condition, to which he smiled and replied that he was fine. The third act was uneventful, but the tenor's singing voice was uninspired and lacked its typical color and clarity. Although concerned, the tenor, his manager, and the conductor excused the problem as fatigue. This role was a career opportunity that the tenor did not wish to "blow." Unfortunately, his voice "blew" before the end of the week. When a medical examination was finally conducted, indirect laryngoscopy revealed a hemorrhage of the right vocal fold, which likely occurred at the first sign of trouble. His continued singing had threatened permanent damage.

Khambato[1] paralleled the experiences of professional singers and actors with those of professional athletes. Because of their physical work demands, athletes are at greater risk than the general population for developing muscle and joint injuries. Likewise, because singers and actors demand more from their voices than an average person, they are at greater risk for developing laryngeal disorders. Despite these similarities, the mentality for seeking treatment for injuries, as shown in the foregoing examples, is often different for the two professional populations. The prized athlete generally is required by management to seek treatment for injury promptly

so as to quickly promote healing and reduce the possibility of further or permanent damage. Singers and actors, however, often minimize the disability to avoid canceling even one engagement. Granted, the financial ramifications may be huge, but permanent injury certainly would be worse. Professional actors and singers often fear developing a reputation for unreliability and continue using the damaged voice, often risking permanent vocal disability. Even nonperformance professional voice users, such as teachers, clergy, and lecturers, typically behave in the same manner as their more elite counterparts. In the face of vocal difficulties, teachers continue to teach, lecturers continue to lecture, and preachers continue to preach rather than risk loss of income and damage to their reputations or because they simply see no other alternative.

Who, then, are professional voice users? Professional voice users are those individuals who are directly dependent on vocal communication for their livelihood. Koufman and Isaacson[2] suggested a "vocal usage" classification system comprised of four levels. Level I is the elite vocal performer. Professional singers and actors for whom even slight vocal difficulty may cause serious consequences belong in this level. Level II is the professional voice user, for whom even moderate vocal difficulty would prevent adequate job performance. Clergy, public speakers, lecturers, call center operators, airline reservationists, and so on are examples of Level II.

Level III is the nonvocal professional. This level is comprised of doctors, lawyers, businesspersons, salespersons, and others who could not perform their work properly if suffering with severe dysphonia. Mild or moderate dysphonias may be inconvenient but would not preclude adequate job performance. Level IV is the nonvocal nonprofessional. This is the factory worker, laborer, and clerk who would not be prevented from doing his or her work if experiencing vocal disability. The history and vocal needs of each patient will ultimately determine his or her own personal vocal level.

This chapter deals with the management of voice disorders in the elite vocal performer, the professional voice user, and those seeking to reach such a status (Level I or II). A voice disorder in this population has a dual impact. Not only does it cause the interfering vocal symptoms characteristic of the disorder, it also carries with it a high level of emotional strain and anxiety. The anxiety is caused by the disorder's potential impact on the person's reputation, ability to meet professional commitments, and ability to perform and make a living. The interdisciplinary voice team is the recommended standard of care for all voice disorders. The team approach is even more essential for the professional voice user. Individuals who comprise the voice team must all work together to remediate all aspects of the voice disorder. These aspects include management of general and emotional health, vocal hygiene counseling, symptom modification, and retraining of the artistic voice. Team members may include the professional voice user, the otolaryngologist, the voice pathologist, the singing voice specialist, the vocal coach, and the singing teacher. Occasionally, the voice user's manager and producers also must be included in the rehabilitative process. Successful rehabilitation may depend on the abilities of these professionals to compromise and work together with the patient's long-term vocal health as the primary consideration. Ideally, the professional voice

user will ultimately assume responsibility for the well-being of his or her own voice.[3]

It is commonly assumed that, because of the intimate dependency that professional voice users have with their voices, they would know how their laryngeal mechanisms work and understand general concepts of good vocal hygiene. This assumption is not always correct. In our practice, we often find professional voice users with only a vague awareness of the anatomy and physiology of the vocal mechanics who do not understand the consequences of poor vocal hygiene or follow unusual vocal practices based on "old wives' tales." Therefore, education becomes an important part of any remediation program.

Many factors may contribute to voice disorders in this population. Causative factors include:

- Phonotrauma
    poor singing or speaking technique
    singing out of range
    chronic coughing or throat clearing
    smoking
    poor hydration
    overuse of the voice

- Chronic medical problems
    laryngopharyngeal reflux (LPR)
    allergies
    sinusitis
    upper respiratory infections
    prescription drug use
    poor diet
    fatigue
    illicit drug use
    alcohol

■ Environmental factors

    performing in smoky, dry, musty environments

    exhaustive schedules

    dry environments, such as airplanes and hotel rooms

    loud backup music

    cast parties

    poor acoustics

■ Emotional factors

    stage fright

    anxiety

    self-confidence

    depression

    performance stress

The professional voice user also is susceptible to any and all causes of voice disorders common to the general population. The case studies in this chapter examine many of these etiologic factors. The studies also illustrate the advantages of the multidisciplinary management team for the remediation of voice disorders in the professional voice user.

Voice Team Care of the Elite Vocal Performer

Robert T. Sataloff, MD, DMA

Case: Study: Patient LL

> *In the following case study, Robert T. Sataloff combines medical treatment with voice therapy and voice teaching to successfully remediate the threatening voice problems of a legitimate "rock star."*

Patient LL, a 24-year-old rock music star, was seen emergently during the second month of his first world tour promoting an album. Initially, he complained only of a sore throat and upper respiratory infection that had been present for 2 days. Inquiry revealed several other problems that were of greater concern to him, however. He reported a 3-week history of hoarseness and neck pain following singing, breathiness, decreased ability to sing softly, and diminished range (especially upper). When the symptoms first appeared, they were noticeable primarily following performances, but his voice was normal the following day. For the previous 2 weeks, his voice had remained hoarse and breathy all the time, although it became considerably worse during performances. He also had a long history of morning hoarseness, halitosis, prolonged warm-up time, and frequent throat clearing; these symptoms seemed to have become more pronounced in the past few weeks, which also had been characterized by extreme stress.

He was known for clear, balladlike high singing, and he had already been forced to cut some of his most famous songs from his concerts. He was performing 3 or 4 nights per week in large halls and stadiums. He had had no formal training for speech or singing, although he was extremely intelligent and well educated in other disciplines. He had no other medical illnesses, used no medications or recreational drugs, and was highly motivated and cooperative.

Physical examination revealed normal ears and hearing, mild nasal congestion, moderate pharyngitis, and no neck masses. His speaking voice was hoarse and breathy. Indirect laryngoscopy showed marked erythema of the arytenoids, with no significant erythema or edema of the true vocal folds except at the junctions of the anterior and middle thirds where there were small nodules. Strobovideolaryngoscopy confirmed that glottic closure was impaired anterior and posterior to these soft masses. There were no hemorrhages, mucosal disruptions, or adynamic segments. Flexible fiberoptic laryngoscopy revealed supraglottic hyperfunction with decreased anterior-posterior diameter during speaking at his habitual pitch. Laryngeal architecture returned to normal with a slight voluntary increase in pitch.

Objective voice analysis revealed normal pulmonary function, with increased laryngeal mean airflow rate. Perturbation, jitter, and shimmer were mildly increased, and the harmonic-to-noise ratio and percent voiced speech were decreased. Formal evaluations by a certified speech-language pathologist and a singing voice specialist confirmed the vocal problems noted, analyzed them in greater detail, and included trial therapy that showed the patient's excellent ability to modify voice technique quickly. He had an excessive number of harsh glottal attacks. He spoke English with a British accent, although he was from a northern European country, and English was not his native tongue.

Examination of his singing technique revealed an unbalanced stance, with weight over his heels; ineffective abdominal support; thoracic breathing; alteration in laryngeal position with pitch changes; and excessive tension in his neck, jaw, and especially the tongue. Similar problems were present to a lesser degree in his speaking voice. The hoarseness and breathiness were present throughout his range but less apparent on lower notes. There was a poorly controlled break at his passagio.

Discussion

Professional singers frequently have complex, multiple medical problems. This patient's difficulties included (1) acute upper respiratory infection, (2) chronic gastroesophageal reflux laryngitis, (3) improper vocal technique, and (4) nodules.

The management of acute upper respiratory infection in professional singers depends on the severity of the infection, skill of the singer, importance of upcoming performances, and long-term performance schedule. In this case, pharyngeal cultures were taken, and the patient was started empirically on an antibiotic. Cultures later revealed that the antibiotic choice (ampicillin) was appropriate for his infection with *Haemophilus influenzae*. Corticosteroids have a place in the management of upper respiratory infections, but they must be used with great caution. In a technically excellent singer who has a particularly important performance followed by a period of rest, a short course of steroid medication may be extremely valuable for inflammatory or even infectious laryngitis. In the case presented here, however, signs of infection were limited to the pharynx. The arytenoid edema was caused by gastroesophageal reflux, and the nodules were caused by voice abuse. There was no significant vocal fold edema except the traumatic response around the nodules, and steroids were not used. Absolute voice rest (silence) rarely is necessary except following submucosal hemorrhage or mucosal disruption (traumatic tear), and it was not used in this case. Relative voice rest is always helpful, however. The patient was counseled regarding voice conservation and hygiene and instructed to use his voice only when he was being paid to do so.

Hydration is a particularly important consideration, but singers with reflux should not consume large quantities of water immediately prior to singing because upright reflux during performance is common and is worsened with a stomach full of clear liquids. Morning hoarseness, chronic sore throat, frequent throat clearing, excessive phlegm, prolonged warm-up time, a sensation of a "lump in the throat," and night coughing are common signs of gastroesophageal reflux laryngitis. Typical dyspepsia (heartburn) usually is absent. Reflux is common among singers for several reasons. First, they frequently perform on an empty stomach late at night, and then eat immediately before retiring. This induces reflux by generating acid secretion and mechanically stressing the lower esophageal sphincter. Second, abdominal support necessarily includes increased intra-abdominal pressure, which tends to compress the stomach, causing its contents to reflux into the esophagus and throat. Third, performing careers are stressful. Stress is commonly believed to aggravate problems associated with gastric acidity, including reflux and ulcer disease. Gastroesophageal reflux is a chronic source of vocal fold irritation that frequently underlies other vocal problems. In this case, it was treated with elevation of the head of the bed, antacids, an H_2 blocker (ranitidine), and avoidance of nighttime eating. The patient was willing to modify his habits, eating a larger breakfast and lunch, a light supper a few hours before performance and nothing for 3 hours before going to sleep.

Small, early vocal nodules should not be diagnosed on the basis of one examination. "Physiologic swellings" that resemble nodules occur in many singers but disappear after 24 to 48 hours of voice rest. They are not believed to be significant clinically. This patient was asked to remain silent except when absolutely necessary for 24 hours and was re-examined. Slight edema around the nodules had resolved, but they were still clearly present. The proper treatment for vocal nodules is voice modification, not surgery or silence. Because of this patient's compelling professional commitments (documented by the fact that his insurance company paid $250,000.00 for every performance canceled), only two performances were canceled for medical reasons.

Emergency voice therapy and singing lessons were instituted. He received 1-hour sessions of each, once or twice daily for 1 week. Voice therapy concentrated on development of abdominal breathing and support, connection of breath support with vocal production, and relaxation of hyperfunctional muscles in the head and neck. Speaking pitch was not addressed specifically, but it increased spontaneously by approximately three semitones when the excessive tongue, jaw, and neck tension were eliminated.

Because English was not the patient's native language, he had no particular need to continue the dialect of British English (Liverpool area) he had acquired, an accent characterized by a high percentage of harsh glottal attacks. His native northern European language did not have a similar pattern, and his speech initially was much better in his mother tongue than it was in English. A limited amount of accent training ameliorated this problem. The speaking voice training was extremely helpful to him not only in daily life, but also during radio and television interviews. Traditional voice therapy was coordinated with singing voice training. This also concentrated on development of abdominal support and relaxation of head and neck muscles. He was trained rapidly to produce the sounds he needed without vocal strain and without sounding "operatic." The voice therapy team attended his first concert in Philadelphia and subsequent concerts elsewhere over the next few weeks. He was able to incorporate the speaking and singing modifications into his performances quickly. His ability to sing his customary repertoire began returning within 2 weeks, and his nodules resolved in approximately 6 weeks.

Summary

This patient's upper respiratory infection resolved promptly. He was able to complete his tour without difficulty. He has continued to use trained speaking and singing technique, and antireflux therapy. He has had no further voice problems.

High-Risk Vocal Performer

Bari Hoffman Ruddy, PhD, Jeffery Lehmann, MD, and Christine Sapienza, PhD

Case Study: Patient MM

High-risk performers produce their singing or theater voice at their maximum vocal effort level. Typically working in such venues as major theme parks, dinner theaters, and summer repertory, the high-risk performer does not find it uncommon to complete a minimum of five shows per day in a 5-day work week. The environments in which they work are not optimum for producing healthy voice. Factors contributing to their voice problem(s) include the performance demand, physical interference with costumes, and inferior placement of their microphone for amplification.[4]

The consequences to the laryngeal anatomy include vocal fold edema and increased vascularity. Permanent disruption to the vocal fold edge can be observed as vocal fold nodules, polyps, or polypoid changes. Among some of the more prevalent functional consequences experienced by high-risk performers are dehydration, chronic laryngitis, and chronic laryngeal muscle tension.

More generally, Sataloff has described common causes of dysphonia in professional voice users.[5] Typically, performers present with a combination of these factors. They include

- overcompensation of the speech production mechanism as a result of infection and irritation to the larynx
- compensatory strategies stemming from inadequate respiratory dynamics and excessive muscle tension
- engaging in vocally abusive behavior, such as yelling, screaming, or talking too loudly
- improper vocal training
- environmental constraints and physical compensation
- emotional reaction stemming from the stresses of one's daily lifestyle.

This case study focuses on a performer engaged in street theater within a major theme park. Street theater is a unique setting. The performance site is outside with no covering or barrier walls. The performers are required to project their voices with no amplification. They perform five to nine shows daily. Hoffman et al[4] showed that street theater performers present with environmental conditions that have a great negative impact on facilitating healthy voice production. Analysis of environmental variables found external noise levels to be 82 dB with vocal output levels ranging from 107 to 114 dB SPL at 3 inches.

Patient History. Patient MM's referral course to our clinic was by report from the stage manager to the theme parks in-house health service center. The medical personnel at the health center, as routinely done, placed the performer on vocal rest for 1 week. Following persistence of the vocal disturbance, the performer then was referred to our clinic for an evaluation by an otolaryngologist. Following completion of an indirect examination of the vocal folds via laryngeal mirror, the patient was referred to a team of speech-language pathologists for videolaryngostroboscopy and vocal function studies.

The patient was a 31-year-old female. She reported a successful 10-year history performing in street theater and musical theater in a theme park setting. She had formal coaching in musical theater and majored in theater during her undergraduate education over 12 years prior. Past medical history was unremarkable. Her schooling included studies in music theory, music performance, and theater. During the clinical interview, she reported an awareness of voice and respiratory strategies used in performance for projecting and maintaining a "good" voice. She stated "I have learned about diaphragmatic support for belting and placement of the head voice." Our interpretation of the patient's knowledge of voice production was that it was adequate but not focused on the physiologic mechanisms necessary for developing the pressure for her specific performance style.

Time Line. Patient MM reported a normal voice until September 2007. She experienced one incident of vocal disturbance occurring in September when she screamed for about 10 minutes and strained her voice. Although she experienced some acute voice difficulties following this incident, she did not perceive any long-standing voice problems. She continued with her daily activities and performance following this event without modifications.

Early the next year, in January 2008, the patient recalled a particular performance during which she was not warmed up, had "no real support" during loud vocalization, and "pushed through her throat" to perform. She stated that during one of nine performances that day, it "felt like a muscle was pulled in my neck." Although she struggled, she stated that she was able to complete all nine shows but experienced intermittent aphonia and vocal strain. She also reported concurrent emotional stress from caring for a family member who was extremely ill. She stated that she had extensive periods of crying and "high amounts of tension in her throat."

Voice Evaluation. Voice evaluation included the patient interview as described above, assessment of performance site and demand, videolaryngostroboscopy, perceptual assessment of vocal characteristics, and acoustic recording and analysis of the voice signal prior to intervention.

Perceptual Impressions. At the initial office visit, Patient MM's speaking voice was perceived as moderately breathy and slightly strained with frequent glottal fry occurring throughout conversation. There were repeated episodes of hard glottal attacks at voice onset. Vocal pitch was perceived to be within normal limits, and vocal loudness was perceived as too loud. Occasional voice breaks were perceived during conversation, which appeared to be related to the degree of vocal strain. Laryngeal muscle tension was determined to be moderate based on external laryngeal palpation. The patient reported mild soreness with palpation of the hyoid and midthyroid area.

A maximum phonation time of 12 seconds was measured during sustained vowel production of /a/. Evaluation of the singing voice revealed the highest pitch easily sung was E above middle C and the lowest was C below middle C with a 17 semitone (limited) range; pitch control during this task was fair.

Acoustic Evaluation and Results. The KayPentax Computerized Speech Lab (CSL), Model 4300 and Multidimensional Voice Program (MDVP; KayPentax, Lincoln Park, NJ) were used to document vocal features both prior to and following intervention. This analysis was used to document and objectively define the frequency, intensity, and temporal characteristics of the patient's voice. Recordings were obtained using an omnidirectional headset microphone and digital audio recorder. The voice signal was digitized and analyzed for the selected parameters of fundamental frequency (average, high, and low), standard deviation of fundamental frequency, and noise-to-harmonics ratio. These parameters were selected because they provide information about the voice

source and its variability during phonation. Fundamental frequency indicated the number of cycles of vocal fold vibration, and noise-to-harmonic ratio compared the spectral energy with the energy of noise existent in the voice signal.

Phonatory tasks included a sustained vowel phonation at both comfortable and loud phonation, pitch glides, and oral reading of the Rainbow Passage.[6] The same tasks were evaluated posttreatment. (Table 7–1 presents the results of the acoustic analysis for only the sustained vowel /a/ and reading passage prior to intervention.)

Videolaryngostroboscopy Results Prior to Intervention. The KayPentax RLS 9100 70-degree Endo-Stroboscope with Computer integrated System Model 9195, CCD camera Toshiba (Model 9110) was used for imaging the larynx. Following topical anesthesia with ponticaine spray, a complete view of Patient MM's vocal folds was obtained. The patient was compliant and tolerated the procedure well. Using the Hirano and Bless[7] rating form as a general guide, rating of the stroboscopic image was completed. Results were as follows:

■ *Vocal fold edge:* A wide-based polyp on the left true vocal fold was identified at the junction of the anterior one third and the posterior two thirds of

Table 7–1. Acoustic Characteristics of Patient NN's Voice During Sustained Vowel and Oral Reading Pre- and Posttreatment

	F_0 (Hz)	STD (Hz)	Jitter (%)	Shimmer (%)	NHR	F_0 (Hz)	Fhi (Hz)
Pretreatment	201	4.3	3.23	5.18	0.18	145	239
Posttreatment	223	1.4	.35	2.38	0.11	142	269

the membranous vocal fold with moderate vascularity noted. On the contralateral vocal fold, a moderate degree of edema with a small reactive nodular change was identified, presumably secondary to irritation from the left vocal fold pathology.

■ *Glottic closure:* Hourglass
■ *Phase closure:* Open-phase predominated
■ *Vertical level:* Equal
■ *Amplitude:* Moderately decreased in both vocal folds, slightly more on the left vocal fold
■ *Mucosal wave:* Moderately decreased in both vocal folds, more on the left
■ *Vibratory behavior:* Partial absence always, more on the left
■ *Phase symmetry:* Mostly irregular
■ *Hyperfunction:* Present.

Behavioral Intervention. Treatment for this patient involved a behavioral approach that focused on modifying behaviors and factors that appeared related to the vocal pathology. The general strategies at the onset of the behavioral program included identifying and eliminating any form of phonotraumatic behavior, initiating a modified voice rest program (no more than 2 hours of talking per day for approximately 1 week), and modified work duty,, which meant performance duties were stopped. This patient maintained some income by working in a job that did not require any voicing (filing, etc).

Most individuals are taken out of their performance role when vocal dysfunction arises, but complete voice rest was not recommended because of the nature of this performer's personality, and performance demands. The likelihood of a performer going back to the same performance schedule and producing the same phonotraumatic behaviors is high without strategies in place to reduce strained, back-focused voicing.

Consequently, in the first therapy session with this patient, the concept of the therapeutic voice was introduced. Soft voice (low-impact), relaxed voice production (without strain), and use of a breathy voice characterized the therapeutic voice. Clinicians may recall that these techniques share similarities to the Confidential Voice program.[8] With these recommendations, we attempted to reduce overadduction of the vocal folds, reduce the collision force during vocal fold closure, and prolong the open phase of vocal fold vibration. The main goal was to preserve the normal tissue properties, prevent more damage to the vocal fold mucosa, and restore the vibratory characteristics of the damaged area.

For this high-risk performer, complete restoration of fluid balance after vocal exercise was also an important consideration to the recovery process. She performed in an outside environment that ranged on average from 70 to more than 90° F with high humidity. Within the recovery process, we required the performer not only to hydrate with water, but also to replace electrolytes. Exercise performance becomes impaired when complete rehydration is not achieved.[9] It has been estimated that approximately 3 oz of water should be replaced per 20 minutes of moderate exercise. [10]

With this patient, water intake was recommended at between eight and ten 8-oz glasses of water per day with electrolyte replacement from over-the-counter juices. This patient drank 2 to 3 cups of juice per day.

A general overview of the patient's nutrition also was reviewed to identify any potential contributions to vocal fold irritation or diminished drive. We discussed overall general body health and its relationship to the health of her larynx. Additionally, external sources of stress and tension were discussed. For Patient MM, this included performance demand, financial reliance on her job, strategies in coping with her ill family member, sleep difficulties, and her motivation for participating in the voice therapy program. None of the difficulties mentioned above necessitated referral to other medical professionals. The patient's awareness of these factors was noted to be elevated based on her compliance with recommendations for change as well as her ability to learn how to monitor her vocal behaviors that were not conducive to vocal health.

To relax the laryngeal musculature and reduce laryngeal height and stiffness, circumlaryngeal massage was employed.[11] To further facilitate a lower laryngeal position an open-mouth posture was used during voice production when articulatorily feasible. Although lung volume levels were not measured, the patient was instructed to take an adequate breath prior to initiating voicing. Breathing to higher lung volumes assists in lowering laryngeal position.[12] Also, approaches similar to the yawn-sigh technique[13] were implemented. These techniques concentrated on the inspiratory and expiratory phases of the breathing cycle and slow and controlled expiration for correspondence with the onset of voicing.

Performers spend many hours in rehearsal perfecting the show voice and placing it properly. Nonetheless, we have found that when the rehearsal or performance is over, the forward focus falls to the back of the throat, the breathing techniques become more lax, and

little attention is paid to the amount of vocal use. Forward placement of the voice focuses on relaxing the tongue musculature, using nasal resonance to "move" the tone to the upper vocal tract rather than the lower vocal tract, and paying close attention to the relationship between what is produced and what is heard. A forward focus is achieved by implementing strategies that incorporate humming (/m/, /n/, and /ng/), short resonant words and phrases, conversational voicing, chanting, and singing.

This patient was encouraged to explore both the sensory and the physiologic components of these exercises.[14] Self-auditory perception was developed by contrasting the forward resonant production to the back focus production (negative practice). Back focus production is where the tongue is elevated high in the back of the mouth. It was described as if the voice were deep in the throat and focused on the anatomic site of the problem.[15]

Results of Behavioral Voice Therapy Program. After 7 weeks of voice therapy, Patient MM's vocal folds were reexamined using oral endoscopy and videostroboscopy. The patient was compliant with the voice therapy, and review of the videostroboscopic examination revealed improvement in the movement of the right vocal fold, increased mucosal wave on the left side and a decrease in the overall generalized edema and vascularity of both vocal folds. Unfortunately, polypoid changes and dysphonia persisted. Surgery was recommended.

Surgical Procedure and Result. The patient was brought to the operating room and placed under general anesthesia via oroendotracheal intubation with a small diameter tube. A Dedo laryngoscope was inserted and suspended, and the endolarynx visualized with a binocular operating microscope under high magnification. Bilateral vocal fold polyps were noted at the junction of the anterior and middle thirds of the vocal folds, the left being larger than the right. Both polyps were removed by retraction with Bouchayer forceps and precise excision with curved microscisssors. Excised tissue was sent for pathology evaluation, confirming the clinical impression of benign, traumatic vocal polyps. The patient tolerated the surgical procedure well and recovered uneventfully.

Perceptual Impressions and Acoustic Analysis of Voice Following Surgery.

Recall that the initial perceptual impressions of the patient's speaking voice were characterized as moderately breathy, slightly strained, with glottal fry and frequent episodes of hard glottal attacks, occasional voice breaks, and a vocal loudness that was perceived as too loud. Posttreatment perceptual impressions of the patient's voice were characterized as appropriate vocal pitch and loudness without any perceived strain, breathiness, glottal attacks, or phonatory breaks. A maximum phonation time of 23 seconds was measured during sustained vowel production of /a/. Evaluation of the singing voice revealed the highest sung tone without strain to be A, one octave above middle C; the lowest was G, one octave below middle C with a 27 semitone range.

Table 7–1 shows the results of the acoustic analysis for the sustained vowel /a/ and reading passage following behavioral and surgical intervention. All acoustic parameters were within the normal range posttreatment.

Videolaryngostroboscopic Results Following Surgery

- *Vocal fold edge:* Smooth bilaterally; free of laryngeal lesion and no edema
- *Glottic closure:* Complete
- *Phase closure:* Normal
- *Vertical level:* Equal
- *Amplitude:* Normal
- *Mucosal wave:* Normal
- *Vibratory behavior:* Fully present
- *Phase symmetry:* Regular
- *Hyperfunction:* Not present

Behavioral Voice Therapy Postsurgery. After the pathology was surgically removed and the vocal fold structure and function were observed to be returning to normal, voice therapy was reinitiated. The program focused on retraining, strengthening, and balancing the three systems responsible for voice production and quality; respiration, phonation, and resonance. Principles of vocal exercise physiology, as well as breathing physiology, were used to help the patient maintain an optimum vocal performance. The patient was taught that the muscles in the respiratory and laryngeal system can be trained much as athletes train the muscles that govern movement during a particular type of athletic task. An analogy that we often use is, "A runner would not enter in a track meet without proper training in endurance, strength, flexibility, and muscle toning," neither should a singer return to a high performance work demand without considering the same training principles. We consider singers and actors (or any professional voice user) as "vocal athletes" such that working with respiratory and vocal exercise physiology addresses the issues of strength, flexibility, and endurance as they apply to the voice.

Due to her work demand and style of voicing, expiratory muscle strength training (EMST) was recommended. Several of our studies have examined the use of respiratory muscle strength training as an alternative treatment technique for those patients who have respiratory muscle weakness, high upper airway resistance or performers who encounter high physical demand, excessive laryngeal work loads, and environmental constraints that were not responsive to traditional therapies.[15–18] The EMST paradigm was implemented because it is known that the expiratory muscles are critical for the generation of sounds. Specifically, strengthening the muscles will enhance the performance of the expiratory musculature by providing an increased ability to develop the pressure for sound production with less physiologic effort. This type of training is applicable to those who are required to develop high pressures and for sustaining a given pressure for a long duration (ie, a vocal performer).

Patient MM was issued an EMST device and participated in a 4-week training program. She was seen for a baseline evaluation two times before the training began and her maximum expiratory pressure (MEP) was averaged at 72 cm H_2O. She was seen in our office weekly to reestablish her training threshold pressure based on her new MEP measurement. After 4 weeks of EMST training, her MEP averaged at 156 cm H_2O. Subjective assessment revealed that her perception of her voice quality and "support" for singing had substantially improved.

The application of therapy with this patient involved training the laryngeal and expiratory musculature as well as avoiding improper use of the mecha-

nism. A secondary effect of these methods was to train the proper mechanics of breathing to utilize the natural recoil forces of the respiratory system to facilitate voice production. This provided the patient with a mechanism of producing her voice in an efficient, low-risk manner for meeting her performance and lifestyle demand.

The schedule for Patient MM included a return to work on a gradual basis. It is important to note that, although her vocal pathology was eliminated and her vocal function restored, the training strategies needed to be maintained prior to returning to the performance environment. The patient successfully engaged in practicing these strategies. She understood that vocal warm-ups and cool-downs were mandatory prior to and following a performance and that the vocal exercises were tailored to fit her individual needs.

Returning to Work. The patient's gradual return to work 5 weeks postsurgery progressed as follows. She completed one show per day in a 5-day workweek, incorporating modification strategies and carrying out various laryngeal strengthening exercises to increase vocal endurance throughout this week. In addition, the patient implemented laryngeal relaxation strategies on a regular basis and particularly right after vocal performance. The patient returned to our clinic weekly for reevaluation and voice therapy.

The results of the videostroboscopic evaluation after her first day back to work revealed straight vocal fold edges, slight edema bilaterally, and slight limitations in vibratory amplitude. It was recommended that she continue increasing the time involved working. The second week she completed two shows per day for 3 days and three shows for the remaining 7 days. In Week 4, the patient began feeling comfortable with her performance and was able to incorporate modification strategies to meet the demand of her performance schedule. On reevaluation, the vocal fold structure and function were deemed to be within normal limits. The vocal fold edges continued to be straight with an absence of the generalized edema. It was recommended that she return the next week to perform four shows per day. Intervention continued throughout this time period two times per week. As she moved into her regular work schedule, therapy focused on maintaining the training strategies outlined above with her actual script.

Final Thoughts. We find that high-risk performers are unique compared with general vocal performers. At a minimum, this conclusion can be based on the supported evidence of a high environmental demand. Consequently, clinicians must understand the relationship between the environmental demand and the structural and functional deviations presented to them.

As with many types of rehabilitation, there is no single therapeutic technique that fits all individual needs, although the underlying pathology, structure, and function may share common traits. Most typically, the treatment program for the high-risk performer is based on occupational, social, and behavioral needs.

We have found ourselves advocating for management issues related to performance scheduling and believe it is critical for speech-language pathologists who are involved in the care of the professional voice to advocate for improved training and management.

The Developing Performer

Barbara Jacobson, PhD

Case Study: Patient NN

> *In the following case study, Barbara Jacobson reports the case of a young "top-40" singer who presented with multiple medical and voice misuse factors causing hoarseness and reduction in singing ability.*

Patient NN, a 21-year-old female aspiring singer/songwriter, was referred to the Voice Center for complaints of hoarseness in her speaking voice, diminished control of her singing voice, decreased vocal range for singing, and loss of "head register" (ability to produce singing voice for high notes). She experienced vocal fatigue in both her speaking and singing voice. She was seen in the multidisciplinary clinic by a speech-language pathologist, otolaryngologist, and singing voice specialist, all on the same day. She was planning to have songwriting appointments and participate in singer showcases and this was the impetus for seeking help.

Patient NN gave the following voice history. She had been singing since she was very young. She was a cheerleader in high school. She sang in school choirs as an alto/tenor and began singing contemporary country repertoire with a band during her late teens. She attended college for 2 years. After she left school, she typically sang 4 nights per week, with multiple sets (at least three) per night. She often sang in smoky environments. At age 19, she developed significant problems with her voice, particularly after an episode in which she had a particularly bad bout of bronchitis. At that time, she was diagnosed with vocal nodules. The physician also suspected gastroesophageal reflux. After a period of total voice rest (including singing), treatment with steroids, and a course of a proton pump inhibitor, the nodules appeared to go away. She did not receive voice therapy at that time. Her voice became somewhat clearer, but over the past year, she began to have problems with both her singing and speaking voice.

Patient NN had formal voice training during her college years. She acknowledged that she had difficulty applying knowledge from these lessons to her singing technique. Her voice teacher categorized her as a soprano, although Patient NN struggled to produce her voice in the higher voice range. She believed her singing style was most consistent with a "belting" technique. Her current singing range was approximately one-and-a half octaves, which was significantly below her potential range. Any attempts to reach high notes resulted in a breathy, "weak" sound.

The patient's medical history was remarkable for temporomandibular joint dysfunction with bruxism, hiatal hernia, and suspected allergies (which were not documented). The patient described bulimic and anorexic behavior that had occurred approximately 6 years previously and lasted for 1 year. She did not seek medical or psychiatric assistance. The patient currently was taking no medications. She did not use antihistamines or aspirin. Hydration was adequate. She drank two to three beers per week. She occasionally drank a caffeinated beverage. She had a 2-year history of one pack per day cigarette smoking but had quit 3 years ago. She complained of occasional feelings of heartburn.

Patient NN was employed as a waitress. She described her daily voice use as heavy. She frequently had to raise her voice to be heard at work. She would often go out with friends to bars or music venues after her shift on the nights she was not performing. Her informal songwriting appointments often lasted several hours at a time, and she did the demo work for the songs written during these sessions.

Otolaryngologic evaluation revealed slightly dry nasal mucosa. Oral cavity, oropharynx, and nasopharynx were normal. Indirect laryngoscopic examination was remarkable for bilateral vocal fold focal edema. Vocal folds were vascular. There was increased pain on palpation of the thyrohyoid space with some discomfort on palpating her strap muscles. There was marked popping in her temporomandibular joints on jaw opening.

Voice analysis included videostroboscopy which demonstrated an hourglass closure configuration. There was compression of the ventricular folds on phonation onset. This increased supraglottic activity, which included anterior to posterior compression, increased as the patient approached her register break, at the transition from her middle to head voice. During stroboscopy, it was noticed that her mucosal wave was moderately decreased bilaterally, especially over the area of midfold swelling. The open phase of vibration predominated. These videostroboscopic results indicated that the patient had a significant amount of air wastage due to decreased glottic efficiency during phonation. She also exhibited increasing extralaryngeal tension in her higher singing range. There was a characteristic "hyperfunction/underclosure" glottic configuration evident at higher pitch productions. The patient's acoustic analysis is shown in Table 7–2. Acoustic measures indicated a decreased habitual pitch and reflected her rough voice quality. The results of her aerodynamic analysis are shown in Table 7–3.

Normally, we might expect that airflow values would be low at all pitches and even across all pitches for singers. Phonation time should be significantly longer than the average 18 to 20 seconds we expect for nonsingers. Results for this patient reflected inefficient laryngeal valving during phonation at her habitual and high pitches.

Perceptual analysis of the patient's voice revealed a mild dysphonia characterized by roughness and breathiness. There was a slight strained voice quality. Habitual speaking pitch was perceived as being low. Habitual loudness

in conversation was increased. Abusive voice production behaviors included throat clearing. The patient was able to sustain /i/ for only 11 seconds. Her s/z ration was 1.57 (normal = 1.4). An oral peripheral examination revealed normal oral structures for voice production. There was significant neck musculoskeletal tension with withdrawal on palpation and manipulation. Muscle tension was also apparent in the shoulders and upper back. The patient sat with a chin/neck forward posture. Her Voice Handicap Index (VHI) score was 54 (range = 0–120; reflecting a moderate self-perceived handicap). Singing Voice Handicap Index (SVHI) was 95 (range = 1–144; reflecting a severe self-perceived handicap). The patient rated her voice problem as "moderate to severe." Her ASHA NOMS score was Level 4 ("Voice

Table 7–2. Pretreatment Acoustic Analysis for Patient NN

	Mean F_0 (Hz)	Jitter (ms)	Shimmer (%)	SNR (dB)
Habitual pitch	173.5	.114	4.02	25.50
High pitch	624.5	.020	2.86	20.34
Low pitch	148.3	.080	3.02	27.22
Oral reading	178.7			26.09

*Mean values are shown. Semitone range = 33.4.

Table 7–3. Pretreatment Aerodynamic Analysis for Patient NN

	Mean Flow Volume (mL)	Maximum Phonation Time (sec)	Peak Flow Rate (mL/sec)	Airflow Rate (mL/sec)
Habitual pitch	3630	12.26	390	244.35
High pitch	3360	14.05	240	220.80
Low pitch	3245	13.67	225	130.25

Mean values are shown.

is functional for communication, but sometimes distracting. Individual's ability to participate in vocational, avocation, and social activities requiring voice is occasionally affected in low-vocal demand activities, but consistently affected in high-vocal demand activities").

Assessment by the voice teacher was significant for reduced vocal range. There were some excessively tense jaw and tongue postures observed during singing. In addition, the patient had difficulty dissociating jaw and tongue movements while singing. Breath support appeared to be normal. Tension was apparent during all aspects of singing.

Consensus by the voice team was that the cause of the patient's voice disorders was multidimensional. There appeared to be influences from both her speaking and her singing technique and speaking voice use. Her medical history (bruxism and bulimia) also contributed. She was referred to a gastroenterologist for assessment with pH probe and manometry. This was determined to be normal. Responsibility for day-to-day management was assigned to the voice pathologist and voice teacher.

Patient NN immediately began voice therapy and voice lessons. Coordination between the voice pathologist and voice teacher was close, and treatment goals were developed to be parallel. We were struck by the patient's motivation and commitment to achieving improvement in her voice and felt that this reflected favorably on her prognosis and eventual outcomes.

In speaking voice therapy, treatment goals were established to educate the patient regarding vocal hygiene (in particular, to reduce loud voice use, throat clearing, and the amount of time spent in aversive, loud environments), to decrease laryngeal area muscle tension,

and to increase the use of oral resonance and efficient airflow during voice production. In addition, to optimize vocal fold closure, a low-impact adductory exercise (see Vocal Function Exercises, Chapter 3) was implemented to produce improved vocal fold closure. She simultaneously underwent treatment with a singing voice clinician. Our overarching goals for modifying her voice production were to decrease the phonotrauma due to excessive muscle effort and increase coordinated appropriate airflow and resonance for better efficiency in overall use.

Weekly visits were scheduled, and the patient demonstrated compliance with vocal hygiene recommendations. Areas of treatment emphasis were coordinated with the singing voice specialist. For example, structured tasks specifically focused on reducing musculoskeletal tension were timed to correspond with work in relaxing jaw and tongue and increasing supraglottic "space" during voice lessons. We determined that myofascial release treatment would be beneficial and the patient was referred to the Integrative Health Center for physical therapy.

After four sessions, the patient's laryngeal status was monitored with videostroboscopy. At that time, there was a reduction in the size of the bilateral vocal fold swellings. Also evident at that time was an increase in mucosal wave. Subjectively, the patient was beginning to notice an increase in her vocal range. She remarked that she did not feel as though she had to "push" as much to produce voice for either speaking or singing. She noted less roughness in her voice quality. Perceptually, we noticed an increase in her habitual pitch.

Over the course of treatment, Patient NN was able to increase times for sustaining notes C through G on Vocal Function Exercises. Gradually, she lost the breathy quality on a sustained tone, inferring increased vocal efficiency. In particular, the patient found these exercises to be most helpful for monitoring the status of her voice. If she had used her voice too strenuously on the previous night, then on the following morning she noticed a decrease in the amount of time she was able to produce an engaged, sustained tone. This served to reinforce her ability to self-monitor vocally abusive behaviors.

In addition to Vocal Function Exercises, cup bubble and gargle exercises were used to help the patient overtly maintain continuous airflow during sustained phonation and increase oral resonance. She was able to use the change in sensation and awareness of extraneous effort at the laryngeal level as a monitoring device to know when she was "pushing" her voice. She gradually transitioned into nasally loaded syllables, words, phrases, and sentences using these facilitators.

Progress in both her speaking and singing voice production was rapid. The patient reported that the coordinated focus of treatment goals in both voice therapy and voice lessons helped her to understand concepts more quickly, even though the vocabulary might be somewhat different. In voice therapy, the patient was asked to associate consciously techniques and principles for speaking with those for singing. Her voice clinician reported that as she worked during voice lessons, a soprano vocal range was emerging.

Voice therapy continued for eight sessions. At the end of that time, posttreatment objective measures were made, as was a reanalysis of perceptual features. Significant changes were evident in airflow rate at habitual pitch, in fundamental frequency at habitual pitch and while reading, in vocal quality, and in perceived habitual pitch and loudness. Comparison of pretreatment and posttreatment measures is shown in Tables 7–4 and 7–5.

Perceptually, the patient's speaking voice was more resonant. Loudness in conversation was at a suitable level. There was a reduction in laryngeal area muscle tension. Overall, the patient reported that producing a voice for speaking was easier. The effort to produce voice with clearer voice quality was more automatic and less conscious.

The most telling result of treatment was demonstrated in comparison of recordings of her singing voice at three difference stages: 1 year previously, just

Table 7–4. Posttreatment Aerodynamic Analysis by Vowel for Patient NN

Condition	Flow Volume (mL)	MPT (sec)	Airflow Rate (mL/sec)
/a/	3480	28.4	122.53
/i/	3740	29.7	125.93
/u/	3610	29.1	124.23

Table 7–5. Posttreatment Airflow Rates (mL/sec) for Patient NN

Condition	Pretreatment	Posttreatment	% Change
/a/	235.4	122.5	52
/i/	253.3	125.9	49
/u/	244.3	124.2	51

prior to treatment, and at the end of treatment. In the last recording, the patient reported an overall increase in ease, clarity, and efficiency in use, which translated to a maximum phonation time that was within expected limits, a "brighter," more resonant tone, decreased effort in managing dynamics (moving from a quiet tone production to a louder one), notes produced on pitch, and stronger, clearer notes at the high end of her singing range, creating more of a "one voice" sound throughout her range. Voice therapy was ended with follow-up to be maintained by telephone contact. Patient RR continues to receive voice lessons.

The Patient on Tour

Wendy LeBorgne, PhD, CCC-SLP

Case Study: Patient OO

> *How does one treat a national performing artist who is in town for a brief period of time? Wendy LeBorgne offers her insight on the matter with the case of a musical theater actor in the midst of a national tour.*

Patient OO, a 31-year-old woman, was a self-referred performer in town during a national Broadway tour. Patient OO came to the voice center after several weeks of vocal fatigue following performances. She found particular difficulty in maintaining "clarity" in her upper range and found that her singing voice was quite fatigued after a show. In addition, she reported difficulty traversing her passagio or transition into her head voice, but she did not believe that it was audible to her audience. She reported feeling a general tiredness in her voice after a show and that she had no desire to sing or speak. No particular change was noted in the quality of her speaking voice. On the day of examination, a complete voice evaluation was conducted, including laryngeal videostroboscopy and laryngeal function testing, including aerodynamic and acoustic measures.

History. Because Patient OO traveled to a new city every 3 to 4 weeks, she was unable to see her regular otolaryngologist for this particular problem. Therefore, a thorough history was taken, and the videostroboscopic examination was reviewed by an otolaryngologist. A case history revealed that, 3 weeks prior to her arrival in Cincinnati, she had developed a mild upper respiratory infection, which was treated with 10 days of antibiotics. She reported that she continued to sing during the infection, although she was coughing significantly at the time. She reported that her cough subsided within 4 days of being placed on the antibiotics but that her voice had not felt "quite right" since that time.

Currently, Patient OO had a supporting role in the show and performed that role six times per week. A typical day included arising around 11 AM, going to rehearsal from noon until 2 PM, relaxing or napping in the afternoon, and reporting back to the theater by 6 PM. Following the show, she typically went out to dinner with friends and returned to her hotel by 2 AM. The typical length of the show was approximately 2.5 hours. She had been performing professionally for 13 years and had rarely missed a performance because of illness or vocal problems. This was her sixth national tour of a Broadway show.

Patient OO was in excellent physical shape and had approximately 17 years of formal voice training and coaching. Early in her career, she reported having vocal fold nodules, which resolved with rest, therapy, and continued vocal training. She was concerned that the nodules may have recurred with all of the recent harsh coughing. She did not smoke but was often exposed to passive smoke in restaurants and bars, and she also had to perform several scenes with fog on the stage. This patient had no complaints of gastroesophageal reflux or dysphagia. Current medications included Zoloft for treatment of mild depression, and Claritin for seasonal allergies. Patient OO was well versed in vocal hygiene issues and attempted to follow the recommendations faithfully. She religiously drank 8 to 10 glasses of water per day and only 1 cup of coffee. She reported being a "vocally enthusiastic" person but attempted to use her voice conservatively on days of shows and when in noisy environments.

This singer was single, and most of her close friends were scattered across the country. Unfortunately, the current national production with which she was touring was planning to close after the next city, and she was taking all of her free time traveling to auditions for her next job. She was hoping to get a role in a nontouring company because she needed a "break from the road."

During the intake, the voice pathologist noted a slight "edge" to Patient OO's speaking voice, with some back focus and glottal fry phonation. She did not demonstrate any observed tongue or jaw tension. Breathing and rate of speech also were within normal limits for conversational speech.

Videolaryngostroboscopic Examination. Under direct light, this patient presented with grossly normal-appearing true vocal folds bilaterally. Some mild vascularity was noted on the superior surface of the vocal folds, but the medial edges appeared smooth and straight bilaterally. While sustaining the vowel /i/, stroboscopic lighting was employed, and it was observed that this patient presented with a small anterior glottal gap, which was present at all pitches tested. The amplitude of vibration and mucosal wave appeared mildly decreased bilaterally, but the overall system was quite flexible. The open phase of the vibratory cycle was slightly dominant, whereas the symmetry of vibration was irregular at low pitches only. No mass lesions, paralysis, or paresis were noted. Mild pachyderma was noted in the interarytenoid area suggestive of possible laryngopharyngeal reflux.

Acoustic Findings. This patient first was asked to read the "Rainbow Passage" in a normal conversational voice. Her attempt at this task revealed a mean fundamental speaking frequency of 185.3 Hz with a standard deviation of 13.6. Second, this patient was asked to describe a picture. Her attempt at this task revealed a mean fundamental frequency of 186.9 Hz and a standard deviation of 16.4. Both reading and conversational samples of speech were considered to be within normal limits.

Next, the patient was asked to glide to her highest and lowest pitches in two separate attempts to attain her physiologic frequency range. She peaked at a frequency of 1244 Hz, and her lowest tone was measured at 164 Hz. No audible pitch breaks were noted in her voice. She maintained an adequate range for her age and voice type.

A final acoustic measure taken was a modified voice range profile. Tables 7–6 and 7–7 show the Hz, semitones, and decibel levels across 11 pitches encom-

passing her vocal range. It is evident from these results, Patient OO had excellent dynamic control of her voice, with the exception of the extremes of her range, and the passaggio into her head voice (at about 698.5 Hz). At that point, she was only able to achieve a dynamic difference of 18 dB. Unfortunately, the solos that she sang in the show were in that general area of her voice difficulty.

Aerodynamic Results. Following acoustic testing, this patient completed laryngeal function testing using the Nagashima Phonatory Function Analyzer (Kelleher Medical, Richmond, VA). Tables 7–8 and 7–9 show the resultant flow volumes, maximum phonation times, and airflow rates. All aerodynamic measurements were within normal limits, with the exception of low sustained pitches. At these pitches, Patient OO demonstrated an increased airflow rate and decreased

Table 7–6. Pretreatment Voice Range Profile for Patient OO

Semitone	Hertz	Minimum dB	Maximum dB
40	164.8	59	76
43.5	207.6	60	86
47	246.9	57	91
50.5	311.1	58	91
54	370	58	93
57.5	466.2	65	98
61	554.4	67	102
64.5	698.5	82	100
68	830.6	74	111
71.5	1046.5	77	113
75	1244.5	81	105

Table 7–7. Posttreatment Voice Range Profile for Patient OO

Semitone	Hertz	Minimum dB	Maximum dB
40	164.8	58	76
43.5	207.6	57	85
47	246.9	58	93
50.5	311.1	58	92
54	370	58	95
57.5	466.2	62	98
61	554.4	67	101
64.5	698.5	69	104
68	830.6	71	113
71.5	1046.5	77	112
75	1244.5	79	105

Table 7–8. Pretreatment Aerodynamic Analysis for Patient OO

Frequency (Hz)	Flow Volume	Flow Rate	MPT
185	3220	102	33.3
165	3430	160	21.5
500	3370	102	33.1

Table 7–9. Posttreatment Aerodynamic Analysis for Patient OO

Frequency (Hz)	Flow Volume	Flow Rate	MPT
185	3360	100	33.7
165	3410	103	33.3
500	3380	101	33.4

maximum phonation time. This was consistent with the anterior glottal gap observed on stroboscopy, particularly at low pitches, indicating a possible intrinsic laryngeal muscle weakness. [19,20]

Diagnosis and Treatment. Based on the above information, it was determined that this patient was experiencing a mild laryngeal myasthenia, which most likely resulted from singing during an upper respiratory infection and severe coughing. At the time of the evaluation, the upper respiratory infection and the coughing had resolved completely, and it was advised that this patient enroll in a formal voice therapy program. The voice therapy program included Vocal Function Exercises (VFE), designed to condition and balance the laryngeal musculature, and Resonant Voice Therapy (RVT), designed to promote a frontal, oral, open focus during conversational speech. Both approaches have the goal of rebalancing the three subsystems of voice production, respiration, phonation, and resonance.

Voice therapy began immediately. Initially, therapy focused on proper technique of both the VFE and RVT. Patient OO was also counseled regarding vocal hygiene and the importance of recognizing when she needed to take a day off from singing during times of infections. Because of her skill as a singer, she was engaging in proper technique for both exercise programs almost immediately.

The VFE program that was used for this singer included the musical notes C through G. In the first portion of the exercise program, she was asked to sustain the vowel /i/ on the musical note F for as long as possible. Special attention was drawn to the fact that the /i/ sound was to be produced in a nasal, overly forward-placed tone. Patient OO expressed concern that this was not the way in which she would sing an /i/ vowel. It was explained to her that these were not "singing exercises" and that she would hopefully never sing with the amount of nasality required for this particular exercise. The second part of the exercise program, designed to stretch the vocal folds to maximal length, was to have Patient OO glide from her lowest pitch to her highest pitch on the

word "knoll" using an extremely forward focus. Her first attempt at this exercise resulted in a beautiful glide to her highest note, and then she started to glide back down again. This is a common mistake seen in many singers because it is similar to a vocalise often called the "siren," in which one glides from the lowest note to the highest note and back down again in one breath. The importance of stretching only to her highest note and then stopping was impressed on Patient OO. She was also reminded to use proper abdominal breathing through all exercises. Step 3 of the exercise program was to glide from her highest note to her lowest note, again on "knoll." She was extremely proficient at this but needed a word of caution not to initiate the tone with a hard glottal attack or go into glottal fry phonation at her lowest notes. Finally, the exercises designed to build adductory efficiency and stamina of the intrinsic laryngeal musculature were taught. These consisted of the patient sustaining the musical notes C, D, E, F, and G, on the word "old" without the /d/, for as long as possible and as softly as possible, but with an engaged tone. Special care was taken to ensure Patient OO began with a *coup de glotte* phonation, meaning that she initiated the phonation at the precise moment the vocal folds adducted and the resonators were perfectly tuned to the vowel. It is important to be extremely precise with singers' onset of phonation and not allow them to cheat themselves on a less than optimal onset. Several attempts were made with this patient to ensure precise onset of the tone and breath. She was an extremely astute patient and performed the exercises with accuracy after minimal instruction. She was asked to do the Vocal Function Exercises two times per day, no less, no more. She was given a log sheet, to keep track of her phonation times on the exercises and was asked to bring it back during each return visit.

A modified regimen of RVT was employed with this patient because she progressed through the steps quickly. As with most singers, this patient had an excellent sense of vocal tract resonance. The first step of RVT was to have her hum on a comfortable pitch in her speech range. She was asked to note where she felt any vibrations while phonating. She reported a general sense of "buzzing" in her cheeks and nose. This was repeated several times. Next, the patient was asked to maintain this "buzz" while chanting, then doing a messa di voce (slow-soft, gradually increasing to loud-fast, and then gradually decreasing back to slow-soft), then overinflecting voiced syllables. (See Patient OO Appendix for a complete description of modified RVT as presented by Stemple, Glaze, and Klaben, 2009.)

She was extremely proficient at this, and therapy continued into chanted sentences. The sentences (see Patient OO Appendix) were used to maintain a frontal, oral, open focus during connected speech. The patient was asked to first chant the sentences with a nasal, forward tone, then she was to overinflect them with the same tone, and then to speak them in a normal voice while maintaining the forward (not nasal) resonance. Minimal difficulties were found when doing Stage 1 of RVT. She reported that her voice "felt good" when doing RVT. She was advised to do these exercises at least twice a day.

During the next session, she was able to progress with Stage 2 of RVT, which entailed warming up with Stage 1 and then moving to the list of voiced-voiceless syllables and then sentences

(See Patient OO Appendix for a complete outline of the therapy stages and steps). They were performed in the same fashion as the voiced exercises. The only difficulty that Patient OO had was during the speaking portion of the sentence level. She had the tendency to drop her voice at the last syllable into a glottal fry phonation pattern. When she was made aware of this, she was able to immediately correct it. Patient OO found RVT easy to do on her afternoon break and was able to do the exercises three times daily.

Finally, during the third session, the patient was proficient enough in the RVT exercises that Stage 3, the "Any Phrase" Stage, was skipped and paragraph reading was added. The same principles of maintaining a frontal, oral, open focus was applied at this level. By this time, however, Patient OO was well aware of any glottal fry phonation and essentially was able to eliminate it from all reading and conversational speech.

Because of the limited amount of time she was in town, the patient was seen two times per week, for the 2 weeks that remained of her stay. She was extremely compliant with all recommendations, and rapid progression was noted with therapy. Her Vocal Function Exercise times (MPT) improved from an average of 22.4 seconds at the initiation of therapy to an average of 35.2 seconds by the fourth therapy session. She particularly enjoyed doing the resonant voice therapy and found that her voice was "lighter and easier" after only a few days of doing them.

At the end of the 2-week period of therapy, Patient OO felt her voice was markedly improved but opted to continue doing both Vocal Function Exercises and Resonant Voice Therapy. Posttherapy voice range profile and aerodynamic results may be seen in Tables 7–7 and

7–9. Note the marked improvement in her airflow rates at low pitches, as well as an increase in dynamic range at the 698.5 Hz frequency. A follow-up stroboscopic evaluation also was done, and it revealed only a small posterior glottic gap. No anterior glottic chink was present at any pitch on stroboscopic evaluation.

Patient OO received word that following the closing of this Broadway tour, she would begin rehearsing for the New York premiere of a new Broadway musical in a supporting role. Although we were not permitted to spend the ideal amount of time in therapy with her, she had such a strong underlying vocal mechanism, it only took minimal guidance to see dramatic improvement.

Patient OO Appendix
Materials for Use with Resonant Voice Therapy (RVT)

Basic Training Gesture for RVT

■ holm-molm-molm-m-molm . . . As a sigh
■ Extreme forward focus is required with appropriate breath support.
■ Make the connection from the abdominal muscles to the lips.
■ Patient should feel very relaxed at the end of this gesture.

RVT Hierarchy: Stage 1 All Voiced

1. molm-molm-molm . . . (sustained pitch) _____

   ■ Vary the rate only.
   ■ Discover the vibrations; experiment with broad and narrow vibrations.
   ■ Increase the ease of production by reducing the effort by half and half again.
   ■ Increase "lift" (as if pitch were increasing).

2. molm-molm-molm . . . slow-fast-slow
   soft-loud-soft on _____

3. molm-molm-molm . . . as speech

   ■ Use nonlinguistic phrases; vary the rate, pitch, and loudness; make the connection from the abdominal muscles to the lips.

4. Chant the following voiced phrases on the musical note _____

   ■ Mary made me mad.
   ■ My mother made marmalade.
   ■ My merry mom made marmalade.
   ■ My mom may merry Marv.
   ■ My merry mom may marry Marv.
   ■ Marv made my mother merry.

5. Overinflect these phrases as speech

RVT Hierarchy: Stage 2 Voice-Voiceless Contrasts

1. mamapapa . . . vary the rate on _____ (musical note)

2. mamapapa . . . slow-fast-slow
   soft-loud-soft on _____ (musical note)

3. mamapapa . . . As speech

   ■ use non-linguistic phrases; vary the rate, pitch, and loudness; make the connection from the abdominal muscles to the lips.

4. Chant the following voiced/voiceless phrases on the musical note _____

   ■ Mom may put Paul on the moon.
   ■ Mom told Tom to copy my manner.
   ■ My manner made Pete and Paul mad.
   ■ Mom may move Polly's movie to ten.
   ■ My movie made Tim and Tom sad.

5. Overinflect these phrases as speech

RVT Hierarchy: Stage 3 Any Phrase

1. Chant five to seven syllable phrases on the note _____.

2. Overinflect the same phrases with an extreme forward focus.

3. Repeat the same phrases in a more natural forward speech/voice production.

RVT Hierarchy: Stage 4 Paragraph Reading

1. Read a paragraph with phrase markers. Separate each phrase only by the natural inhalation of air.

2. Exaggerate focus and then repeat with a more normal speech and voice production.

3. Repeat the above without phrase markers.

RVT Hierarchy: Stage 5 Controlled Conversation

■ Practice forward speech placement in conversation.
■ Do not permit glottal attacks, glottal fry, etc.

RVT Hierarchy: Stage 6 Environmental Manipulations

■ Simulate actual speaking environments consistent with patient's needs (actual and simulated).
■ Use tapes of background noise.
■ Go to noisy cafeteria.

RVT Hierarchy: Stage 7 Emotional Manipulations

■ Use materials and topics that increasingly engage and challenge the patient.

RVT Hierarchy: Home Exercises

■ The critical portion of the exercises for each week is tape recorded as a home exercise example. The home program involves 15- to 20-minute sessions, two times per day with "minis" as needed.
■ Basic RV gesture
■ Selected level of hierarchy

From Stemple J, Glaze L, and Klaben B. *Clinical Voice Pathology: Theory and Management.* 3rd ed. San Diego, CA: Singular Publishing Group; 2009. Reprinted with permission.

Intervention for Bilateral TVF Nodules in a Praise and Worship Leader

Martin L. Spencer, MA, CCC-SLP

Case Study: Patient PP

> *In the following case, Martin Spencer illustrates two levels of voice therapy directed at rehabilitation of an active praise and worship leader and educator diagnosed with "nodules." The first level was intended to promote awareness and calibration of basic vocal dynamics. The second level, to promote awareness of singing technique freed from hyperconstrictive phonation. Both levels promote lesion abatement and advance vocal insight.*

Background: Singer-Related Pathology.
Typical contributing factors to pathologic occurrence in singers include:

- Excessive predominance of high-pitched, chest register phonation
- Consistent mismatch of voice part, intensity, tessitura, or fach with innate physiologic capacity
- Excessively sustained primary or secondary muscular tensions. (Primary tensions proceed from intrinsic laryngeal musculature, and secondary tensions from associated elements such as the jaw, tongue, pharyngeal constrictors, extrinsic laryngeal musculature, strap muscles, and torso.)
- Lack of awareness to "mark" or rest when vocally fatigued
- Lack of vocal warm-up before rehearsals or performances
- Insufficient amplification or feedback monitoring in enhanced acoustic environments

- Poor vocal hygiene via factors such as smoking, excessive alcohol intake, excessive social voice usage, physical deconditioning, poor hydration, and unattended reflux or allergy control
- Ignoring early warning signals of vocal injury:
  - ☐ Loss of phonatory ease thereby incurring compensatory strain
  - ☐ Asynchronous tonal onset with breath unintentionally preceding phonation
  - ☐ Diminished breath control
  - ☐ Loss of intensity control
  - ☐ Curtailment of pitch range or loss of register
  - ☐ Loss of smooth passaggio transition
  - ☐ Persistently undesirable quality such as voice breaks, burring or diplophonia
  - ☐ Excessive delay of vocal recovery after performance.

Singers who have not received formal vocal instruction may be unaware of these factors.

Gospel singers, praise and worship singers, music theater performers, and rock musicians are a commonly encountered clinical population. These art forms require a high level of vocal engagement, which consistently may tax the voice and strain and stress laryngeal tissues beyond usual recovery patterns. Phonotrauma may develop over months or years before clinical intervention is sought—with correspondingly complex clinical intervention required. A major thrust in rehabilitation of singing-related injury focuses on patient education about usage and care of the vocal "instrument."

Therapy alone may be effective in voice restoration, and should always be considered as an initial phase of intervention. Note, however, that lesion type may militate against therapeutic effectiveness, and therefore vocal rest (eg, as in TVF hemorrhage) or surgery may be indicated (eg, as in a cyst or significant polyp.) Surgical prognosis, without therapy, may be diminished if phonotraumatic etiology is not identified, and, ideally corrected before surgery.

Client History. Patient PP presented to our clinic with moderate to severe dysphonia that was impairing both speaking and singing voice ("My voice cuts out . . . I've lost my falsetto."). The patient was 26 years old and very active in her denomination as a praise and worship leader, and bible school teacher. Patient PP sought intervention as her dysphonia was not resolving and she was planning on being the primary praise and worship leader for a large church convention in several months. Her clinical goal was "to get my voice back to where it used to be."

She had received several months of vocal training at college and was classified as a soprano. Subsequent song leading frequently required alto range transposition (author's note: this may imbalance head to chest register dominance and be a catalyst for phonotraumatic injury.) Patient PP never warmed up before singing.

In the summer months preceding her fall clinical exam, Patient PP had actively led worship at a youth conference and several youth camps; she felt that her dysphonia dated from this time. Since the summer she had returned to work as a gregarious Starbuck's barista. Patient PP continued active involvement with her church through leading bible studies three evenings per week. Her high level of activity and progressive loss of voicing had led to severe life stressors in response to which she suffered loss of dietary control and weight gain of approximately 20 lbs over the preceding year. At the time of examination, Patient PP noted that she had started work with a personal trainer to improve fitness and lose weight.

Singing voice impairments included loss of head register ("falsetto"), inability to vary dynamics (particularly toward softer intensity), and loss of tonal clarity with increased breathiness.

On initial presentation, associated symptoms included frequent throat clearing, intermittent aphonia, and increased morning hoarseness. She was avoiding going out socially to reduce her vocal loading. Prior medical history was otherwise unremarkable, with no medications or tobacco usage.

SLP and Medical Evaluation. VLS observation revealed small but clearly formed, translucent, symmetric, bilatero-medial TVF "nodules" consistent with phonotraumatic etiology. The lesions appeared to be soft and nonfibrous; it was possible, but unlikely, that they were polypoid. Mild to moderate postcricoid edema likely was consistent with chronic reflux irritation and complaints of chronic throat clearing.

As a result of the VLS and ensuing ENT diagnosis, it was recommended that Patient PP receive voice therapy and start on Protonix 40 mg qam. Educational materials regarding laryngopharyngeal reflux were supplied. Patient PP was advised that compliance with therapy directives would be the key component of recovery.

Perceptual and Acoustic Measures. Patient PP's voice was rated perceptually with CAPE-V[21] administration. Results indicated moderate to severe roughness, strain, and overall dysphonia. Loudness was moderate to severely elevated, possibly to attempt compensatory stabilization of voice quality due to elevated phonation threshold pressures incurred by lesion presence. Speaking fundamental frequency (SF_0) was in atypical alto range. In conversation, Patient PP demonstrated an aphonic syllable every several sentences.

Pitch glides indicated severe impairment of singing voice with loss of head register, soft intensity, and crisp onset. (Further detailing of singing impairment at the first therapy session revealed intact pitch range of a major tenth; from Ab3 to C5. Head voice could not be produced in spite of multiple probes. Average maximum phonation times (MPTs) progressively decreased from 9.3 seconds at C4 to 4.4 seconds at G4.

On VHI[22] and V-ROQL[23] indices, Patient PP noted that her most significant problems outside of church performing and lecturing activity were "frustrating" repetitions of speech to make herself understood. Her voice would constantly "give out," and conversational partners would frequently ask "What's wrong with your voice?"

Acoustic analysis of the Rainbow Passage[6] indicated mean fundamental frequency (F_0) of 225 Hz (A3 with a SD of 3.34 semitones.)

Behavioral Intervention: Treatment Approaches for the Singing Voice. In her barista work, Patient PP had started relative vocal conservation with usage of a head-mounted microphone. She was using head nods to indicate "yes" or "no" responses to fellow employees. It was difficult for her to implement voice conservation as Starbucks was a "fun environment." (She was advised that increasing transglottic airflow could potentially ease hyperadductive phonation and decrease associated fatigue.)

She had found substitute teachers and guest speakers for her current bible classes. The author was impressed with these patient-generated strategies.

Patient PP noted that she had a recurring loss of her head voice prior to the current period of complaint and therefore had favored transposition of songs down into her chest register so that she could guarantee a level of consistency in her singing. She liked the resulting richness in her voice when singing in a lower pitch range. To the author, these details raised the possibility of lesion presence before the current period of complaint.

Patient PP's history and medical diagnosis of bilateral TVF nodules corroborated two primary causes of phonotrauma: voice overuse and ill use. Therapeutic approach would implement greater awareness of vocal care in both speaking and singing, expand basic knowledge of singing technique, and certain exercises were hypothesized to reduce lesion presence.

Probable laryngeal irritation stemming from reflux irritation was treated with Protonix 40 mg qid. Subsequent necessity for qid PPI usage was bolstered by Patient PP reporting heartburn when off of the PPI for 1 day.

Patient PP was started on the Hybrid Voice Therapy (HVT)[24] protocol, which was developed by the author in response to the specific requirements of voice professionals occupationally reliant on sustained, projected voicing. Once HVT goals of respiratory and phonatory regulation were assimilated, it was expected that therapy would more directly address integration of singing into a voice therapy. These two stages of rehabilitation, and their component goals and rationales, are addressed in detail below.

1. Description and Rationale for Hybrid Voice Therapy (HVT). The impetus for HVT arose from the author's desire to integrate related aspects of voice rehabilitation and performing arts training protocols into a single practical program. In particular, it was recognized that current voice therapy methods might not sufficiently address the demands of professional voice users who, posttreatment, would continue to be at high risk for phonotrauma. It is significant that many of these nonperforming professionals seldom, if ever, receive vocational training in the development and usage of projected voice. Therefore, rehabilitation of the "conversational" speaking voice alone may not suffice to prevent pathologic recurrence. It was proposed that further preventative training drawn from the arts might promote better technical management of vocal resources.

The HVT program is divided into four stages that address the three subsystems of voice production, respiration, phonation, and resonance. It was hoped that Patient PP would experience these essential voice components in both relative isolation and combined output. Educational materials were provided to increase awareness of therapy objectives. Her home therapy schedule was advised to be approximately 10 minutes per session, or 20 minutes when performed on a recommended twice-daily basis. An accompaniment CD was provided to increase compliance.

Goal 1. *Lower abdominal breathing.* "Sit or stand erectly, and place your hand frontally over the belly to monitor respiratory movement. Inhale deeply through your nose and blow out through pursed lips. Avoid superfluous upper chest involvement." (10×)

Rationale. Separated respiratory attention is a fundamental and powerful precursor to vocal rehabilitation. This is especially so in the treatment of professional voice users as projected voice usage requires active respiratory engagement in advance of the demands of conversational speech.

In theory, this initial HVT exercise addresses the controlled delivery of aerodynamic energy that subsequently fuels phonatory transduction into acoustic energy. Inadequate or perturbed subglottal driving pressures provide poorly for source energy generation. Such pressure irregularities may necessitate compensatory, adductory hyperfunction to regulate equivalent acoustic output, and be factorial in the pathogenesis of "nodules."

When Patient PP was asked to inhale deeply, she modeled a high proportion of upper thoracic, rather than diaphragmatic, engagement. This localized hyperfunction typically leads to extrinsic and intrinsic laryngeal constrictions. She was quickly stimulable to the rationale and implementation of lower abdominal respiratory primacy.

The clinician and patient stood to fully reveal and explore the circumferential nature of lower abdominal breathing. Patient PP's compliance was increased with hand placement over the belly. The lungs were slowly filled "from the bottom up," and exhalation accomplished in one sustained pulse seemingly driven by elastic abdominal contraction. Patient PP was advised that thinking "80% full to 20% empty" may reduce undesirable hyperfunction.

It was hoped that respiratory exploration prior to the introduction of phonation would facilitate greater awareness of respiratory activity during actual phonation. The author feels that phonation appears to attract chief cognitive focus during voicing, possibly depriving sensation of "auxiliary" respiratory and resonant contributions.

Goal 2. *Forward resonant placement/ vocal fold stretching*: "Lightly siren up and down on a "mmmmm" which stimulates vibration behind the upper lip. Do not force the sound. Release the sound over an entire breath, and try to span from the lowest to highest pitches currently in your range." (10×)

Rationale. This exercise is based on standard vocal arts protocols, and is supported by integration of vocal fold stretching/contracting components from Vocal Function Exercises and resonant/ adductory elements from Resonant Voice Therapy variants.

True vocal fold (TVF) stretching and contracting exercises (*andanti portamenti*) allow fine dynamic calibration of laryngeal muscular activity to related airflow requirements. It was hoped that portamento usage would facilitate smoothed muscle activity without the subtle hyperfunction that may be incurred by relatively static change between scale pitches. In this exercise it was hoped that a physiologic model for eased phonation, initiated by the moderately low-pitched onset, would be more easily maintained when the gliding rise and descent from a pitch maximum was continuously performed across one breath.

Patient PP was encouraged to traverse register transitions and release, rather than force, her voice into the higher pitches. Unfortunately, the presence of "nodules" completely dampened head register. Still, she was encouraged in home practice to spend a brief period of time each day attempting to "open up" her head voice; any tendril of sound could be indicative of lesion or edema abatement. She was encouraged to explore other resonant humming loci through nasal phonemes such as /n/ and /ŋ/.

Goal 3. *Voice release/projection*: "Fully inhale, and sigh on a long and unforced 'haaaa' which falls from a medium-high pitch down through your lowest range (3×). Float your voice on a column of breath."

Rationale. A yawnlike sigh is widely used in the performing arts to promote pharyngeal expansion, vocal freedom, and emotional release. Ideally, the tone should be suspended on the breath, free of laryngeal constriction, and confident in delivery. To avoid trailing hyperfunction, the voice should naturally diffuse into breath, rather than glottal fry on a low-pitched offset.

The /hə/ was produced with a relaxed tongue and gently dropped jaw. When freed from the relatively sharper occlusions necessary to produce / e, i, a, o, u/, the "neutralized" vocal tract may facilitate more rooted contact with an abdominal "center," widely described in the dramatic arts as the imaginary source of vocal vibration. The artistic notion of a deeply rooted voice source appears to encourage a desirable distribution of loading into the thorax and abdomen so that the larynx is less pointedly exposed to the demands of projected quality.

Goal 4. *Conditioning and balancing:* Typically, the first five pitches of a C major scale will be used (eg, C3–G3 in adult males, and C4–G4 in females and children). Note transposing the series down a minor third may better suit Patient PP's capacity.

Comfortably sustain the final /w/ in "mow" on each target pitch. Close your lips sufficiently to generate a light buzzing sensation. Pause to breathe when you feel excessive tightening in the neck or body. Sustain each pitch for a cumulative total of about 90 seconds.

Rationale. Sustained phonation may be a key component in the rehabilitation of organic and behavioral pathology:

■ Phonatory and respiratory musculature may be more efficiently synchronized and conditioned to fatigue resistance.
■ Systematic sustaining of vocal fold oscillation may decrease stiffness associated with scarring and fibrosis, and may encourage optimal phenotypic expression of new vocal fold tissue.

The gently pouting /w/ (as in "mo<u>w</u>") may direct patient attention to combined bilabial and anterior maxillary resonant placement. Lip closure should be characterized by light buzzing. This kazoolike effect may facilitate vocal fold oscillation due to increased acoustic top-down loading on the vocal folds. Sympathetic allowance of cheek inflation may reduce the potential hyperfunction required for labial occlusion in buccal and perioral musculature.

Hybrid Voice Therapy does not specify that tone duration should utilize the maximum lung inspiratory and expiratory reserve volumes necessary to produce an optimal maximum phonation time. Rather, it is recommended that the inspiratory and expiratory reserve volumes, augmenting basic tidal volume, be more moderately taxed (the "80% full to 20% empty" maxim.)

The exercise goal of approximately 90 seconds of accumulated phonation time per pitch was chosen on the basis of excellent nonpathologic Vocal Function Exercise performance (eg, two MPTs × 45 seconds for each pitch). Five pitches, cumulatively sustained for approximately 90 seconds each, should result in roughly 7.5 minutes of accumulated phonation time. Stages 1 through 4 of the HVT program therefore should take approximately 10 minutes *in totum*, or 20 minutes when considered on the recommended twice-daily basis. This 20-minute span could be comparatively viewed as the minimum amount of time required to keep a singing voice in a basic state of conditioning, or a daily therapy interval typically recommended by physical therapists.

Within one month of 1-hour weekly sessions and excellent program compliance, Patient PP demonstrated understanding of rehabilitation objectives and was moving toward vocal health (although head voice was still dampened). Therapeutic focus was then directed towards concurrent rehabilitation of the singing voice. HVT goals 1, 2, and 3 were used as brief warm-ups at the start of all subsequent therapy sessions.

2. Integration of Singing into Voice Therapy. Singing is a valuable tool in the treatment of voice disorders. Its range of clinical utility includes behavioral voice dysfunction, neuropathy, atrophy, lesion presence, and phonosurgical recovery. In the sense that singing heightens speech, singing also may heighten the rehabilitative potential of voice therapy. The following text outlines a rehabilitative method that places singing exercises in the context of therapy.

The rationale for inclusion of singing into voice therapy may touch numerous bases for both singers and nonsingers:

- Musical notation provides accurate targeting of pitch zones of therapeutic interest. It also facilitates objective documentation of changing vocal capacity across treatment.
- Exercise variations are limitless, fun, and adaptable to changing phases of recovery.

Each exercise was sequentially transposed by semitones so that a completed series taxed the patient's usable compass. The gist of such therapy was to preserve quality as pitch borders were gently extended. Each series was initiated with a lower midrange pitch that elicited optimal baseline performance. Notes were made of pitch versus quality correlations when either parameter was challenged by the pathology.

Unison humming was used to introduce tasks, stimulate resonant proprioception, and dispel patient self-consciousness.

Goal 5. Chanting facilitates movement of airflow, tone, and intensity objectives towards conversational speech.

Rationale. Chanting is valuable for:

- Stabilizing undesirable pitch-related voice change (eg, elevating the excessively lowered SF_0 demonstrated at times by PP.)
- Promoting forward resonant placement through transalveolar "buzzing."
- Minimizing perturbations induced by voiced to unvoiced switching in speech.
- Providing an easily grasped transitional mode from prosaic therapy tasks to conversational speech.

The author frequently returned to chanting when tasks were inconsistently transferred into a higher level of techni-

cal difficulty. It was recommended that Patient PP use chanting as an easily implemented minitherapy to stimulate better voicing outside of the clinic.

The following protocol outlines a rehabilitation model toward this goal:

- Each pitch was initially sustained as a hum sensed through buzzing resonance above the upper lip.
- Nasalance was released through an opening vowel series such as /mu/, /mo/, and /ma/ (Fig 7–1).

The logic of the /mu mo ma/ sequence was that acoustic impedance and aerodynamic inertance induced by lip closure may stabilize phonation. Consequently, an open-most /ma/ could be regarded as the series endpoint most prone to perturbation, a pattern consistently observed in clinical practice.

The syllabification process moves toward more varied speech tokens continued through tasks such as:

- Continuant-laden monotone chants in which the nasals were slowly and deliberately accented; "mmanny mmenn onn the mmoonn."
- Continuously voiced, but unsung, sentences first with natural prosody, and then with natural phrase breaks (eg, "My-mom-may-marry-Marv" leads to "My-mom/may-marry-Marv.")

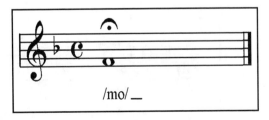

/mo/ _

FIGURE 7–1. Nasalance release.

- Monotone chants of rote sets with jumbled articulatory features: "January, February, March . . . December," leading to spoken iterations.
- Conversational sentence lists of progressively greater length.

Goal 6. A major tetrachord is hummed or sung on the vowel sequence /mu mo ma/.

Rationale. A major tetrachord is one symmetric half of an octave scale, either *"doh re mi fa"* or *"soh la ti doh "* as noted in Figure 7–2.

The author favors tetrachord structure for several reasons:

- Rising transposition of the semitone interval between the top two pitches permitted creeping exploration of recovery margins during the rehabilitation process.
- The semitone advancement ensured accurate documentation of changing Patient PP's capacity across time, and was more reliable and accurate than a pitch glide. (Descending P5 or octave scales were useful for determining lower boundaries.)
- The narrow range of the scale provided an accurate gauge of register boundaries, which in turn facilitated focus on voice production without the complication of register change.
- The several seconds required for each iteration fit comfortably within

the brief time span dictated by pathology.
- Controlled, gentle stretching of the vocal folds may serve to dissipate "nodules," or teach range extension while minimizing habitual strain.

Seldom is the tetrachord useful beyond a mezzo piano or mezzo forte dynamic. There was great value in the author tightly controlling an innate tendency for Patient PP to progressively push intensity as rising transpositions entered higher pitch range. Phonation should proceed from a balance of energized, but not hyperfunctional or uncontrolled, production.

Goal 7. Eased phonation and focus on resulting quality is promoted by sliding scales between two sustained boundary pitches.

Rationale. A *portamento* is a sliding scale (without discrete pitches) activated primarily by continuous differential engagement of the cricothyroid and thyroarytenoid muscles in conjunction with finely tuned respiratory control. This physiologic underpinning makes the *portamento* an ideal vehicle for increased vocal control.

Each exercise iteration was as follows:

- Eased, deep, transnasal inhalation with diaphragmatic primacy, pharyn-

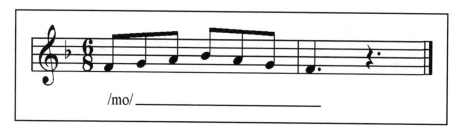

FIGURE 7–2. Major tetrachord.

geal expansion, and spinal elongation. Patient PP was asked to direct her awareness to the quality of the initial sustain (fermata), conceptualized as a referent "marker."

■ The marker glided upward to a fermata on the upper boundary pitch. The ensuing quality ideally matched similar flow phonation characteristics to the starting tone (even if registers were crossed). Once the highest pitch was accepted for quality, there was a gentle return to a pause on the starting pitch (which should have had a matching quality to the two previously held markers.)

Two intervals function well in portamento therapy: the perfect fifth and octave. It was discerned via initial probes that Patient PP was unable to comfortably phonate across an octave range, hence perfect fifth portamenti were used to implement objectives (Fig 7–3).

Across time, as greater healing and vocal control were consolidated, octave portamenti were used to tax greater phonatory and respiratory control, particularly in her area of primary register

transfer from chest into head register (Fig 7–4).

Note that the subtle onset of inhibitory hyperfunction was masked in traditional scales as Patient PP's senses were dulled by habitual acceptance. Early recognition and release from these insidious tensions was more fully realized through portamenti. Hand placement on the sides of the neck, mirror usage, and clinician mimicry are other useful sensitization tools.

The author conducted each exercise movement with hand gestures. Without this direction, Patient PP generally sustained the fermati for too long, which correspondingly rushed the *portamenti*. This defeated the objective of finely graduated muscular and respiratory coordination.

Results of Voice Therapy Program. At the time of writing this article, Patient PP had completed six sessions of voice therapy across a 7-week period. It was expected that the full course of therapy might last from 3 to 4 months, and ultimately forestall medical management. In the chance that surgery ultimately was

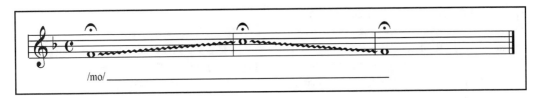

FIGURE 7–3. Perfect fifth portamenti.

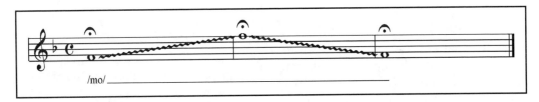

FIGURE 7–4. Octave portamenti.

deemed necessary by an ENT, Patient PP would have gained new understanding of vocal technique and personal performance limits that would work preventively against lesion recurrence.

A VLS performed at the midterm therapy interval revealed a decrease in the sloping of the lesions, which still remained morphologically symmetric. In therapy, Patient PP demonstrated a consistent ability to produce head register phonation and produced good quality tone up to E5. The significant remaining problem was of equalized register transfer from chest to head registers, and vice-versa. Speaking voice characteristics included more stabilized SF_0, forward resonant placement, and no aphonic segments. MPTs increased from a baseline average of 6.4 seconds to 8.8 seconds; it was hoped that eventual times of more than 15 seconds would indicate significant lesion abatement.

At the conclusion of midterm therapy Patient PP provided a requested copy of historic recordings from a time when her voice was functioning without pathologic interference. In these college recordings, she was an energetic soloist riding on top of a gospel chorale. Pitch center was in a high alto range with frequent easy extensions into head voice. Current intervention status allowed some duplication of these abilities and Patient PP was given permission to participate in her hoped for worship conference. It was strategized that she would use a forewarned team to handle the bulk of song leading, and that she would participate on a noninjurious basis. Vocal warm-ups were deemed essential.

The author was privileged to work with this patient toward vocal restoration. More weekly therapy sessions were scheduled, and therapy compliance was re-emphasized. The author was curious as to how worship conference participation might affect her voice via pitch range and MPT probes in the immediately ensuing time period.

Conclusion. It is hoped this case study provides rationale for procedures that may be effective across many areas of voice rehabilitation. Of course, it is expected that such goals and rationales will become increasingly effective as tissue research further illumines pathologic and curative processes. It is important for clinicians and voice scientists to work together to consolidate this work.

In acute injury there is a fine line between helping or hindering the injured performer with active therapeutic adherence. A clinician must develop a sensitivity as to when compliance with protocols is warranted, or when treatment may better proceed with a period of voice conservation.

There are overlapping zones between poor vocal performance and vocal pathology and between rehabilitation and habilitation. As successful intervention concludes, it is hoped that a voice pathologist with experience in singing pedagogy, or singing voice specialist will continue toward restoration of artistry.

Collaborative Voice Team Services Prove Effective in the Treatment of Dysphonia in an Elite Operatic Singer

Brian E. Petty, MA, CCC-SLP and Miriam van Mersbergen, PhD, CCC-SLP

Case Study: Patient QQ

In the process of treating a 45-year-old professional operatic singer, described in the following case study, Brian Petty and Miriam van Mersbergen use a behaviorally aggressive and surgically conservative approach to maximizing laryngeal structural and functional efficiency in a professional voice user with very specific vocal needs. Using a team-based approach, this singer exceeded his premorbid baseline in both vocal quality and stamina.

Patient History. Patient QQ, a 45-year-old lyric tenor, self-referred to the Voice and Swallowing Clinic with a 1- to 2-year history of vocal quality and stamina changes. He described instability in the passaggio (the transition range between modal and high pitch ranges), as well as significant difficulty maintaining controlled vocal production in the top two notes of his range, around B4 and C5. He reported that he was able to phonate in these pitches, but "it requires so much mental concentration and physical effort to stay on this very narrow path ... I've never had a super strong extreme high range, but it's always been easier than this."

Patient QQ's medical history was significant only for a remote history of chronic bronchitis, which in recent years had been well-controlled. There was no history of head or neck injury. Patient had no history of vocally phonotraumatic activities. Hearing acuity was within normal limits. No chronic medical problems were appreciated other than seasonal allergies, which were well-controlled using fexofenadine prn. Water consumption was within normal limits, 5 to 7 glasses daily.

History of the Problem. Patient QQ self-referred to the Voice and Swallowing Clinic after approximately 6 months of noticing the aforementioned symptoms. Patient description of his vocal demands revealed a full teaching load consisting of studio instruction of undergraduate and graduate level singers, as well as classroom and seminar instruction. The patient also maintained a busy performance schedule, particularly in the spring and summer months. His professional specialization was in baroque cantatas, which he performed extensively every year during international concert tours. The vocal ease and agility required in this type of literature were becoming progressively more problematic for this patient, prompting his presentation to the clinic.

Evaluation Procedures. The speech-language pathologist visualized the larynx using 70-degree rigid oral endoscopy without anesthetic, revealing bilaterally mobile vocal folds. Adduction of the vocal folds during modal and high pitches was characterized by a minimal gap extending along the length of the glottis. The left vocal fold showed decreased mucosal wave propagation at modal and high pitches associated with a groovelike lesion along the vibratory margin extending from the anterior commissure to the vocal process, although propagation resumed on the superior surface. Mild phase asymmetry was noted through the modal and high pitch ranges. Supraglottic hyperfunction was noted with variable severity throughout the examination.[7]

Subsequent evaluation and interpretation of stroboscopic data with the laryngologist revealed a left sulcus vocalis (type II), as well as evidence of vocal fold scarring.

As is often customary in highly trained professional singers, acoustic and aerodynamic measures all were within functional limits. Therefore, the evaluation of the patient's reported vocal change was necessarily completed using careful perceptual and patient self-report processes.

Patient QQ's voice quality was judged perceptually by the speech-language pathologist during informal conversation as well as singing tasks, using the 4-point GRBAS scale measuring overall (general) voice performance (G), roughness (R), breathiness (B), weakness or aesthenia (A), and strain (S).[25] Patient showed mild breathiness and strain in the passaggio. Some mild pitch instability was noted in the passaggio and the upper range, with a perceptually delayed voice onset time. In conversation, the patient was perceptually normal compared to age- and gender-matched nonsinging peers; however, he presented with a mildly pressed vocal quality with a slightly higher modal pitch.

Description and Rationale for Therapy Approach. Treatment for high-level vocal performers can be a daunting task, particularly when the degree of change that is sought consists of subtle improvement that would be considered within the range of normal variability. After collaborative discussion regarding possible treatment options, the team decided together to offer a behaviorally aggressive and surgically conservative approach. With the patient's extensive history of classical Italianate vocal training, maximizing behavioral change before considering structural alteration was thought to be preferable. The patient was in agreement with this approach. The patient was seen for behavioral voice treatment by two speech-language pathologists over a 2-year period. Both speech-language pathologists had extensive experience as classically trained singers and singing teachers, and were members of the National Association of Teachers of Singing.

Goal 1. Patient QQ will complete Vocal Function Exercises with 95% to 100% accuracy independently.

Rationale. Vocal Function Exercises have been shown to be effective in treating a variety of voice disorders,[26] and have been shown to be a useful tool in the practice regimen of trained singers.[25] The patient was trained in this protocol over four 1-hour sessions of behavioral voice treatment over 8 weeks. The patient adhered to home practice recommendations with remarkable consistency. After 8 weeks, the patient reported improvement of vocal stamina and range access to within his normal baseline. Repeat videostroboscopy of the larynx revealed improved vocal fold adduction during modal and high pitch phonation, as well as decreased supraglottic hyperfunction. Patient QQ continued to use Vocal Function Exercises at home as a daily warm-up, and returned to his teaching and performance work without difficulty.

Approximately 1 year after his initial visit, Patient QQ returned to the voice and swallowing clinic for follow-up. He reported initial success using Vocal Function Exercises, but had noted a slight return of the previous symptoms of decreased access to and control of the high range as well as pitch instability and increased vocal effort. He stated that he felt that this return of symptoms may have been related to a decrease in overall vocal load that summer, resulting in deconditioning. A repeat videostroboscopy of the larynx revealed findings that were consistent with the previous images, with slightly increased supraglottic hyperfunction compared to baseline. The patient was remanded to speech-language pathology for continued behavioral treatment, focusing on the following two goals:

Goal 2. Patient QQ will perform resonant hum in the absence of extralaryngeal resistance and strain to facilitate optimal laryngeal configuration during a simple phonatory task, with 100% accuracy independently.

Rationale. The purpose of this goal was to reacquaint Patient QQ with phonation in the absence of vocal "pressing," a quality consistently observed in the patient's speech and singing, albeit mild compared to nonsinging peers. The focus on a highly sensory-based technique was used to facilitate self-awareness in habitual vocal techniques. The patient demonstrated excellent acquisition of resonant hum and excellent awareness of the difference between pressed and relaxed voicing.

Goal 3. Patient will produce Estill "twang" during singing tasks throughout and above the passaggio to facilitate singer's formant in the absence of vocal pressing, with 90% accuracy independently.

Rationale. Patient QQ continued to express concerns regarding the unpredictability of certain notes throughout and above his passaggio, particularly at the top of his functional singing range. During observations of vocal behaviors during singing tasks, he presented with accessory behaviors characterized by chin-jutting and shoulder-raising before these notes. These were indicative of the anticipation of vocal difficulty. Estill "twang" techniques were used primarily as a distraction technique to eliminate anticipatory accessory behaviors. In addition, the patient was familiar with this form of resonance facilitation from past training. This served to reacquaint him with successful technique used in the past.

The patient did well and achieved goals 2 and 3, reporting that during performances these techniques worked well for him. However, the patient began to experience heightened levels of anxiety during practice and prior to performance, which inhibited his ability to focus on behavioral strategies. The cognitive load necessary to apply learned strategies appeared to interfere with the other tasks required to perform as a high-level musician. Essentially, the patient reported that his musicianship suffered under the weight of the cognitive and emotional effort needed to execute specialized behavioral techniques.

After an intensive counseling session with one of the treating speech-language pathologists, Patient QQ decided to meet with the voice team to discuss further options. Until this time, the patient had been understandably resistant to exploring more invasive medical and surgical options. Behavioral treatment had been effective in alleviating initial complaints (unpredictability in voicing and poor vocal power) but it also exposed deeper underlying difficulties (the increased cognitive effort to vocally excel after the reduction of previously employed, habitual compensatory strategies). The treatment team included the treating speech language pathologists, a specialist in high-speed imaging, and the otolaryngologist. The patient underwent additional evaluation using high-speed imaging with an integration of past medical and behavioral training. High-speed imaging elucidated the impairment of vocal fold stiffness, which resulted in a confirmed diagnosis of sulcus vocalis. During this process, Patient QQ appreciated his anatomic deficit, which resulted in a concrete realization of his vocal limitations.

As a result of this meeting, Patient QQ decided to undergo the recommended exploratory direct microlaryngoscopy, which resulted in confirmation of left vocal fold type II sulcus, left vocal fold scar, and left vocal fold type III sulcus in the infraglottic space. The otolaryngologist decided to employ subepithelial infusion of saline and injection medialization of the left vocal fold using a conservative 0.3 mL of Restylane. The patient was scheduled for postoperative voice therapy.

One-Week Postoperative Treatment. The patient employed total voice rest for 3 days, with very gradual onset of voicing using resonant hum after that. The patient understandably was anxious regarding the surgical results and presented to his first postop therapy session with significant agitation because of pitch breaks and hoarseness in his speaking voice. After counseling and reestablishment of optimal technique in resonant voice, the patient's vocal quality was markedly improved and his emotional well-being was mollified. A subsequent therapy session 4 days later was scheduled to enhance clinician support for the patient. The patient arrived at the second session in an improved emotional state, which was facilitated by the understanding that balanced oral-nasal resonance could be attained using resonant voice techniques regardless of whether his speaking was normalized. A secondary goal of this session was to bring resonant voice techniques to unstructured connected speech. After positive and negative practice and awareness building, Patient QQ demonstrated excellent awareness of how his behaviors contributed to postoperative vocal instability. Subsequently, he obtained conversational resonant voice quickly after establishing self-monitoring strategies. Further post-

operative goals included continuation of behavioral strategies learned in preoperative treatment. Home practice guidelines were assigned and followed scrupulously.

Results of Therapy. By the 1-month postoperative date, the patient reported that he had experienced a significant improvement in his vocal quality and stamina, describing his ability to control his high range as "better than ever." He had returned to his teaching and performance activities with much-improved ease. Videostroboscopy and high-speed imaging of the larynx showed improvement in glottic closure pattern, vibratory symmetry, and tissue pliability.

Follow-up at 1 year postop revealed continued functional success. Patient QQ had managed a busy performance schedule that summer, and reported that he had been able to continue his easy and effective vocal production without significant difficulty.

This report at 1-year postop revealed that the patient's success was due not only to his enthusiastic compliance with home programming but also to the careful and collaborative planning of behavioral and surgical intervention and management of the understandable emotional factors that potentially could have interfered with an otherwise solid plan. By allowing this patient to pursue perioperative behavioral management before surgical intervention, he was able to improve his initial vocal quality and function, identify underlying technical issues that might not have been identified otherwise, and facilitate quicker recovery of optimum vocal function. A collaborative team approach to voice care was therefore optimal for this patient, particularly given the special nature of his vocal needs.

Use of Estill Voice Training in the Rehabilitation of the Injured Singing Voice

Mary McDonald Klimek, MM, MS, CCC/SLP

Case Study: Patient RR

> *In relating her treatment of a 23-year-old grade school teacher, graduate student, and amateur solo singing performer, Mary McDonald Klimek discusses how the Estill Voice Model informs and guides decision-making within the recognizable framework of a treatment program for dysphonia with phonotraumatic lesions.*

Patient History. Patient RR, a 23-year-old female elementary school teacher, graduate student in education, and singer was referred by her otolaryngologist to the Voice and Speech Laboratory (VSL) for evaluation and treatment. Referring diagnoses were hoarseness and nodules. In excellent general health, she was taking Zantac at the time of her initial evaluation. Past medical history was unremarkable. She was a nonsmoker with rare alcohol consumption. Hydration was inadequate (1 to 3, 8-oz servings of water daily).

History of the Problem. She reported problems with her voice in the past, working summers as a lifeguard during high school and college, when she would experience a recurring hoarseness in the second half of her week. The current voice problem had been evolving gradually over the past 2 years and reached the point where she sought medical attention 5 months prior to her initial evaluation at the VSL. During these years,

she entered the classroom and joined a jazz standards band as vocal soloist. An active amateur singer and alto, she studied voice formally for about 3 years during high school and played guitar and piano. She did not have an established vocal warm-up nor cool-down routine, nor did she use her singing voice on a regular basis outside of the twice weekly 2- to 3-hour sessions with the band. She had approached a voice teacher who worked with her twice before recommending medical assessment. She was forced to stop singing because she simply could not hit her notes nor last out a rehearsal.

Presenting complaints at the time of her initial evaluation included hoarseness in speaking voice several days a week with no associated events nor patterns, and once weekly episodes of pain in throat, throat irritation, and frequent throat-clearing associated with increased voice use that would persist for several hours. Singing voice symptoms included problems hitting high notes, throat irritation while singing, feelings of tightness in throat and straining while singing, and loss of endurance (voice fatiguing after 1 hour of singing). By the time she reported for her first treatment session a month later, she would add complaints of limitations in the dynamic range of her speaking voice, speaking voice breaks, and more frequent throat clearing. She presented with a friendly, outgoing personality, quick to smile, but also expressed concerns surrounding her voice problem. Although she spoke enthusiastically about her new teaching career and her enjoyment of singing, it was obvious that her voice problem was weighing her down with its "general discomfort that quietly (nagged at her) all day long."

Evaluation Procedures. Patient RR received a Complete Voice Evaluation at the Voice and Speech Laboratory. Assessments included:

■ *Speech-language pathology evaluation.* Detailed case history, patient and clinician subjective assessments of voice quality and associated symptoms, hearing screening, oral mechanism assessment, and trial of voice therapy techniques to assess stimulability.

■ *Laryngeal function studies testing.* Acoustic analyses of connected speech, sustained vowels, maximum frequency range, and maximum phonation time; aerodynamic analyses of comfortable and loud phonation.

■ *Endoscopic evaluation of laryngeal function.* Transnasal examination of vegetative and respiratory tasks, connected speech, singing, and sustained phonation with stroboscopy; transoral examination of sustained phonation with stroboscopy; presentation of case and exam videos to weekly conference of VSL clinicians and Dr. Ramon A. Franco, Jr., Medical Director of the Voice and Speech Laboratory, for diagnosis and treatment recommendations.

1. *Laryngologic findings.* Examination revealed normal arytenoid mobility with periarytenoid and postcricoid edema. Broad-based and bilateral true vocal fold nodules were seen in the mid-musculomembranous region creating premature contact with a small persistent posterior chink and occasional/intermittent anterior chink. She was noted to have minimal ventricular compression. There were varices over the superior surfaces bilaterally, more pronounced over the right true vocal fold. The right true vocal fold

also was stiffer than the left vocal fold; moderate decreases in amplitude and magnitude of mucosal wave were noted. Diagnoses: bilateral fibrovascular changes, varices, stiffness, laryngopharyngeal reflux with associated findings of periarytenoid and postcricoid edema, and vocal hyperfunction.

2. *Acoustic analysis.* Digital recordings were analyzed with Multi-Dimensional Voice Program running on the Computerized Speech Lab. Selected results are reported and interpreted in reference to the norms that have been used at the VSL since 1992.

■ Connected speech (reading sample):

Average intensity: 64.0 RMS dB SPL (below normal limits, "soft")

Average frequency: 186.2 Hz (within normal limits, but low in the normal range)

■ Maximum performance testing:

Frequency range: 36 semitones: 132 Hz to 1047 Hz (well within normal limits).

Phonation Time: 22 seconds (well within normal limits)

■ Perturbation Measures:

Jitter: 1.24% (elevated, slightly over the norm of ≤1.0%)

Shimmer: 3.87% (elevated, very slightly over the norm of ≤3.8%)

3. *Aerodynamic measures.* Indirect estimates of sub glottal air pressure and glottal airflow were obtained during comfortable and loud phonation of /pæ/ syllables using a pneumotachograph mounted in a facemask and a catheter placed between the

lips, with data recorded and analyzed on the Kay Aerophone II. Results are reported and interpreted in reference to the norms used at the VSL since 1992.

- Comfortable phonation

  Intensity: 70 dB SPL

  Pressure: 7 cm of water (within normal limits, but well above the mean of the norming samples at this relatively low average intensity)

  Airflow rate: 1.3 liters/second (within normal limits, but low in normal range)

- Loud phonation

  Intensity: 85 dB SPL

  Pressure: 17 cm of water (abnormally high, with significant elevation)

  Airflow Rate: 1.25 liters/second (within normal limits, but low in normal range)

4. *Audio-Perceptual.* Her voice was judged by the evaluator to be consistently mildly strained, intermittently mildly breathy and gravelly, with intermittent hard glottal attacks, and vocal fry. Vocal pitch was consistently too low, whereas vocal loudness was adequate. Tension was visible in jaw, tongue, and shoulders. Respiratory behaviors exhibited included intermittent shallow inhalations. She also exhibited consistently mildly decreased oral resonance. A brief examination of the oral/facial mechanism revealed normal structures and functions; however, Patient RR reported pain during palpation of the larynx with increased sensitivity in bilateral thyrohyoid spaces and cricothyroid visor.

The evaluator's subjective impression of mild strain was supported by the objective aerodynamic measure of increased subglottal air pressure in loud phonation, by Patient RR's complaint of pain during laryngeal palpation, and by the visual assessments of multiple tension sites and minimal ventricular supraglottal compression during video-endoscopy. Impressions of intermittent breathiness and gravelly voice quality were supported by objective acoustic findings of increased perturbation measures (jitter and shimmer) and videoendoscopic findings of a persistent posterior and intermittent anterior glottal chinks. The perception of gravelly voice quality also corresponded with objective acoustic findings of relatively low speaking pitch (although within normal limits) and observations of intermittent glottal fry.

A 12-session course of once-weekly hour-long individual voice therapy sessions was recommended, with goals for patient education, hygiene, and increasing efficiency in both speaking and singing voice production through reducing musculoskeletal tension and direct modification of breath, tone, and resonance. Prognosis was seen to be good to excellent given objective acoustic findings of normal frequency/pitch range in maximum performance testing and reductions in both jitter and shimmer to well within normal limits during voice therapy technique trials—in this case, lip trilling into vowels.

Description and Rationale for Therapy Approach. Patient RR's past history, diagnosis of nodules, and findings during the evaluation suggested that long-standing vocal strain was at the root of her pathology and that protective "restraint" was contributing to her dysphonia. Although impossible to verify, it was likely that the fibrovascular changes so recently identified actually had been evolving over the past decade. Given laryngeal pathology, it was of interest to note that so many objective measures of vocal function were within, or just slightly outside, normal limits. Vocal demands in the classroom, vocal demands in social settings, and vocal demands singing with the band appeared to have conspired to overwhelm an inefficient and vulnerable system. Overuse and inappropriate body mechanics were reflected in symptoms of discomfort and fatigue.

Improved vocal hygiene and reduction of vocal load would have been included in the treatment plan; however, Patient RR had already been switched to a classroom with older and more attentive students and she was on hiatus from the jazz band, not singing at all. Yes, she was social and talkative, but not excessively so. Increasing her water intake was identified as an appropriate hygiene intervention. The major focus of treatment would be development of a training program that would improve efficiency and stamina in speaking and singing voice. Education would be included to support Patient RR in becoming independent with exercises and strategies.

Estill Voice Training maneuvers and exercises were chosen to repattern vocal behaviors for a number of reasons. The clinician had been using the theoretical principles of the Estill Voice Model for over 10 years and was comfortable using auditory, tactile, and visual cues to analyze physiologic imbalances within the voice production system. Given the athletic training principles of Estill Voice Training, analysis of an "imbalance" would immediately suggest a physiologically contrastive or complementary motor-based solution. Furthermore, with 20 years of voice teaching experience prior to encountering Jo Estill and subsequently becoming a voice therapist, the clinician was comfortable translating the anatomic and kinesthetically dominant terminology of this approach into whatever terms or images Patient RR might find most productive given her own processing and learning style preferences. In addition, any effective concept, principle, and/or posture/gesture of Estill Voice Training would apply to any vocal application: the rules for vocal efficiency and economy would not change when Patient RR moved from speaking to singing, from crooning to belting. Moreover, exercises would develop a "working vocabulary" of sensory experiences during "primal" vocal activities (when the voice production system "defaulted" to naturally elegant and economical biomechanical vocal behaviors), that could later be applied to improve the efficiency of speaking and singing. This experiential learning, framed within education regarding relevant power-source-filter physiology, would help to reform faulty "internal models" of voice production that led the patient to persist in the voice-use patterns that were breaking her voice down over the past couple of years.

Goal 1 (Hygiene). Patient RR will maintain daily water intake of more than 64 ounces throughout the treatment period. Patient RR's related personal goal was to reduce and/or eliminate throat clearing. Initial short-term goal was to have patient purchase a water bottle she could carry with her and use throughout the school day.

Rationale. Frequent throat clearing, and complaint of general throat discomfort could be associated with dehydration and/or laryngopharyngeal reflux.

More frequent sipping might result in the following benefits: short-term desensitizing of the larynx to sensations prompting throat clears, "up and out" clearance of phlegm during laryngeal closure during the swallow, washing away of stomach secretions within the pharynx, and long-term improvement in systematic hydration and possible thinning of mucus.

Treatment Course Toward Goal 1. Patient RR did purchase her water bottle, and, in the course of coming months, she would increase her water intake. Her referring otolaryngologist did not feel her LPR symptoms merited more than OTC Zantac, and Patient RR was medication-averse and had discontinued the medication by the time she started treatment. The decision was to keep the focus on hydration. She never reached the 64-oz criterion of the clinical goal; however, her personal goal was met in that complaints of throat clearing subsided and were not reported in her post-therapy re-evaluation.

Goal 2 (Reduce Musculoskeletal Tension). Patient RR will perform relaxation exercises at least three times a day to increase awareness of fluctuations in tension and stress throughout the day and reduce the impact of same on the free/flexible response of larynx and articulators to the demands of speech and song. Patient RR's related goals were to feel comfortable using her voice even at the end of a difficult week and to be able to speak and sing with her old expressive range in pitch and volume. Short-term goals were memorization and adequate performance of the "McClosky Six," massages and stretch/releases for face, jaw, tongue, geniohyoid (and other muscles along midline

beneath the tongue), infrahyoid strap muscles, and muscles to side and back of neck (see: David Blair McClosky, *Your Voice at Its Best*).

Rationale. Muscle tension restricts and/or offers resistance to normal movement patterns throughout the body. Chronic tension can pull bone and cartilaginous structures out of optimal alignment, with consequences to "resting" muscle morphology and strain on joints. Chronic tension frequently results in symptoms ranging from discomfort to pain. Muscles and structures in the head, neck, and torso are responsible for the efficient adjustment and coordination of subsystems in Power, Source and Filter domains. This means that tension just about anywhere in the body will have a negative impact on voice production.

Reduction of tension is important, but total relaxation is not the ultimate goal. In context of Estill Voice Training, speaking and singing are seen as athletic activities in which a certain amount of muscle contraction is required. In pure application of Estill Voice Training, muscle effort (contraction) is controlled kinesthetically via use of self-calibrated "effort numbers." Careful effort number monitoring and specific relaxation maneuvers are used in an attempt to confine effort only to the muscle(s) where it is needed and to prevent the nearly inevitable spread of muscle contraction to other muscles in the anatomic neighborhood. Sometimes the flow-on effects of muscle contraction are beneficial; sometimes the overflow is left unattended and becomes habituated into tension, undermining future activity/mobility. The coaching and training of elite athletes offers a model of the requirements that must be met by an elite singer who sustains a successful career over decades without injury or loss of functional capacity. Often, both athlete and singer make their performances look easy! Injured singers can be deceived by this appearance of ease, and often take for granted their own level of athletic conditioning when things were going well. One clinical challenge is to provide patients with the skills to assess muscle contraction and determine whether it is the energizing exertion of a job being well done or the depleting tension of muscle strain that will result in a loss of stamina. The starting point is the reduction/elimination of tension and its associated pain and discomfort.

Treatment Course Toward Goal 2. Some interesting insights were gained during introduction of the McClosky Six, during which Patient RR volunteered to be trained in strap muscle/laryngeal massage through clinician demonstration. Crepitance was noted during lateral displacement of larynx during single-sided massage. Palpation revealed a small thyrohyoid space and Patient RR reported pain during massage of the thyrohyoid muscle. Discussion of strenuous closure of the larynx had been included in the overview of normal anatomy and physiology that preceded introduction of these massages, with specific discussion of the false vocal folds, given observations of supraglottal compression and high subglottal air pressures during loud phonation. Voluntary control of the false vocal folds is an Estill Voice Training exercise, and clinician was able to demonstrate three false vocal fold positions—constricted, mid, and retracted—while Patient RR pressed into the clinician's thyrohyoid space. Patient RR was able to recognize a similar elevation of the larynx and tightening of the thyrohyoid space during the constricted

condition. In order to work through/release some of the tension in the thyrohyoid muscle, Aronson-style deeper pressure massage and manipulation were introduced, with 8 to 12 dime-sized circles of firm pressure into the thyrohyoid muscle in attempt to widen the space, followed by 6 to 8 seconds of firm downward pressure on the superior border of the thyroid cartilage over the prominence at the top of the oblique line. Although the musculature did not "release" in response to the downward press, the larynx did descend and the thyroid space enlarged during spontaneous laughter between manipulation task sets. "Laugh posture" is one of the natural activities used in Estill Voice Training to retract the false vocal folds, and this observation was filed away for future reference.

Patient RR would remain compliant with multiple daily administrations of these massages throughout her treatment course, even when she was ill with an upper respiratory infection and unable to do much else. Tension in her masseter/pterygoids would prove resistant to release, but strap musculature would relax and soften, and both sensitivity in thyrohyoid muscle and crepitance during massage would decrease over time. Neck, shoulder, and torso stretches also would be included in her program.

Goal 3 (More Efficient Speaking Voice Production). Patient RR will increase vocal efficiency as demonstrated by use of relaxed, "easy" abdominal breaths in support of clear tone with oral resonance in 90% of conversational speech. Patient RR's related goals were to feel comfortable using her voice even at the end of a difficult week and to be able to speak with her old expressive range in pitch and volume.

Rationale. Patient RR's breathiness, gravelly voice quality, fatigue, reduced dynamic ranges, and vocal fold pathologies all were seen in relation to constrictive closure of the complex valve that is the larynx. Simple overuse and minimal strain can increase the impact stress of the true vocal folds during vibration and lead to true vocal fold edema. Vocal fold edema can stiffen the vocal folds, increasing glottal resistance. Reaction to glottal resistance is often the urge to "press' through it. It is not unusual in the evolution of fibrovascular changes to find patients who notice themselves becoming hoarse and discovering that making their voices louder clears up the tone. Often, this making-the-voice-louder is accomplished by an undifferentiated increase in effort throughout the voice production system. Strenuous closure of the false vocal folds, pressing at the true vocal folds, and increased expiratory force are all triggered in no particular sequence and end in excessive subglottal pressure and increased impact stresses to vocal fold tissue. A vicious cycle ensues and vocal fold tissues begin to react with formation of scar tissue.

It is very common to hear from singers with evolving or established voice disorders—students, amateurs, or professionals—that their problems arise from a lack of "support." Already out of balance with breath-tone relationship, they act out of a belief that more "support" will solve their problems. This internal model of how the voice functions prompts more and more effortful inhalation to higher and higher lung volumes. The increased respiratory drive inherent in relaxation pressure at high lung volumes, coupled with the popular misconception that "singing from the diaphragm" means using the abdominal muscles to propel the breath at whatever lung volume, drives the singer further from the most efficient breath-tone balancing point. Speakers who need to "raise their voices," be they teachers or actors, will act on similar impulses. Even if Patient RR had not had complaint of speaking voice problems, treatment would have begun with speaking voice training to probe for and adjust her internal model of how the voice works.

Estill Voice Training embraces dynamical systems theory. Power-source-filter relationships are not seen as linear, nor is power (breath) seen as the wide foundation of the voice production pyramid. In Estill Voice Training, the ideal is breath responding to what it meets on the way out. "Most Comfortable Vocal Effort" results from careful balancing of all of the down- and upstream interactions of breath, tone, and resonance.

By the time Patient RR presented for evaluation and started treatment, she was demonstrating protective voicing behaviors, fearful of speaking too loudly for fear she would do more damage to her voice. Her pendulum had swung to too little breath flow, low pitch, low intensity, and frequent glottal fry. This "holding back" was in itself a strain, and she often was on the edge of fry, experienced as raspiness.

Treatment Course Toward Goal 3. During her second session, following a review of the McClosky and Aronson exercises, Patient RR was moved through systematic exploration of muscle activity associated with inhaling and exhaling to and from different lung volumes. With minimal corrections to less-than-ideal postural alignment, she was able to fall back into abdominal breathing patterns she had learned in voice lessons without difficulty. She was able to observe for herself the recruitment of accessory muscles in neck and shoulders at highest lung volumes and the abdominal "squeeze" below resting expiratory level (REL). She was then oriented to the resting tidal volume and the concept of a "comfortable" inhalation slightly above this volume, with exhalations "coasting" down to REL on relaxation pressure alone. She monitored with hand on belly to resist temptation to engage abdominal muscles. Deliberate and steady breath flow rate throughout this excursion of lung volume change was practiced on monoloud "sh" prolongations, with acknowledgment that relaxation pressure alone would not be sufficient to meet the monoloud condition when approaching REL, and that "nurture" would be required to compensate for the decline in relaxation pressure.

Calm and comfortable breathing have a flow-on effect of reducing muscle tone in the larynx and vocal tract. Building on this foundation, humming was introduced as a basic training gesture for forward placement. Patient RR found herself pressing at the larynx and pushing with the breath, recognized as familiar habits when "trying" to do anything with her voice. After a bit of exploration, "Laugh Posture" was identified as the most effective intervention to promote sensations of vibrations up and out of the throat, to the front half of the mouth. Time was taken to train Patient RR in the principles of effort number monitoring via a hand clasp, with waving and shoulder shrugging as foils to challenge isolation of effort to the hand and forearm. These principles were applied to the variable effort that can be invested in retraction of the FVFs

using a laugh posture continuum. Explorations included holding the number of the subtle experience of abduction of the true vocal folds during a nasal inhalation into the onset of the hum, to the feeling a "secret smile" or "smile behind the eyes," to the impulse of resisting a giggle, to the effort involved in suppressing hysterical laughter—as a child might do playing hide and seek and hearing his or her clueless seeker standing next to the hiding place. Having something active to "do," rather than focusing on the "don't" of pressing or pushing appeared to make sense to her, and variable practice ensued. Speaking range pitch glides, CVCVCVs, and carrier phrase practice drills were all introduced in this second session. CVCVCVs provided the opportunity to make connections between the work of nurturing a respiratory gesture of steady breath flow rate in the "sh" to the similar "work" required in not letting airflow rate drop in final syllables. Patient RR was encouraged by the clarity and ease of her voice during practice phrases.

In the following weeks, there would be setbacks due to holiday celebrations, inconsistent practice, and frustration with breathing. On closer inspection, posture came into question as the culprit, leading us to work backed up against the wall, blowing imaginary birthday candles, which was effective in what singing teachers describe as "freeing up" the breath. In terminology used by Janice Chapman (see: *Singing and Teaching Singing: A Holistic Approach*) in a workshop at the Voice Foundation Symposium in 2006, Patient RR was able to access "SPLAAT" breath—"Singers (or Speakers) Please Let Go-of All Abdominal Tension"—during inhalation. Away from the reinforcement of the wall, posture waivered and this feeling of release during inhalation was lost. Postural exercises for "upper-crossed syndrome" developed by Barbara Wilson Arboleda, MS-CCC/SLP, and Arlette Frederick, PT, were introduced in the following session.[28]

By session 6, Patient RR was able to work herself through her exercise routine into what clinician described as "gold standard voicing" in the context of reading aloud, at which point she could use reading aloud in the classroom as a daily opportunity to refine and improve her voice production. The next weekend a birthday party at a bar resulted in voice loss the following morning and discouragement, even though voice bounced back later in the day. In session 7, another Estill exercise was introduced into the mix: aryepiglottic narrowing, the cardinal feature of "twang quality." This "nyae-nyae" adjustment in the epilarynx boosts high-frequency energy around 3 kHz, making comfortable voice production much louder (literally, as in the Fletcher Munson curve) to project over background noise. (See and listen to Klimek exercise contribution in Behrman and Haskell, *Exercises for Voice Therapy*.) This physiologic strategy to boost projection was practiced through phrases and then in mock social encounter with loud background noise provided by a radio tuned just off the frequency of a station with music.

Goals for speaking voice would be met by session 9 as demonstrated by clear and resonant speaking voice on entry to clinic and by patient report of positive experiences with her voice through the week in the classroom. This trend would continue in spite of an upper respiratory infection that would plague her for nearly a month during the treatment period. Establishment of a more efficient speaking voice production allowed Patient RR's voice to begin putting itself back together functionally. We began singing voice work well before her new speaking patterns were truly established, and some insights and observations from her singing work fed back to speech in beneficial ways. It was vital that she to get to the point where she could be in the classroom all day, all week, and actually felt like singing afterward. In this sense, efficient, nonfatiguing speaking voice use was seen, in and of itself, as a "warm-up" for singing voice. Again, the priming of the system with "laugh posture" and the "balance" of breath and tone developed motor skills that would apply directly to singing voice.

Goal 4 (More Efficient Singing Voice Production). Patient RR will demonstrate appropriate balance of effort and relaxation in singing voice production as demonstrated by singing two songs in contrasting styles without visible/audible signs or symptoms of strain. Patient RR's related goals were to sing with her old expressive range in pitch and volume.

Rationale. The rationale implied in the "balance" language of this goal has been discussed in support of earlier goals. Given her style of singing in particular (jazz standards vs opera), singing was seen as an extension of speaking voice. Further, singing voice work attempting to restore stable vibration of the vocal folds through the range might soften/revise scar tissue over time through the stretch of true vocal folds at higher pitches. Singing voice work over time also would settle the question lurking at the back of most singers' minds when they hear "nodules": will surgery be required?

Treatment Course Toward Goal 4. The official start of singing voice rehabilitation would begin in Session 4 with assessment via the Estill Siren (which will remain capitalized to distinguish it from other pitch gliding tasks that share the label). The Estill Siren has a very particular physiologic "recipe" in terms of Estill Voice Training voice production system structural component options, were you to build it bottom-up. Luckily, it is generally accessible top-down through its primal, emotive prompt: softly "whimper" (or "whine") an "ng" as in the word, "sing."

As the singer feels his or her way through the not-always-so-simple "whimper," attention is directed to various sensations associated with vocal tract configuration. There is the "high" tongue posture with dorsum forward along the hard palate and margins of the tongue to either side of the dorsum touching the upper teeth, usually in the region of the 6 or 12 year molars, and the "low" position of the velum as it comes into contact with the back of the tongue opening the velopharyngeal port and closing off the oral cavity from participation as a resonator. Given the close association of "whimpering" with "crying," there is often automatic retraction of the false vocal folds ("laughing," "crying," and "sobbing" will all tend to retract the false vocal folds — with varying degrees of larynx lowering). Given our auditory memories of small children and animals "whimpering" or "whining," the singer often will start at a relatively high pitch, where careful body scanning of the neck will reveal some of the sensations associated with cricothyroid muscle (CT) activity and a forward tilting of the thyroid cartilage. The instruction to make the tone soft, together with the stretch on the true folds from CT activity will tend to promote a "thin" true vocal fold edge (as opposed to the "slack" edges in fry, the "thick" edges in modal vibration, or the "stiff" edges of the falsetto register in the male voice and the "head register" of many female voices). All of these features of the Siren can be isolated and used in other vocal contexts. In direct Estill lingo, the recipe as related so far is: Thin TVF: Body-Cover, Retracted FVFs, Tilted Thyroid Cartilage, High Tongue, and Low Velum. In addition, there might be Smooth TVF: Onset/Offset and there definitely would be Wide Aryepiglottic Sphincter (the sound is not "twangy"). Vertical Cricoid Cartilage, Mid Lips, Mid Jaw, Relaxed Head and Neck, and Relaxed Torso likely would go unappreciated. Larynx Height (the only Estill Voice Training structure not mentioned in this paragraph) would vary as the Siren moved to the extremes of the pitch range.

The Siren presents several specific challenges to the disordered voice, not the least of which is negotiation through the total pitch range without shifting vibratory mode. In Estill Voice Training there are no "registers." Qualities (Speech, Falsetto, Sob, Twang, Opera, and Belting) are narrowly defined by the options mixed in their "recipes" and maintained throughout the range with recognition of range-associated advantages-disadvantages, stabilities-instabilities, and benefits-risks. The development of the concept of "registers" can be explained in terms of frequency-related biomechanical and aerodynamic "attractor states" for various qualities (eg, the untrained singer will tend to be in Speech quality low in the range and flip into Falsetto quality high in the range).

In any case, the Siren is a "fussy" task, easily disrupted, and, for that reason, very valuable as an assessment of true vocal fold vibratory function. Even a bit of phlegm will undermine the task. Trying too hard, or not hard enough, also will cause it to break down. It is an excellent "Vocal Barometer," a term used by this clinician to represent an exercise done daily to see how the voice is doing. If the voice can make it in the Siren, it likely can make it anywhere, and along the way the singer will learn that singing through the range at a bare minimum requires different locations and degrees of effort in different frequency regions.

In this case, Patient RR was able to Siren down to C3 (consistent with self-classification as an alto) and, with moderate cues, up to G5, albeit with an increase in breathiness above the Eflat5. Some counseling was required to accept that a 2½ octave range was a good start, even if tone in upper reaches was breathy. In the next session, she would Siren up to A5, with cues to engage Head and Neck Anchoring and recruitment of muscle activity high in the vocal track (superior pharyngeal constrictors) nicknamed, with gestures added, as "tightening the tuning peg between the ears." This center-of-the-head locus of effort high in the range, and the sensations of downward pull in the neck low in the range, generally require some getting used to. Distraction from pushing the breath is seen as very useful. Patient RR was coached through some simple scales and triads (chords) morphing the Siren into "cry" quality by closing the velopharyngeal port and sustaining thyroid cartilage tilting to promote improved adduction. Adding some effort in AES narrowing (twang) cleared the tone further. As the tone became less breathy, Patient RR became less defensive/sensitive about her voice quality and commented that singing felt much easier.

Even in the first session with 15 minutes to work on singing voice, she was able to apply the feelings associated with "whimper" and "twang" in a simple song, "The Lady Is a Tramp."

We would stabilize some of these adjustments over the next couple of weeks, then introduce exercises for Speech and Falsetto qualities through the middle of her range, experiencing the natural limitations of each moving out of its attractor state range. Working on microphone, even when the voice "weakens" beyond an attractor state boundary, the tone is still very useful for dramatic effect.

Generally speaking, thyroid tilt made the most powerful contribution to clearing her singing voice quality. She was a singer who tended to surrender CT activity as she moved lower in the range. When she began to acclimate to the effort required to hang on to thyroid tilt, outside of its upper range attractor state, her lower range took on a "sweeter" tone, closer to the croon appropriate to the songs she was singing. Ascending vocal lines became much easier to negotiate. Constantly thinking about "cry" and "whimper" had the beneficial side effect of retracting the false vocal folds, significantly reducing resistance to breath flow. During her treatment course, she would successfully return to the band, recovering her stamina and find options in vocal color/timbre she had never experienced before.

Goal 5 (Patient Education). Patient RR will demonstrate basic understanding of vocal physiology in insightful commentary during sessions and in choice of appropriate solutions to vocally problematic situations as encountered or posed. Patient RR's related personal goals were to better understand how to take care of her voice and to know what she was doing when she "belted" in her singing.

Rationale. Knowledge is power, and sharing knowledge with patients—in terms and exercises appropriate to their learning styles and needs—makes them feel like partners in the therapeutic relationship rather than students. When working with singers, this is particularly important, as experiences in the singing voice studio often are structured by the right/wrong auditory judgments of the teacher. In this case, Patient RR, a teacher herself, came into therapy with a goal to better understand how her voice broke down and how to fix it. (In the interest of full disclosure, it would turn out that her use of the term "belting" was not literal, and so the quality was never addressed.)

Treatment Course Toward Goal 5. Providing Patient RR with explanations that corresponded to her sensory and kinesthetic experience did in fact promote the development of independent problem solving. Some of her struggles along the way were seen as crucial in forcing her to puzzle through things on her own. Driven out of her head (intellect) and into her experience (sensations), she came to her own conclusions regarding the options for voice production modification provided to her. By session 13, she was able to propose and test out her own proposals to fix sounds and sensations in her singing voice that she did not like, revealing a productive revision in her inner model of how her voice worked. She left voice therapy feeling confident that she could continue with the exercises.

Posttreatment Reevaluation. A Complete Voice Evaluation was re-administered after 13 sessions of voice therapy to assess the benefit of treatment. Patient RR summarized her progress as follows: "My voice feels much healthier and more under control. I haven't lost my voice since (4 months ago), and I am able to sing a little bit everyday because my voice is no longer tired from school." Her only complaint was raspy voice quality occurring once a week and resolving within an hour. She was practicing vocal exercises 5 days a week and practicing songs every day.

1. *Visual-Perceptual/Laryngologic Findings.* Dr. Franco's dictation and diagnoses for the re-evaluation were strikingly similar to his reading of the initial examination, with the small exception that the varices over the superior surfaces of the folds were not commented upon. Indeed, the folds were generally much whiter in this exam, particularly the right fold, even though the nodules and their hourglass closure patterns appeared virtually the same in side-by-side exam comparisons.

2. *Acoustic Analysis*

   ■ Connected Speech (reading sample):

     Average Intensity: equipment malfunction during the calibration process prevented collect of this data point during re-evaluation

     Average Frequency: 212 Hz (within normal limits, and a couple of semitones higher than the 186.2 Hz average where she started)

   ■ Maximum Performance Testing:

     Frequency Range: 37 semitones: 123 Hz to 1000 Hz (well within normal limits and essentially unchanged).

Phonation Time: 23 seconds (well within normal limits and essentially unchanged from the 22 seconds recorded during the initial evaluation)

- Perturbation Measures:

Jitter: 0.82% (well within normal limits and reduced from 1.4%)

Shimmer: 2.56 (well within normal limits and reduced from 3.8%)

3. *Aerodynamic Measures*

- Comfortable Phonation:

Intensity: 73 dB SPL

Pressure: 6 cm of water (within normal limits, and closer to the Mean of norming samples despite the increase of intensity over previous samples)

Airflow Rate: 0.9 liters/second (within normal limits towards the bottom of the range)

- Loud Phonation

Intensity: 82 dB SPL

Pressure: 12 cm of water (within normal limits and reduced from 17 cm)

Airflow Rate: 0.6 liters/second (within normal limits, low in normal range)

4. *Audio-Perceptual.* Her voice was judged by the evaluator to be intermittently mildly breathy and mildly strained, with intermittent vocal fry. Vocal pitch and loudness were judged to be adequate. Tension was intermittently visible in the neck. Respiratory behaviors exhibited included intermittent shallow inhalations.

Patient RR did not have the happy ending of smaller lesions, and the improvements in objective measures were gratifying, but subtle. The striking turnaround she experienced in her symptoms and functional capacity were out of proportion to more "objective" measures and observations. Her thank you note cartoon of a smiling woman riding a bicycle down a hill with a stream of musical notes in her wake pretty much summed up her feelings at discharge. Perhaps the bicycle was no accident? Recovering her coordination and balance was really all it took. Estill Voice Training offers a comprehensive model with simple exercises to restore balance between the components of voice production.

Voice Treatment Following Medical Management for a University Vocal Performance Major

Barbara Weinrich, PhD

Case Study: Patient SS

In the next case presentation, Barbara Weinrich describes some of the issues involved in treating the voice problems of a singer in training. Youthful university students often have other issues involved in maintaining the health of the vocal mechanism. Indeed, this patient presented a significant challenge to the voice pathologist.

Patient History. Patient SS was a 19-year-old female, who was referred to our university speech and hearing clinic by a local otolaryngologist for a voice evaluation and videostroboscopic examination. She was beginning the first semester of her second year as a vocal performance major at the university. The otolaryngologist diagnosed "a nodule on the right true cord and possibly early one on the left side." Patient SS also had a medical diagnosis of laryngopharyngeal reflux (LPR) and described her voice as "becoming hoarse and raspy." The patient's chief complaint was tension and pain while singing, especially in her upper range, and frequent throat clearing.

Patient SS noted that she began experiencing problems with her voice approximately 3 months prior to this evaluation. During that time, she was quite active in summer theater productions and camps for children with special needs. She "constantly used mints in an attempt to control the need to throat clear," talked excessively throughout the day, ate late night snacks (such as pizza or chips with salsa) before lying down, and typically had 5 to 6 hours sleep at night. She usually drank two glasses of tomato juice, twp cups of coffee, one glass of water, and three Cokes daily throughout the summer. She noted that people often asked her if she "was getting a cold," and her singing voice became "very airy." In her upper range, the vowel /i/ was more easily produced than the vowels /a/ or /æ/. Patient SS stated that her voice fatigued while singing and her singing was laborious. She often required a long warm-up before she could sing. Currently, her voice quality changed throughout the day and she cleared her throat frequently.

Patient SS reported no previous hospitalization or surgery. She had a history of asthma and allergies, with a recent diagnosis of laryngopharyngeal reflux. Currently, she did not take any medications for asthma or allergies, other than Nasonex. She was given prescriptions for medical management of the reflux (Prilosec), but had not yet obtained the medication. She reported that she was a nonsmoker and attempted to avoid smoky environments. She continued to drink comparable amounts of tomato juice, coffee, water, and Coke that she consumed during the summer. She did not drink alcohol. She was beginning to notice a globus sensation in her throat. She described her general health as "good" on a daily basis.

Patient SS completed a self-assessment of her voice handicap using the Voice Handicap Index scale. She obtained the following scores: *Functional* subscore equaled 7, *Physical* subscore equaled 15, and *Emotional* subscore equaled 5, yielding a total score of 27, which was within the mild classification of self-perceived voice rating.

Social History. Patient SS had studied voice for 5 years, and her career goal was to become a vocal music high school teacher. Her current weekly vocal use consisted of (a) 3 hours vocal ensemble weekly, (b) three 1-hour vocal lessons weekly, (c) 2 hours play rehearsals daily, and (d) 1 hour church choir practice weekly. She frequently sang solos in the church choir. She served as an officer in a campus music organization, which entailed one weekly meeting and leading campus recitals. Additional singing occurred in vocal music classes. She lived on campus in a dormitory. She indicated that she often was sleep deprived due to the typical stresses associated with university life.

Oral-Facial Examination. The structures and functions of the oral mechanism appeared to be well within normal limits for speech and voice production. The patient reported a sensation of tightness in the throat, especially after singing.

Neck muscle tension was not observed, but the thyroid cartilage was resistant to movement, and the patient reported some laryngeal area muscle discomfort. No other laryngeal sensations or swallowing difficulties were noted. Hearing acuity was normal bilaterally.

Voice Evaluation

General Quality. This vocally enthusiastic patient presented with moderate dysphonia, characterized by moderate roughness/breathiness in conversational speech. Using the Consensus Auditory-Perceptual Evaluation of Voice (CAPE-V), the clinician's perceptual analysis of the patient's overall severity was 45/100 (moderate).

Respiration. A supportive, thoracic breathing pattern was demonstrated. The patient was able to sustain the /s/ for 30 seconds and the /z/ for 10 seconds. This yielded an abnormal ratio of 3:1.

Phonation. Using the CAPE-V perceptual analysis, the patient scored a 45/100 (moderate) for roughness, 45/100 for breathiness (moderate), and 20/100 (mild-moderate) for strain.

Pitch. The patient's pitch was perceptually rated as mildly low (12/100), using the CAPE-V. Her average speaking fundamental frequency was 185 Hz, while reading the CAPE-V sentences, with mild intermittent glottal fry at the end of phrases/sentences. Her highest fundamental frequency was 587 Hz, lowest fundamental frequency was 139 Hz, and comfortable sustained /a/ was 196 Hz.

Loudness. Patient SS's loudness was rated as a 10/100 (mild/loud) on the CAPE-V perceptual analysis. Comfort-

able intensity measures averaged 78 dB, with loud intensity measures at 98 dB.

Rate. The patient spoke with a normal rate of speech.

Aerodynamic Measures. Using the Phonatory Aerodynamic System (PAS; KayPentax Model 6600), mean airflow during voicing was high (560 mL/s), as was mean peak air pressure at 12.83 cm H_2O.

Videostroboscopic Evaluation. Under direct light, the patient presented with an irregular gap in glottic closure of the vocal folds. The left fold was characterized with a smooth, straight edge, but the right fold had a moderately rough edge. There was erythemic, granular-appearing swelling in the midsection of the right vocal fold. The patient displayed no supraglottic activity. Under simulated slow-motion stroboscopy, the mobility of the both vocal folds appeared to be normal. The amplitude of the vocal folds, as well as the mucosal wave pattern, appeared normal for the left fold, but moderately decreased on the right side. The open phase of the vibratory cycle was mildly dominant, whereas phase symmetry was irregular during onset of the phonatory tasks. Overall, the larynx was functioning normally. Pachydermia was noted in the interarytenoid space.

Impressions. The patient exhibited moderate dysphonia, characterized by roughness and breathiness. The right vocal fold edge was moderately irregular, with the amplitude of vibration and mucosal wave moderately decreased on the right side. Airflow and air pressure measures were high. She presented with an imbalance in the subsystems of voice production. The primary etiology of this voice disorder was a vocal fold lesion, which was attributed to voice misuse/abuse, including the following causative factors:

- Persistent throat clearing
- Straining while singing
- Excessive talking
- Laryngopharyngeal reflux
- General fatigue of the laryngeal mechanism.

Prognosis, Recommendations, Medical Treatment. Prognosis for regaining normal voice characteristics was regarded as good, with medical treatment and voice therapy. The results of this evaluation were given to the otolaryngologist to re-examine his medical diagnosis. The physician revised his diagnosis to a "right vocal cord polyp, granuloma." The patient was scheduled for surgery. The postoperative specimen was diagnosed as a "laryngeal nodule."

It was recommended that Patient SS be enrolled in voice therapy following medical treatment/recovery.

Voice Therapy/Treatment Approach. The multidimensional treatment approach selected for this patient consisted of three treatment plans designed to manage the etiologic factors contributing to the hyperfunctional voice problem. The three management approaches included (a) vocal hygiene counseling and education, (b) Vocal Function Exercises, and (c) Resonant Voice Therapy. Progressive portions of these three treatment strategies were presented to the patient in each of the eight 45-minute, weekly treatment sessions. After the initial instructional session, the remaining seven sessions began with a review of the patient's recorded data for the weekly treatment goals that were established at the conclusion of the preceding session. Following the review, the prototype of the sessions consisted of didactic clinical instruction, with clinician-modeled vocal behaviors when appropriate, followed by patient performance.

The etiologic component to this therapeutic process entailed vocal hygiene counseling and was a significant portion of each treatment session. Although the patient was enrolled as a vocal performance, music education major, her cognitive awareness of the vocal mechanism appeared to be scant. Therefore, the initial session began with a verbal description of the laryngeal anatomy and physiology with accompanying pictures and videos. The edema and erythema produced by vocal misuses and abuses were discussed in relation to the specific behaviors demonstrated by the patient. The abusive "banging" of the vocal folds during throat clearing episodes was described. The patient reported that her throat clearing behaviors had subsided considerably in comparison with the initial attack about 3 months prior to therapy, but she noted that some residual behavior remained. She stated that she had begun to consistently use the prescribed medication for LPR. Also, she was adhering to her patient-relevant dietary/behavioral precautions for LPR, such as eliminating the use of mints in an attempt to control the need to throat clear; late night snacks (such as, pizza or chips with salsa) before lying down; and, drinking tomato juice, caffeinated coffee, and colas daily. She had increased her daily water intake to 60 ounces.

The patient indicated that she had not decreased any of her weekly vocal performances following the first 4 weeks of treatment. She continued to manage her leadership role in the various organizations and was "vocally productive" throughout her daily functions. She commented that she was not a person who required much sleep and felt she had mastered the management of stress associated with performances, academic assignments, and examinations. The clinician praised the student for her successful accomplishments, while noting that excessive use of her vocal mechanism may need to be targeted as a behavior to be modified. The patient agreed and was asked to delineate the "vocally challenging" events that would occur each day until her next therapy session. Each event was analyzed, and a written plan for modification was made. The patient was instructed to note her actual performance for each event and return with the written assignment. In addition, she agreed that her body would benefit from some additional sleep on a nightly basis. Therefore, she would also record her amount of sleep.

The second component to this eclectic voice therapy was direct physiologic exercises. Vocal Function Exercises and Resonant Voice Therapy were used to improve the coordination, flexibility, and stamina of the laryngeal musculature, as well as to balance the airflow, laryngeal muscle activity, and resonance. The rationale for the Vocal Function Exercises was explained to the patient. She readily identified the purpose as being similar to physical therapy she had received after injuring her leg skiing. A description of the exercise program was presented to the patient verbally, as well as in a written format. As each exercise was demonstrated with a soft volume by the clinician and followed by the patient's performance, the data were recorded on a record form. The exercises consisted of:

■ *Warm-up exercise:* sustaining /i/ on musical note F4

■ *Stretching exercise:* gliding to highest note
■ *Contracting exercise:* gliding to lowest note
■ *Power exercises:* sustaining /ol/ on five notes (C4 through G4)

Each exercise was performed twice. As the patient demonstrated the ability to perform a particular vocal task, the clinician would enthusiastically "coach" the patient to perform the task again to reach mastery of a preset maximum phonation time (MPT) goal. The patient was instructed to perform each task two times each, two times per day, preferably morning and late afternoon or early evening. She was given the record form to track her performance and was asked to return the form at the next session. Goals were established for the Vocal Function Exercises based on the patient reaching an airflow rate of approximately 80 mL/s for 25 to 30 seconds during sustained tones.

The Resonant Voice Therapy program was utilized in conjunction with the Vocal Function Exercises. The patient was told that the purpose of Resonant Voice Therapy was to develop a forward-focus to the voice and eliminate any back-focused, intermittent glottal fry and hard glottal attacks during conversation. It was stressed that all phonatory exercises were in the context of easy phonation. The program was presented in detail with clinician modeling for the "Basic Training Gesture," and all the steps of the "All Voiced," "Voice-Voiceless Contrasts," and "Any Phrase" portions of the program.

Results. The patient was seen weekly for eight 45-minute treatment sessions. She was highly motivated and extremely compliant with all assignments in her daily routine. During the treatment period, she was able to eliminate the throat clearing behavior and reflux symptoms, monitor the excessive talking, and improve her daily amount of sleep and antireflux behaviors.

The patient made significant vocal improvement throughout the treatment period. Her conversational voice improved from moderate dysphonia to a voice that was perceptually normal with appropriate resonance. The aerodynamic measures changed dramatically from mean airflow during voicing of 560 mL/s to 160 mL/s and mean peak air pressure of 12.83 cm H_2O to 8.13 cm H_2O. The acoustic measures and videostroboscopic findings were normal. The patient had achieved a balance in the subsystems of voice production.

The patient's lowest performance time for the Vocal Function Exercises' warm-up exercise was noted during the first treatment session when she was able to sustain the /i/ using the musical note F4 for 9 seconds. Her performance during the 10th treatment session for /i/ was 30 seconds. During the treatment period, her highest and lowest notes on the stretching/contracting exercises expanded to a 2.5 octave range, with primary expansion in her upper range. The patient's pre- and posttreatment performance for the Vocal Function adductory power exercises consisted of the following data:

Session 1	Session 10
C4 10 seconds	C4 23 seconds
D4 9 seconds	D4 28 seconds
E4 9 seconds	E4 26 seconds
F4 8 seconds	F4 27 seconds
G4 8 seconds	G4 26 seconds

The patient completed all phases of the Resonant Voice Therapy program. She did not demonstrate any back-focused, glottal fry productions for utterances during reading exercises or controlled conversation tasks. The patient's chief complaint when enrolled in therapy was tension and pain while singing, especially in her upper range. She indicated that she was no longer experiencing these sensations while singing, nor did her voice fatigue, and she was satisfied with her progress.

Summary. Although the description of this patient and her treatment paradigm is representative of many university students majoring in the vocal arts and demonstrating vocal hyperfunction, the results will vary based on the patient's willingness to comply with the treatment program in nontherapy settings. With compliance that includes modifying the etiologic factors and performing the direct physiologic exercises, the laryngeal pathology will resolve and normal voicing will be restored. However, as was the case for this patient, there are medical conditions that require surgical intervention and medical management prior to voice treatment to ensure successful outcomes.

The Music Educator: A High-Risk Professional Voice User

Sharon Radionoff, PhD

Case Study: Client TT

The music educator is one of the most "at-risk" vocal professionals. The daily demands on the voice are great enough to challenge even the healthiest vocal mechanism. Sharon Radionoff, a singing voice specialist, shares her experiences in dealing with this population and presents direct voice and whole body exercises that she has found helpful in maintaining the vocal health of these professionals.

The field of music education requires high-end voice use that starts when the bell rings and continues to the end of the day without any real voice off or voice rest time. Music educators can have up to 8 classes back-to-back per day (including double class loads of 60 to 70 students). There may be a scheduled lunch hour, but they often have to "serve" lunch duty. Other voice use requirements can include bus duty after school or hall duty as well. The potential is high for breeding muscular tension dysphonia (hyperfunction).

Music educators use voice for instruction, demonstration, and discipline. Therefore, they switch back and forth between speaking and singing many times during a single class period. Unfortunately, the luxury of possessing one larynx for singing and one for speaking is not available. What does this mean for the music educator? It means that speaking habits must be as pristine as possible to ensure vocal survival. However, this is usually not the case.

It is common for music educators to demonstrate the following speaking habits during conversational speech:

- excessively low pitch
- low airflow
- harsh glottal attacks
- laryngeal resonance
- pushed or pressed voice.

These technical faults often occur as a result of the teacher trying to sound more authoritative and stern. These speaking habits then bleed into even the best singing techniques. Common singing problems include:

- loss of range (usually upper)
- pushed or pressed chest voice
- strained head voice
- loss of flexibility
- hoarseness.

Remember, people have only one larynx. Therefore, what we do when we do not sing directly affects what we do when we do sing. It is critical to career survival that a music educator who experiences vocal difficulty undergo both speech therapy and singing voice training. This is necessary so that the voice can be "rebalanced" to allow for efficient use.

Client History. Client TT was a 40-year-old female elementary music educator who taught general music in grades K through 5. She had been teaching for 15 years. She taught single classes of kindergarten, first, and second grades, but the third, fourth, and fifth grade classes were double classes with no teaching assistant available. The single classes had from 20 to 28 students and the double classes were as large as 60 to 70 students. Client TT reported that she used hand signals, checks on charts, and musical sounds to keep classroom discipline and behavior under control.

Client TT is also a professional singer and songwriter and a recording artist. During the week, she sings with a praise and worship team, and on weekends she travels throughout the nation singing at church services and retreats. Because of this, she could not use the weekends to "recuperate" from a hard teaching week. It was imperative that she use both excellent speaking and singing techniques while teaching because she had little or no "down time" during the weekend.

Client TT reported that she did not have bus or hall duty but that she had to alternate with other teachers for lunch duty. She further reported that she tried to drink six to eight glasses of water a day, but that it was difficult because she often could not leave the classroom to use the restroom. Her caffeine intake was minimal at one cup of coffee in the morning before school started. The client also reported that she had two teenagers at home, one boy and one girl, but that they were well behaved and she did not need to shout at them. She reported normal conversational speaking at home with minimal background noise from television, stereo, dishwasher, and so forth. She further reported that she had a studio set up at home where she practices, writes music, and records.

Client's Description of the Problem. Client TT reported that she got hoarse very quickly. She stated that "my voice is shot after 45 minutes of singing and also after 30 to 45 minutes of talking." She also reported that she has a loss of high range, loss of vocal clarity, and loss of vocal power.

Medical Diagnosis. Viewing under videostrobolaryngoscopy by an ear, nose, and throat physician specializing in care of the professional voice revealed bilateral prenodular swelling and muscle tension dysphonia (medial-lateral compression). She was examined with both the rigid telescope and the flexible endoscope.

Singing Voice Evaluation. Client TT was taken through a five-note ascending-descending scale on /a/ up and down by half steps to find her current range and to examine her technique (Fig 7–5). (The goal was to get maximum information in the minimum amount of time.) After going through scales, she was instructed to choose two songs of varying styles from her tour repertoire to sing while holding a microphone. She reported that she does not sing and play an instrument simultaneously while on stage.

During her initial evaluation, Client TT demonstrated the following technical deficits:

- a collapsed upper torso and sternum position
- tension in the neck and jaw
- manipulation of the vertical laryngeal position (varying between being pulled too high and pressed too low)
- head-neck protrusion and elevation
- tongue retraction, elevation (upper range) and depression (lower range)
- thoracic breathing
- insufficient breath support
- decreased airflow
- decreased oral resonance

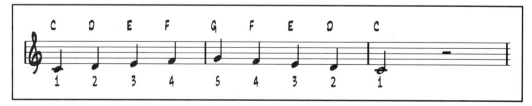

FIGURE 7–5. Five-note ascending/descending pattern on /a/.

■ laryngeal-posterior tone placement and focus.

She presented with a generally covered, tight sound. Her approximate physiologic frequency range of phonation was E3 to D6. She stated that her current useable singing range is approximately Bb3 to Eb5. During conversational speech, she used vocal fry, harsh glottal attacks, and overall poor breath management.

Classroom Singing Evaluation and Treatment Approach. Following the initial singing voice evaluation, Client TT was asked to give some mock teaching lessons. She was instructed to sit on the floor as she would with her kindergarten class and to sit at the piano as with her other classes using songs that she is working on with her students.

Scenario 1. While sitting on the floor, Client TT demonstrated a collapsed upper torso and sternum position, arched small of her lower back, and elevated and protruded head-neck position. The head and neck at the base of her skull were compressed. Because of this, she had to compensate to achieve her desired sound. The client used excessive muscular tension in the extrinsic laryngeal muscles to compensate for poor breath support and control caused by her postural problems.

Scenario 1 Solutions. She was advised to practice her lesson plans while sitting on the floor and to monitor her posture, breath flow and support, and resonance.

Scenario 2. While sitting on a piano bench behind an upright piano, Client TT demonstrated an elevated and protruded head-neck position (which would allow her to see her students over the piano), collapsed upper torso and sternum position, and an arched small of her lower back. She stated that she often taught songs by rote to the students from behind the piano while she played.

Scenario 2 Solutions. Client TT was advised to sit on a stool because this would allow her to have a good line of vision with her students while also allowing her to use a healthy head-neck position and better upper torso and sternum and back position. In turn, she would be able to release and use her abdominal muscles for breath support. She also was advised to have the students come around the piano for small classes.

Scenario 3. Client TT reported that she felt more like an entertainer than a teacher while teaching a double class without an assistant. She further reported that no microphone was available. She stated that she had to work to project her voice over the classroom full of students. Client TT also stated that it was difficult to keep class discipline and teach music at the same. Finally, she stated that she was absolutely exhausted after teaching a double class because of the high energy level of excitement that she must exude to keep the students involved.

Scenario 3 Solutions. Client TT was advised to monitor her behavior and to ask herself the following questions when teaching a double class:

■ In an effort to create energy, am I tensing my abdomen and contracting the most important muscles for active exhalation even before using them for breath support?

■ Is my energy dispersing up and out instead of keeping body weight centered down and using my abdomen as the "control panel?"

She also was advised to monitor rate of speech, length of talking and singing phrases (too long for healthy vocal technique?), enunciating habits (does she use a myriad of harsh glottal attacks?), and voice projection (does she push from the throat instead of using a balance of airflow, phonation, and resonance?).

Client TT was advised to practice her lesson plans specifically for pacing, breath flow, resonance, and energy level. She also was advised to use a microphone when teaching and to write reminders on index cards for posture and breathing to put in the classroom and in the car and around the house. The more senses one uses, the quicker things go into long-term memory.

Treatment Approach for the Singing Voice. The entire body is the singing instrument. The skeleton is the frame of the singing instrument. When the body is tight, tense, and out of alignment, the singing voice also will be tight, tense, and out of balance or alignment. Client TT had gotten into the habit of trying to use her extrinsic laryngeal musculature to manage airflow and to produce loudness. This compensational behavior was largely the result of poor postural habits, which in turn reduced her air capacity and breath control. Therefore, it was necessary to help Client TT release her extra stress and tension before addressing posture and sound production. After relaxation and stress release, a sequence of exercises called "building blocks" was used. This logical "building block" sequence of exercises included:

■ airflow management
■ phonation
■ resonance.

Sound production must be balanced before a variety of changing consonant-vowel patterns, pitch variation, and vocal agility exercises are used. After the voice is balanced, then one can begin to work on songs.

Following the voice evaluation and testing, a treatment plan was proposed. The plan included:

■ stress release exercises
■ relaxation exercises
■ postural alignment monitoring
■ building block exercises
■ pitch variation exercises
■ melody-text separation exercises
■ cool-downs.

Stress Release Exercises. Client TT was advised to use stress release exercises between classes that she taught, as well as at the end of the teaching day. These exercises included:

■ passive and active head-neck stretches (passive meaning using one's own body weight with hands clasped together and resting at the base of the back of the head-neck with elbows hanging in toward the center of the body. Active meaning actually physically moving the head in various slow patterns—left to right in a frontal half moon. The individual must breathe while moving the head!)
■ shoulder rolls
■ body stretching
■ full body movement.

Other exercises for stress reduction are jaw release exercises. These include:

- letting the head roll back and allowing the mouth to relax into a "duh" feeling and then slowly roll the head forward while keeping a relaxed mouth;
- opening and closing the mouth with the jaw freely "flapping," making fish-like shapes with the lips; and
- on a comfortable pitch with good airflow management, complete repetitions of "bubb bubb bubb bubb bubb."

Relaxation Exercises. Client TT was advised to do the following exercise at least once daily either sitting while at school or lying down at home after teaching:

Lying Down

- Make sure that the legs are uncrossed.
- Put a book or small pillow under the head to make sure that posture is in line.
- Close the eyes (if desired) and put the hands on the lower abdomen.
- Knees may be bent up, or legs may be straight.
- Cues for body relaxation:

From the top of your head to the bottom of your toes you are going to allow your body to relax. This relaxation will start at the top of your head and move down your neck, shoulders, arms, elbows, wrist, abdomen, thighs, kneecaps, shins, ankles, and all the way out your toes (thinking/saying one word per second).

As you are lying there, I want you to notice what happens as breath goes in and out of your body. As breath comes into your body, your body expands, and as breath leaves your body, it contracts because you no longer need that space. It's almost as if you have an inner tube that goes all the way around your body, and when

air comes in it fills up and when air leaves it deflates. Abdomen and ribs (side, front, back) expand as inhalation occurs, and contract as exhalation occurs.

Postural Alignment Monitoring. Next came the process of the alignment of Client TT's body posture while teaching, whether she was sitting on the floor, sitting at the keyboard, or standing. As discussed previously, postural recommendations were made for Client TT in the classroom setting. To improve alignment when standing to perform with a microphone, Client TT was advised to practice in front of a mirror and specifically watch her head and neck position to be sure that it is not elevated and protruded.

Building Block Exercises. The sequence of building block exercises is (1) airflow management, (2) phonation, and (3) resonance (Fig 7–6).

Exercise 1 (Lying Down, Sitting, Standing): Blow and Relax

1. Make sure that the upper torso and sternum are slightly raised. It should feel as if the chest is slightly tipped up (not with a backward shoulder rotation).
2. Relax the abdomen.
3. Blow all the air in the lungs out on /sh/.
4. Release and relax the abdomen and allow the body to fill up with air. Abdomen and ribs (side, front, back) expand as inhalation occurs.

Client TT was advised to do the exercise in a series of five repetitions as often as possible. It is realistic to do this lying down at home or sitting and standing while at school and at home. Most singers work too hard for inhalation. By

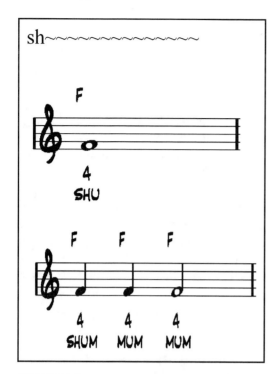

FIGURE 7–6. Sequence example of building block approach (vowels in IPA).

starting this exercise on exhalation, inhalation must occur. Therefore, the singer will be able to get out of the habit of "working" for a breath.

I advised Client TT to do blow-and-relax exercises between classes. This would help to keep her stress level down and also to keep a lower center of breath, which will result in better supported sound with less vocal fatigue.

Exercise 2: Phonation. Prepare the body as in Exercise 1. Start with one or two blow-and-relax exercises on /sh/. On the next blow instead of just /sh/, phonate with /sha/ on a comfortable single pitch. Hold it for as long as comfortably possible. Take this exercise up and down by half steps. Keep it in a comfortable range. Do not push the upper and lower limits of the range. Repeat 3 sets of 10 repetitions per day, using both /shu/ and /sha/.

Reminders: Be sure that the tongue tip is forward, touching the back of the bottom teeth, and do not press the jaw down.

Exercise 3: Resonance. Prepare the body as in Exercises 1 and 2. Start with one or two blow-and-relax exercises on /sh/. On the next blow, phonate with /sha/ on a comfortable single pitch and then close the lips for /m/. Hold /m/ for as long as comfortably possible. Take this exercise up and down by half steps. Keep it in a comfortable range. Do not push the upper and lower limits of the range. Repeat 3 sets of 10 repetitions per day. Vary the speech samples using /shum/ and /sham/ (see Fig 7–6).

Resonance 2

1. Make sure that the body is in line.
2. Relax the abdomen and fill the body with air.
3. Exhale slowly through the nose.

Think of the sound that is made when people are "huffy" or irritated about something and they blow airflow through the nose (teenagers do this a lot!).

Resonance 2a. Begin with the same three steps as Resonance 2 exercise. After a small amount of air is exhaled through the nose, proceed with a gentle vocal /hm/ on a single pitch. Just think about closing the lips for the /m/. Be sure that the tongue tip is forward and touching the back of the bottom teeth and that the jaw is relaxed, not clenched.

All of the building block exercises may be done lying on the floor (back or side), sitting, and standing. There are pros and cons for each position. Lying on the back is beneficial for getting the body to relax quickly, but gravity works against the tongue position, and one must work harder to keep the tongue forward. The position of lying on the side is also beneficial for getting the body to relax quickly. It is better for the tongue position, but it can be difficult for the jaw. It is beneficial to go from lying down to sitting before moving to a standing position. There are not as many postural considerations allowing the individual to concentrate on voice production and technique in an intermediary posture before trying the exercises standing.

Pitch Variation Exercises

Exercise 4: Small Pattern. Begin producing voice in the same manner as Exercise 3 on /sham/ plus /mam - mam/ while moving down one half step and then back up to the original note. (1 - 7 - 1 or C - B - C). /Shum - mum - mum/ may also be used (Fig 7–7).

Exercise 5: Small Pattern. Begin the same as Exercise 4 on /sham - mam - mam/ but go up one whole step and then back down to the original note. (1 - 2 - 1 or C - D - C). /Shum - mum - mum/ may also be used (Fig 7–8).

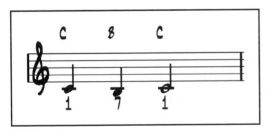

FIGURE 7–7. Stepwise pattern 1 – 7 – 1.

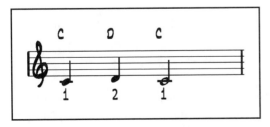

FIGURE 7–8. Stepwise pattern 1 – 2 – 1.

Exercise 6: Larger Patterns. For the beginning of larger patterns, add the two previous patterns together. 1 - 7 - 1 - 2 - 1 (C - B - C - D - C) or 1 - 2 - 1 - 7 - 1 (C - D - C - B - C). Do these on /sham - mam . . . /, /shum - mum . . . /, or other consonant/vowel combinations (Fig 7–9).

The next step is to use a larger descending patterns such as 3 - 2 - 1 (3 blind mice) and add the previous pattern 1 – 7 – 1 to become 3-2-1-7-1 before moving to either ascending or skip-wise motion patterns (Fig 7–10).

Melody and Text Separation Exercises. Singing a song is a complex activity because a singer must not only execute excellent technique, but also musically and textually interpret the song. Before interpreting a piece of music as a song, the elements of the music must be broken down. The specific musical elements that will be broken down with regard to technique are rhythm, melody, and text. To transfer into song the newly balanced systems produced by the previous exercises, it is necessary to separate the text and the melody of the songs.

Exercise 1: Rhythm. Clap or tap the rhythm of the melody. Speak the rhythm of the text in conversational speaking voice. Break the melody into small rhythmic patterns as difficult passages demand.

Exercise 2: Text. Starting on either /sham/, /shum/, or /mum/, chant the words of the text on a comfortable single pitch. Chant the words of the text on the beginning note of the melody. Chant the words of the text in rhythm.

Exercise 3: Melody. Break down the melody of the song into small patterns and phrases. Sing the patterns on a single consonant vowel combination. Start with /sha/, /shu/, /sham/, /shum/, or

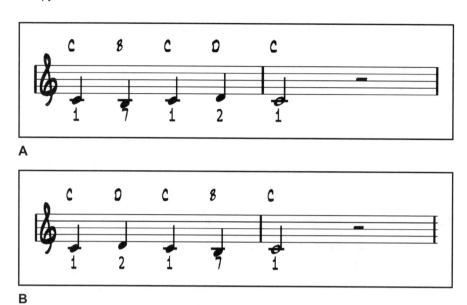

FIGURES 7–9. A and **B**. Stepwise patterns 1 – 7 – 1 and 1 – 2 – 1 combined in two orders.

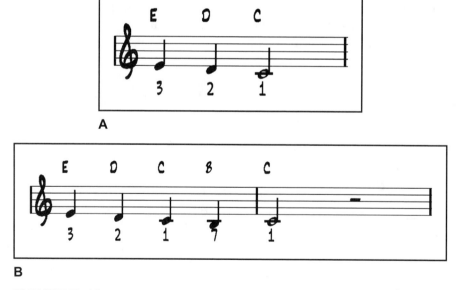

FIGURE 7–10. A and **B**. Descending pattern 3 – 2 – 1 and descending pattern 3-2-1 added with pattern 1 – 7 – 1.

another combination of choice. After practicing with these consonant-vowel combinations, begin using consonant-vowel combinations found in the music. After singing the patterns and phrases, sing the entire melody.

Exercise 4: Whole Song. Put the words and melody back together, practicing patterns and phrases. Practice first for a "technique run" through the entire song before beginning on interpretation.

Cool-Downs. Music educators must release vocal tension after a strenuous day of teaching or after singing a concert. Cool-downs are designed to aid in release of vocal tension. Often, excessive tension and pressure puts the larynx in an unusually pulled, high position or an unusually pressed, low position. To bring the larynx back to a "natural," at-rest position, use descending slides. Start on a comfortable pitch with either /shu/ or /hm/ and slowly descend using easy airflow and a medium volume level. After a few descending slides on /shu/ or /sha/, add the /m/ onto the end. Do two sets of 5 to 10 repetitions

For additional exercises and further explanation consult chapters 2 and 4 of "The Vocal Instrument."[1]

Results. Client TT reported that after the first week of using her new technique, she was able to teach through Wednesday before vocal fatigue set in. By the second week, she was able to see the effects of tension release exercises because she was not as tired vocally after singing in church on Sunday; she was able to get through the entire week of teaching. By the fourth week, Client TT reported that other people mentioned she sounded better and she sang four songs in concert without any vocal fatigue. By the sixth week, the client reported that she noticed an improvement in increased range, ease of singing, and clarity of quality. After seven sessions of working on balancing the voice and releasing tension, Client TT was beginning to integrate healthy technique into performance songs. The eighth session began a vocal strengthening and stamina routine of singing more sessions during the day for longer periods of time. Also the break time between the sessions continued to decrease. She started with two early-afternoon sessions (one 5-minute and one 7-minute with a 45-minute break in between) and worked up to two 30-minute sessions with a 15-minute break in between. By the 11th session, Client TT was able to sing through an hour-long concert and still be able to talk afterwards. She continues to do well vocally and comes in for maintenance checkups every 6 to 8 months or as the need arises.

Suggested Reading

Radionoff, SL. *The Vocal Instrument.* San Diego, Calif: Plural Publishing Inc; 2008.

Hyperfunctional Voice in an Actor

Bonnie N. Raphael, PhD

Case Study: Patient UU

> *In the following case study, Bonnie Raphael uses her skills as a voice coach and speech-language pathologist to treat the voice disorder of a fine actor.*

As resident coach for a regional professional theater, my goals include enabling each actor to meet the needs of the role being played, the directorial concept, the acquisition of requisite skills the role demands (eg, dialects, singing, dancing), the locations in which the play will be rehearsed and performed, the rehearsal and performance schedule, and associated tasks such as recording sessions and publicity interviews (live and recorded) without cannibalizing his vocal mechanism or his voice in the process. A production of "Blue Door" by Tanya Barfield presented by PlayMakers' Repertory Company in the fall of 2008 provided an opportunity to deal with all of these challenges.

"Blue Door" tells the story of an African American college teacher who, on the day his wife leaves him, is confronted by his insufficiently acknowledged history and ancestry in the form of dreams and memories during the course of one night. It is written for two African American actors who play multiple roles (black-white, young-old, male-female, slave-slave owner, uneducated-college professor): some recurring, some involving a capella singing and dance in the course of a nearly 2-hour show with no intermission and virtually no offstage time for either actor. An extremely physically and emotionally demanding undertaking, this play includes instances of a slave being chased by dogs and whipped and chained, the physical abuse of a child by his father and of a young black slave by the son of a slave owner, drunkenness, and despair. As such, it required strategizing, execution, consistency and self-preservation on the part of both actors throughout the 5-week rehearsal period and 2½-week run (including one, 2-show day).

Fortunately, both actors were in excellent physical condition and in the habit of visiting a gym to work out each day, and neither actor was a smoker. Their physical alignment was very good, so they were up to the demands of the physical blocking of the show (which included each of them physically climbing a 15-foot tall, architectural "tree" upstage and getting onto and off one of the "branches"). Both had undergone some voice training as part of their

respective graduate acting programs and had some noteworthy professional acting experience on their resumes before doing this show. Because they were hired on Equity contracts (Actors' Equity Association or "Equity" is the professional actors' national union), theirs was an 8-hour workday 6 days a week, in which their voice and dialect coaching sessions had to be included. What follows is a brief description of some of the exercises and strategies that were employed with the actor playing the ancestors under these highly demanding but certainly not atypical rehearsal and performance conditions.

Techniques for Voice Building and Lessening Vocal Fold Trauma

Warming Up, Warming Down, and Rebalancing the Vocal Mechanism. A customized *warm-up* regimen was designed by the voice coach in collaboration with the actor and modified during the course of rehearsals and performances. Priorities included keeping the chosen exercises clear, efficient, relatively undemanding and short so that the actor could preserve his energy for the demands of any given day.

1. Lowering the center of breathing activity in the body (rather than allowing it to move up into the chest, especially during emotionally demanding sequences)—exercises included holding a chair with some weight to it overhead while phonating on "HAAAAAAAAH" and then while speaking the speech and/or panting lightly in the area of the diaphragm between lines of an emotionally demanding speech;
2. Loosening neck, shoulders, jaw, tongue and soft palate muscles to

make it easier to initiate and sustain both phonation and articulation-related activities;

3. Connecting outgoing breath with phonation (ie, vocal support) via breathing through, then phonating through, then expanding range through, and then speaking directly behind loosely flapping lips before removing this "obstacle" and releasing fully voiced text;

4. Increasing specificity and ease of articulation via speaking text as clearly and communicatively as possible over a relaxed tongue tip lying loosely on the bottom lip for at least a minute before allowing it to drop back into the mouth to resume its articulatory duties;

5. Finding a "trigger" phrase or sentence for each different vocal characterization in the play, so that tone placement and rhythm could be more easily recalled and sustained.

In addition, the actor was taught to *warm-down* or to reestablish balance and relaxation in the vocal mechanism as soon as possible after rehearsals or performances. This regimen did not take more than 5 or 10 minutes but was essential to preserving the health and stamina of the voice:

1. Restoring adequate hydration by sipping some room-temperature water, swishing it around in order to relubricate the mouth, the tongue, and the throat;

2. Relaxing the breathing mechanism by enjoying a series of ten relatively deep breaths, taken in through the nose, down into the area of the back ribs and spine and out through the mouth (accompanying yawns were encouraged);

3. Restoring balance in the muscles of the upper body, neck and face via gentle head rolls (half or full) in both directions, gentle shoulder rolls, rolling down through the spine until it elongates due to gravity while feeling extra blood circulating in the head by sustaining that full bend-over position for a few minutes; gentle humming and moving the tongue around in the mouth as if chewing midrange before rolling back up the spine incrementally, bringing the head up last;

4. Singing or humming quite softly but not breathily midrange to allow the vocal folds to revert to their more usual function;

5. Massaging of shoulders, neck and jaw muscles (particularly the masseters) while gently vocalizing midrange, alternating between /u/ and /i/ to get the lips and face muscles moving.

This play is constructed in such a way that, while onstage, there are times when each actor is out of the light and quietly listening to the other actor, who may be speaking a monologue as much as a minute or two in length. The actor found it very helpful to use just a few hidden warm-ups, unnoticed by audience members (even in a thrust-stage theatre), while the other actor was speaking:

1. Gently, slowly, and unobtrusively moving the head around into profile and back, tipping each ear down to the shoulder on the same side or dropping the chin onto the chest to relax the involved muscles;

2. Sharply biting the tongue tip and/or moving the tongue unobtrusively inside the mouth in order to produce some saliva to relubricate the

mucous membranes of the mouth and throat (there was no water available to the actors onstage, although there was a vessel of "emergency water" available to them if necessary);

3. Slowly and unobtrusively breathing in through the nose and out through the mouth to rebalance the breathing mechanism, even incorporated some subtle closed-mouth yawns when facing upstage and standing or sitting out of the lights; and

4. Mentally reviewing the "trigger" or target phrase or sentence for the next character being played to prepare the voice to function in that pitch vicinity, with that particular resonance and/or that particular dialect.

Making Less Vocally Demanding Acting Choices. To enable this actor to succeed artistically without abusing his voice, he was encouraged to make several vocal choices that were potentially less taxing and therefore more easily sustainable:

1. Using techniques advocated by Arthur Lessac and Kristin Linklater, the actor was encouraged to keep tone placement solidly connected to the hard palate as opposed to the soft palate or the throat whenever possible in both rehearsal and performance;

2. The actor was taught how to link directly into initial vowels in order to minimize hard glottal initiation (see the last part of Arthur Lessac's chapter on "Consonant Action"); he was also coached to initiate grunts (eg, when miming the chopping of wood, when fighting) and screams (eg, when being whipped as a slave or attacked by dogs) with /h/, again to minimize hard glottal initiation;

3. The actor was taught to minimize extra-verbal vocalization and stridor whenever possible. For example, to simulate a coughing spell referred to in the script, the actor was encouraged to make choices far easier on his throat than the ones he had thought of initially;

4. When the actor wanted to "rough up" his tone in order to portray a mean and abusive prisoner, he was encouraged to do so midrange rather than working near the limits of his habitual pitch range;

5. The actor was encouraged to find alternatives to loudness and speed when communicating anger and other emotionally heightened states —the exploration of the use of different keys and different rhythms and different relatively safe vocal qualities in which to play different characters as well as the exploitation of opportunities to rest his voice within the context of performance provided very good strategies for increasing ease inside of demanding characterizations;

6. The actor was taught the concept of *minimum loudness level* (ie, the level below which the loudness must never go if one is to retain intelligibility in the theater). Attention to phrasing, to silent catch-breaths, to unstressed syllables, and to final consonants made his words far clearer onstage without his obviously "enunciating" or "projecting" the voice; and

7. The actor was encouraged to carry some of his good singing habits (eg, lengthening vowels, fully voicing softer phonation, sufficiently energizing and specifying consonants, linking directly into initial vowels) over into his speaking voice throughout the show.

Offstage Behavior Modification and Strategies. In addition to the above methodology, the voice coach reminded the actor to "save demanding voice use for the paying customers" by practicing some basic vocal hygiene:

1. *Adequate hydration*—the actor was instructed to pay attention to both frequency and quantity of water consumption, as well as the consumption of diuretics such as coffee;
2. *Steam inhalation*—the actor was provided with the company steam inhaler to use during both rehearsals and performances and was extremely compliant in this regard because he liked its effects;
3. *Limiting cell phone use and postrehearsal visits to noisy places*—the actor was strongly encouraged to limit his cell phone usage, especially immediately following rehearsals or performances. When he had to make a call, he was encouraged to set a timer, so that his phone conversations would last no longer than 5 to 10 minutes. Even at the opening night postperformance reception, the actor was reminded to step into a quieter space to have any long conversations, because the reception room was very noisy and the actor had a matinee performance on the following day;
4. *Adequate sleep and rest*—the actor was strongly encouraged not to shortchange himself on sleep, especially during the couple of weeks it took him to memorize a great deal of text for this particular role; and
5. *Healthful habits*—the actor was discouraged from using alcohol or any other recreational drugs and from lifting heavy weights as he worked out daily at the gym.

Further Considerations. In addition to ongoing sessions with the actor and vocal notes taken and communicated throughout the rehearsal process, the voice coach took responsibility for *advocating for the actor* with both the play's director and other members of the production team:

1. Occasionally, the voice coach spoke with the director during rehearsal breaks or immediately afterward, making her increasingly aware of the potential dangers lurking behind some of the behavior she had the actor using; and
2. The voice coach spoke with the publicity and marketing departments' personnel, asking them to spare the actor, as much as possible, from long hours of interviews and recording sessions, and so forth. These people were asked to keep the audience "talk backs" from going longer than about 30 minutes because longer sessions might deprive the actor of much needed postperformance voice rest.

Assessment. Even when using the above strategies, exercises, and techniques, the coach considered her efforts only a qualified success despite the considerable critical and popular success enjoyed by this production. Actors, and not just young ones, are people-pleasers by nature and may be insufficiently assertive when it comes to protecting themselves or preserving their physical and vocal health. They do not wish to be thought of as fragile or as divas or as poor team players, especially when working with a director for the first time. It is useful for the vocal coach or teacher or therapist to keep this in mind and to intervene or represent his or her client's best interests whenever possible. By the end of the run of "Blue Door," I was pleased that this actor had played every performance he was contracted to play and that he walked away with his voice in better shape than it was when he began rehearsals. Impressing performers with the importance of making sustainable choices while educating directors regarding ways to avoid vocal injury in actors might just be two of the most important functions of the voice coach, voice teacher, or therapist.

Suggested Readings

Lessac A. *The Use and Training of the Human Voice*. 3rd ed, rev. Mountain View, CA: Mayfield Publishing Company; 1997.

Linklater K. *Freeing the Natural Voice*. 2nd ed, rev. Hollywood, CA: Drama Publishers an imprint of Quite Specific Media Group, Ltd; 2006.

Raphael B. A consumer's guide to voice and speech training. In: Hauptman M, Acker B. *The Vocal Vision*. New York, NY: Applause Books; 1997:203–213.

Raphael B. The sounds of violence: vocal training in stage combat. *Theatre Top.* 1991;1(1):73–86.

Raphael BN. Carryover: bringing skills acquisition from studio to life. *Voice Speech Rev.* 2003;3(1)72–76.

Raphael BN. Dancing on shifting ground: Voice coaching in the professional theatre. *Voice Speech Rev.* 2000;1(1):165–170.

Rodenburg P. *The Right to Speak*. Portsmouth, NH: Heinemann; 1992.

Rodenburg P. *The Need for Words*. Portsmouth, NH: Heinemann; 1993.

Rodenburg P. *The Actor Speaks*. London, UK: Methuen; 1997.

References

1. Khambato A. Laryngeal disorders in singers and other voice users. In: Ballantyne GJ, ed. *Scott Brown's Diseases of the Ear, Nose, and Throat*. Vol 4. London, England: Butterworth; 1979.

2. Koufman J, Isaccson G. *The Spectrum of Vocal Dysfunction*. Philadelphia, PA: WB Saunders; 1991.

3. Stemple JC, Glaze L, Klaben BG. *Clinical Voice Pathology: Theory and Management*. San Diego, CA: Singular; 2000.

4. Hoffman, B, Lehman, J, Sapienza CM, C. *High-risk performers: laryngoscopic and acoustic characteristics*. Presentation at the 28th Annual Symposium: Care of the Professional Voice; June, 1999; Philadelphia, PA.

5. Sataloff, R. *Vocal Health and Pedagogy*. San Diego, CA: Singular Publishing Group; 1988.

6. Fairbanks G. *Voice and Articulation Drill Book*. 2nd ed. New York, NY: Harper and Brothers; 1960.

7. Hirano M, Bless, D. *Videostroboscopic Examination of the Larynx*. San Diego, CA: Singular Publishing Group; 1993.

8. Colton R, Casper J. *Understanding Voice Problems: A Physiological Perspective for Diagnosis and Treatment*. Baltimore, MD: Williams & Wilkins;1996.

9. Maughan RJ, Shirreffs, SM. Recovery from prolonged exercise: restoration of water and electrolyte balance. *J Sports Science*. 1999;5:297–303.

10. Newton Wellesley Primary Care. Dehydration: common facts. Retrieved June 25, 1999 from http://www.nwpcmd.com/dehydration.html.

11. Roy N, Bless DM, Heisey D, Ford CN. Manual circumlaryngeal therapy for functional dysphonia: an evaluation of short- and long-term treatment outcomes. *J Voice*. 1997;11(3):321–331.

12. Iwarsson J, Sundberg J. Effects of lung volume on vertical larynx position during phonation. *J Voice*. 1998;12(2):159–165.

13. Boone D, McFarlane, S. *The Voice and Voice Therapy*. Englewood Cliffs, NJ: Prentice-Hall: 1994.

14. Verdolini, K, DeVore, K, McCoy S, Ostrem J. *National Center for Voice and Speech's Guide to Vocology*. Iowa City, IA:

University of Iowa, National Center for Voice and Speech; 1998.

15. Baker S, Davenport P, Sapienza C. Examination of strength training and detraining effects in expiratory muscles. *J Speech Lang Hear Res.* 2005;48(6): 1325–1333.

16. Sapienza C, Hoffman-Ruddy, B, et al. *Acoustic and physiologic characteristics of high-risk vocal performers following expiratory pressure threshold training.* Presentation at the 17th International Conference on Acoustics; 2001; Rome, Italy; 2001.

17. Sapienza CM. Respiratory muscle strength training applications. *Curr Opin Otolaryngol Head Neck Surg.* 2008;16(3):216–220.

18. Sapienza CM, Davenport PW, Martin AD. Expiratory muscle training increases pressure support in high school band students. *J Voice.* 2002;16(4):495–501.

19. Eustace CS, Stemple JC, Lee L. Objective measures of voice production in patients complaining of laryngeal fatigue. *J Voice.* 1996;10(2):146–154.

20. Stemple JC, Stanley J, Lee L. Objective measures of voice production in normal subjects following prolonged voice use. *J Voice.* 1995;9(2):127–133.

21. American Speech Language Hearing Association. *Consensus Auditory-Perceptual Evaluation of Voice (CAPE-V): Purpose and Applications.* Bethesda, MD: Author; 2002.

22. Jacobson B, Johnson A, Grywalski C, Silbergleit A, Jacobson G, Benninger MS. The voice handicap index (VHI): Development and validation. *Am J Speech Lang Pathol.* 1997;6:66–70.

23. Hogikyan ND, Sethuraman G. Validation of an instrument to measure voice-related quality of life (V-RQOL). *J Voice.* 199913(4):557–569.

24. Spencer, ML. Hybrid voice therapy. *J Singing.* 2004;61(2):127–135.

25. Hirano M. *Clinical Examination of Voice.* New York, NY: Springer-Verlag; 1981.

26. Stemple JC, Lee L, D'Amico B, Pickup B. Efficacy of vocal function exercises as a method of improving voice production. *J Voice.* 1994;8(3):271–278.

27. Sabol JW, Lee L, Stemple JC. The value of vocal function exercises in the practice regimen of singers. *J Voice.* 1995;9(1): 27–36.

28. Wilson Arboleda BM, Frederick AL. Considerations for maintenance of postural alignment for voice production. *J Voice.* 2008;22(1):90–99.

8

Management Approaches for Neurogenic Voice Disorders

Introduction

Neurogenic voice pathologies are voice disorders caused directly by an interruption of the innervation to the larynx, including both central and peripheral insults. Some of these disorders are confined to voice and laryngeal manifestations, such as vocal fold paralysis (discussed in Chapter 4). Others may reflect a larger deterioration of many motor control systems, including broader impairment of respiration, resonance, swallowing, and other functions beyond the head and neck where a voice disturbance is only one of many impairments (eg, progressive neurogenic disease). This chapter offers a discussion of treatments for a sampling of neurogenic disorders including adductor and abduc-

tor spasmodic dysphonia, oromandibular dystonia, Parkinson's disease, and Tourette's syndrome.

Spasmodic Dysphonia

Imagine developing a condition so insidious that it may cause loss of self-respect and confidence; a disorder so negative as to cause depression, reclusivity, and thoughts of suicide; a condition that can ruin careers, marriages, and friendships. This disorder is spasmodic dysphonia.

Spasmodic dysphonia is a term that describes a family of strained, strangled voices. Perceptually, the voice symptoms are classified in two primary groups: adductor and abductor spasmodic dysphonia. Adductor spasmodic dysphonia, which is the most common, is characterized by strained, strangled phonation with occasional intermittent stoppages of voice. The severity may range from very mild, intermittent symptoms to a very severe, persistent struggle to produce phonation. The abductor type is characterized by abductor vocal fold spasms causing sudden, intermittent explosions or escapes of air. Abductor spasms appear to occur most frequently during the transition from voiceless consonants to vowels.

Although the incidence of this disorder is thought to be relatively low, the extreme negative effects that it brings to many individuals suffering with the disorder highlight the importance of appropriate professional care. Most researchers agree that the onset of spasmodic dysphonia generally occurs during middle age (although clinical reports include children and older adults).[1,2] The exact ratio of female to male cases is unknown, but most agree that the majority of cases seen are women. Some patients experience a rapid onset of symptoms, whereas others experience a gradual onset over many years.

Researchers and clinicians have debated the cause of spasmodic dysphonia for many years. Early descriptions linked the disorder to psychoneurosis.[3] Indeed, Aronson[3] commented that one type of strained, strangled voice has a psychological cause and can be treated as a functional aphonia or a disorder of musculoskeletal tension. An argument could be made that classifying these disorders as spasmodic dysphonia may not be appropriate. Others have advocated a neurologic origin.[1,4,5] Blitzer et al[6] offered the first evidence that spasmodic dysphonia is a focal dystonia specific to the larynx and similar to other dystonias, such as blepharospasm and torticollis.

Symptom relief as a result of voice therapy has been minimal at best. Until recently, most patients treated in our clinic have had the disorder for many years prior to diagnosis. They have sought treatments from many laryngologists, speech-language pathologists, psychologists, and psychiatrists. They have been prescribed various drugs and have gone through relaxation therapy, biofeedback, hypnosis, and acupuncture. Some patients have sought the services of a faith healer. All patients have been consistent in their frustrations over the lack of relief.

Until 1976, most patients with spasmodic dysphonia remained untreated, that is, until Herbert Dedo[7] suggested a fairly radical prophylactic treatment for symptom relief. This treatment was to create a unilateral vocal fold paralysis. Dedo and Izdebski[8] reported that creation of the unilateral paralysis proved successful in relieving the adductor spasmodic dysphonia symptoms 4 years postoperatively in 90% of 306 patients. Dedo and Shipp[9] reported that spasmodic dysphonia returned in 10% to 15% of their patients within 1 month to 2 years following recurrent laryngeal nerve (RLN) resection. Aronson and De-Santo[10] followed 38 patients and reported that 64% had worse voice quality after 3 years postoperatively.

The current treatment for spasmodic dysphonia is prophylactic as well. It involves creating a paretic or weakened vocal fold condition. This is accomplished by injecting botulinum toxin (BOTOX) into the thyroarytenoid muscle (for adductor spasmodic dysphonia) and the posterior cricoarytenoid muscle (for abductor spasmodic dysphonia), creating a temporary paresis of the muscles.[11] The weakened muscles do not permit the spasms to occur, and thus the vocal symptoms are relieved.

Functional Voice Therapy for Spasmodic Dysphonia

Joseph C. Stemple, PhD

Case Study: Patient VV

> *Some patients certainly do benefit from a direct symptom modification approach of voice therapy. Indeed, as a result of the physical struggle inherent in attempting to push the voice through the spasmodic occurrences, many patients develop secondary behaviors that make the voice quality worse than the baseline spasmodic condition. For example, patients develop extreme neck, shoulder, and thoracic tension; lowered pitch and glottal fry phonation; and monotonous phonatory patterns. The first case study in this chapter involves an individual who developed these secondary behaviors. The study describes functional voice therapy that subsequently improved the symptoms significantly, albeit without eliminating the spasms.*

Patient VV, a 57-year-old high school English and drama teacher, was referred to the voice center by the speech-language pathologist serving her school. Her history was typical of many individuals with this disorder. Although she had been symptomatic for 3 years and had consulted three laryngologists and one speech-language pathologist, the diagnosis of spasmodic dysphonia had never been made.

Patient VV had never married and was extremely independent and outgoing. She had taught for 34 years and stated that she "lived to teach." By the time of the initial evaluation, she was extremely upset, confused, and full of self-doubt. She had independently sought the counsel of a psychologist who, unfortunately, was not familiar with spasmodic dysphonia and who supported the notion that the problem was "all in my head." She had developed lesson plans and techniques that minimized her own speaking, but she suffered with these teaching modifications. Previously, she had been honored as an outstanding educator, and she was convinced that she had become less than effective in the classroom.

Away from school, this normally outgoing individual had withdrawn and, for at least 18 months, lived a reclusive existence. She refused to see friends and totally avoided the telephone. Several weeks into our treatment, she admitted to having had thoughts of suicide. The two things most dear to her, teaching and friendship, had been taken from her as a result of her voice disorder.

The voice pathologist performed three roles during the initial session: evaluator to confirm the presence of spasmodic dysphonia; educator to teach the patient what was known about the disorder; and treatment planner to attempt to remediate the disorder. Patient VV presented with adductor spasmodic dysphonia of moderate severity. Phonation was characterized by intermittent glottal stops and glottal fry phonation as well as a flat, monotonous inflection pattern. It was evident from the physical appearance of neck and shoulder tension and facial expression that she was very tense, nervous, upset, and depressed.

The voice problem began in the Fall 3 years prior to the examination. It manifested as hoarseness that persisted following an upper respiratory infection. Much probing regarding other possible psychosocial issues yielded nothing related to the onset. When the hoarseness persisted for several weeks, she sought the opinion of an otolaryngologist who prescribed antibiotics three times over a 4-month period. As the symptoms worsened, hesitations began "shutting off" her voice, requiring her to force to speak. She reported that teaching was actually causing her to be physically fatigued because of the effort it took to speak. She was exhausted at the end of a school day. Some days, her abdominal muscles would become sore from straining to produce voice. During the 2 subsequent years, she sought the opinion of two more physicians, one of whom prescribed more medication, with the other recommending psychological counseling. A speech-language pathologist, new to Patient VV's school, heard her speak and thought the patient presented with the symptoms of spasmodic dysphonia. She then suggested that the patient come to our center for evaluation. Desperate for help, she complied.

It was determined through examining voice quality characteristics, abilities and lack of abilities, that she indeed had adductor spasmodic dysphonia. The diagnosis of spasmodic dysphonia is a diagnosis of perception. She demonstrated normal phonation when humming or singing, or when speaking in lilting accents. She loved to read aloud from the writings of the American dramatist Tennessee Williams because the higher pitched rhythm of the U.S. southern dialect reduced her effort to talk and improved the voice quality. She could

laugh normally and felt that her voice was "near-normal" when she talked to her cat. The patient also thought that her voice quality was improved following ingestion of wine. This led her to try tranquilizers, which did not improve her voice quality.

Following identification of the problem, Patient VV was given much information, regarding spasmodic dysphonia. This included written information provided by the National Spasmodic Dysphonia Association (NSDA).[12] She was greatly relieved that she suffered from a "recognized" disorder and that the problem was not necessarily psychologically induced. (In retrospect, Patient VV also had a very mild head tremor, which is not an unusual co-occurrence with spasmodic dysphonia.) The possibility of a nonspecific central nervous system disorder was discussed. The differences between vocal symptoms of organic tremor and spasmodic dysphonia were discussed because of the patient's observation of her vocal likeness to a popular actor.

Treatment options were then discussed. As with many patients, Patient VV was distressed to learn that treatments would produce only symptom relief and not cure the disorder. Recurrent laryngeal nerve resection and BOTOX injections were described. Functional voice therapy designed to eliminate secondary tension, inappropriate pitch, and inflection was discussed. The decision was made to initiate treatment with functional voice therapy.

It was interesting to note the change in Patient VV's entire persona from the initial session to the second session. From a tense, depressed, and beaten individual emerged an encouraged, determined, and resolute person. During the first session, we identified the vocal tasks that she could perform well with fair consistency. These included:

- humming and singing
- speaking at a higher pitch
- speaking with a slight Southern dialect.

It was discovered that she could speak well to her cat because she was speaking in a higher pitched, "baby" voice.

She had developed the habit of producing voice with muscle tenseness, back focus, and at low pitch in an effort to overcome the intermittent spasms. Because the patient had no idea when the spasms would occur, she postured her phonatory and respiratory systems in a manner that produced constant tension and pressure. The first step of therapy was to introduce relaxation techniques to demonstrate the degree of tension. Progressive relaxation as well as electromyographic (EMG) biofeedback was successfully utilized for this purpose.

Phonatory tasks then were added to this newly relaxed state, utilizing a slightly higher pitch and phrases controlled by length. Although the spasms persisted, the therapist and the patient noted that frequency and severity decreased. Phrases were lengthened, and the patient was trained to breathe more normally. A midtone focus permitting a slightly breathy phonation was deemed acceptable by the patient. In addition, she felt comfortable in slightly overinflecting her phonation patterns of pitch and loudness, which also seemed to decrease the severity of the spasms.

Longer phrases utilizing these techniques were then expanded into paragraph readings with and without phrase or breath markers and finally into practiced conversational speech. Because of Patient VV's background in drama, the

entire therapy program was completed within 6 weeks. The spasms persisted of course, but were heard only as occasional hesitations during speech production. The patient learned to permit her voice to flow through and past the hesitations without redeveloping the previous strained postures. Eliminating the secondary behaviors proved adequate for this patient. She did not then choose to pursue BOTOX injections. Prior to discharge, the patient was advised that her voice may continue to decline in the months and years to come and that she should seek follow-up care and reconsider the possibility of BOTOX injections when concerns arise in the future.

Medical and Behavioral Management of Adductor Spasmodic Dysphonia

Edie R. Hapner, PhD, and Michael M. Johns, MD

Case Study: WW

In the next case study, Edie Hapner and Michael Johns discuss an interdisciplinary comprehensive medical and behavioral management approach for a patient presenting with adductor spasmodic dysphonia.

Patient History. A 56-year-old female teacher presented with a 5-year history of dysphonia. Recently, she had noticed that people asked her if she was upset when she talked. She noted that her voice was better when she was singing. It also improved slightly with a glass of wine. Using the phone made her voice worse, and she had stopped ordering in restaurants because of her voice. She had seen multiple otolaryngologists and had been diagnosed with hoarseness and reflux. She had been treated with several full courses of antibiotics, steroids, proton pump inhibitors for laryngopharyngeal reflux (LPR), and a 14-week course of voice therapy. In voice therapy, she was able to achieve a clearer tone but frustrated both herself and the speech-language pathologist when she was unable to carryover the clear voice outside of therapy. Both the speech-language pathologist and otolaryngologist had suggested that perhaps there was some unconscious stressor in her life that she was not dealing with, and they had recommended that she see a psychiatrist. During her own Internet search, she came across information about a multidisciplinary voice center in her area and made an appointment to be seen.

Evaluation

Overview. The patient was seen and evaluated in a multidisciplinary voice clinic. Both a speech-language pathologist and an otolaryngologist evaluated the patient on the same day, separately and together. Recognizing that there was significant overlap, the otolaryngologist largely obtained the medical history described above, and the speech-language pathologist obtained the voice history. The otolaryngologist performed the general and otolaryngology examination, and the speech-language pathologist performed the endoscopic laryngeal imaging. A perceptual voice screening was completed in the presence of both the otolaryngologist and speech-language pathologist asking the patient to complete the following tasks while observing for phonation breaks, voice-voiceless transitions, and the presence of vocal tremor: (a) Prolong the vowels /i/ and /a/; (b) Produce vowelloaded sentences and; (c) Count from 60 to 65 and 80 to 85.

General Examination. On physical examination, the patient appeared healthy and was breathing comfortably in no acute distress. Vital signs showed that the patient was afebrile. The pulse was 82, respirations were 14, and blood pressure was 146/91. The patient had normal gait. Upper and lower extremity examination demonstrated full muscular strength and normal sensation. No hand tremor or joint cogwheel rigidity was noted. Reflexes were 2+. Respiratory examination showed clear breath sounds with full inspiration and normal forceful expiration.

Head and Neck Examination. The patient's voice had a severe strained and strangled quality, making her difficult to be understood. The neck was supple without skin lesions, thyromegaly, lymphadenopathy, or masses. There was moderate tenderness to palpation in the thyrohyoid region that was symmetrical. Cranial nerves II through XII were grossly intact, eye movements were full, and head and neck muscle strength was normal. Otoscopy demonstrated clear external auditory canals, and intact tympanic membranes with aerated middle ear spaces. Hearing was grossly normal. Anterior rhinoscopy showed healthy mucous membranes without masses or obstruction of the nasal cavities. Oral cavity and oropharyngeal examination demonstrated moist mucous membranes without lesions. Palatal rise and gag reflex were normal. Indirect laryngoscopy was somewhat limited by the gag reflex, but there were no gross masses and vocal fold mobility appeared normal.

Laryngeal Imaging. Detailed laryngeal imaging was performed using both rigid transoral examination with a

70-degree telescope for detailed mucosal examination and transnasal flexible imaging using a distal-chip videolaryngoscopy for dynamic assessment of the larynx and pharynx. These endoscopic examinations were performed by the speech-language pathologist using both plain and stroboscopic light. The rigid 70-degree stroboscopic assessment was the first laryngeal imaging examination to be completed. The stroboscopic examination yielded: symmetrical vocal process approximation in the midline, complete glottal closure, symmetrical entrained vibration of the membranous vocal folds without asymmetry, normal mucosal waves bilaterally (propagating to 50% of the superior surface of the vocal folds), and intermittent vibratory aperiodicity.

Flexible transnasal imaging was performed to assess motion and symmetry of the vocal mechanism. A mixture of topical ponticaine and oxymetolazine was applied to the nasal mucosa by the clinic nurse for the flexible examination. During the flexible examination, the patient's voice improved significantly, which considerably increased the overall intelligibility of her communication. Palatal closure was complete and without fatigue. Pharyngeal squeeze was normal. No pharyngeal or laryngeal masses were noted. The laryngeal mucosa appeared healthy with mild interarytenoid pachydermia and postcricoid edema observed. Arytenoid motion showed full adduction and abduction that was symmetrical and brisk bilaterally.

Behavioral Voice Assessment. Following the office evaluation, the patient was seen by the speech-language pathologist for a comprehensive voice evaluation including: (a) perceptual voice assessment, (b) acoustic assessment, (c) aerodynamic assessment, and (d) assessment of the impact of the voice disorder on quality of life.

Perceptual Assessment. The Consensus-Auditory Perceptual Evaluation of Voice (CAPE-V)[13] was administered. The patient had an overall score of 84/100, indicating a dysphonia of a severe nature. Aberrant perceptual features identified in the voice included roughness, pitch breaks, phonation breaks, and strain. There was laryngeal/pharyngeal focused resonance with base of tongue tension that dampened the intensity of voice output. Respiration appeared to be primarily abdominal/thoracic. There was evidence of breath holding during conversational speech indicating poor coordination of respiration and phonation for efficient phrasing in running speech and increased tension in the neck and chest.

A motor speech evaluation indicated a normal oral mechanism with normal articulatory precision. On vowel prolongation, there were audible voice stoppages with a strain-strangled harshness to the tone though no tremor was noted. Laryngeal diadochokinesis indicated phonation breaks.

Aerodynamic Measures. Aerodynamic measures of syllable repetition have been suggested for use in differential diagnosis. To complete this task, the patient was fitted with a standard face mask connected to a commercially available pneumotachograph and pressure transducer. She was asked to produce repetitions of the syllable /pa/. Results indicated a lower than normal phonatory flow rate of 130 mL/sec (norms = 177–187 mL/sec) and phonatory airflow was interrupted with seven instances of airflow perturbations in the task (norms = 1–2 instances).

Acoustic Assessment. A headset microphone was placed at a 45-degree angle at 2 cm from mouth for acquisition of acoustic information per standards recommended by Titze and Winholtz[14] in their 1993 article about standards for acoustic assessment of voice. The patient was placed in a soundproof booth for testing. The results of the assessment were abnormal including: (a) decreased maximum phonation time of 5 seconds; (b) speaking fundamental frequency (sF_0) was abnormally low at 165 Hz; (c) standard deviation of sF_0 was abnormally high (= 29 Hz); (d) restricted physiologic pitch range across the entire physiological frequency range of phonation; (e) abnormally high pitch perturbation (jitter) = 1.05%; (f) abnormally high intensity perturbation (shimmer) = 3.85%; (g) elevated noise to harmonic ratio >0.12; and (h) elevated degree of voice breaks = 1.01. Results of the testing indicated a voice type 3, with chaotic or random signal acquisition and relative average perturbation high. This indicates that the acoustic data are not a reliable source of information and that perceptual ratings of voice should be used.

Trial Therapy. During trial therapy, the patient was stimulable for improvement in voice quality using chant talk, high-pitched productions, vegetative vocal tasks, and whispering.

Voice Quality of Life. Voice-Related Quality of Life (VRQOL)[15] was administered to assess the patient's perception of the impact the voice disorder on quality of life. VRQOL raw score was 34/50, which converts to 35/100. [Higher QOL scores correlate with higher quality of life.] These scores indicate that the patient perceives her voice disorder as having a significant impact on her quality of life.

Diagnosis. After the evaluation above, the otolaryngologist and the speech-language pathologist conferred and reviewed the patient's presentation. A diagnosis of spasmodic dysphonia—adductory type was rendered. Together, the clinicians shared the diagnosis with the patient. They explained that the problem was a focal dystonia, a benign neurologic condition that results in uncontrolled spasm of the laryngeal muscles responsible for vocal fold adduction (primarily the thyroarytenoid and lateral cricoarytenoid muscles). The patient asked what caused the condition and was told that the exact cause is unclear, but that it is felt to result from an abnormality in the basal ganglia (a center of movement control in the brain). The patient was then told of the alternate diagnoses that can present similarly to or simultaneously with spasmodic dysphonia, such as muscle tension dysphonia and benign essential vocal tremor. The patient was given written and online (http://www.dysphonia.org) information about spasmodic dysphonia and watched a video produced by the National Spasmodic Dysphonia Association. The otolaryngologist and speech-language pathologist answered all the questions that the patient had regarding the diagnosis and then a detailed discussion regarding treatment ensued.

Treatment

Medication. The patient asked about medications that could be used for treatment. She was told that there are no medications that have been demonstrated to provide any long-term benefit. Benzodiazepines, such as diazepam, help some patients for short periods, but the risk of dependency from chronic use was discussed as well as the goal of avoiding the routine use of such medications. Some medications have limited utility for vocal tremor, such as beta blockers (eg, propranolol), and anti-epileptics (eg, primidone), but these have not been shown to be effective for isolated spasmodic dysphonia.

Surgical Options. The history of surgical procedures for spasmodic dysphonia was reviewed with the patient including recurrent laryngeal nerve section, recurrent laryngeal nerve avulsion, and the newer selective laryngeal adductory denervation and reinnervation (SLAD-R). The former two are limited by frequent recurrences of voice breaks, typically do not have long-term benefits, and may be complicated by permanent breathiness to the voice. The latter is a newer procedure that may be effective in patients who respond well to botulinum toxin injections, but it has not become widely utilized for spasmodic dysphonia, largely due to lack of long-term data regarding its effectiveness. The patient was encouraged to take an initial therapeutic approach with botulinum toxin injections.

Speech Therapy. The patient asked about returning to voice therapy as a treatment for ADSD. She was counseled that, as she had experienced with her previous attempts at voice therapy, research supports that voice therapy is not the most effective treatment for patients with ADSD. She was told that there are speech-language pathologists who believe that they are able to cure ADSD through the use of inhalation phonation targeting the abductor muscles or a method using a traditional symptomatic voice therapy approach requiring the patient to attend 5 hours of voice therapy 5 days a week for 4 to 5 weeks.

However, there is limited evidence for either treatment technique's effectiveness in permanently curing ADSD.

Botulinum Toxin Injections. The patient was told that the most widely utilized treatment for spasmodic dysphonia is botulinum toxin type-A injection into the laryngeal adductory muscles. Botulinum toxin is neurotoxin that blocks the ability of nerves to make muscles contract. When injected into a target muscle, it impairs the release of neurotransmitter from nerve endings at the neuromuscular junction. This effectively paralyzes or significantly weakens the muscle and prevents muscle contraction. Botulinum toxin acts temporarily, with effects from 3 to 6 months. Because of this, repeated injections are necessary for long-term treatment.

She was counseled that botulinum toxin injections for spasmodic dysphonia have been shown to be effective in reducing voice breaks and improving quality of life for patients both in the short- and long-term. The injections usually are given to an awake patient in the outpatient setting, utilizing laryngeal electromyography for accurate guidance into the laryngeal adductory muscles. Less commonly, injections are guided by flexible transnasal laryngoscopy, and, rarely, by injection under anesthesia using direct laryngoscopy. Usually a starting dose of 1.25U to 2.5U is used, either unilaterally or bilaterally, in the thyroarytenoid muscles.

The expected results of treatment were reviewed and she was given the following summary: The effects of injection appear after 24 to 48 hours. There is a fairly typical clinical course following injection that is important for her to understand. Once the botulinum toxin takes effect, patients typically notice a very weak and breathy voice. This is occasionally accompanied by mild dysphagia for liquids. This period usually lasts for 1 to 2 weeks, based on the amount of toxin injected. Patients usually can manage the dysphagia with conservative techniques such as slower rate of drinking, especially thin liquids, using a nectar thick consistency for liquids, slight chin tuck on drinking liquids, and an effortful swallow. After 1 to 2 weeks, the patient's voice begins to return and gradually gains strength with dramatic improvement in the voice breaks, fluency, effort, and understandability. This therapeutic period typically lasts 2 to 3 months. Following this, the patient will begin to notice voice breaks returning, and a repeat injection is scheduled.

The physician went on to explain to the patient that dosing for spasmodic dysphonia is an art and is based on individual patient's needs and results from treatment. The breathy period following injection can be very bothersome to patients. This can be minimized by using lower dose (0.625U to 1.25U) bilateral injections, or by performing unilateral injections. Although the weak and breathy voice period is minimized, patients should be counseled that the therapeutic effect might be lower. Alternatively, patients may travel long distances to receive their injections and they may want to maximize the duration of the effect. In these situations, higher doses can be used (5.0U bilaterally or more). Repeated dosing can be performed for long periods of time. He told her that many patients have had successful treatment with botulinum toxin for nearly 2 decades. He reviewed the possible complications from treatment. He also told her that, aside from the side effects of breathy voice and mild dysphagia, the possibility of breathing problems

existed following any procedure on the vocal folds. She was told to seek immediate medical attention if this occurs.

This patient received a starting dose of 2.5U into each thyroarytenoid muscle. She experienced a weak and breathy voice with very mild dysphagia for liquids that was most noticeable in the first week following treatment and waned during the second week. She returned to clinic 1 month following injection with a significantly improved voice. She did notice some vocal strain and occasional voice breaks that were still causing some voice fatigue. She was pleased with the result, but asked whether any adjunctive treatment was possible.

Adjunctive Voice Therapy. Voice therapy was initiated adjunctive to the botulinum toxin injection. It was explained to the patient that a brief course of voice therapy after injection has been found to increase the time between injections by teaching the patient to utilize an open pharyngeal tract and reduce compensatory muscle tension, especially when the toxin begins to wear off in 3 to 4 months. Therefore, the following goals for therapy were established:

Goal 1 and Rationale. The patient will increase kinesthetic awareness of compensatory muscle tension in the chest, shoulders, jaw/face, and laryngeal/pharyngeal areas of the vocal mechanism. The rationale for this goal lies in the frequency of extralaryngeal muscle tension utilized by those with ADSD in an attempt to overcome the excessive strain of sound production. Despite the use of botulinum toxin, the patient continued to utilize preinjection compensatory muscle tension. Treatment techniques used were specific to the area of the body targeted. To increase awareness of compensatory tension in the chest and shoulders, the patient was taken through lower abdominal focused breathing exercises and stretching exercises, and was encouraged to meet with the Feldenkrais practitioner in the multidisciplinary center. To target tension in the jaw/face, the patient was instructed in stretching exercises used in the Lessac-Madsen Resonant Voice Therapy (LMRVT). (The LMRVT method is described in full for readers in a case study by Katherine Verdolini Abbott in Chapter 3.)

To increase awareness of tension in the pharyngeal/laryngeal area, the patient was taken through a series of exercises comparing voiceless and voiced productions of fricatives. The use of voiceless productions of fricatives allows the patient to experience an easy sound production. Once the target sensation of easy sound production in voiceless fricatives was achieved, the patient was moved on to voiced fricatives and was instructed to maintain the open kinesthetic sensations in the throat felt during voiceless sound productions.

Goal 2 and Rationale. The patient will reduce effortful production of speech. Despite the use of botulinum toxin injection and the reduced glottal closure, the patient continued to use preinjection effortful voicing behaviors. The rationale for this exercise was to teach the patient to use less subglottal pressure and more of a continuous flow phonation during sound production. Treatment began with use of semioccluded vocal tract exercises to balance the resonators in the pharynx and amplify the sound intensity of phonation. Once the patient realized that she could produce phonation of a normal loudness by using an open pharyngeal/laryngeal tract, she

was able to implement a speaking style with less phonatory effort, thus decreasing vocal fatigue and encouraging a smoother phonatory style.

Goal 3 and Rationale. The patient will improve coordination of respiration and phonation. Preinjection, the patient had a tendency to breath-hold in an attempt to overcome the vocal spasm. After injection, the patient continued to utilize breath holding, often producing words on expiratory reserve volume of breath support. Additionally, with the increase in glottal gap due to the effects of botulinum toxin, the patient actually had less glottal valving and to efficiently coordinate respiration and phonation. Therefore, another goal was to encourage the patient to use shorter breath groups. The rationale for this goal was to increase awareness of coordinated respiratory phonatory support for speech. Treatment began with low abdominal breathing, stressing awareness of the onset of abdominal muscles contraction during exhalation. The next step was to add phonation to the low abdominal breathing, encouraging the patient to use voiceless fricative prolongation to avoid the laryngeal valve effort. Next, she was instructed to do pulsed productions of voiceless fricatives. She was then instructed to repeat the tasks with voiced fricatives. The task progression continued with use of sentences of increasing length and instructing the patient to use shorter breath groups with brief replenishing breaths in conversation.

Quality of Life. Impact of the use of botulinum toxin injections on quality of life is very personal and usually is dependent on the effectiveness of the injections, the vocal demands of the patient, and the environmental support of the patient. As a teacher, the patient often was plagued with balancing the breathy, whispered immediate postinjection voice and the vocal demands of teaching. She tried to coordinate injections a few days before the winter semester break, right before spring break, during the quieter months of summer when she did not teach, and a few weeks before the school year begins. But, even with all the planning, she often felt her life was ruled by her injections. The speech-language pathologist encouraged her to attend a local National Spasmodic Dysphonia Association support group. In the group, the patient found camaraderie, support, and wealth of resources from people who had lived with ADSD, undergone botulinum toxin injections, and tried a plethora of adjunctive treatments.

This case highlights the need for comprehensive care of patients with adductory type spasmodic dysphonia. Proper diagnosis, effective treatment, and close monitoring to ensure that the treatment meets the needs of the patient are hallmarks in the care of these patients.

Management of Adductor Spasmodic Dysphonia and Oral Mandibular Dystonia

Celia F. Stewart, PhD, and Andrew Blitzer, MD, DDS

Case Study: Patient XX

Spasmodic dysphonia can occur as an independent disorder or can be part of a cluster of symptoms associated with dystonia in other parts of the body. In the following case, Celia Stewart and Andrew Blitzer describe the treatment of a patient who presented with both adductor spasmodic dysphonia and oral mandibular dystonia.

Patient XX was a 38-year-old Jamaican-born male who had immigrated to the United States as an adult. He led a normal life and worked as a carpenter in New York until he had a motor vehicle accident. In January of 1985, he was visiting Jamaica and was crossing the street when he was hit by a car, lost consciousness, and was hospitalized in Jamaica for a prolonged period. His loss of consciousness lasted for about 2½ weeks and when he woke up, his left side was "dead." A brain scan revealed general brain damage with specific damage to his cerebellum. His left-side function slowly returned and his left arm slowly improved. He noted that as his arm improved, his speech deteriorated.

Mr. XX was discharged from the hospital in March 1985 and by April 1985, he returned to New York and was speaking normally. However, by the end of April, his articulation deteriorated and his speech was unintelligible. He went to speech therapy for 2 years with no significant improvement. He went to three prestigious hospitals and had a number of scans to his brain and spinal cord, but the results were not available. His articulation slowly improved, and he began to communicate again in July 1991. However, after about a year, he reported that his voice began to "tighten up." His voice symptoms progressed for about a year and then gradually stabilized. His speech symptoms fluctuated from day to day, and he reported a severe strangle in his throat.

In 1993, he was assessed in the Department of Neurology at Columbia Presbyterian Medical Center in New York. Mr. XX complained that it was very difficult for him to speak and to be understood. He experienced marked effort when speaking, and he was unaware of any activity, food, or medicines that improved his voice. He reported that on a scale of 0 to 100%, he was functioning at about 45% of normal. He reported having several nonspeech symptoms. He noted that his movement in his left arm had improved slightly. His arm shook during movement and he needed, at times, to hold it to keep it still. At times, his fingers were stiff. Occasionally, he felt the feeling of an electric current going through his legs and a tingling in his foot and left hand. He could not walk for long, or run up and down steps because of pain in his knee joints.

During the assessment, Mr. XX was diagnosed with adductor spasmodic dysphonia and generalized dystonia. His conversational speech was characterized by a moderate-to-severely decreased intelligibility, a severe degree of strain and strangle in his voice, and effortful respiration and voice production. His voice was decreased in loudness, breathy, and produced in constant vocal fry. This production persisted throughout all of his conversational speech, and it was clear that he had glottal obstruction during speaking. However, when sitting at rest, his respiratory pattern was normal. Sustained /a/ and /i/ and sentences "He saw half a sea shell" and "ambling along rainy Island Avenue" were similarly strangled. In addition, he had a mild dysarthria and a Jamaican accent. His consonants were slightly prolonged but had the proper rhythm, but his overall speech intelligibility was poor. Singing and laughing did not improve his condition.

On examination, he had generalized dystonia that affected his left side. At rest, his neck was straight and the left hand was comfortably relaxed on his thigh. Sitting at rest, he had a left facial droop, but had good symmetrical elevation of the eyebrows. His extraocular movements were full and he did not have nystagmus. During speech, his

facial muscles were tight with clenching of the masseter muscle, excessive stiffness in his lips and tongue, and overflow of muscle activity to his upper face. Tongue movements were imprecise on the left side with slightly decreased range of motion, but he did not have a palatal droop. He had involuntary movements on the left side of his body and an occasional almost ticlike jerk of his left thigh and left arm. Rapid alternating successive movements of the right arm and leg were normal, but on the left side, finger and foot taping was mildly uncoordinated with a mild degree of dysdiadochokinesia and mild ataxia. He performed tandem walking with some difficulty and exhibited mild ataxia. Writing with his dominant right hand was normal but was tremorous in his left hand. Sensation in his face was normal, and tone, posture, and strength in the upper and lower extremities was normal.

In 1993, Mr. XX began receiving bilateral injections into the thyroarytenoid muscle of botulinum toxin type A (BoNT-A), a purified protein produced by the bacterium *Clostridum botulinum* that, when prepared for medical use, can be injected into muscle to provide a graded muscle relaxation. He had some improvement in his speech but continued to have difficulty with communication and severely impaired intelligibility. The toxin relieved some, but not all, of the strangled quality of his voice and larger doses of toxin resulted in breathy voice quality or aphonia. He continued to receive BoNT-A injections for treatment of the excessive vocal muscle contractions, even though the results did not improve his speech intelligibility. He reported that the injections reduced his feeling of effort during speech. On examination, his intelligibility was moderately to severely impaired. His voice was moderately decreased in loudness, breathy, and he produced frequent vocal fry. He used increased expiratory effort during all speech. His articulation was imprecise, and his speech rate was slow. In addition, he had excessive stiffness in his face, lips, tongue, and chest during speech. This muscle stiffness disappeared when he stopped talking.

A re-evaluation in 2004 revealed that his speech intelligibility had deteriorated, his speech was severely impaired, and he complained of discomfort in his facial muscles during speech. Mr. XX participated in voice therapy focused on decreasing expiratory drive, coordinating voicing with expiratory drive, and decreasing extraneous muscle stiffness. In response to the combination of BoNT-A and voice therapy, his speech improved in structured settings and his speech intelligibility improved to moderately impaired. Nevertheless, he was unable to transfer the improvement to his everyday speech. Examination during therapy revealed that masseter, platysma, levator labii superioris, and risorius were stiff and his face was severely asymmetrical. In an attempt to decrease the stiffness in his face, small bilateral injections of BoNT-A were made into each of these muscles bilaterally. The injections decreased the muscle stiffness in his lips and cheeks and the result of decreasing his facial stiffness had a synergistic effect on his voice production. Following injection, not only did his articulation become more precise, but his voice production also improved. His intelligibility improved from severely impaired to moderately impaired in conversation.

Concluding Thoughts. This patient's disorder illustrates the additive effect of dystonia symptoms. Reassessment of individuals with recalcitrant spasmodic dysphonia may reveal dystonia in other parts of the body. Therefore, it is important to identify all symptoms of dystonia in the patient and to determine if the dystonia in the other parts of the body is impinging on the production of voice. Reduction of dystonia outside of the larynx can result in a synergistic effect and improve the laryngeal function and consequently improve overall intelligibility of speech.

Dystonia frequently is misdiagnosed because the clinical symptoms are unusual and the disorder is rare. Dystonia is a syndrome characterized by sustained muscle contractions that can cause twisting and repetitive movements or abnormal postures and can involve any voluntary muscle.[16,17] These dystonic movements are abnormal and involuntary and usually are triggered by a volitional action. The body part usually appears to be normal at rest, but functions abnormally during action. Common areas where dystonia emerges include the eyelids, and the action that triggers the symptoms is consciously looking at something during reading or driving. Dystonia in the mouth, jaw, and tongue is elicited by speaking or chewing. However, cranial dystonia may be present in the absence of specific animation with symptom aggravation with voluntary use of the muscles. Furthermore, the dystonic movement can be ameliorated for brief periods by sensory tricks such as gently touching the chin, pinching the nose, or touching the throat.

In spasmodic dysphonia, the vocal folds typically appear to be normal during quiet breathing and the skilled movement that initiates the dystonic voicing is speech. Nonspeech voice tasks like sustaining vowels, crying, moaning, singing, laughing, coughing, and yawning usually do not often bring out the symptoms and so performance of nonspeech sounds typically remain unimpaired.[2,11,18] During speech, the vocal folds move inappropriately with an inappropriate *add*uctor or *abd*uctor movements.[19]

*Add*uctor movements are more common. These result in increased expiratory effort, and the prominent vocal symptoms are a strained-strangled, rough voice quality with sudden intermittent voice arrests and decreased loudness. *Abd*uctor movements result in a breathy or whispered voice quality with sudden intermittent voice arrests and a mild rough voice quality.

Dystonia can be focal, segmental, or generalized. Focal dystonia involves one small group of muscles in one body part, segmental dystonia involves a contiguous muscle group, and generalized dystonia is widespread.[17] Common focal dystonias include uncontrolled eye blinking (blepharospasm); movements of the jaw, tongue, and mouth (oromandibular dystonia); spasms twisting the neck (spasmodic torticollis); and spasms of the hand and forearm during writing ("writer's cramp").[17,20] Segmental dystonia involves two regions and includes Meige's disease, which is a combination of blepharospasm and oromandibular dystonia. Generalized dystonia is an impairment of most of the body, frequently involving the legs and back.[16] All of these dystonias can co-occur with spasmodic dysphonia.

Dystonia can be the primary symptom or secondary to another disorder. Whereas primary dystonia is idiopathic either with a hereditary pattern or without a hereditary pattern,[21] secondary dystonia develops as a symptom of another

neurologic disorder, psychologic disorder, or exposure to environmental cause such as trauma, infections, tumors, toxic chemicals, or medication.[16]

The emergence of dystonia can be a consequence of central and peripheral trauma.[22] Dystonia is not present immediately following head trauma but emerges during the period of 1 month to 9 years following the trauma.[22,23] Traumatic head injury can result in focal or diffuse dystonia. The dystonia may start as a focal dystonia and then spread over time for several months. In some cases, it remains focal.[22] Focal lesions to the basal ganglia, thalamus, subthalamus,[22] brainstem lesions,[24] caudate, and putamen[23] have been identified with the onset of dystonia. Peripheral trauma also has been associated with the onset of dystonia.[25] Trauma to the larynx has been related to the emergence of spasmodic dysphonia when it emerges within 12 months of the event.[25]

When dystonic movements outside the larynx accompany spasmodic dysphonia, it is important to use the identification of these dystonia symptoms for both the diagnosis of SD and its treatment. Treatment of the dystonia in the larynx is generally well managed with local injections of botulinum toxin. However, when dystonia exists in other parts of the body, treatment of the larynx alone may not be enough to elicit the best result. At times, patients may need concurrent treatment of the concomitant dystonias. In this particular individual, treatment of his facial dystonia by injecting BoNT-A into the masseter, platysma, levator labii superioris, and risorius muscles allowed him the freedom to produce more precise articulation and less effortful voice production resulting in enhanced speech intelligibility.

Management of Abductor Spasmodic Dysphonia

Andrew Blitzer, MD, DDS, and Celia F. Stewart, PhD

Case Study: Patient YY

> *Although injection of BOTOX into the thyroarytenoid muscle has proved beneficial for relieving symptoms of adductor spasmodic dysphonia, these injections have not proved helpful for patients with abductor spasmodic dysphonia. Andrew Blitzer and Celia F. Stewart present a case study describing a technique for injecting the only intrinsic abductor muscles, the posterior crico-arytenoid muscles (PCAs). Injections of the PCA muscles are effective for minimizing the symptoms of this disorder.*

Patient History. Patient YY was representative of the typical patient with abductor spasmodic dysphonia. He was a 40-year-old, right-handed, Irish-Presbyterian radio announcer. Twelve years prior to his examination, he noticed a weakening of his voice near the end of his broadcasts. The weakening progressed, and he developed breaks in phonation, especially during broadcasts. He also had an increased number of breaks during telephone conversations. He had learned to avoid certain words to avoid the breaks. His voice also was worse when he was fatigued or had ingested caffeine. During the examination, his laugh was normal, as was his singing, humming, and yawning. He did not have signs of dyspnea or dysphagia. Ethanol ingestion did not produce any change in the character of his symptoms. He did not have any sensory tricks to make his voice better.

Patient YY had a normal birth and normal childhood growth and development. He was otherwise healthy and did not take any medications. He was told previously that his disorder was psychogenic and was referred to a psychiatrist. Confident that he did not have a mental disorder, he never went to the psychiatrist. He had a normal MRI, ceruloplasmin level, and normal results of routine serum chemistries.

His conversational speech was characterized with moderate-to-severe, breathy, abrupt voice termination; breathy voice quality; and reduced voice loudness. The aphonic breaks in his voice reduced the smoothness and intelligibility of his speech. He frequently produced short, quick, one-word responses with normal voice quality, but the voice quality was not sustained in conversational speech. He sustained /a/ and /i/ in modal and loft register without phonation or pitch breaks. He produced a clear cough and shout. No vocal tremor was observed.

Fiberoptic laryngoscopy revealed a synchronous and untimely abduction of the true vocal folds, exposing an extremely wide glottic chink. These spasms were triggered by consonant sounds, particularly when consonants were in the initial position in words. Stroboscopy revealed a normal mucosal wave during voiced segments, with intermittent opening of the posterior glottis.

Characteristics of Abductor Spasmodic Dysphonia. Spasmodic dysphonia or laryngeal dystonia (LD) is a speech disorder characterized by breaks in speech fluency. The abductor type is caused by intermittent abduction of the vocal folds, resulting in a reduction of loudness, breathy breaks, aphonic whispered segments of speech, or a combination of these features. Aronson's description was "a voice in which normal or hoarse voice is suddenly interrupted by brief moments of breathy or whispered (unphonated) segments."[3] The voice may begin to manifest nonspecific hoarseness or breathiness and, over a period of days or weeks, begin to show signs of intermittent breathy breaks.

Some patients have a mixed abductor-adductor type, with a mixture of breathy breaks and tight, harsh sounds. Cannito and Johnson[26] proposed that both conditions exist in all the patients, and the symptoms depend on whether there is more adductor or abductor activity. The disability from abductor LD may be profound. Telephone calls and stress exacerbate the disorder and make the speech pattern more unintelligible.

As with other types of focal dystonia, most of the symptoms begin in adulthood.[20] The average age of onset for primary laryngeal dystonia is 38 years, with a range of 3 to 85 years.[20,27] Spasmodic dysphonia occurs more frequently in women (58%) than in men.[20] The cause of laryngeal dystonia is unknown, but the onset has been associated with trauma, exposure to phenothiazine drugs, head colds, flu, laryngitis, upper respiratory infections, and a genetic predisposition.[27,28] In addition, no geographic, environmental, or occupational patterns have been associated with the onset of spasmodic dysphonia.

The family history is also important because 12.1% of the patients with spasmodic dysphonia have a family history of dystonia.[16] Over the past decade, our understanding of genetics of dystonia has improved through family and linkage studies that have identified several genetic locations and may prove to be a link to a cure or better treatment. Family linkage studies have identified

several subtypes of dystonias with different genetic bases. In most cases of childhood onset, idiopathic dystonia, family studies have shown autosomal dominant inheritance with reduced penetrance. A marker for some cases of childhood-onset dystonia has been found on human chromosome 9q34.[29-31] Other genes have been mapped for other phenotypes of the disease including an autosomal dominant dopa-responsive dystonia (DRD) on chromosme 14q, X-linked Filipino torsion dystonia (XLTD), and an autosomal dominant (nondopa responsive) idiomatic torsion dystonia not mapping to the DYT1 gene on chromosome 9q34.[31-37] Both the DTR and the XLTD are rare forms of idiopathic torsion dystonia associated with Parkinsonism. Identification of the genes and understanding their function eventually may lead to better treatment or cure for dystonia.

Evaluation of Abductor Spasmodic Dysphonia. Diagnosis and treatment of this difficult-to-diagnose voice disorder requires a team approach, including a speech-language pathologist, an otolaryngologist, and a neurologist. The four components of the evaluation include the case history, the voice and speech signs and symptoms, the evaluation and observation of the structure and function of the vocal folds, and the neurologic evaluation of the movements of the body.

Speech-Language Evaluation. The speech evaluation encompasses collecting a thorough case history, perceptual evaluation of speech symptoms, acoustic and aerodynamic analysis, and screening for other communicative and swallowing disorders.[38] The severity and types of perceptual voice symptoms can be rated on the Unified Spasmodic Dysphonia Rating Scale (USDRS), a standardized evaluation for spasmodic dysphonia.[38] On the USDRS, the severity of the voice symptoms is rated along several parameters, including overall severity, breathy voice quality, voice arrests, aphonia, voice tremor, and expiratory effort. We have been rating patients on a 7-point scale on which 1 = no instance, 2 = mild, 3 = mild to moderate, 4 = moderate, 5 = moderate to severe, 6 = severe, and 7 = profound. The USDRS has been used for both the initial evaluation and for measuring change following treatment. It is recommended that patients be evaluated with the USDRS and video-recorded at the initial evaluation and at intervals following treatment so that adequate records can be maintained to evaluate changes over time.

Voice and speech tasks on the USDRS include reading aloud, spontaneous speech, and voice tasks that test the patient's ability to use voice at the limits of the voice and speech mechanism. The tasks are easier to perform when a patient has mild spasmodic dys-

phonia and more difficult when a patient has severe spasmodic dysphonia. Evaluating a patient's ability to perform all the tasks and describing the voice and speech symptoms on the tasks helps to identify the severity of the dysphonia, the effectiveness of the patient's response to therapy, and the need for further treatment.

Descriptions of voice function and changes in voice production with treatment can be further documented through acoustic evaluation. The acoustic aspects of vocal tremor and voice breaks are observed through waveform analysis and narrow-band spectral analysis (Fig 8–1). Tremor can be visualized to determine its consistency, its relative frequency, and any changes with various levels of breath support. The frequency and length of voice breaks also can be visualized utilizing electroglottography (Fig 8–2).

Otolaryngologic Examination. All patients should have a detailed history, with particular attention to other abnormal cervicocranial function. A thorough head and neck examination is per-

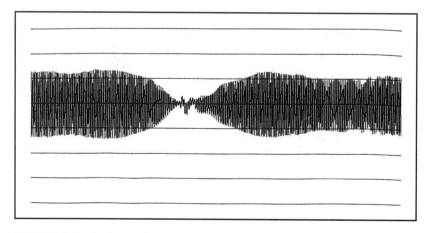

FIGURE 8–1. Acoustic waveform from the DSP Sono-Graph model 5500 (KayPentax, Lincoln Park, NJ) visually displays a breathy voice break.

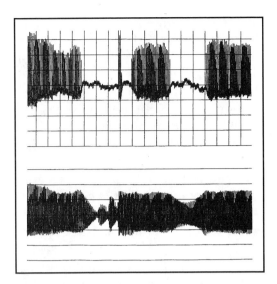

FIGURE 8–2. Simultaneous recordings of /a/ as detected by electroglottography (*upper tracing*) and an air conduction microphone (*lower tracing*).

formed. Fiberoptic direct laryngoscopy is performed to allow observation of the larynx while the patient speaks words and sentences, thus permitting the detection of the abductor or adductor spasms causing dysfluency. The movements can be recorded and analyzed in slow speed or stop action modes. This cannot be performed easily with rigid (ie, transoral) indirect laryngoscopy, in which anterior tongue traction limits the speaking ability. Most of these patients usually can perform pure phonation of vowels without disclosing the dysphonia that produces breaks between voicing onsets and offsets.[16]

Videostroboscopy is also useful in assessing dysphonia. The strobe allows analysis of the regularity and symmetry of the mucosal wave, the presence of tremor, and the degree of glottic closure. The videorecorded version of this examination can be reviewed to help differentiate abductor, adductor, and the compensatory laryngeal dystonias.[39]

Laryngeal electromyography is performed in many patients. It allows analysis of the motor unit potentials as well as localization of active parts of the laryngeal muscles. In our initial EMG study of adductor SD patients, we found some patients with a diagnosis of spasmodic dysphonia who had other disorders, including tremor, myoclonus, and pyramidal and extrapyramidal diseases.[40]

Neurology Examination. A complete history is mandatory for patients with dystonia. A family history of other members with dystonia; history of head trauma, perinatal or developmental abnormalities; history of other neurologic disease; or exposure to drugs known to cause dystonia (eg, phenothiazines) is imperative. Examination should find the intellectual, pyramidal, cerebellar, and sensory examinations normal. The clinical phenomenology often will be the clue to etiology. Primary dystonia typically is action induced; symptoms are enhanced with the use of the affected body part and the region may appear normal at rest. Secondary dystonia frequently results in fixed dystonic postures. The presence of extensive dystonia limited to one side of the body suggests a secondary etiology. Dystonia may involve the muscles of the oral cavity, larynx, pharynx, tongue, and jaw. An MRI scan, SMAC, complete blood count, ceruloplasm concentration, erythrocyte sedimentation rate, electromyogram, EEG, and antinuclear antibody assay all may be useful to rule out a metabolic or neurodegenerative disease etiology.[16]

Therapy for Abductor Spasmodic Dysphonia. Speech therapy and relaxation therapy may help to moderate the symptoms, but provide little, if any, long-term benefit. Pharmacotherapy provides little for the long-term relief of symptoms. Our group reported early benefit from anticholinergics in some patients,[11] but the early success was not maintained.

Our group and others have reported impressive success in the treatment of adductor laryngeal dystonia with localized injections of botulinum toxin (BOTOX) into the thyroarytenoid muscle(s).[20] In our series of more than 400 patients, voice recovery to an average of 90% of normal function was reported by patients. The injections could be given comfortably via a percutaneous route in an ambulatory setting. The side effects from such injections were minimal. The injections lasted an average of 4 months.

In abductor spasmodic dysphonia, we believed the posterior cricoarytenoid (PCA) muscle was most responsible for the breathy voice, but initially we were reluctant to treat the PCA muscle with BOTOX because of our concern of airway compromise. A severely disabled patient urged us to try treating his PCA muscle, however, even if it meant performing a tracheostomy.

After receiving approval from our institutional review board, one of the authors (AB) performed a direct laryngoscopy and an attempt at injecting one PCA directly through the laryngoscope. This attempt proved difficult for the patient, had no EMG control, and did not improve voice quality. We therefore developed an EMG-guided percutaneous technique. The larynx is manually rotated, and the Teflon-coated hollow EMG recording needle is placed posterior to the thyroid lamina through the inferior constrictor muscle until it reaches the cricoid cartilage. This directly impales the PCA. Another technique in which injection is given through the cricothyroid membrane across the airway is

effective in some young individuals. A small amount of xylocaine is first injected into the airway to cause topical anesthesia. Once this is accomplished, the EMG needle is placed through the cricothyroid membrane and angled off the midline. The needle is advanced until it hits the rostrum of the cricoid. The needle is further advanced through the cartilage until it impales the posterior cricoarytenoid muscle. Once the muscle is engaged, the patient is asked to sniff, which yields maximum abduction of the vocal folds. The EMG signal is observed for correct needle placement, and the BOTOX is given when the needle is in an area of brisk electrical activity.

In the 1990s, we reported the results of our first 9½ years of BOTOX treatments.[25,41] In those discussions, we shared the findings of 154 cases where BOTOX had been used to treat abductor laryngeal dystonia.[25,41] Initially, we attempted to weaken or paralyze one PCA muscle with an injection of 3.75 U in .15 mL into the most active posterior cricoarytenoid muscle. After 1 week, a fiberoptic laryngoscopy was performed to observe the vocal fold function. In 20% of the cases (31 patients of 154), weakening or paralyzing just one PCA produced a good voice without breathy breaks. In general, such patients had less severe pretreatment symptoms. The others all needed additional toxin injected into the contralateral posterior cricoarytenoid in doses ranging from 0.625 to 2.5 U. The muscles were titrated based on symptoms, fiberoptic evaluation of motion and the airway, and whether the patient developed noisy breathing or stridor. The average onset of effect was 4.1 days with the peak effect at 10 days. The duration of benefit was 10.5 weeks. Patients initially rated themselves at 54.8% of normal function and improved to an average of 66.7% of normal function.

The amount of improvement in voice is related to the types of symptoms. When our group of 154 patients with abductor spasmodic dysphonia is analyzed, 30% have tremor and 4% have adductor spasmodic dysphonia in addition to segmental cranial or axial dystonia. Some of these had respiratory muscle involvement. The highest percentage of improvement was in the group with focal laryngeal involvement without a tremor. They had an average of 43% improvement of normal function with an average best function of 80%. The worst response was the group with combined dystonic abnormalities with only 30% improvement.

If both PCAs were been treated and the voice was still breathy despite weakening of both PCAs and narrowing of the glottal chink, additional treatments were provided. Nine patients received injections of 2.5 U in each cricothyroid muscle in addition to the posterior cricoarytenoid injections. These were patients who, despite significant limitations of abduction, still had breathy breaks or tremor. This technique was based on the work of Ludlow, Naunton, Terada, and Anderson[42] who found significant abnormal activity in the cricothyroid muscle on EMG. Of these nine patients, five had benefit with louder voice and fewer breaks. One patient's symptoms worsened with the CT injection, and we postulated that the cricothyroid actually was involved in compensatory strategy and that, with the muscle weakened, the abductor spasms were less well controlled. In addition, 10 patients had unilateral type 1 thyroplasty to mechanically limit the amount of abduction of one vocal fold. This combination of BOTOX and thyroplasty raised the best average percentage of function to 82% of normal. Some of the patients received adjunctive systemic therapy including clonazepam, trihexiphenidyl, or baclofen to enhance their response to BOTOX and to prolong their period of improved voice.

Transitory adverse experiences include four patients who developed exertional wheezing or stridor when going up stairs or jogging and 10 patients who reported some dysphagia. The dysphagia probably was related to some of the toxin diffusing into the inferior constrictor muscle. These side effects have been transient, usually resolving within 1 week.

In reviewing the graphs of data from our standardized vocal rating scale (Figs 8–3 and 8–4, Table 8–1), a clear improvement is seen in all cases in overall rating, breathy voice quality, and aphonia. When reviewing tremor, it was noted that several of the patients had worsening of their tremor. The reason for this is that the tremor existed before, but was visual and not voiced; as phonation improved with PCA weakening the tremor became audible and the quality of speech was improved but still disabling in some cases.

Therefore, we have devised a staging system for abductor LD patients (see Table 8–1) in which stage 1 consists of those patients with focal symptoms; stage 2, those with segmental cranial or axial symptoms; stage 3, those with a tremor; and stage 4, those with a tremor with segmental axial-cranial symptoms, respiratory dyssynchrony, or both. This staging system will allow better pretreatment counseling with patients. They can be prepared for the type of response expected and the possibility of other injections or procedures to achieve a functional voice.

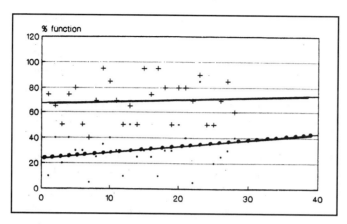

FIGURE 8–3. Overall severity of abductor laryngeal dystonia as % function plotted for each patient. Upper and lower grids provide the same information, but the upper grid is presented in a linear plot to demonstrate the average improvement. Series A (pretreatment) = bulleted line; series B (after BOTOX) = solid line.

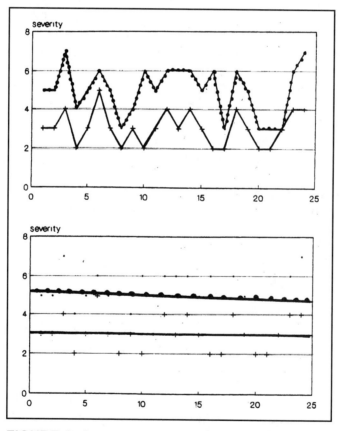

FIGURE 8–4. Upper grid = aphonia in abductor laryngeal dystonia; Lower grid = breathy voice quality in laryngeal dystonia. Series A (pretreatment) = bulleted line; series B (after BOTOX) = solid line.

Table 8–1. Abductor Laryngeal Dystonia Staging System

Stage 1	Focal disease
Stage 2	Segmental cranial or axial
Stage 3	Tremor
Stage 4	Tremor with segmental dystonia and/or respiratory dysynchrony

Speech therapy is helpful following injections of BOTOX to improve voice quality and prolong the response to the toxin. Therapy should focus on decreasing expiratory drive and coordinating respiration, phonation, resonance, and articulation. Improving the patient's posture and decreasing extraneous muscle activity in the head, neck, shoulders, and chest can improve control of the expiratory drive and decrease tension levels in the larynx. The patient also can modify environmental noise to enhance communication.

Botulinum Toxin Treatment for a Patient with Tourette Syndrome

Celia F. Stewart, PhD, Andrew Blitzer, MD, DDS, and Stephen Salloway, MD

Case Study: Patient ZZ

In 1885, Guilles de la Tourette first described a syndrome of recurrent motor and phonic tics and obsessive-compulsive behavior.[43] Tics are brief involuntary movements or sounds superimposed on the background of normal motor activity.[44] Tics can be classified in several ways. Simple motor tics involve only one group of muscles, causing a brief, isolated, jerklike movement, whereas complex motor tics are coordinated, sequenced movements resembling motor acts or gestures that are inappropriately intense and timed.[43] Simple phonic tics consist of inarticulate noises such as sniffing, throat clearing, grunting, squeaking, screaming, coughing, blowing, and sucking sounds.[44] Complex phonic tics usually are linguistically meaningful such as coprolalia, echolalia, and palilalia.[45] Jankovic[45] further categorized tics into clonic, tonic, and dystonic types. Clonic tics are produced by brief abrupt muscle contractions; tonic tics are isometric muscle contractions with no movement; and dystonic tics are briefly sustained movements with abnormal postures. All these tics can be observed in patients with Tourette syndrome.[45]

Neuroleptic and other medications can suppress tics at multiple sites through their central mechanism of action. High potency neuroleptics effectively treat tics in 78% to 91% of patients with Tourette syndrome.[43,46] Other medications such as clonidine also can be helpful. Nonetheless, 25% of patients with Tourette syndrome on haloperidol therapy are considered treatment failures because of limited response or intolerable side effects.[45,46] Botulinum toxin (BTX) has been used to treat debilitating refractory focal tics because BTX treats only the muscle injected.[47]

BTX is a potent toxin that acts presynaptically to prevent the release of acetylcholine from the nerve endings.[48,49] It has been approved for the treatment of blepharospasm, hemifacial spasm, and strabismus. It has been used widely to treat facial, cervical, laryngeal, and limb dystonias; to cosmetically smooth wrinkles; to ameliorate headaches; and to reduce focal tics, including eye blinking and movements in the neck and shoulders.[11,16,20,41,45,47,50–54] Jankovic[55] did an open study investigating the efficacy of BTX treatment in 10 patients with Tourette syndrome who had disabling tics. Five of his patients had frequent blinking and blepharospasm, and the other five had severe, painful, repetitive dystonic tics of the neck or shoulder muscles. Marked-to-moderate functional improvement and reduction in amplitude and frequency of tics were noted in all patients. Jankovic concluded that BTX was an effective treatment for patients with focal, partially dystonic tics.[55]

This case study describes the use of BTX for alleviating simple and complex phonic tics associated with Tourette syndrome. Patient ZZ was a 28-year-old man with long-standing refractory Tourette syndrome with vocal tics. His father also had Tourette syndrome and obsessive-compulsive disorder. The patient had a normal birth and early developmental history. At age 5, he developed involuntary blinking, lower facial tics, and shrugging movements in his upper extremities. At age 8, he developed jaw movements and phonic tics, including loud brief screams and coprolalia. Tourette syndrome was diagnosed at age 11, and at that time he had frequent eye blinking, shoulder shrugging, hyperactivity, oppositional behavior, and attention deficit problems. He was educated in a number of residential schools for children with behavior problems.[56]

At the time of his examination, he continued to have shoulder shrugging and eye blinking, but his most disabling symptoms were simple and complex phonic tics including loud screams, grunting, shouting vowels and words, coprolalia, and loud talking. He made approximately 100 to 180 loud screams per day, lasting 3 to 7 seconds each. His conversational voice was characterized with a severely rough strident voice quality and moderately to severely increased voice loudness that improved. He used moderately to severely increased effort during speech, and effortful piercing screams frequently interrupted his speech. His pitch range was severely reduced at both ends, and his voice became aphonic when he attempted to decrease the loudness of his speaking voice. His laugh and sigh were rough, and his cough and shout were excessively loud.

Patient ZZ was 6 feet, 2 inches tall and weighed 285 pounds; his screaming could be heard from a considerable distance. He had held a few jobs for short periods but had to quit because of the phonic tics. He also had minimal social relationships. When his vocal tics were severe, he became seriously depressed, requiring frequent inpatient or day hospital psychiatric care.

His medications at the time of the evaluation were haloperidol 5 mg/qid and benzotropine mesylate 2 mg/qid to decrease neuroleptic side effects. This regimen provided only partial relief for the tics. In the past, haloperidol at a dose of 40 mg/qid caused sedation and only mild improvement. Adequate trials of pimozide, clonidine, clonazepam, diazepam, alprazolam, lorazepam, buspirone, fluoxetine, and clomipramide were either ineffective or caused intolerable side effects.

He was evaluated by a team of professionals including a speech-language pathologist, otolaryngologist, neurologist, and psychiatrist. Voice measures were recorded in a quiet room during the evaluation and prior to each BTX injection for 14 months. Three types of voice samples were collected: The subject provided brief biographical information, previewed the Rainbow Passage[57] and read it aloud, and described the

Cookie Theft picture.[58] His voice samples were rated on a 7-point scale for overall severity, rough voice quality, stridency, voice loudness, and speech effort. In addition, the loudness of his screams was rated.

Tic severity was rated using the Yale Global Tic Severity Scale (YGTSS)[59] at baseline and before each BTX injection. The YGTSS rates the number, frequency, intensity, complexity, interference, and impairment of tics using a 6-point scale for each dimension.

The vocal folds were visualized at baseline and once after completing four BTX injections using a flexible fiberscope laryngoscopy. Evaluation was performed while Patient ZZ produced sustained vowels, sentences, and automatic speech. The vocal folds were rated for forceful adduction and for pathology.

Following the evaluations, bilateral BTX injections were performed while he was awake. During the procedure, the thyroarytenoid and lateral cricoarytenoid muscles were identified under electromyographic guidance (EMG), which added precision to the procedure.[5,60,61] Increased EMG activity in the muscles was observed during phonation to ensure the correct placement of the BTX. He received 1.25 units of BTX into each thyroarytenoid muscle with a 27-gauge, Teflon-coated, hollow-bore needle.[20] The injections weaken the contraction of the thyroarytenoid muscle and lateral cricoarytenoid muscles to decrease hyperadduction and hyperfunction of the vocal folds. Injections were repeated approximately every 3 months for 14 months.

From week 1 to week 10 after each injection, Patient ZZ had a moderate reduction in the loudness of the phonic tics. The loudness score for his screams decreased 2 points on the 7-point voice scale, and the intensity rating on the YGTSS decreased from marked-severe to moderate. Patient ZZ and his father reported a 50% decrease in tic loudness, and he rated himself as "much better." Phonic tic frequency decreased from "almost always" to "frequently" on the YGTSS, and the patient reported that the frequency of the phonic tics decreased by approximately 10% overall, but at times he noticed as much as a 40% decrease. His overall and rough voice quality ratings improved from "severely" to "moderately" impaired and voice loudness decreased from "moderately to severely" loud to "moderately" loud as rated on a 7-point scale. The increased effort score decreased 2 points from "moderate to severe" to "mild to moderate" and his pitch range expanded by five semitones. Table 8–2 lists voice quality before and after BTX injection.

Table 8–2. Voice Quality Rating Scale Before and After BTX Injection

Voice Symptoms	Before BTX Injection	After BTX Injection
Overall voice quality	Severe (6)	Moderate (4)
Rough voice quality	Severe (6)	Moderate (4)
Excessive loudness	Moderate-to-severe (5)	Mild-to-moderate (3)
Breathy voice quality	Normal (1)	Moderate (4)

All ratings were performed on a 7-point scale.

Transient side effects from the BTX included a passing moderately breathy speaking voice and minor difficulty swallowing liquids. The breathy quality of his speaking voice gradually improved over 6 weeks following treatment. The average duration of improvement was 9 weeks, whereas the screaming tics remained decreased in intensity. The reduction of phonic tic loudness was greater than the reduction in loudness of the speaking voice. The intensity of the speaking voice gradually improved after 6 weeks and remained improved from week 7 through week 10, whereas the screaming tics remained diminished in intensity.

Fiberoptic laryngoscopy at the baseline revealed laryngeal nodules and erythema with hyperadduction during speech and screams. Gross adduction and abduction of the vocal folds was synchronous. Repeated fiberoptic evaluation after 14 months of treatment revealed decreased erythema, normal adduction, and a one-third reduction in the size of the nodules.

During treatment, he was better able to socialize with people, he felt a greater sense of control, his sense of well-being improved, and his number of psychiatric hospitalized days decreased by 50%. Following BTX treatments, his ratings for interference and impairment on the YGTSS decreased from marked-severe to moderate. He reported feeling less isolated and more comfortable going out in public. He said he had an increased sense of well-being and considered doing volunteer work. Inpatient and day hospital psychiatric care decreased from 45 days in the 14 months prior to initiation of BTX therapy to 23 days in the 14 months after starting BTX.

The treatment was discontinued when the insurance company refused reimbursement claiming that the treatment was experimental. The patient's vocal tics returned to baseline after discontinuation of the BTX treatment. The fact that his symptoms returned to baseline when the treatment was removed provides further evidence for the efficacy of BTX in this case.

Botulinum toxin is not recommended as the first line of treatment for Tourette syndrome because neuroleptics treat a spectrum of symptoms, whereas BTX treats only focal symptoms. Nonetheless, loud phonic tics that are refractory to medication treatment may respond well to BTX treatment protocol used for spasmodic dysphonia. Loud simple and complex phonic tics are repetitive, forceful contractions of vocal folds that provide a specific anatomic site for injection. BTX injections decrease the intensity of muscle contractions and may decrease the premonitory symptoms of tension and discomfort. In this case, the weakness of the thyroarytenoid muscle had a more profound effect on the shouting tics than on conversational speech. Therefore, it appears that the increased subglottic pressures needed to generate shouting could not be produced with the adductor weakness caused by the BTX that resulted in decreased loudness and frequency of shouting tics.

Parkinson Disease

Parkinson disease often results in characteristic changes in the voice relatively early in the disease process. The condition, secondary to the progressive loss of dopaminergic cells in the substantia nigra, results in increased vocal fold stiffness and bowing along the vocal fold edge. A monopitch voice with reduced loudness typically results. Unfortunately, patients may show little awareness of the extent their voice limitations. Progressive deterioration of articulation abilities frequently accompanies the voice changes.

> The following section shares the case stories of two individuals with Parkinson disease. In the first case, Lorraine Ramig discusses the use of Lee Silverman Voice Treatment® in a 78-year-old male with idiopathic Parkinson disease. The final case by Lyn Tindall shares how she used telehealth services to deliver the LSVT program to a patient with Parkinson disease who was unable to travel in for regular services.

Use of LSVT® LOUD (Lee Silverman Voice Treatment) in the Care of a Patient with Parkinson Disease

Lorraine Olson Ramig, PhD-SLP, and Cynthia Fox, PhD, CCC-SLP

Case Study: Patient AAA

> In this case study, Lorraine Ramig and Cynthia Fox describe how one component of voice production, healthy vocal loudness, positively affects all subsystems of speech production including respiration, phonation, resonance, and articulation. This single cognitive focus makes improving speech feasible in individuals with neurologic conditions who often have limitations in cognition and learning.

Background on LSVT LOUD

Nearly 90% of the 8 million individuals with Parkinson disease (PD) worldwide have a speech or voice disorder that significantly diminishes quality of life.[62] Over the past 20 years, LSVT LOUD has been developed and advanced as the first efficacious speech treatment for PD.[63,64] LSVT LOUD is organized around a simple but powerful therapeutic principal: to increase vocal loudness (targeting amplitude of respiratory-laryngeal movement) in individuals with PD while retraining the sensory motor processes involved in disordered speech communication.[65] The training mode of LSVT LOUD requires high effort (self-perceived effort) and intensive training (16 individual 60 minutes treatment sessions in 1 month), consistent with principles of motor learning, skill acquisition, and neural plasticity.[66–68] Furthermore, LSVT LOUD results in long-lasting improvements (out to 2 years[63]) that are correlated with brain reorganization as revealed by recent neural imaging studies.[69,70]

Improvements following LSVT LOUD extend beyond the respiratory-laryngeal focus to include enhanced articulation, facial expression, swallowing, and communicative gestures.[71–75] The positive treatment effects of LSVT LOUD also have been observed in individuals with stroke, multiple sclerosis, ataxic dysarthria, and children with Down syndrome and cerebral palsy.[65,76,77]

Patient History. Patient AAA was a 49-year-old man employed as a family physician. He had been diagnosed with idiopathic Parkinson disease (PD) for 2 years and was in stage 2 (out of stages 1–5, with stage 5 being the most severe) on the Hoehn and Yahr Scale.[78] His medications for PD included Sinemet and Eldepryl. Neuropsychologic testing revealed some mild attention difficulties. Initial clinical speech examination revealed an oral peripheral mechanism that was normal in both structure and function, with no characteristics atypical of PD; hearing was within normal limits.

History of the Problem. Patient AAA reported that during the past year his voice had become soft and raspy. He had associated the raspy voice with frequent upper respiratory infections. He reported that he felt people "could understand" him most of the time. In contrast, his spouse and coworkers reported that it was "often difficult to understand" him. It is not unusual for individuals with PD to have reduced awareness of their speech problem. In fact, the soft-spoken individual with PD often is heard to report "My spouse complains that I am too soft, but she/he really needs a hearing aid!"

Pretreatment Evaluation. Patient AAA participated in assessment procedures spanning a range of tasks and measures designed to provide insight about the physiologic bases of the disorder, as well as its impact on speech production. The goal was to sample treatment-related

changes across the speech mechanism (respiratory, laryngeal, and oral articulation) to evaluate system-wide effects of treatment accompanying an impact on functional communication. Select pretreatment data are summarized in Table 8–3.

Perceptual Measures. Patient AAA's speech was judged to be reduced in loudness and to be monotone, hoarse, and breathy. He was described as having some reduction in articulatory valving. Stimulability testing for increased loudness revealed that he easily was able to increase loudness (to within normal limits) and improve voice quality. This was viewed as a positive sign for potential treatment success.

Stroboscopic Measures. Pretreatment videostroboscopic images were rated as bowed (lack of medial glottal closure).

Acoustic and Aerodynamic Measures. Vocal sound pressure level (SPL),

Table 8–3. Select Pretreatment Data for Patient AAA

	Pre 1 X	Pre 1 SD	Pre 2 X	Pre 2 SD	
Duration /a/, in seconds	24.3	2.5	23.3	2.9	(n = 6)
SPL /a/	61.1	0.6	63.0	0.4	(n = 6)
Jitter /a/	0.45	0.15	0.48	0.20	(n = 6)
SPL "Rainbow"	60.5	2.8	60.7	2.7	
SPL Monologue	59.1	3.3	58.5	1.9	
SPL /pae/	62.3	0.8	63.4	0.4	(n = 3)
Psub (cm H$_2$O)	4.8	0.8	5.0	0.4	(n = 3)
Rlaw (cm H$_2$O/cc/s)	0.02	0.003	0.02	0.002	(n = 3)

All SPL data are dB at 50 cm.

duration, fundamental frequency, and variability of the fundamental were measured from maximum duration sustained vowel phonation, reading, conversational monologue and dual tasking. Measures of phonatory stability (jitter, shimmer, harmonics-to-noise ratio) were obtained from sustained vowel phonation. Select articulatory acoustic measures (frication duration, rise time, and vowel duration to whole-word duration ratio together with second formant trajectory extent and duration and rate) were measured to assess laryngeal-oral interarticulatory coordination and vocal tract movement. Estimated subglottal air pressure and laryngeal resistance were measured to assess respiratory laryngeal interaction.

Course of Treatment. Patient AAA participated in sixteen 1-hour individual sessions of the LSVT LOUD within 1 month (4 days/week for 4 weeks). LSVT LOUD differs from traditional voice/speech therapy three major areas: *target* of treatment, *mode* of delivery, and *calibration*. There is a single *target* of improved vocal loudness. The treatment improves vocal loudness by increasing respiratory drive, vocal fold adduction, and vocal tract opening. It is never the goal of the LSVT LOUD to teach a pressed, hyperfunctional voice, but rather a voice with maximally efficient vocal fold closure. Individuals with PD frequently have reduced vocal fold closure and thus need to increase adduction to achieve optimum voice production.[79,80] The treatment is delivered in an intensive, high effort *mode*. This intensity involves more than dosage (4 days/week for 4 weeks) as it is the intensity and effort required within each treatment session (multiple repetitions of tasks, increasing complexity) that is also

required for lasting changes. Finally, *calibration* addresses the sensory, internal cuing and neuropsychological impairments in people with PD that may limit generalization of treatment effects outside of the treatment room.

Treatment sessions are divided into two halves. The first half of the session is spent on three "Daily Tasks." The purpose of these tasks is to rescale the amplitude of vocal output required for within normal limits loudness. These tasks include multiple repetitions of: (1) Sustain "AH" with increased loudness as long as you can; (2) Sustain "AH" while going high/low in pitch; and (3) Repeat a list of 10 self-selected functional phrases. The second half of the session (25–30 minutes) is spent on a speech hierarchy. The purpose of the speech hierarchy is to train the voice that was achieved during the daily tasks into functional communication. As the weeks of therapy progress, the clients are required to maintain loudness for longer periods of speaking and in more complex speaking situations (eg, progressing from words to conversational speech). The speech hierarchy material is tailored to be salient to each individual consistent with principles that drive experience-dependent neural plasticity.[66] In addition to the above treatment tasks, clients are required to complete daily homework practice (all 30 days of the month of therapy) and daily carry-over exercises (daily assignment to use LOUD voice with another person outside of the therapy room).

Throughout all tasks, *calibration* was addressed. The patient was encouraged to "Feel that effort, feel that loudness. That is what it needs to feel like when you talk so that people understand you." The treatment was administered in a *mode* consistent with principles of motor learning and muscle training (eg, frequent repetitions, intensive, high-effort exercise, simple focus, and progressive resistance).

In addition, the treatment tasks and target behaviors were trained with simplicity and redundancy to facilitate learning in a population with potential neuropsychological problems. Although Patient AAA generated increased loudness in sustained phonation and speech with relative ease, he was resistant to use this louder voice outside of the treatment room. As is the case with many individuals with PD, he would "perform" increased loudness tasks in the therapy room but would complain that "I can't speak like this outside. I feel like I am shouting." LSVT LOUD sensory retraining activities (*calibration*), which include carryover, homework, and education, were administered daily. By the end of the 16 sessions of treatment, Patient AAA was convinced and comfortable with the concept that "when he feels like he is 'talking loud,' he is speaking at a normal volume and people will understand him." He was encouraged

to continue to keep practicing his homework every day and return in 6 months for a follow-up assessment.

Posttreatment Evaluation. Select posttreatment data are summarized in Table 8–4.

Perceptual Measures. The speech of Patient AAA was judged to be louder and stronger posttreatment. His voice quality was clear and the magnitude and precision of his articulatory gestures increased. His wife reported that he now had regained the resonant voice he had when they first met in college, in fact she told him "that's the voice I fell in love with!" His coworkers reported that they now could understand him most of the time. Patient AAA reported that he initiated conversations more and was asked to repeat much less often than before treatment. He reported with confidence that he knew what to do to make people understand him.

Stroboscopic Measures. The videostroboscopic examination revealed no vocal fold bowing.

Table 8–4. Select Posttreatment Data for Patient AAA

	X	SD	X	SD	
Duration /a/, in seconds	38.6	2.2	41.8	2.2	(n = 6)
SPL /a/	82.8	1.7	83.7	1.3	(n = 6)
Jitter /a/	0.26	0.16	0.30	0.11	
SPL "Rainbow"	73.1	3.79	72.8	3.67	
SPL Monologue	65.2	4.00	63.7	4.24	
SPL /pae/	70.9	0.5	71.2	0.6	(n = 3)
Psub (cm H$_2$O)	7.7	0.2	6.6	0.9	(n = 3)
Rlaw	0.037	0.005	0.037	0.005	(n = 3)

All SPL data are dB at 50 cm.

Acoustic and Aerodynamic Measures. Significant increases were measured across tasks in sound pressure level, maximum duration of phonation, and fundamental frequency variation. Measures of phonatory stability were consistent with improved voice quality and vocal fold closure. Articulatory acoustic measures supported improved valving and precision, consistent with increases in effort and coordination across the speech mechanism accompanying increased loudness. Estimated subglottal air pressure and laryngeal resistance support increased respiratory drive and vocal fold valving posttreatment.

Follow-Up Recommendations. A key element in long-term treatment success with any disorder and particularly progressive neurologic conditions, is continued practice. All patients who receive LSVT LOUD are encouraged to continue practicing their LSVT exercises after treatment is over. During the month of treatment, homework practice routines are well-established so that the patient is easily able to maintain these routines on their own. In addition, various new materials (eg, LSVT practice videos/DVDs) and delivery systems (eg, software supported LSVT delivery (LSVT-Companion,[81] and telehealth delivery of LSVT (eg, LSVT®eLOUD) as well as patient support groups (eg, LOUD Crowds) enhance feasibility of ongoing practice.

Application of the LSVT LOUD to this individual with PD was successful immediately posttreatment; positive treatment effects were maintained up to 12 months follow-up. These observations are consistent with previous outcomes on larger numbers of individuals with PD. Patient AAA demonstrates the importance of early intervention in an individual who was employed and was dependent on his oral communication for his livelihood. The greatest challenge to a successful outcome for Patient AAA, and for many individuals with PD, is the need for sensory retraining (LSVT LOUD: concept of calibration). Research data support a breakdown in sensory proprioception in individuals with PD that must be addressed to have successful voice treatment outcomes. As was the case with Patient AAA, it is critical to differentiate "performance" in the treatment room from evidence of generalized "learning" outside of the treatment room. The mode of treatment administration (4 times a week for a month of high effort in individual treatment) also appears to be a key element in retraining both the sensory and motor speech systems in PD. Patient AAA also demonstrates the positive system-wide effects of increased loudness. One simple goal, "be loud," resulted in multiple improvements across the speech mechanism, generating a significant improvement in intelligibility. This global effect of "loud" can be particularly beneficial in individuals whose learning may be facilitated by reduced cognitive load. The simplicity and redundancy of the LSVT LOUD also may be particularly valuable in such individuals.

It can be a challenge to make lasting improvements in speech and voice in individuals with progressive, neurologic disorders who may also have cognitive impairment. Nonetheless, improved functional oral communication can make a significant impact on the quality of life of these individuals, as it did in the case of Patient AAA.

Disclosure Statement: Dr. Ramig receives a lecturer honorarium and has ownership interest in LSVT Global, LLC. Dr. Fox receives a lecturer honorarium and has ownership interest in LSVT Global, LLC.

Use of Telehealth Technology to Provide Voice Therapy

Lyn R. Tindall, PhD

Case Study: Patient BBB

Individuals with Parkinson disease (PD) usually develop a speech disorder characterized by reduced loudness, hoarse and breathy voice, monotony of pitch, short rushes of speech, and imprecise consonants. The inability to effectively communicate negatively impacts their ability to function in society and maintain quality of life. A successful program developed to improve speech in these individuals is the Lee Silverman Voice Treatment (LSVT)®.[82] A critical component of this treatment is intense daily therapy for 4 weeks, a regimen that is difficult for many elderly clients to accomplish. Videophones placed in the homes of individuals with PD may offer a way to provide treatment that might otherwise be inaccessible.

Patient Medical History. Patient BBB was a 78-year-old male who was referred to speech pathology for low vocal intensity by the neurologist who had diagnosed him with idiopathic Parkinson disease 5 years prior to the referral. His medications included Pramipexole 0.5 mg three times daily plus Carbidopa 25/Levodopa 100 1/2 tab three times daily. He had occasional mild hallucinations in the evening, upper extremity resting tremor that was worse in the morning, and stiffness and tightness in muscles that cause difficulty walking. Patient BBB managed his activities of daily living (ADL) and remained active by assisting his sons on their cattle farm. However, he stated that many of his friends and family members could not understand his speech anymore and

that it was getting progressively worse. His voice problem restricted his personal and social life and made him feel handicapped.

Evaluation Procedures. Patient BBB received a battery of vocal function tests in the voice laboratory that included:

1. *Videostroboscopic examination of the larynx.* This examination was completed using the Kay-PENTAX 70-degree rigid endoscope. Observations revealed incomplete glottal closure, no supraglottic hyperfunction, and normal mucosal wave, bilaterally.
2. *Acoustic analysis of sustained vowels and conversation.* Patient BBB's mean fundamental frequency was 133.30 Hz with low and high range of 101.83 to 255.10 Hz. His mean intensity for vowel prolongation was 59.95 dB, and for conversation it was 58.90 dB with his maximum intensity of 63.60 dB.
3. *Mini-Mental State Examination.*[83] This tool was used to systematically assess mental status. The maximum score is 30 and a score of 23 or lower is indicative of cognitive impairment. Patient BBB scored 25, indicating that he had the ability to process information and follow directions in order to participate in voice therapy.
4. *Voice Handicap Index-10 (VHI-10).*[84] The VHI-10 was developed as an abbreviated voice handicap assessment compared to the Voice Handicap Index (VHI).[85] The VHI-10 is designed to give an indication of a client's perception of voice handicap before and after treatment. This patient scored 35 on the VHI-10, indicating his voice disorder was almost always a handicap to him.

5. *Pretreatment probes of sound pressure level (SPL) measures of vocal tasks including vowel prolongation, reading passage, picture description, and monologue.* Recordings of SPL were obtained in a sound-treated room three times prior to initiation of therapy. The following tasks were used for analysis: (1) sustaining vowel /a/ phonation, (2) reading the "Rainbow passage,"[57] (3) speaking freely on a self-chosen topic, and (4) describing the "Cookie Theft Picture."[58] Instruction to the patient for the first task was "take a deep breath and say "ah" for as long as you can." Then, he was asked to read the "Rainbow passage." For the third task, he produced a one minute monologue on a topic of his choice. Finally, he was given the "Cookie Theft Picture" and told to "describe everything that is happening in the picture." During each probe task, SPL was recorded from the digital hand-held sound level meter. An integrated average sound pressure level (SPL) was calculated for these tasks using digital output of the sound level meter placed 30 cm from the patient's mouth. The digital sound level meter was set to average the total duration of the speech signal. The sound level meter averages the speech signal; pauses during connected speech are not calculated from the sample. Pretreatment averages for these tasks were:

Vowel prolongation	62.9 dB and 8:53 seconds duration
Reading	67.3 dB
Monologue	64.6 dB
Picture description	62.6 dB

Results of this evaluation were consistent with moderate hypokinetic dysarthria associated with PD. Treatment goals were targeted to increase vocal loudness and endurance using LSVT® including: (1) *maximum duration of a sustained vowel by the participant* to improve glottal competence and respiratory/laryngeal coordination; (2) *practice of pitch range* to improve range of motion of the cricothyroid muscle; and (3) *practice of maximum functional speech loudness drill* to increase phonatory effort.[86] Administration of LSVT® requires therapy four times a week for 4 weeks; such massed practice is consistent with principles of motor learning, skill acquisition, and muscle training. Nonetheless, the high intensity that makes this program successful also is associated with a tendency to decline initiating therapy or to miss therapy appointments. For patient BBB, travel to this facility to receive treatment involved driving 160 miles round trip and 4 hours of time, including travel, to provide a 1-hour treatment session. Additionally, patient BBB's wife, who is his primary caregiver, had to take 6 hours off from her job to transport him and wait for the treatment session to conclude. It should be noted that these typically are non-reimbursable expenses. Therefore, in order to provide this treatment in the manner prescribed, a videophone was issued to patient BBB to enable him to receive therapy at home. The Televyou TV 500SP® from Wind Currents Technology was installed in his home to receive therapy. The TV 500SP® is a standalone plug-and-use videophone with duplex speakerphones that use plain old telephone service (POTS) lines. It has a 5-inch active matrix display with adjustable color and brightness and transmits and receives voice and simultaneous video.

Goals for Therapy. The LSVT® prescribes three treatment tasks for each therapy session to improve vocal intensity, including:

Goal 1: Maximum duration of a sustained vowel. The rationale for this goal was to improve glottal competence and respiratory/laryngeal coordination. The goal for patient BBB was to increase vowel prolongation from 8.53 seconds to 15 seconds and intensity from 69.2 dB to 75 dB. For this task, patient BBB was instructed to "take a deep breath and say /a/ for as long and loud as you can." This task was performed 15 times daily during each treatment session.

Goal 2: Improve range of motion of the cricothyroid muscle. To achieve this goal patient BBB produced /a/ at his highest and lowest pitches 15 times each for a total of 30 trials. For this task, he started at his approximate midfrequency range and sang up to his highest pitch 15 times, and then, starting again at his midfrequency range sang down to his lowest pitch for 15 trials. The highest and lowest pitches were sustained for 2 to 3 seconds each.

Goal 3: Practice of maximum functional speech loudness drill to increase phonatory effort. This goal was accomplished by having patient BBB produce 15 functional phrases/sentences during each session. These phrases and sentences were identified by him prior to therapy for use in his individual daily conversation. He read each phrase/sentence 5 times each for a total of 75 productions per session. In addition to 15 functional phrases, the protocol for LSVT® instructs clinicians to provide additional words the first week, sentences the second week, paragraph reading the third week, and conversation the fourth

week in a task that encourages loud speech when producing these stimulus items. These stimulus items were provided by the patient with examples from the LSVT® handbook.

Patient BBB was encouraged to complete homework assignments each day during the course of treatment. Homework included performing the same tasks used during treatment but with fewer repetitions. For example, he produced /a/ as loud and long as he could for 6 trials on the days he had treatment and 12 trials on the days no treatment was scheduled. Using the same procedure utilized during a treatment session, patient BBB produced his highest pitch and then lowest pitch 6 times each on the days of treatment and 12 times each on days with no treatment. Additionally, he read his 15 functional phrases 5 times each on the days of treatment and once each on no treatment days. Patient BBB completed one homework page each day while in treatment.

After sixteen 1-hour speech therapy treatments over 4 weeks were completed, patient BBB returned to the speech clinic within 1 week and underwent posttreatment data collections previously described. After the posttreatment assessment, he again completed the VHI-10, a Telemedicine Satisfaction Questionnaire (TSQ),[87] and cost analysis comparing videophone delivered therapy to traditional delivery of speech therapy.

Results of Treatment. Patient BBB's performance on voice tasks following therapy were as follows:

Vowel prolongation	79.1 dB and 11.56 seconds
Reading	76.5 dB
Monologue	72.0 dB
Picture description	72.0 dB

Results of treatment indicated that post-treatment improvements were achieved in vocal intensity leading to functional speech for Patient BBB.

His score on the VHI-10 reduced from 35 to 26 post treatment indicating that he no longer perceived his voice disorder "almost always" a handicap, but that it was "sometimes" a handicap. Patient satisfaction reflects values and expectations regarding aspects of healthcare. Therefore, a match between care expected and care received result in user satisfaction. The TSQ was developed to measure user satisfaction with telemedicine. Patient BBB's responses to the TSQ indicated that he was highly satisfied with the quality of service provided via videophones. In terms of cost comparison of videophone delivered voice therapy to traditional delivery for patient BBB, round trip mileage was 160 miles for a traditional visit compared to none for the videophone visit, 4 hours time compared to 1 hour, $96.80 compared to no cost per visit (Table 8–5).

The significant change in pre- to posttreatment measures of vocal loudness, cost savings, and client satisfaction with the technology combine to make videophone-delivered voice therapy an efficacious method of service delivery of speech services. Speech pathology services appear to be well-suited for telehealth technology; hence, speech-language pathologists looking for alternative ways to provide effective, less expensive care should consider telehealth technology as an option for individuals who would otherwise receive limited or no speech therapy services.

Table 8–5. Cost Comparison for Outpatient Versus Videophone Delivered Therapy for Patient BBB.

Per Visit Costs	Out-patient Visit	Video-phone Visit
Round trip mileage	160 miles	0 miles
Amount of time involved including travel time	4 hours	1 hour
Monetary costs (gas + meal)	$96.80	0

References

1. Aronson AE, Brown JR, Litin EM, Pearson JS. Spastic dysphonia. I. Voice, neurologic, and psychiatric aspects. *J Speech Hear Disord.* 1968;33(3):203–218.
2. Brodnitz FS. Spastic dysphonia. *Ann Otol Rhinol Laryngol.* 1976;85(2 pt.1):210–214.
3. Aronson A. *Clinical Voice Disorders: An Interdisciplinary Approach.* 3rd ed. New York, NY: Thieme Medical Publishers; 1990.
4. Aminoff MJ, Dedo HH, Izdebski K. Clinical aspects of spasmodic dysphonia. *J Neurol Neurosurg Psychiatry.* 1978;41(4): 361–365.
5. Blitzer A, Lovelace RE, Brin MF, Fahn S, Fink ME. Electromyographic findings in focal laryngeal dystonia (spastic dysphonia). *Ann Otol Rhinol Laryngol.* 1985;94(6 pt 1):591–594.
6. Blitzer A. Letter to the editor. *Laryngoscope.* 1986;96:1300–1301.
7. Dedo HH. Recurrent laryngeal nerve section for spastic dysphonia. *Ann Otol Rhinol Laryngol.* 1976;85(4 pt 1):451–459.
8. Dedo HH, Izdebski K. Intermediate results of 306 recurrent laryngeal nerve sections for spastic dysphonia. *Laryngoscope.* 1983;93(1):9–16.
9. Dedo H, Shipp T. *Spastic Dysphonia: A Surgical and Voice Therapy Treatment Program.* Boston, MA: College-Hill Press; 1980.
10. Aronson AE, De Santo LW. Adductor spastic dysphonia: three years after

recurrent laryngeal nerve resection. *Laryngoscope.* 1983;93(1):1–8.

11. Blitzer A, Brin MF, Fahn S, Lovelace RE. Localized injections of botulinum toxin for the treatment of focal laryngeal dystonia (spastic dysphonia). *Laryngoscope.* 1988;98(2):193–197.

12. Dystonia Foundation: National Spasmodic Dysphonia Association. Retrieved January 20, 2000 from http://www.dystonia-foundation.org. .

13. Kempster GB, Gerratt BR, Verdolini Abbott K, Barkmeier-Kraemer J, Hillman RE. Consensus auditory-perceptual evaluation of voice: development of a standardized clinical protocol. *Am J Speech Lang Pathol.* 2009;18(2):124–132.

14. Titze IR, Winholtz WS. Effect of microphone type and placement on voice perturbation measurements. *J Speech Hear Res.* 1993;36(6):1177–1190.

15. Hogikyan ND, Sethuraman G. Validation of an instrument to measure voice-related quality of life (V-RQOL). *J Voice.* 1999;13(4):557–569.

16. Brin M, Fahn S, Blitzer A, Ramig L, Stewart C. Movement disorders of the larynx. In: Blitzer A, ed. *Neurologic Disorders of the Larynx.* New York, NY: Thieme Medical Publishers; 1992.

17. Fahn S. The varied clinical expressions of dystonia. *Neurol Clin.* 1984;2(3):541–554.

18. Arnold GE. Spastic dysphonia. *Logos.* 1959;2(1):3–14.

19. Aronson AE. *Clinical Voice Disorders.* New York, NY: Thieme; 1985.

20. Blitzer A, Brin MF. Laryngeal dystonia: a series with botulinum toxin therapy. *Ann Otol Rhinol Laryngol.* 1991;100(2):85–89.

21. Marsden CD. Investigation of dystonia. *Adv Neurol.* 1988;50:35–44.

22. Lee MS, Rinne JO, Ceballos-Baumann A, Thompson PD, Marsden CD. Dystonia after head trauma. *Neurology.* 1994;44(8):1374–1378.

23. Krauss JK, Mohadjer M, Braus DF, Wakhloo AK, Nobbe F, Mundinger F. Dystonia following head trauma: a report of nine patients and review of the literature. *Movement Disord.* 1992;7(3):263–272.

24. Loher TJ, Krauss JK. Dystonia associated with pontomesencephalic lesions. *Movement Disord.* 2008;7(3):157–167.

25. Brin MF, Blitzer A, Stewart C. Laryngeal dystonia (spasmodic dysphonia): observations of 901 patients and treatment with botulinum toxin. *Adv Neurol.* 1998; 78:237–252.

26. Cannito MP, Johnson JP. Spastic dysphonia: a continuum disorder. *J Commun Disord.* 1981;14(3):215–233.

27. Brin M. Movement disorders of the larynx. In: Blitzer A, ed. *Neurologic Disorders of the Larynx.* New York, NY: Thieme Medical Publishers; 1992.

28. Gordon F, Brin F, Giladi N, Hunt A, Fahn S. Dystonia precipitated by peripheral trauma. *Movement Disord.* 1990;5:67.

29. Ozelius L, Kramer P, Moskowitz C. Human gene for torsion dystonia located on chromosome 9q. *Ann Neurol.* 1990;27:114–120.

30. Ozelius LJ, Hewett JW, Page CE, et al. The gene (DYT1) for early-onset torsion dystonia encodes a novel protein related to the Clp protease/heat shock family. *Adv Neurol.* 1998;78:93–105.

31. Ozelius LJ, Kramer PL, de Leon D, et al. Strong allelic association between the torsion dystonia gene (DYT1) and loci on chromosome 9q34 in Ashkenazi Jews. *Am J Hum Genet.* 1992;50(3):619–628.

32. Bressman SB, de Leon D, Kramer PL, et al. Dystonia in Ashkenazi Jews: clinical characterization of a founder mutation. *Ann Neurol.* 1994;36(5):771–777.

33. Bressman SB, Heiman GA, Nygaard TG, et al. A study of idiopathic torsion dystonia in a non-Jewish family: evidence for genetic heterogeneity. *Neurology.* 1994;44(2):283–287.

34. Fahn S, Moskowitz C. X-linked recessive dystonia and Parkinsonism in Filipino males [abstract]. *Ann Neurol.* 1988;24:179.

35. Kupke KG, Lee LV, Muller U. Assignment of the X-linked torsion dystonia gene to Xq21 by linkage analysis. *Neurology.* 1990;40(9):1438–1442.

36. Nygaard TG, Marsden CD, Fahn S. Dopa-responsive dystonia: long-term treatment response and prognosis. *Neurology.* 1991; 41(2 pt 1)):174–181.

37. Wilhelmsen KC, Weeks DE, Nygaard TG, et al. Genetic mapping of "Lubag" (X-linked dystonia-parkinsonism) in a Filipino kindred to the pericentromeric region of the X chromosome. *Ann Neurol.* 1991;29(2):124–131.

38. Stewart C, Brin M, Blitzer A. Spasmodic dysphonia. In: Ferrand C, Bloom R, eds. *Introduction to Organic and Neurogenic Disorders of Communication.* Boston, MA: Allyn & Bacon; 1997.

39. Hirano M. Stroboscopic examination of the normal larynx. In: Blitzer A, ed. *Neurologic Disorders of the Larynx.* New York, NY: Thieme Medical Publishers; 1992.

40. Brin MF, Fahn S, Moskowitz C, et al. Localized injections of botulinum toxin for the treatment of focal dystonia and hemifacial spasm. *Adv Neurol.* 1988;50:599–608.

41. Blitzer A, Brin MF, Stewart CF. Botulinum toxin management of spasmodic dysphonia (laryngeal dystonia): a 12-year experience in more than 900 patients. *Laryngoscope.* 1998;108(10):1435–1441.

42. Ludlow CL, Naunton RF, Terada S, Anderson BJ. Successful treatment of selected cases of abductor spasmodic dysphonia using botulinum toxin injection. *Otolaryngol Head Neck Surg.* 1991; 104(6):849–855.

43. Kurlin R. Tourette's syndrome: current concepts. *Neurology.* 1989;39:1625–1630.

44. Pauls DL, Towbin KE, Leckman JF, Zahner GE, Cohen DJ. Gilles de la Tourette's syndrome and obsessive-compulsive disorder. Evidence supporting a genetic relationship. *Arch Gen Psychiatry.* 1986; 43(12):1180–1182.

45. Jankovic J, Schwartz K, Donovan DT. Botulinum toxin treatment of cranial-cervical dystonia, spasmodic dysphonia, other focal dystonias and hemifacial spasm. *J Neurol Neurosurg Psychiatry.* 1990;53(8):633–639.

46. Shapiro A, Shapiro E, Young J, Feinberg T. Studies of treatment. *Guilles de la Tou-rette Syndrome.* 2nd ed. New York, NY: Raven Press; 1988.

47. Clark CE. Therapeutic potential of botulinum toxin in neurological disorders. *Q J Med.* 1992;82:197–205.

48. Binz T, Blasi J, Yamasaki S, et al. Proteolysis of SNAP-25 by types E and A botulinal neurotoxins. *J Biol Chem.* 1994; 269(3):1617–1620.

49. Blasi J, Chapman ER, Link E, et al. Botulinum neurotoxin A selectively cleaves the synaptic protein SNAP-25. *Nature.* 1993;365(6442):160–163.

50. Blitzer A, Brin M. Spasmodic dysphonia (laryngeal dystonia). In: Gates G, ed. *Current Therapy in Otolaryngology-Head and Neck Surgery.* Vol 4. Toronto, Canada: Brian C Decker; 1990.

51. Grillone GA, Blitzer A, Brin MF, Annino DJ, Jr., Saint-Hilaire MH. Treatment of adductor laryngeal breathing dystonia with botulinum toxin type A. *Laryngoscope.* 1994;104(1 pt 1):30–32.

52. Jankovic J, Brin MF. Therapeutic uses of botulinum toxin. *N Engl J Med.* 1991; 324(17):1186–1194.

53. Schneider I, Thumfart WF, Pototschnig C, Eckel HE. Treatment of dysfunction of the cricopharyngeal muscle with botulinum A toxin: introduction of a new, noninvasive method. *Ann Otol Rhinol Laryngol.* 1994;103(1):31–35.

54. Whurr R, Lorch M, Fontana H, Brookes G, Lees A, Marsden CD. The use of botulinum toxin in the treatment of adductor spasmodic dysphonia. *J Neurol Neurosurg Psychiatry.* 1993;56(5):526–530.

55. Jankovic J. Botulinum toxin in the treatment of tics. In: Jankovic J, Hallett M, eds. *Therapy with Botulinum Toxin.* New York, NY: Dekker; 1994.

56. Salloway S, Stewart CF, Israeli L, et al. Botulinum toxin for refractory vocal tics. *Movement Disord.* 1996;11(6):746–748.

57. Fairbanks G. *Voice and Articulation Handbook.* New York, NY: Harper & Row; 1960.

58. Goodglass H, Kaplan E. The cookie theft picture. *The Assessment of Aphasia and Related Disorders.* Philadelphia, PA:

Williams & Wilkins, Lea and Febiger, and Harwal; 1983.

59. Leckman JF, Riddle MA, Hardin MT, et al. The Yale Global Tic Severity Scale: initial testing of a clinician-rated scale of tic severity. *J Am Acad Child Adolesc Psychiatry*. 1989;28(4):566–573.

60. Blitzer A. Laryngeal electomyography. In: Gould W, Rubin RJ, Karovin G, Sataloff R, eds. *Diagnosis and Treatment of Voice Disorders*. New York, NY: Igaku Shoin; 1994.

61. Castellanos PF, Gates GA, Esselman G, Song F, Vannier MW, Kuo M. Anatomic considerations in botulinum toxin type A therapy for spasmodic dysphonia. *Laryngoscope*. 1994;104(6 pt 1):656–662.

62. Sapir S, Countryman S, Ramig L, Fox C. Voice, speech, and swallowing disorders. In: Factor S, Weiner F, eds. *Parkinson Disease: Diagnosis and Clinical Management*. 2nd ed. New York, NY: Demos Publishing; 2008:77–98.

63. Ramig LO, Sapir S, Countryman S, et al. Intensive voice treatment (LSVT) for patients with Parkinson's disease: a 2 year follow up. *J Neurol Neurosurg Psychiatry*. 2001;71(4):493–498.

64. Ramig LO, Sapir S, Fox C, Countryman S. Changes in vocal loudness following intensive voice treatment (LSVT) in individuals with Parkinson's disease: a comparison with untreated patients and normal age-matched controls. *Movement Disord*. 2001;16(1):79–83.

65. Fox C, Morrison C, Ramig LO, Sapir S. Current perspectives on the Lee Silverman Voice Treatment (LSVT). *Am J Speech Lang Path*. 2002;11:111–123.

66. Kleim JA, Jones TA. Principles of experience-dependent neural plasticity: implications for rehabilitation after brain damage. *J Speech Lang Hear Res*. 2008; 51(1):S225–239.

67. Schmidt RA, Lee TD. *Motor Control and Learning: A Behavioral Emphasis*. Champaign, IL: Human Kinetic Publishers; 1999.

68. Verdolini K, Hess MM, Titze IR, Bierhals W, Gross M. Investigation of vocal fold impact stress in human subjects. *J Voice*. 1999;13(2):184–202.

69. Liotti M, Ramig LO, Vogel D, et al. Hypophonia in Parkinson's disease: neural correlates of voice treatment revealed by PET. *Neurology*. 2003;60(3):432–440.

70. Narayana S, Zhang W, Franklin C, Vogel D, Lancaster JL, Fox PT. Changes in speech motor network following speech therapy in Parkinson's hypophonia: evidence from TMS-PET. *Org Human Brain Map*. 2006.

71. Duncan S. Preliminary data on effects of behavioral and levodopa therapies on speech-accompanying gesture in Parkinson's disease. *ICSLP-2002*. 2002: 2481–2484.

72. El Sharkawi A, Ramig L, Logemann JA, et al. Swallowing and voice effects of Lee Silverman Voice Treatment (LSVT): a pilot study. *J Neurol Neurosurg Psychiatry*. 2002;72(1):31–36.

73. Sapir S, Spielman J, Countryman S, et al. Phonatory and articulatory changes in ataxic dysarthria following intensive voice therapy with the LSVT: a single subject study. *Am J Speech Lang Pathol*. 2003;12:387–399.

74. Sapir S, Spielman JL, Ramig LO, Story BH, Fox C. Effects of intensive voice treatment (the Lee Silverman Voice Treatment [LSVT]) on vowel articulation in dysarthric individuals with idiopathic Parkinson disease: acoustic and perceptual findings. *J Speech Lang Hear Res*. 2007;50(4):899–912.

75. Spielman JL, Borod JC, Ramig LO. The effects of intensive voice treatment on facial expressiveness in Parkinson disease: preliminary data. *Cogn Behav Neurol*. 2003;16(3):177–188.

76. Mahler LA. *Intensive behavioral voice treatment of dysarthria secondary to stroke*. Doctoral dissertation, University of Colorado-Boulder, UMI 3239406; 2007.

77. Sapir S, Pawlas A, Ramig L, Seeley E, Fox C, Corboy J. Effects of intensive phonatory-respiratory treatment (LSVT) on voice in two individuals with multi-

ple sclerosis. *J Speech Lang Path.* 2001; 9(2):35–45.

78. Hoehn M, Yahr M. Parkinsonism: onset progression and mortality. *Neurology.* 1967;19:427–442.

79. Perez KS, Ramig LO, Smith ME, Dromey C. The Parkinson larynx: tremor and videostroboscopic findings. *J Voice.* 1996; 10(4):354–361.

80. Smith ME, Ramig LO, Dromey C, Perez KS, Samandari R. Intensive voice treatment in Parkinson disease: laryngostroboscopic findings. *J Voice.* 1995;9(4): 453–459.

81. Halpern A, Matos C, Ramig L, Petska J, Spielman J, Will L. Technology supported speech treatment for Parkinson's disease. *Movement Disord.* 2005;20(10): S134.

82. Ramig L, Bonitati C, Lemke J, Horii Y. Voice treatment for patients with Parkinson disease: development of an approach and preliminary efficacy data. *J Med Speech Lang Path.* 1994;2(3):191–209.

83. Folstein MF, Folstein SE, McHugh PR. "Mini-mental state." A practical method for grading the cognitive state of patients for the clinician. *J Psychiatr Res.* 1975;12(3):189–198.

84. Rosen CA, Lee AS, Osborne J, Zullo T, Murry T. Development and validation of the voice handicap index-10. *Laryngoscope.* 2004;114(9):1549–1556.

85. Jacobson B, Johnson A, Grywalski C, et al. The voice handicap index (VHI): development and validation. *Am J Speech Lang Pathol.* 1997;6(3):66–70.

86. Ramig LO, Countryman S, Thompson LL, Horii Y. Comparison of two forms of intensive speech treatment for Parkinson disease. *J Speech Hear Res.* 1995;38(6): 1232–1251.

87. Yip MP, Chang AM, Chan J, MacKenzie AE. Development of the Telemedicine Satisfaction Questionnaire to evaluate patient satisfaction with telemedicine: a preliminary study. *J Telemed Telecare.* 2003;9(1):46–50.

9

Successful Voice Therapy

Introduction

The chapters of this text have focused on the successful management of a wide range of voice disorders by clinical, medical, and surgical methods. Each contributor demonstrated techniques and approaches that proved successful in improving voice quality of patients with various laryngeal disorders. These successful cases, however, may set an unrealistically high standard for the beginning voice clinician and may not adequately reflect the many management pitfalls that are encountered even by experienced voice clinicians. Such pitfalls may lead to delayed success in treatment, less than totally successful results, or failure to resolve the voice problem. In many of the preceding case studies, it was shown that the clinician and the patient share equally in the success or failure of voice therapy. In this chapter, Joseph Stemple examines in detail some determinants of successful voice therapy followed by a thorough discussion of patient compliance issues by Eva van Lear.

Clinical Preparation

To manage voice disorders successfully, voice pathologists must be well grounded in anatomy, physiology, etiologic correlates, laryngeal pathology, and the psychodynamics of voice production. They also must possess outstanding skills in human interaction. Without a complete grasp of these areas of clinical knowledge, their efforts to provide successful voice therapy may be sabotaged by some or all of the factors discussed in this chapter.

Interview and Counseling Skills

The ability to talk to people—to skillfully and systematically divine the important aspects of the voice disorder and then to counsel appropriately—is a skill that must be mastered. For some, it is natural and easily applied in clinical use. For others, it is developed only with practice and experience. Most clinicians continue to hone this skill throughout their careers. The initial patient interview and subsequent counseling are the most important components of a voice evaluation. When these are conducted poorly, successful resolution of the patient's voice problem is in doubt. The following is but one example.

Case Study: Patient CCC

During her second year of graduate training, a student was assigned to intern at the voice center. Following appropriate observation, she was given her first case in which she was to conduct the patient interview portion of the voice evaluation. Patient CCC was a 38-year-old man who had been experiencing 6 weeks of persistent hoarseness. Laryngeal examination revealed only mild erythema of the bilateral folds. Voice quality was only mildly dysphonic, with a dry, strained hoarseness. The patient also complained of a "thickness" feeling in his throat that he tried to eliminate with throat clearing. Other than throat clearing, the patient denied all aspects of voice overuse or trauma, and his medical history was unremarkable as related to this problem. The interview broke down when the intern began questioning the patient regarding his social his-

tory. It was obvious throughout the interview that the intern was nervous, which is certainly understandable in a new clinician. Unfortunately, she became even more uncomfortable when asking questions regarding the patient's personal life. Every interview provides the clinician with either several little "ahas" or one big "aha" as the diagnosis becomes clearer; however, this intern was more attentive to her scripted questions than to the answers she received. The exchange between the student (S) and patient (P) went something like this.

S: "Are you married, single, or divorced?"

P: (Heavy sigh) "I was married until 2 months ago." (Tear in eye; face turned red.)

S: (Assuming divorce, with face down in her prepared questions) "How many children do you have?"

She missed it! She missed the most important moment during the interview and moved right along to the next question. To that point, only one etiologic factor had been identified: throat clearing. Because of the intern's lack of experience, she failed to "tune in" to the patient. She listened to what the patient said but not to how he said it. This breakdown was later pointed out to her as part of her internship training.

In a follow-up discussion with the patient, it was discovered that his wife had been fatally injured in an automobile accident just prior to the onset of his voice disorder. The patient was suffering from an emotional dysphonia. Learning this, the intern was then able to adequately explain the relationship of emotions to voice quality. In this patient, the voice problem was not resolved until he received psychological support along with voice therapy.

It is not adequate to simply ask the right questions. Successful voice evaluation, and thus voice therapy, is determined by the clinician's ability to apply the questions appropriately during the interview, together with the ability to listen to what is said and how it is said and to respond appropriately.

Clinical Understanding of the Problem

The clinician who does not fully understand all aspects of voice disorders may not grasp the less obvious nuances of various pathologic conditions. Certainly, if the clinician does not understand the problem, then successful resolution will either be by luck, or it will be doomed. I've received many secondary referrals from speech pathologists who obviously did not have a complete understanding of the clinical problem. These cases have included lack of recognition of functional dysphonia, functional falsetto, and functional ventricular phonation, among others. In all cases, the clinicians were attempting direct symptom modification without recognition of the true diagnosis.

Clinicians also may have unrealistic expectations of therapy results if they do not grasp the effects of neurologic or surgical changes of the vocal folds. Patients with vocal fold paralysis may become frustrated when effort closure therapy is continued for a lengthy period of time. Our experience has demonstrated that if this management approach is at all helpful, positive results are seen within 2 to 3 weeks of daily exercise. Continued exercise appears to yield little,

if any, benefit. Large glottic gaps often do not improve significantly, although we have secondarily seen patients in our clinic who have had months of voice therapy for "vocal fold compensation."

I recall also a postsurgical case in which, because of the clinician's lack of understanding regarding surgical treatment, both the patient's and clinician's expectations for improvement were unrealistically high. The patient was identified through indirect laryngoscopy as having bilateral edema and erythema with a suspicious lesion located on the superior surface of the middle third of the left true vocal fold. The patient underwent a microlaryngoscopy and biopsy of both vocal folds. The biopsy was positive for the suspicious lesion, but biopsies taken in a wide area around the lesion and on the right fold were negative. The decision was made to treat the lesion aggressively through surgical excision. In 9 months of postsurgical voice therapy during which the patient stopped smoking, she improved from a severe to a moderate dysphonia. The patient was very frustrated, however, because her presurgical voice, although low pitched, was not nearly as dysphonic and "hard to push out." The clinician fed this frustration by indirectly accusing the patient of "doing something" to maintain the hoarseness.

The clinician should have understood that aggressive surgery of a cancerous lesion might permanently damage the mucous membrane of the vocal fold. The trade-off for this conservative treatment of cancer most likely would be some level of permanent hoarseness. Indeed, stroboscopic examination of this patient's vocal folds revealed severe stiffness of the mucosal wave and amplitude of vibration of the left vocal fold. The clinician simply did not understand the consequences of surgery.

428 Voice Therapy: Clinical Case Studies

Countless examples could be given regarding clinicians' lack of understanding about some aspect of the voice disorder affecting treatment. Indeed, even the most experienced voice clinicians always are learning new information to add to their bank of clinical knowledge, and the most successful possess the largest "bank accounts" of knowledge.

Misapplied Management Techniques

One of the problems in preparing a text of this nature is the fear that it will be used as a voice management "cookbook": Look up the recipe, stir in this and that ingredient, use this and that technique, practice for 8 weeks, and create a lovely normal voice. No! Voice therapy cannot be successful with a cookbook approach. Every patient is an individual with different problems requiring individual interventions. People with similar voice disorders will not necessarily respond to the same management approaches. For example, some patients with vocal nodules may require and respond well to a progressive relaxation therapy, whereas this approach may be totally inappropriate for others. Some patients with unilateral vocal fold paralysis may benefit from effort closure exercises whereas others already are spontaneously using too much effort closure. The voice clinician cannot and should not arbitrarily apply certain management techniques to certain voice disorders.

Successful voice clinicians are aware of and ready to use any and all management techniques as deemed appropriate, but, again, the appropriateness of the chosen technique is dependent on the clinician's knowledge and expertise of all aspects of the voice disorder. Knowledge of the voice disorder will dictate the use of the various therapy approaches. The management technique does not dictate its own use.

Lack of Patient Education or Understanding of the Problem

Most patients have little concept of why they sound dysphonic. Voice production, like speech production, is just one of those bodily functions that we all take for granted, that is, until a problem arises. Education is one key to successful management. The more information patients have regarding their voice disorders, the more likely it is that they can successfully remediate the problem. For patients to "buy" the concept of voice therapy, they must understand why they were referred to a speech pathologist. Once this is adequately explained, the nuances of their particular disorder must be described in detail. With this information, the patient should be able to understand the purpose behind the management techniques (some of which seem silly unless fully understood).

Without a full understanding of the problem, the total management burden remains with the clinician. The clinician must use education to shift the burden to the patient. The patient must become an equal, if not greater than equal, partner in the process of voice improvement. For patients to be motivated to change vocal behaviors, they must understand why the change is required. The successful voice clinician will take great care in educating the patient in all aspects of the voice disorder.

Recognition of One Philosophical Orientation or One Etiologic Factor

Successful voice therapy is eclectic. We need not say more regarding the folly of subscribing to one management philosophy. Another potential cause for a poor management result is failure to identify and treat all of the etiologic correlates. For example, much of the emphasis of management for children with vocal abuse problems is placed on eliminating or modifying shouting, screaming, and loud talking. The more subtle causes, such as throat clearing and noises of vocal play (mimicking cars, guns, and so on), may not be identified. I have had the experience of meeting with frustrated speech-language pathologists who are consulting about children who they "know" are no longer shouting. "But he's not getting any better!" Without modifying or eliminating all contributing factors, the voice disorder is likely to continue. The following is an example from my case files.

Case Study: Patient DDD

Patient DDD, a 36-year-old woman, presented with small bilateral vocal fold nodules, as well as mild bilateral vocal fold edema. The abusive behaviors of shouting at her three adolescent children, shouting at sporting events, straining her voice while singing in a gospel choir, and chronic throat clearing were identified. All of these problems were either modified or eliminated through therapy, and her voice quality improved. During each Monday appointment, however, Patient DDD was more dysphonic than when seen for a Thursday appointment. As a result of this quality fluctuation, the problem was not totally resolving. What was going on? What had I missed?

Although Patient DDD was not singing in the church choir at that time, she attended a church that apparently was verbally and vocally enthusiastic to the pastor's message. Patient DDD admitted to many loud vocal outbursts over a period of 2 hours every Sunday. As it turned out, the patient chose not to control her vocal enthusiasm in church, and she remained mildly dysphonic.

The successful voice clinician realizes that voice problems do not just happen. There is always a reason for the dysphonia. Seeking and modifying all of the etiologic factors are essential for the successful remediation of the problem.

Premature Discontinuation of Therapy

One of the most difficult stages of therapy for any communication disorder is the carryover phase. Voice therapy is no exception. Many aspects of the communication process are modified during voice therapy. These aspects include the patient's own perception of vocal image, voicing habits, and behaviors, as well as the direct anatomic and physiologic modifications that often must occur in the laryngeal, respiratory, and resonance systems. In addition, new skills acquired in the therapy setting will not automatically be applied outside of this setting. The carryover phase of therapy must not be isolated from the changes demonstrated in the office. The new behaviors must occur in all situations.

I recall the difficulty I had with one young man who presented with the classic "pseudoauthoritative" voice:

Case Study: Patient EEE

The patient was a recent college graduate in business who, in his new job, had been made supervisor of a small auditing department. Being young, and even younger in appearance, he had affected a low-pitched voice with intermittent glottal fry phonation. This behavior had led to irritation (not yet ulcerated) of the vocal processes of the arytenoid cartilages. He was noticeably hoarse, with the chief complaint of voice fatigue.

Interestingly, the patient was readily able to modify the inappropriate vocal properties during the initial session. I assumed carryover would be rather easy to accomplish. At one point (at about 4 weeks), he was discharged from therapy only to return 1 month later with recurring symptoms. This young man was so involved in his perceived need for a different vocal image at work that he continued his abusive vocal behaviors. As his clinician, I had not ensured carryover of his improved vocal habits to the offending environment and had discharged him from therapy prematurely. We then worked more diligently on his vocal image with the appropriate counseling, and the problem was successfully remediated.

The successful voice clinician will ensure carryover of the improved vocal condition to all environments before discharging the patient. Follow-up rechecks also are advisable to guarantee habituation of the vocal improvement.

The Clinical Ear

Sometimes a clinician's clinical training cannot account for all the skills necessary to conduct successful voice therapy. In some instances, natural talent plays a role. One of these skills is the musical "ear." In a clinical study, we gave 30 speech pathology graduate students pre- and posttreatment phonatory function tests, including acoustic and aerodynamic analyses. During the posttest, subjects were required to match pretest frequency levels. I was amazed at the number of students who could not readily match pitch. Empirically, the number exceeded 50%. Possession of a clinical-musical ear is necessary in voice therapy to recognize quality deviations and changes, to model inappropriate and appropriate voice productions, to recognize pitch deviations, and to work on pitch matching exercises. The successful voice clinician must possess a clinical-musical ear.

Patient Realities

Assuming adequate preparation of the voice clinician, failure to achieve success in voice therapy may be related to the patient. The patient must bring to the therapy process a level of cooperation necessary to permit change. Voice change and developing habits of good vocal hygiene are not always easy, and the process often is frustrating for the patient. Several situations, described in the following sections, may occur that could lead to therapeutic failure.

Lack of Patient Motivation

Any therapeutic change requires the individual to perceive that a problem exists and that the problem needs to be changed. The voice pathologist will determine the patient's level of motivation. The next task is, through education and counseling, to induce the patient to have the incentive to follow through and comply with the management suggestions. Most patients are motivated and require little encouragement to improve their voices. Some patients, however, are simply not interested in voice therapy.

Case Study: Patient FFF

Patient FFF was a 56-year-old male insurance agent who had become dysphonic 4 months prior to the laryngeal examination. He sought the opinion of a physician only after much encouragement from his wife. Because of the publicity regarding hoarseness as a sign of cancer, this patient, a smoker, was frightened and delayed going to the doctor. Examination by the laryngologist revealed the presence of diffuse polypoid degeneration. When informed that he did not have cancer, Patient FFF was obviously relieved.

Patient FFF was referred to the voice center for laryngeal videostroboscopy, a phonatory function test, and a voice evaluation. During the interview, it became evident that the man no longer was concerned about the hoarseness. Although he submitted to the voice evaluation, he lacked the motivation to improve voice quality. He was satisfied that he did not have cancer and chose not to accept the argument that his current vocal condition was a sign of negative tissue change. Patient FFF did not seek further treatment.

The voice clinician should always try to motivate the patient to seek improvement of the voice, but, as illustrated, will not always be successful. Successful voice therapy depends on a well-motivated patient who has the incentive to work toward positive vocal change.

Resistance to Share Information

Information gathered during the patient interview is valuable only if it is complete and accurate. The patient must be willing to share all pertinent information. Even the most skilled clinician has experienced situations in which, several sessions into therapy, a patient finally releases information critical to management decisions. Some patients are reticent to talk about personal or family problems that may be directly related to the voice disorder (such as tension, shouting, or crying). Certain behaviors such as drug use, smoking, and alcohol consumption are inaccurately reported. An eating disorder (such as bulimia) or an emotional problem requiring medication may not be mentioned.

Successful voice therapy is dependent on an open and honest relationship between patient and clinician. The clinician must establish credibility and a positive, relaxed therapeutic atmosphere. The patient must be made aware of the importance of answering all questions honestly and accurately. Ultimately, the patient has final control over the information he or she is willing to share.

Perceived Need for Negative Vocal Behavior

The young man previously described in this chapter as having a "pseudo-authoritative" voice perceived a need to produce a low-pitched voice with glottal fry phonation. He was resistant to vocal change, even though he was dysphonic and uncomfortable, and he maintained the inappropriate vocal symptoms in his work environment. He wanted to project a more mature image and chose voice modification as a means of accomplishing this task.

The gospel-singing, vocally enthusiastic parishioner decided that her abusive vocal response to the pastor's message was more important than her vocal health. Her Sunday response was a deeply religious experience that she chose not to modify, and as a result, she remained dysphonic.

Over the years, I have had several patients who had another motive for maintaining negative vocal behaviors. I recall the case of a woman who, during the evaluation, exhibited body language signaling that she did not want to participate in the process. She refused to remove her coat, gave monosyllabic responses, and gave little effort to produce her "best" voice during testing. We learned later that she was seeking disability for a work-related injury (inhaling toxic fumes) and therefore it was in her best interest not to improve her negative vocal behavior. She did not.

Voice therapy is composed of a series of choices by both the clinician and the patient. One choice is to follow the management suggestions of the clinician. Successful voice therapy is dependent on the patient recognizing negative vocal behaviors and choosing the need to modify those behaviors.

Need to Identify with the Problem. Vocal image has a strong psychological influence on many people. Patients often find it difficult to modify even moderate to severe vocal disturbances because of the effect this change may have on their image. Individuals close to or related to the patient also may object to vocal change. For example: "Matthew has always sounded a little husky. We think it's cute." In this case, the parent so strongly identifies the voice problem with the child that cooperation for modification may prove difficult.

Occasionally, patients may say something such as, "My husband likes my voice; he thinks it's sexy," or "I don't want to change very much. I won't sound like me," or "But to me I'd sound like I'm shouting if I talk like that." All of these comments are legitimate concerns to the owners of these voices. Our auditory feedback systems dictate to us what we are *supposed* to sound like. The feedback system may become accustomed to even the most dysphonic voice. Some patients become resistant to vocal change either because they like or approve of the dysphonic voice or because they dislike the new feedback they are receiving. Occasionally, this resistance is powerful enough to make the therapy program unsuccessful.

Many voice disorders may be a symptom of emotional or psychological disorientation. In this circumstance, the need to maintain a voice problem may far outweigh the benefits of vocal improvement. An obvious sign of emotional well-being is voice quality.

Case Study: Patient GGG

Patient GGG, a 38-year-old woman, was identified as having an "emotional dysphonia" (MTD) caused by a recent divorce and other serious family problems. As efforts were made to modify the problem, the patient continually sabotaged the proceedings. The sabotage came in the form of new ailments ("My chest hurts when I do these exercises") or lists of rather bizarre questions

("Do you think this all started when the horse bit my ear?") that monopolized much management time. At that moment in her life, this patient needed to sound ill. Family counseling was suggested, and voice therapy was postponed. Subsequent voice therapy was not needed because Patient GGG's vocal problem spontaneously cleared as her life's problems resolved.

Patients may feel the need to project poor voice quality as a means of subconsciously demonstrating emotional upheaval in their lives. Successful voice therapy therefore is dependent on the patient's willingness and ability to identify with a different, and, it is hoped, an improved voice quality. To accomplish this, the patient often must override the auditory feedback system and yield to a new vocal image.

Finances

Unfortunately, a patient's finances may play a role in the successful remediation of a voice disorder. As with all medically related services, the costs of providing vocal rehabilitation are rising. When prioritizing the use of funds, some patients will find other areas for spending that they deem more important than voice therapy. When finances prove to be a factor in the patient's decision to participate in therapy, the clinician must be willing to provide the patient with a reasonable estimation of the number of sessions, time frame, and cost of services. Third-party payors often support the cost of voice therapy services. Voice pathologists should learn as much as possible about funding services to assist patients in their decision to seek treatment. Successful voice therapy may be dependent on the patient's willingness

to assume financial responsibility for the services provided.

Personality Issues

"He never met a person he didn't like." In a Pollyanna world, maybe this statement could be made, but, I must admit, the statement does not apply to me. I have worked with a few patients with whom I had a difficult time appreciating their personalities. (To be blunt, I did not like them.) This being the case, I am sure some of these patients, and others, did not necessarily appreciate my personality and skills. Being a professional, however, I usually have been able to recognize the problem and to work through it, and the patients have successfully remediated their voice disturbances.

Occasionally, when it becomes evident that a clinician and patient cannot work well together, modifications must be made. With some patients, I always felt that we were on different pages of the same book. We could not communicate well, and progress was not made. Successful voice therapy is dependent on excellent communication between clinician and patient. This may require constant adjustment in the mindset of the clinician from patient to patient. When personality conflicts arise and communication breaks down, they must be handled with frank discussion of the problem and with referral to another clinician reserved as an option.

Can All Voices Be Improved?

Most voice disorders can be improved. Through the many management approaches now available, most vocal systems, and the personalities that own them, can be manipulated, modified, medicated, undergo surgical intervention, or a combination of these, to yield voice quality improvement. The level of improvement will range from dramatic to subtle, but improvement most often is possible.

The patient must be given a realistic expectation of the level of improvement. With this information, informed decisions can be made regarding the advantages of various treatment approaches or whether to be treated at all. Some patients require dramatic change for the treatment to be considered worthwhile. Others relish subtle improvements that increase the effectiveness of their communication skills.

Thoughts on Patient Compliance

The examples above show that voice therapy can fail or be disrupted for a variety of reasons, including poor clinician competence, inadequate patient compliance with the treatment plan, and a patient-clinician personality mismatch. These sources of potential failure can be interrelated. For example, inappropriate/ineffective treatment methods can lower patient motivation despite an initially good therapeutic relationship. Likewise, lack of clinician interest as perceived by the patient can lead to poor compliance despite appropriate treatment. However, for the sake of simplicity, let's examine patient compliance separately, as if clinician competence and personality match are held constant.

Patient compliance is a popular research topic outside of the field of speech pathology.[1] Many illnesses, such as obesity, diabetes, heart disease, depression, hypertension, and back pain, are either behavioral in etiology or respond to behavioral interventions composed of changes in lifestyle (eg, diet and exercise, quitting smoking), changes in thinking, and changes in how we relate to others. Unlike treatments in which patients play a passive role, such as in surgery or massage, behavioral interventions are synonymous with patient action. Because behavioral interventions are only as effective as the extent to which they are carried out, research into patient compliance has sprung up across the fields of medicine, psychology, and public health in an effort to improve treatment outcomes. Even the act of taking a pill—a treatment often requested by our voice patients instead of therapy—can present a substantial compliance problem.[2–5]

Voice therapy contains a unique combination of behavioral elements including motor learning, communication, acoustic-kinesthetic feedback, self-concept, and, at times, diet and medication. As such, improving voice therapy requires dedicated study and practice. Some general principles of patient compliance borrowed from other fields may be useful in framing how we think about compliance in the voice clinic and in directing future research.

The study of patient compliance seeks to answer two questions: (1) Can clinicians (or other outside sources) influence patient compliance? and (2) Can a prospective patient's compliance be predicted? Answering the first question holds implications for both treatment effectiveness and the allocation of health care resources, whereas answering the second question allows for "screening" of potentially noncompliant patients. Like any human behavior, the sources of compliance, as well as the interventions to improve it, can be conceptualized as external (ie, social or environmental), internal (ie, cognitive, emotional, or physical) or behavioral in nature.[6]

Treatment strategies to improve compliance continuously are being devised and tested in various areas of behavioral medicine. Some examined strategies have included reminder phone calls, client-centered or problem-solving oriented counseling and goal setting, peer self-management groups, increased treatment intensity (ie, frequency of appointments), simplification of treatment, financial commitments, and written contracts.[3,7–12] Qualitative and correlational work has demonstrated that amount and quality of clinician feedback[13] has a positive effect: this was also noted in a modest qualitative study of voice therapy adherence.[14] Although it is known that human behavior can be influenced, compliance behavior has proven to be quite resistant to intervention. Variable effects achieved in experimental studies speak to the difficulty of measuring and affecting compliance, but also may indicate the limitation of the "group averaged" research design of the randomized controlled trial (RCT).[15] This design, borrowed from drug trials, applies nonindividualized treatments across the board to groups of patients. Yet, as illustrated in this book, individualization of treatment strategies may be paramount to success in behavioral therapy. It is likely that individualization plays a role in compliance interventions as well; the effectiveness of compliance strategies might depend on the adequacy of the match between the intervention strategy and the individual characteristics or problems of the patients. Our patients' behavior confirms that patient preferences differ: some patients like to schedule their home practice whereas others practice "randomly," some need external reminder systems (sticky notes, alarms, friends) to self-monitor their

voice and to practice; others appear to have an internalized self-monitoring sense; some focus on their breathing whereas others prefer to focus on resonance; and so on. With regard to the clinician's choices, a directive discussion of the importance of treatment may positively inspire one patient but instill anger in another. We may do well to look toward the counseling-psychotherapy literature, in which treatment outcomes have been found to be determined largely by the extent to which the patient likes or has confidence in both the treatment and the therapist.[16–18] No single treatment approach has been found to be more effective than others in ameliorating most of the problems for which individuals seek outpatient counseling, although some clinicians are more effective than others.[19,20] Similarly, investigation into "what works" to improve compliance in voice therapy may prove to be a matter of identifying "what works *for whom*."

The question of influencing compliance is well worth exploration in voice therapy. If it is determined that compliance can be influenced in a practical fashion in the clinic, treatment strategies can be implemented to improve compliance. If it is found, however, that compliance is determined largely by patient factors that are beyond clinician control, it may be prudent to discharge noncompliant patients from therapy without exhaustive clinician efforts. Both approaches (exhaustive efforts versus early discharge) can be found in the current practice of voice clinicians, but have not been studied empirically. The best approach may lie somewhere in the middle, or once again depend on individual characteristics of the patient.

Answering the second question—can we predict compliance—may allow us to determine the best intervention approach at the earliest opportunity. But there is another reason to pursue an answer to this question in voice therapy. Outside of our field, research into predicting compliance has identified some factors that determine compliance. When all things are held equal, the most powerful determinant of patient success in behavioral interventions is self-efficacy: patients' confidence in their own ability to achieve treatment goals and tasks.[21-30] Patient perceived commitment to these goals and tasks also is under investigation.[31]

A Conceptual Framework for Compliance

A clinically useful organizing framework for patient compliance has been proposed by Miller and Rollnick, two clinician-researchers in the field of substance abuse.[32,33] They conceptualize patient motivation to comply with treatment as a combination of patients' perceived importance of therapy goal attainment, and confidence to achieve the goal. Clinicians can sort patients according to four quadrants: high importance/high confidence, low importance/low confidence, low importance/high confidence, and high importance/low confidence. Conceptualizing patients for research purposes is more complex than this, but the four quadrant framework can aid one's clinical thinking.

High Importance/High Confidence. These patients find voice therapy important and are confident that they can meet its demands (ie, voice exercise, vocal behavior change, etc). They make us feel like we are great clinicians, because they do their homework, bring questions and insights, and show progress. In other words they demonstrate personal "agency," the ability to positively affect their own thoughts, feelings, actions, and environment.

Low Importance/Low Confidence. These patients demonstrate features opposite of our "star" patients. They demonstrate neither interest in voice therapy, nor faith in their own ability to improve their voices. We are unlikely to see them after the initial evaluation. If they do return, every aspect of therapy will present a problem.

Low Importance/High Confidence. These patients believe they "could change if they wanted to" but do not want to. They may return for treatment, but never appear "on board" or committed to therapy, because they are not. They may express difficulty completing homework, but it is due to low commitment rather than the difficulty level of treatment. They simply may be uninterested in vocal improvement, or committed to a goal that differs from that of therapy: continuing the voice disorder.

High Importance/Low Confidence. These patients find vocal improvement very important, but are overwhelmed with the demands of treatment. They may express difficulty with any of the aspects of therapy, and they are looking for a real solution.

Discussing Compliance

A discussion can be had with the aim of clarifying the patient's level of interest, and assessing his or her confidence. The clinician's challenge is to differentiate the patient who is failing because of low importance from the one who is failing because of low confidence. The two require a different approach. In a nonjudgmental fashion, the demands of voice therapy can be explained, and the level of patient commitment gauged. Without attempting to convince the patient of the importance of therapy, the clinician can assist the patient in deciding whether he or she wishes to continue in voice therapy or not. In this way, the clinician can remain engaged with the patient, but in the role of helping the patient make a decision, rather than controlling the decision in favor of the larynx. The discussion itself may reveal to the patient that voice therapy is indeed important to his or her life goals or, conversely, that vocal improvement is not a goal for them. In either case, patient and clinician can "get on the same page" by discussing the topic.

When discussing the patient's vocal goals, the client-centered counseling "microskill" of reflecting (ie, restating the patient's thought or feelings) can be useful. Reflecting can help the clinician better understand the patient's perspective and build rapport. I use it to combat my tendency of moving too fast, and to stay out of an argument when a new patient is angry due to factors beyond my control. I recall a patient whose first words upon meeting me were "OK, let's get it over with: just tell me to quit smoking because that's all you white coats ever do so just say it now and I won't have to listen to it again." Taken aback, I muttered "Smoking is very important to you." This reflection initiated a chain of dialogue in which the patient clarified his position ("Well, no, it's not that it's important, it's that I think I need cigarettes") and I would reflect it. I remember saying things such as "Smoking is like a friend to you" and "You just don't believe you can live without cigarettes." Through this conversation, our rapport developed quickly, leading him to dis-

close an extensive substance abuse history to me, and his assessment that cigarettes were by far the hardest to quit. Thus his initial "low importance" impression had been a facade for a lack of self-efficacy! After discussion with our ENT, the patient accepted a referral to the Center for Tobacco Research and Intervention.

Compliance Strategies

If the patient is found to struggle because of low confidence in their vocal and voice-therapy-related abilities, strategies to improve patient confidence can be applied. Voice therapy is hard. The amount of self-regulation involved in successful voice therapy completion is, according to patients, substantial.[14] Patients may experience difficulty in a number of areas of treatment: scheduling and completing home practice, evaluating the accuracy of their practice, improving awareness of vocal behavior in conversation, changing communication habits in child-rearing, using a healthy shout, remembering to use resonant voice, coping with silliness of the exercises, allocating attentional resources to voice use, regulating loudness on the cell phone, and so on. Patients can experience failures that undermine their confidence the moment they set foot outside the clinic, if not within the clinic itself. Any area of difficulty can be targeted for compliance intervention.

One way to improve patient confidence to master a task is to reduce the difficulty or complexity of the task itself. It has been empirically established outside of our field that concrete, short-term goals are inherently motivating and support self-efficacy. The somewhat abstract nature of voice production and kinesthetic/acoustic feedback may be in opposition to the favorable goal characteristic of concreteness. Visual feedback, negative practice, and audio and video examples of target voice production for home practice are strategies that reduce abstraction of the goal. Breaking down the goal to specific, small tasks improves the short-term aspect of the goal. Providing a specific number of times or minutes to practice, and a counter to tally progress, can be as helpful to the voice patient as a pedometer is to the person pursuing exercise.

The patient's response to strategies to improve self-efficacy can aid in the differential diagnosis of noncompliance. I recall a patient who had failed voice therapy with other clinicians three times before seeing me. While verbalizing great commitment to therapy, she expressed overwhelming difficulty dedicating any time to home practice. Most prominently, the renovation of her kitchen proved a barrier to practice. After the kitchen had interfered with home practice for several weeks, I reduced her home practice time commitment to 2 minutes per day, and requested that she not return for therapy should she fail to complete this homework. She did not return, leaving me to assume that her kitchen ranked more important than her voice. In another case, the opposite problem revealed itself. Like the kitchen patient, this patient had difficulty generalizing. She would return week after week in tears, expressing her difficulty in monitoring resonant voice by herself. At session 4, I finally realized that her treatment task needed to be simplified. We experimented with various therapy techniques until we found that she was able to use a breathy voice successfully without much self-monitoring. Having adequate self-efficacy for this task, she successfully generalized breathy voice use across work and social settings, and resolved her vocal fold lesions. Moreover, she learned that friends listen more intently when you reduce your own loudness. She eventually developed what I can only describe as excellent resonant voice, and now teaches 3-hour lectures without any vocal difficulty.

Another "evidence-based" strategy from outside of our field is the use of peer support. Modeling of target behavior by peers with whom one can identify supports patients' beliefs that "they can do it too." Peer modeling and support are entirely unutilized in traditional, directive voice therapy and are worthy of investigation. When, after consent, I arrange a brief meeting between a "model" and a "learning" voice patient, both benefit: the learner receives relevant advice and observes healthy voice use in "real" person (not the clinician), and the model receives validation for her achievement. As a clinician, I cannot provide this type of support, because my role limits me to play the expert.

Last, mastery experiences—the most powerful source of self-efficacy—may be increased by increasing session frequency. Ranging from once-daily therapy to a vocal "boot camp" of multiple sessions per day, increased treatment intensity provides more mastery opportunities in a shorter time frame, thus reducing the possibility of failure between sessions, and supporting the acquisition of motor skills. The "boot camp" approach constructs an environment that is incompatible with noncompliance. However, this approach can not address the self-management of skills that the patient must acquire to be ultimately successful in vocal rehabilitation.

The importance-confidence distinction becomes somewhat fuzzy when we see that the two influence one another.

For example, when goals are simplified, both self-efficacy and importance can increase. The clinician's job is to coach the patient toward the "high importance, high confidence" quadrant, using whatever tools are appropriate and ethical. Aside from "evidence-based" counseling skills, and strategies, these tools may include the clinician's unique personal attributes, such as charm, sense of humor, authority, and physical stature.

Future Compliance Research

Patient compliance is an old topic in voice therapy practice and a new topic in voice therapy research. There is room for basic science research into the factors that affect voice technique goal attainment in non-voice-disordered individuals, qualitative research to describe patient experiences and clinician expertise, correlational research to identify predictors of voice therapy compliance, and experimental research to assess interventions aimed to improve compliance with existing voice therapy regimens. Application of existing knowledge and methods from outside of our field may be helpful in developing this line of research, but we must not hesitate to construct our own, voice-specific, theories and interventions.

Can We Always Expect Success?

What is successful voice therapy? Who determines a level of success? Is the clinician's definition of successful therapy equal to the patient's expectation? Obviously, answers to these questions must be clear for the success of therapy to be determined. As clinicians, our goal is always that the patient should develop the best voice possible. This goal must be made clear to the patient. Otherwise, the patient's goal may be "normal voice" (whatever that is), even when normal voice may not be attainable, or the patient may be satisfied with mild improvement, whereas the clinician continues to push to develop more vocal improvement. This added "push" may require more effort than the patient is willing to give.

As voice clinicians, we should always *expect* success, knowing that many pitfalls exist to sabotage our efforts. Our task is to limit the sabotage and maximize the possibilities through our efforts, experience, and expertise.

References

1. Glanz K, Rimer BK, Marcus Lewis F. Theory, research and practice in health behavior and health education. In: Glanz K, Rimer BK, Lewis FM, eds. *Health Behavior and Health Education: Theory, Research and Practice.* San Francisco, CA: Jossey-Bass; 2002:34.
2. DiMatteo MR. Variations in patients' adherence to medical recommendations: a quantitative review of 50 years of research. *Med Care.* 2004;42:200–209.
3. McDonald HP, Garg AX, Haynes RB. Interventions to enhance patient adherence to medication prescriptions: scientific review. *JAMA.* 2002;288:2868–2879.
4. Robin DiMatteo M, Giordani PJ, Lepper HS, et al. Patient adherence and medical treatment outcomes: a meta-analysis. *Med Care.* 2002;40:794–811.
5. Simoni JM, Pearson CR, Pantalone DW, et al. Efficacy of interventions in improving highly active antiretroviral therapy adherence and HIV-1 RNA viral load: a meta-analytic review of randomized controlled trials. *J Acquired Immune Defic Syndromes.* 2006;43:S23–S35.

6. Bandura A. Health promotion by social cognitive means. *Health Educ Behav.* 2004; 31:143–164.

7. Alexander SC, Sleath B, Golin CE, et al. Provider-patient communication and treatment adherence. In: Bosworth HB, Oddone EZ, Weinberger M, eds. *Patient Treatment Adherence: Concepts, Interventions, and Management.* Mahwah, NJ: Lawrence Erlbaum Associates; 2006: 329–372.

8. Bastian LA, Molner SL, Fish LJ, et al. Smoking cessation and adherence. In: Bosworth HB, Oddone EZ, Weinberger M, eds. *Patient Treatment Adherence: Concepts, Interventions, and Management.* Mahwah, NJ: Lawrence Erlbaum Associates; 2006:125–146.

9. Dominick KL, Morey M. Adherence to physical activity. In: Bosworth HB, Oddone EZ, Weinberger M, eds. *Patient Treatment Adherence: Concepts, Interventions, and Management.* Mahwah, NJ: Lawrence Erlbaum Associates; 2006: 49–94.

10. Yancy WS, Boan J. Adherence to diet recommendations. In: Bosworth HB, Oddone EZ, Weinberger M, eds. *Patient Treatment Adherence: Concepts, Interventions, and Management.* Mahwah, NJ: Lawrence Erlbaum Associates; 2006: 95–123.

11. Konkle-Parker DJ. A motivational intervention to improve adherence to treatment of chronic disease. *J Am Acad Nurse Pract.* 2001;13:61–68.

12. Bosch-Capblanch X, Abba K, Prictor M, et al. Contracts between patients and healthcare practitioners for improving patients' adherence to treatment, prevention and health promotion activities. *Cochrane Database Syst Rev.* 2007;(2): CD004808.

13. Sluijs E, Kok G, van der Zee J. Correlates of exercise compliance in physical therapy. *Phys Ther.* 1993;73:771–782.

14. van Leer E, Connor NP. Patient perceptions of voice therapy adherence. *J Voice.* In press.

15. Tonelli MR. Integrating evidence into clinical practice: an alternative to evidence-based approaches. *J Eval Clin Pract.* 2006;12:248–256.

16. Horvath AO, Symonds BD. Relation between working alliance and outcome in psychotherapy: a meta-analysis. *J Counsel Psych.* 1991;38:139–149.

17. Martin DJ, Garske JP, Davis MK. Relation of the therapeutic alliance with outcome and other variables: a meta-analytic review. *J Consult Clin Psychol.* 2000;68:438–450.

18. Meier PS, Barrowclough C, Donmall MC. The role of the therapeutic alliance in the treatment of substance misuse: a critical review of the literature. *Addiction.* 2005;100:304–316.

19. Wampold BE. *The Great Psychotherapy Debate: Models, Methods, and Findings.* Mahwah, NJ: Lawrence Erlbaum Associates Publishers; 2001.

20. Wampold BE, Minami T, Baskin TW, et al. A meta-(re)analysis of the effects of cognitive therapy versus "other therapies" for depression. *J Affect Disord.* 2002;68:159–165.

21. DiIorio C, Shafer PO, Letz R, et al. Behavioral, social, and affective factors associated with self-efficacy for self-management among people with epilepsy. *Epilepsy Behav.* 2006/8;9:158–163.

22. Ilgen M, Tiet Q, Finney J, et al. Self-efficacy, therapeutic alliance, and alcohol-use disorder treatment outcomes. *J Stud Alcohol.* 2006;67:465–472.

23. Luszczynska A, Sutton S. Physical activity after cardiac rehabilitation: evidence that different types of self-efficacy are important in maintainers and relapsers. *Rehab Psych.* 2006;51:314–321.

24. Brown LJ, Malouff JM, Schutte NS. The effectiveness of a self-efficacy intervention for helping adolescents cope with sport-competition loss. *J Sport Behav.* 2005;28:136–150.

25. Baldwin AS, Rothman AJ, Hertel AW, et al. Specifying the determinants of the initiation and maintenance of behavior

change: an examination of self-efficacy, satisfaction, and smoking cessation. *Health Psych.* 2006;25:626–634.

26. Marks R, Allegrante JP, Lorig K. A review and synthesis of research evidence for self-efficacy-enhancing interventions for reducing chronic disability: implications for health education practice (part II). *Health Promot Pract.* 2005;6:148–156.

27. Dishman RK, Motl RW, Saunders R, et al. Self-efficacy partially mediates the effect of a school-based physical-activity intervention among adolescent girls. *Prevent Med.* 2004/5;38:628–636.

28. Song KJ. The effects of self-efficacy promoting cardiac rehabilitation program on self-efficacy, health behavior, and quality of life. *Taehan Kanho Hakhoe Chi.* 2003;33:510–518.

29. McAuley E, Talbot H, Martinez S. Manipulating self-efficacy in the exercise environment in women: influences on affective responses. *Health Psych.* 1999; 18:288–294.

30. Strecher VJ, McEvoy DeVellis B, Becker MH, et al. The role of self-efficacy in achieving health behavior change. *Health Educ Behav.* 1986;13:73–92.

31. Amrhein PC, Miller WR, Yahne CE, et al. Client commitment language during motivational interviewing predicts drug use outcomes. *J Consult Clin Psychol.* 2003;71:862–878.

32. Miller WR, Rollnick S. *Motivational Interviewing: Preparing People for Change.* New York, NY: Guilford Press; 2002.

33. Rollnick S, Mason P, Butler C. *Health Behavior Change: A Guide for Practitioners.* Edinburgh, UK: Churchill Livingstone; 1999.

APPENDIX

The Smith Accent Technique Protocol

STAGE 1: REST BREATHING

Goals

Develop oral air intake

Be aware of the outward displacement of the abdominal wall during inspiration

Feel the expiratory airflow

Be aware of inward displacement of the abdominal wall during expiration

Position

Supine, sitting, or standing

Breathing Pattern

Slow and rhythmic

Relaxed inspiration with outward abdominal excursion

Relaxed expiration with inward abdominal excursion

Phonation

None

Contract your lips as /w/ or /f/ to hear the expiratory airstream as noise

Turn Taking

Not yet

Body Movements

Supine: Relaxed shoulders, hand on chest and hand on abdomen

Sitting and Standing: Chest and shoulders relaxed, one hand on the chest and one on the abdomen

Standing: Feel your body swaying slightly forward with inbreath, backward with outbreath

---

STAGE 2: ABDOMINO-PHONATORY CONTROL IN LARGO SPEED

Goals

Optimize inspiration for speech (quick, deep and silent oral inbreath)

Develop control of speed and strength of the abdominal muscle contractions (abdominal accents) with phonation during slow largo rhythm

Develop awareness of targeted vocal qualities

Breathing Pattern

Abdomino-phonatory:

Comfortable, quick and silent oral inbreath

Tailored outbreath for phonation

Supportive Voice Production Parameters

Clinician modifies posture, muscle tension (mouth, neck, shoulders and chest), orality, etc . . . as needed in a gentle subtle manner

Largo Tempo

Two to three beats/ accents

Phonation

1. Start by a sustained voiceless fricatives (eg. /sh/, /s/)
2. Short soft unstressed voiceless fricative followed by a longer accentuated (stressed) one that fades away (eg, sh—SH—, f—F—, s—S)
3. Same with voiced fricatives (e.g. z—Z—, v—V—).
4. Proceed to a short unstressed vowel followed by one or two long stressed/accentuated vowel(s) in a 3/4 time signature (eg, /hey yey/, /hoy yoy/, /hey yey yey/, /hoy yoy yoy/).
5. Once mastered→changes in stress, volume, and intonation are introduced.
6. Once mastered→soft and relaxed monosyllabic two-to three-word phrases may be introduced (eg, hey you, he's home)

Predictability

Patient copies predictable modeled stimuli

Turn Taking

Patient starts as soon as the clinician is finished with modeling

Body Movements

Sitting or standing: Chest and shoulders relaxed; one hand on the abdomen.

If standing: Slightly sway forward with inbreath, backward with outbreath.

Arms allowed to hang freely from the shoulders

STAGE 3: ABDOMINO-PHONATORY CONTROL IN ANDANTE SPEED

Goals

Optimize inspiration for speech (quick, deep and silent oral inbreath)

Develop control of speed and strength of the abdominal muscle contractions (abdominal accents) with phonation during medium speed andante rhythm.

Self-monitoring of targeted vocal qualities

Breathing Pattern

Abdomino-phonatory:

Quick, deep, and silent oral inbreath

Tailored outbreath for phonation

Supportive Voice Production Parameters

Clinician modifies posture, muscle tension (mouth, neck, shoulders and chest), orality, etc . . . as needed in a gentle subtle manner

Andante Tempo

Four to five beats/accents

Phonation

1. Short unstressed vowel followed by three to four short stressed vowels in a 4/4 time signature (eg, /hoy ooy ooy ooy/).
2. Short unstressed syllable (consonant–vowel–glide) followed by three to four short stressed/ accentuated syllable in a 4/4 time signature (eg, /toy toy toy toy/).
3. Once mastered→changes in stress, volume, and intonation are introduced.
4. Once mastered→soft and relaxed monosyllabic three-to four-word phrases may be introduced (eg, he came back home)

Predictability

Patient copies predictable modeled stimuli

Once mastered, patient copies unpredictable stimuli

Turn Taking

Patient starts as soon as the clinician is finished with modeling

Body Movements

Sitting or standing: Chest and shoulders relaxed.

Arms allowed to hang freely from the shoulders.

The expressive movements of the arms are observed with the movement of the forearms at the elbow.

STAGE 4: ABDOMINO-PHONATORY CONTROL IN ALLEGRO SPEED AND STABILIZATION OF THE TECHNIQUE

Goals

Optimize inspiration for speech (quick, deep and silent oral inbreath)

Develop control of speed and strength of the abdominal muscle contractions (abdominal accents) with phonation during fast speed allegro rhythm.

Stabilize abdomino-phonatory support during phonation

Self-monitoring and self-correction of abdomino-phonatory control.

Self-monitoring and self-correction of targeted vocal qualities.

Self-monitoring and self-correction of supportive parameters.

Breathing Pattern

Abdomino-phonatory

Quick, deep, and silent oral inbreath

Tailored outbreath for phonation

Supportive Voice Production Parameters

Clinician modifies posture, muscle tension (mouth, neck, shoulders and chest), orality, etc . . . as needed in a gentle subtle manner

Allegro Tempo

Six and more beats/accents

Phonation

1. Six or more short unstressed vowels/syllables in a 4/4 time signature (eg, /hey eey eey eey eey eey/
2. Six or more short unstressed syllable (consonant–vowel–glide)

in a 4/4 time signature (eg, /boy boy boy boy boy boy/)
3. Once mastered→changes in stress, volume, and intonation are introduced.
4. Once mastered→soft and relaxed monosyllabic six or more word phrases are introduced (eg, he said he ate it all)
5. Once mastered→variable rhythms, stress patterns, loudness, and intonation contours are introduced.

Predictability

Patient copies predictable modeled stimuli

Once mastered, patient copies unpredictable stimuli

Turn Taking

Patient starts as soon as the clinician is finished with modeling

Body Movements

Sitting or standing: Chest and shoulders relaxed.

Short rhythmic bouncing movements at the wrist, like someone beating a drum with the hands.

STAGE 5: TRANSFER TO CONNECTED SPEECH

Goal

Continue to increase the dynamic range of voice and speech characters

Habituate the technique in real life situations.

Self-monitoring and self-correction of abdomino-phonatory control.

Self-monitoring and self-correction of targeted vocal quality

Self-monitoring and self-correction of supportive voice production parameters (posture, muscle tension, articulation, oral resonance, voice projection, etc)

Predictability

Patient copies unpredictable stimuli

Patient self-initiates stimuli

Self-Initiation

Patient produces spontaneous performances

Clinician may indirectly modify by modeling a more efficient way of producing the utterance

Phonation

Variable rhythms, stress patterns, loudness, and intonation contours using an interplay between vowel play, nonsense syllables, and meaningful words with the three basic rhythms interchangeably.

The patient practices optimal phrase length, pause location, duration, and speech rate using the following hierarchy:

Automatic series, common or core phrases

Reading (familiar text→unfamiliar text)

Monologue

Dialogue

Challenging conversations/debates

Difference performance modes (as needed)

Different singing styles (as needed)

Index